ORTHOTICS ETCETERA

SECOND EDITION

This volume is one of the series,
Rehabilitation Medicine Library,
Edited by John V. Basmajian,
Originally published as part of the Physical Medicine Library,
Edited by Sidney Licht.

New books and new editions published, in press or in preparation, for this series:

BANERJEE: Rehabilitation Management of Amputees

BASMAJIAN: Therapeutic Exercise, third edition*

BISHOP: Behavioral Problems and the Disabled: Assessment and Management

BROWNE, KIRLIN, AND WATT: Rehabilitation Services and the Social Work Role: Challenge for Change

CHYATTE: Rehabilitation in Chronic Renal Failure

EHRLICH: Rehabilitation Management of Rheumatic Conditions

HAAS ET AL.: Pulmonary Therapy and Rehabilitation: Principles and Practice

INCE: Behavioral Psychology in Rehabilitation Medicine: Clinical Applications

JOHNSON: Practical Electromyography

KHALILI: Management of Spasticity with Peripheral Phenol Nerve Blocks

LEHMANN: Therapeutic Heat and Cold, third edition*

LONG: Prevention and Rehabilitation in Ischemic Heart Disease

ROGOFF: Manipulation, Traction and Massage, second edition*

SHA'KED: Human Sexuality in Rehabilitation Medicine

Originally published as part of the Physical Medicine Library, edited by Sidney Licht.

Orthotics
Etcetera

Second Edition

Edited by

JOHN B. REDFORD, M.D.

Professor and Chairman
Department of Rehabilitation Medicine
University of Kansas Medical Center
Kansas City, Kansas

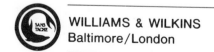

WILLIAMS & WILKINS
Baltimore/London

Made in the United States of America

Reprinted 1981

Library of Congress Cataloging in Publication Data

Main entry under title:

Orthotics etcetera.

   (Rehabilitation medicine library)
   First ed., published in 1966, edited by S. H. Licht.
   Includes bibliographies and index.
   1. Orthopedic apparatus. I. Redford, John B. II. Licht, Sidney Herman, 1907–1979
ed. Orthotics etcetera. III. Series.
RD755.L5 1980   617'.307   79-17729
ISBN 0-683-07197-1

Composed and printed at the
Waverly Press, Inc.
Mt. Royal and Guilford Aves.
Baltimore, Md. 21202, U.S.A.

In memory of Sidney Licht, M.D.
1907-1979
Author, Editor, Historian, Critic, and Raconteur

Series Editor's Foreword

In addition to a new series of books, *Rehabilitation Medicine Library* revives and expands more than a dozen of the most useful volumes in Sidney Licht's Physical Medicine Library. This volume on *Orthotics* is one of those books that has proved to be perennially sought out, even though it has become outdated. Now Dr. Redford and his authors have successfully brought the book up to date while retaining all that was good in the previous edition. Fortunately, they have combined old and new with style and common sense.

The results of a lot of thought and work here represent the state of the art and science, making the book quite unique. Equally important, the writing is easy to follow. Hence, it becomes reasonable to expect that all levels of experts and their students will find the book not only useful but extremely significant in their work and study.

Finally, a word on the editor. John Redford is not only a longtime friend but is also the one person that immediately sprang to mind when this book's future was being considered. He has fulfilled our highest expectations. Sidney Licht would have been proud of this book!

JOHN V. BASMAJIAN

McMaster University
Hamilton, Ontario
1980

Preface to the Second Edition

As related by Doctor Sidney Licht in the "Preface to the First Edition" of *Orthotics Etcetera*, the word orthotic is of recent origin. It was officially adopted in 1960 by the limb fitters and brace makers in America when they formed the American Orthotic and Prosthetic Association from the original Artificial Limb Manufacturers Association. Originally applied to mean the field of straightening deformities by means of external support, the term "orthotics" has taken on a much broader meaning. When the term "orthosis" is strictly defined, it refers to a device applied or attached to the external surface of the body to improve function. However, the field of Orthotics now usually includes such equipment as wheelchairs and environmental control systems, which do not attach to the patient. In this new edition of the original 9th Volume of the Physical Medicine Library, we deemed it very appropriate therefore to keep the term *Etcetera* in the title: many of these "unattached devices" cannot be termed "orthoses," but they still appear to be the "*etcetera*".

In retaining *Etcetera* in the title, we have also retained the format of the first edition. General consideration of orthotic devices is followed by chapters on specific applications of orthoses, and then the remaining half of the book reviews the applications of other assistive devices, and special requirements of disabled persons.

Orthopedic surgery has made remarkable progress in the past decade in the correction of connective tissue disabilities. The outstanding example has been the development of the total hip prosthesis by Charnley, followed by a remarkable number of new prosthetic joint replacements. Development of internal devices has often overshadowed the development of external assistive devices. Nevertheless, there have been some remarkable developments in applying new technology to the solution of age-old problems of crippling diseases, and this book considers a number of these new approaches. We also wish to update current rationale for application of "rehabilitation engineering" in the field of orthotics. Rehabilitation engineering is a new term that recognizes the role of engineers who have pioneered in the field of orthotics, such as Doctor Colin McLaurin, who was one of the first to use this term.

Although engineers have been involved in writing some of this new edition, it was still written primarily by clinicians and for clinicians in the field of rehabilitation medicine. The book cannot completely cover the rapidly expanding field of orthotics, nor does it represent an atlas of available orthoses and details of their manufacture—other books are available for that purpose. It is meant primarily to demonstrate the use of orthotic devices by various experts. We have chosen authors with a reputation for clinical experience and knowledge of the diseases or functional disorders being treated by or assisted by orthotics or other apparatus. Some of the original chapters have been expanded; others have been eliminated but generally, all aspects of *Orthotics Etcetera* that were covered in the first edition are present in this new publication.

This book would be incomplete without a word about the orthotist and his training. In spite of many attempts to improve training and increase the number of teaching programs, there is still a serious shortage of well-trained orthotists throughout the world. Nickel has recently reviewed the development of orthotic education in America.*

Following World War II, a variety of agencies, including the National Research Council, considered means of adapting newer technologies to develop better orthotic devices. Intensive research into kinesiology, biomechanics, and engineering technology was carried out at a number of centers. New concepts and techniques developed that then needed education of medical personnel before the public could benefit from this research. The first courses were in the field of prosthetics but equally important were the needs in the field of orthotics. Therefore, beginning in 1956, short postgraduate courses for training orthotists, physicians, and therapists were offered at New York University, University of California in Los Angeles, and Northwestern University in Chicago. These have been very successful, and these centers are still involved in developing new teaching programs.

Two-year courses leading to an Associate of Arts degree in orthotics were first developed in Cerritos College in Norwalk, California, and later in other programs, such as the Chicago Community College and the Rehabilitation Institute of Montreal. Since 1964, a number of bachelor degrees in orthotics have been developed, the first one at New York University. Other programs are in the planning stage or are evolving. Although there was great debate about the ideal training program, it seems certain that a bachelor's degree consisting of 2 years of general university courses followed by 2 years of intensive education in the field of orthotics and 1 or 2 years of internship is probably the form that will be most acceptable in certifying orthotists in the future.

The American Board for Certification in Orthotists and Prosthetists was incorporated in 1948. It has, as its principal functions, the establishment of professional standards, administration of examinations, and appraisal of orthotic and prosthetic facilities. It also acts as an appeal committee for

* Nickel, V. L., Orthotics in America: past, present and future. *Clllin. Orthop., 102:* 10–27, 1974.

alleged infringements of acceptable standards of the practice of orthotics. In December 1970, the American Academy of Orthotists and Prosthetists was formed to promote scientific conferences for practicing orthotists and prosthetists. The Academy has been particularly influential in improving continuing education in the field. Through its assistance in the publication of the journal "Orthotics and Prosthetics," it has had a wide impact on education and practice.

It is obvious that a medical technology becomes more effective in maintaining life in patients with severe medical problems, orthotists will become more involved not only with greater numbers of patients but also with more complex treatment procedures. As it is recognized that the number of prosthetists and orthotists will probably not increase at the same rate as needed, a more proficient way of fabricating devices must be found. The answer is probably to train more people at subprofessional levels, such as those of orthotic assistants or orthotic technicians, while improving the qualifications of higher education for those orthotists who will work directly with patients, together with the physicians and therapists. This will also probably mean that more professionals in the field of prosthetics and orthotics will be based in medical complexes and will not have immediately at their side an extensive amount of fabrication equipment. They will then rely more on central fabrication laboratories for the supply of required devices, making adjustments on individual patients as the need arises.

Although the above statements are speculative, obviously something has to be done to meet the growing gap between the services required by patients and the shortage of personnel in the field of Orthotics. A recent survey of training programs in the U. S. revealed that of the various specialists associated with rehabilitation services, prosthetists, orthotists, and physiatrists were the group in which there was the highest demand and the lowest supply.

In this new edition of *Orthotics Etcetera*, we have taken a look back by republishing part of the preface from the previous edition. As always in the memorable style of Doctor Sidney Licht, we have been shown how much we are indebted to past developments in this field. Today, we have only a vague glimpse of tomorrow but can safely predict that it will have only a partial resemblance to yesterday and today. New ideas, new materials, and new systems of financing and distribution of orthotic devices will all appear.

To summarize the future position of orthotics, it seems appropriate to quote from an editorial by Thranhardt†:

The days of the "fitter" performing clinical tests part-time and fabricating devices the other part of the time is fading into a bygone era. Tomorrow, the patient care professional in orthotics will rely entirely on a fabrication laboratory for the supply of devices. Fabrication laboratories may spe-

* Thranhardt, T. Tomorrow. *Orthotics Prosthet., 31:* 1, 1977.

cialize in specific services or may offer a complete line of services and appliances. These production experts will have to provide rapid quality service to remain competitive and sustain their business through specialization. The application of modern technology will speed production and reduce costs. The end results are that the patient will receive superior care and a quality appliance at a cost no greater than today.

There are and will be too few practitioners of the orthotic and prosthetic art to possibly handle the treatment of the patients and tomorrow by yesterday's and today's system of delivery of service. Some practitioners are moving in the proper direction everyone must. We cannot stand still while the world moves ahead. Progress is a train; we cannot stop it; we must get aboard."

This latter statement could apply equally well to the physicians who are responsible for prescribing orthotic and prosthetic services. They must be aware of the changes in the field and be constantly alert to new developments. It is hoped that this revised book will contribute that understanding and knowledge.

In preparing this second edition, the editor would like to extend his sincere thanks to all the contributing authors for their contributions and in particular to the late Doctor Sidney Licht and to Doctor Herman L. Kamenetz for their assistance in editing a number of new chapters. We are also most grateful to a number of persons at the University of Kansas Medical Center who assisted with this text, particularly to Mrs. Ellen Roose, Occupational Therapist, for her assistance; to my secretary, Mrs. Beverly Knapp, and the other office staff for their assistance; and to Mrs. Janice Orrick, who assisted with the section on scoliosis. We are also indebted to Mr. Paul Trautman, C.P.O., Director of the Orthotic-Prosthetic Department at the University of Kansas Medical Center; to James E. Smith, Executive Vice-President of the Knit-Rite Company; and to Dr. Serge Zilber, Director of Clinical Technology Corporation in Kansas City for their assistance in reviewing certain chapters. Finally, we would like to acknowledge the aid and advice that has been received from the Williams & Wilkins Company from Mr. James L. Sangston in making the publication of this second edition of *Orthotics Etcetera* possible.

Kansas City, Kansas   JBR
April 1980

From the Preface to the First Edition

Orthotics or orthetics? The proponents of each word have good arguments. Part of the problem of choice stems from the use of two words by the ancient Greeks. According to one classics scholar, *prosthesis* meant both replacement for a part and help for a part. The other word, *orthosis*, meant straightening, or, more accurately, rectitude. Plutarch referred to moral rectitude as *orthosis*. Neither word fully embraces the subject of this book, since in addition to discussing devices to straighten parts and aid function, the book deals with inventions to make life more comfortable, safer, and useful.

According to Professor S. I. Hayakawa of San Francisco, there are two suffixes in English that suggest organized knowledge: *-ology*, which also suggests academic isolation, and the somewhat mysterious *-ics* (art or science), which suggests a method of meeting life's problems. The suffix is well chosen, but what of the root?

Soon after World War II, brace makers began to use the word "orthotics" and in 1965 adopted its usage by vote. In 1955, Dr. Robert L. Bennett of Warm Springs, Georgia, first used the word "orthetics" as the title of an exhibition of braces and other appliances for the increase of the functional capacity of severely disabled persons. He believed that the word should match in sound and sight the long-established word "prosthetics." He defined a prosthesis as an artificial replacement for a missing part and an orthesis as something applied to an existing part.

Everyone seems to accept the Greek root *orthos*, the adjective for straight, for the beginning of the word. The argument is about the second *o* of the root. Some classical scholars insist that when the root ends in *o*, it may not be dropped in ellipses. This argument is untenable, according to Mrs. Ruth Good of Ann Arbor, Michigan, who has pointed out that this very thing was done in the words "arthritis," "hematemesis," "pharyngeal," "rhinencephalon" and many others. A principal objection to the word "orthosis" is that it sounds like many words applied to diseases or disorders, such as "neurosis" and "ptosis." Of course, the most precise word would be "orthothetic" and, although there are many words in the English language as hard to look at and pronounce, the word has no champions.

Few medical dictionaries mention the word "brace." The 1965 edition of *Dorland's Illustrated Medical Dictionary,* the dictionary consulted most in medicine, does not define "brace," but it does mention that orthotics concerns orthopedic appliances. (Orthopedic appliance is the way in which the word is translated into many languages. Just as in English we have more than one word [brace, splint, orthosis], so are there two or more words in several languages. The French use attelle, tuteur, and orthèse.) Our own definition of an orthosis is any device, which, when in contact with the body, improves function. Since this definition will seem too broad to many, we have added a word to the title of the book, *etcetera,* a word of variable spelling. It means, among other things, "other things"—things that we normally associate with the image created by the word immediately preceding it. These *other things* related to orthotics may seem unimportant to ablebodied persons, but the disabled person would ask with Shakespeare, "Are etceteras nothing?" They can mean the difference between total dependence and independence. They are basic to the rehabilitation process for some persons, whereas for still others they are the whole rehabilitation process. How often have we heard of *the rehabilitation of a quadriplegic,* when all that was meant was that he was furnished with an electric wheelchair and an electric arm that could be operated by a set of sensitive switches? It is the position of the editor that there are many aspects of rehabilitation that are mechanical rather than medical and are orthotic *etcetera.* This leads us to the question of the delegation or acceptance of responsibility, sometimes a delicate problem.

During the Civil War there was established in New York City an institution called the Hospital for the Relief of the Ruptured and Crippled. Offhand, that sounds like a peculiar combination and, from a purely medical point of veiw, it was and is. The conjunctive was the appliance maker. The same artisan who made the hernia truss of metal and leather made the limb brace of metal and leather. In the 20th century, the name of the hospital was changed, and so was that of the brace maker (he has become an orthotist). He may still make an abdominal belt, but he has progressed from a leather-and-iron craftsman to a member of the medical team that evaluates and manages disabled persons requiring functional aids—orthoses. As in most vocational and professional groups, progress has meant longer training, more research, improved technology, and higher status. Orthotists no longer wish to be thought of as mechanics but as specialists. In 1966, there were more than 450 certified orthotists in the U.S. To qualify for this rating, the candidate must have had at least 4 years of acceptable experience and must pass written, oral, and practical examinations of the American Board of Certification in Orthotics and Prosthetics, Incorporated. With increased education, the orthotist has come closer to the province of the physician and may one day challenge certain prerogatives and responsibilities of the physicians, as other participants of medical and surgical teams have done from time to time. For example, there are orthotists who believe that the physician who has prescribed an orthotic device does not have the ethical duty to check it out. (A check-out is one of those guild words seldom found in dictionaries, even though hundreds of people use it dozens of times a day. It means inspection. The check-out determines whether the prescription has been followed and whether the appliances fits, is comfortable, and does what it is supposed to do.) Eyeglasses are orthotic devices; they are applied to the body to improve function. An opthalmologist does not consider his prescription for glasses filled until he has checked them himself. A physiatrist who prescribes a brace and does not personally inspect it for fit and function has not fulfilled his obligation to the patient. There are orthotists who feel that the physician should not participate in the check-out. They feel that insistence upon the part of the physician to do this is a demonstration of lack of confidence. However, the government of the United States of American insists upon a check-out by a physician (and his signature) before it will pay for an orthotic device.

SIDNEY LICHT, M.D.
New Haven, Connecticut
April 18, 1966.

Contributors

Marc A. Asher, M.D.
Professor of Orthopedic Surgery, University of Kansas Medical Center, Kansas City, Kansas.

Mary Eleanor Brown, M.A.
Formerly Assistant Professor of Physical Therapy, Supervisor of Continuing Education for Physical Therapists, Case Western Reserve University; Chief Research Associate, Highland View Hospital, Cleveland, Ohio; Former Director of Professional Services, Sunnyview Hospital and Rehabilitation Center, Schenectady, New York; Former Director of Physical Therapy, Institute for the Crippled and Disabled, Rehabilitation and Research Center, New York City, New York.

Michael F. T. Carpendale, M.D.
Chief, Rehabilitation Medicine Service, Veterans Administration Medical Center, San Francisco; Associate Clinical Professor of Orthopedics, University of California, San Francisco, San Francisco, California.

James D. Harris, D.O.
Associate Professor and Chairman, Rehabilitation Medicine Department, Oklahoma Osteopathic Hospital, Tulsa, Oklahoma.

Robert Juvinall, M.S., M.E.
Professor of Mechanical Engineering, University of Michigan; Professor of Mechanical Engineering, Department of Physical Medicine and Rehabilitation, University of Michigan, Ann Arbor, Michigan

Herman L. Kamenetz, M.D.
Chief, Rehabilitation Medicine Service, Veterans Administration Medical Center, Washington, D. C.

Herbert Kent, M.D., F.C.C.P.
Associate Clinical Professor, Department of Physical Medicine and Rehabilitation, University of California (Irvine); Chief, Rehabilitation Medicine Service, Veterans Administration Medical Center, Long Beach, California.

V. Nanda Kumar, M.D.

Director, Rehabilitation Medicine Services, Veterans Administration Medical Center, Kansas City, Missouri; Assistant Professor, Department of Rehabilitation Medicine, University of Kansas Medical Center, Kansas City, Kansas.

Justus F. Lehmann, M.D.

Professor and Chairman, Department of Rehabilitation Medicine, University of Washington, Seattle, Washington.

Sidney Licht, M.D. (Deceased)

Former Curator, Physical Medicine Collections, Yale Medical Library, New Haven, Connecticut.

Charles Long, M.D.

Co-Director, Department of Physical Medicine and Rehabilitation, Cuyahoga Hospitals, Cleveland, Ohio; Associate Professor, Department of Physical Medicine and Rehabilitation, Case Western Reserve University, Cleveland, Ohio.

Becky Monnard Loosen, M.A., O.T.R.

Former Community Consultant, Fred Sammons, Inc., Brookfield, Illinois; Former Assistant Professor, Department of Occupational Therapy, University of Kansas, Lawrence, Kansas.

Donald B. Lucas, M.D.

Professor of Orthopedic Surgery, University of California, San Francisco, San Francisco, California.

Gabriella E. Molnar, M.D.

Professor, Rehabilitation Medicine and Pediatrics, and Director, Pediatric Rehabilitation Service, Albert Einstein College of Medicine, Bronx, New York.

Mieczyslaw Peszczynski, M.D.

Professor Emeritus, Department of Physical Medicine and Rehabilitation, Emory University School of Medicine, Atlanta, Georgia.

John B. Redford, M.D.

Professor and Chairman, Department of Rehabilitation Medicine, University of Kansas Medical Center, Kansas City, Kansas.

Edwin M. Smith, M.D.

Physical Medicine and Rehabilitation, Linden Bristol Medical Center, Flint, Michigan.

Henry H. Stonnington, M.B., B.S., M.Sc., F.R.C.P. (Edin.)
Consultant, Department of Physical Medicine and Rehabilitation, Mayo Clinic and Mayo Foundation; Associate Professor of Physical Medicine and Rehabilitation, Mayo Medical School, Rochester, Minnesota.

George Varghese, M.D.
Assistant Professor, Department of Rehabilitation Medicine, University of Kansas Medical Center, Kansas City, Kansas.

C. Gerald Warren, M.P.A.
Associate Professor, Coordinator of Research, Department of Rehabilitation Medicine, University of Washington, Seattle, Washington.

Wallace H. Whitney, C.O.
Former Director, Department of Prosthetics-Orthotics, University of Kansas Medical Center, Kansas City, Kansas

Marilyn B. Wittmeyer, M.O.T., O.T.R.
Supervisor, Physical Disabilities Unit, Division of Occupational Therapy, and Clinical Associate Professor, Department of Rehabilitation Medicine, University of Washington Hospital, Seattle, Washington.

Isidore Zamosky, C.P.O.
Faculty, New York University Post Graduate Medical School and Former Supervisor, Orthotics Laboratory; Former Director of Prosthetic-Orthotic Laboratory, New York State Rehabilitation Hospital; President, Isidore Zamosky, Inc., Monsey, New York.

Contents

1

Principles of Orthotic Devices[1]

JOHN B. REDFORD, M.D.

Although the indications for orthoses and the principles of orthotics have not changed radically, interest in orthotics and functional aids has increased in this century. Initially, this was because of the attention aroused by paralytic poliomyelitis but lately it is because of increased numbers of patients surviving high spinal cord lesions and other injuries or illnesses with severe paralysis or other handicaps. With the growth of better systems of emergency care and the increased number of intensive care units, more patients are surviving catastrophic illnesses and accidents. This advance in medical care, coupled with the "graying of the population"—the increased proportion of older people—has unfortunately resulted in a proportionate increase in the physically disabled. The growing challenge is being met by much more effective designs of devices to improve function, relieve pain, and make life more useful in the presence of handicaps. The increasing demand for better orthotic appliances has spurred cooperation between engineers, manufacturers, physicians, and allied health professionals in joint ventures that are proving innovative and productive.

Orthotic devices should be prescribed by a physician since he knows best those problems which must be analyzed and correlated to achieve maximum acceptance and use in the daily routine of the disabled. The decision as to whether a joint should be supported or mobilized, or whether a muscle may be injured by overuse or stretching, is medical. The prescribing physician should be able to test muscle strength and range of motion, evaluate all other indications for orthotics, and correlate his findings with the patient's personality and the impact of the device upon him.

Regardless of how knowledgeable the physician is, he will need to work closely with the orthotist to supply the best possible device for each patient.

Introduction of materials that are light, sturdy, and resistant to wear opens possibilities for novel designs but also imposes a greater responsibility

---

[1] We wish to express our thanks to the C. V. Mosby Co. and N. C. McCullough, III, for permission to reprint Figs. 1.1 to 1.6 from *Atlas of Orthotics* (1).

for wise selection. Therefore, orthotic devices should be prescribed by an informed physician. In prescribing, however, the physician must recognize that acceptability and use of the orthosis depends on an interplay among three individuals who are intimately involved: the patient, the physician, and the orthotist. As the need for a mutually acceptable and realistic goal for the device is critical, mutual trust among these three is essential to success. Ideally, orthotic prescription is best accomplished by an orthotic team consisting of a physician with an interest in rehabilitation, a well-trained orthotist, and a physical and an occupational therapist with knowledge of training procedures required with devices. The team should meet so that the prescription and resulting appliance represent consensus. This may only be necessary in the formal way for more complex biomechanical problems. For many patients, close consultation, clearly written prescriptions, and recording the biomechanical and medical data may suffice.

The prescribing physician is responsible for identifying treatment goals, the orthotic purpose, and any precautions to be observed. He makes the decision as to how the orthosis should be used and for what duration. However, if this is done independently of the patient's wishes or the orthotist's advice, chances of success are greatly reduced. The physician should emphasize that the orthosis is only one component of the treatment and not the whole treatment. This is particularly important if an associated physical treatment or learning a functional skill is included in the treatment plan.

The fabricating orthotist knows the devices and the limitations of material at his disposal. Through experience, he knows the factors involved in wearing the orthosis, such as ease of application, cosmesis, comfort and durability, and need for maintenance. He can also advise others on time involved and fabrication costs—the latter a most important factor from the patient's standpoint.

The physical and occupational therapists help in identifying functional problems and orthotic needs. They teach the patients proper use of the orthosis and evaluate its adequacy. Many orthotic devices are discarded by patients because of inattention to this important phase of patient education.

Prescription of Orthotic Devices

Good design of orthotic devices demands a thorough knowledge of pathological anatomy and patient requirements. Frequently, little thought is given to analysis of specific biomechanical defects. A physician may perform an examination, discuss the needs with the patient, and then write a prescription based on a limited knowledge of various orthotic components. Lack of standard terminology for these components has also presented a significant barrier to communication between the physician and orthotist.

To overcome the problem of lack of standard approaches to patient deficits and to develop a more anatomically descriptive orthotic terminology, the Committee on Prosthetics and Orthotics of the American Academy of

Orthopedic Surgeons has developed technical analysis forms for orthotic prescription. These include a checklist and description of the problems, diagrams of bones and joints to be encompassed, and an orthotic recommendation based on the summary of the functional disability and treatment objective (1, 4).

It should be noted that biomechanical deficits are independent of specific disease states present. Bone and joint injuries or infections, varying degrees of paralysis, joint diseases, and congenital deformities all have diverse causes that may present similar biomechanical defects. Even though the underlying disease must always be considered in prognosis and total management, a sound approach is to prescribe from the standpoint of biomechanical deficits. This method can readily be taught to others and fulfills a great need in developing standards of performance and meaningful terminology in a field that has suffered for years from confusing eponyms and individual idiosyncrasies in prescription. Examples of a technical analysis form for the trunk, the upper, and the lower limbs, with the resulting orthotic recommendations, are shown in Figs. 1.1 through 1.6. We have omitted the anatomical diagrams which form an essential part of the description of the problem, but they can be studied in detail in the *Atlas of Orthotics* (1). The *Atlas* gives detailed description of the forms and illustrates cases for practice in using them. All of these forms are available from the C. V. Mosby Co. (St. Louis, Missouri).

Most portions of the forms are self-explanatory; "legend" refers to abbreviations and terms in the limb diagrams. The summary of functional disability should be a concise account of factors producing functional impairment. Treatment objectives may be multiple, and this is indicated by checking the appropriate boxes.

Based on information obtained in the biomechanical analysis, one selects the anatomical involvement and type of orthoses required. Use of the initial letter of the English anatomical term for joints to be encompassed provides a useful abbreviation and anatomical description of the type of orthoses required. Under this system, a "long leg brace" becomes a KAFO, or knee-ankle-foot orthosis, and a "cockup wrist splint" becomes a WHO, or wrist-hand orthosis. Although this terminology has not yet received full recognition, we plan to use it throughout this book wherever possible. In "Orthotic Recommendation," opposite the joint to be encompassed by the orthosis, blanks are provided to indicate each movement to be controlled. Types of control rather than specific components are given by using the "Key." Specific recommendations as to materials, components, etc. can then be given under "Remarks" if necessary.

In summary, the biomechanical approach to orthotic prescription provides a logical method of problem solving, and although the analysis form itself need not be applied in all cases, the concepts and the associated terminology serve to greatly improve communication among members of the orthotic team.

TECHNICAL ANALYSIS FORM　　　　　**RIGHT UPPER LIMB**

Name _____ No. _____ Age _____ Sex _____

Date of Onset _____ Cause _____

Occupation _____ Present Upper-Limb Equipment _____

Diagnosis _____

Hand Dominance:　　　Right ☐　Left ☐

Status of other upper limb:　　　Normal ☐　　　Impaired ☐

1.　Ambulatory status:　　Normal ☐　　　Impaired ☐　　　Walking Aid ☐

2.　Wheelchair ☐　　Sitting Position:　Stable ☐　Unstable ☐　Reclined ☐　Upright ☐
　　Sitting Tolerance:　　Normal ☐　Limited ☐　　Duration _____
　　Propulsion:　Manual ☐　　Motor ☐　　Dependent ☐

3.　Cognition:　　Normal ☐　　　Impaired ☐

4.　Endurance:　　Normal ☐　　　Impaired ☐

5.　Skin:　　Normal ☐　　　Impaired ☐

6.　Pain ☐　　　Location _____

7.　Vision:　　Normal ☐　　　Impaired ☐

8.　Coordination:　Normal ☐　Impaired ☐　　Function:　Normal ☐　Compromised ☐
　　　　　　　　　　　　　　　　　　　　　　　　　　　　　　Prevented ☐

9.　Motivation:　Good ☐　Fair ☐　Poor ☐

10.　Associated impairments: _____

──────── LEGEND ────────

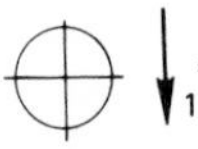

= Direction of Translatory Motion (Grade 1,2 or 3)

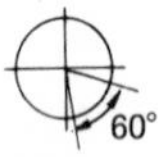

= Abnormal Degree of Rotary Motion　60°

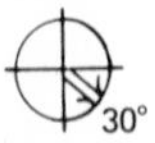

= Fixed Position　30°

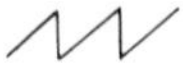

= Fracture

Volitional Force (V)
N = Normal
G = Good
F = Fair
P = Poor
T = Trace
Z = Zero

Hypertonic Muscle (H)
N = Normal
M = Mild
Mo = Moderate
S = Severe

Sensation 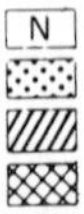
N = Normal
= Hypesthesia
= Paresthesia
= Anesthesia

Proprioception (P)
N = Normal
I = Impaired
A = Absent
D = Distension or Enlargement

Fig. 1.1. Technical Analysis Form with legend—Right Upper Limb.

　　We have stressed that in prescribing orthoses an orthotic clinic, with physician, orthotist, physical therapist, and occupational therapist, will serve the patient best. The clinic is a method of organizing patient management to provide an effective prescription, check-out, and follow-up of

Summary of Functional Disability _____

_____

_____

_____

_____

_____

Treatment Objectives: Prevent/Correct Deformity ☐   Improve Function ☐
Relieve Pain ☐   Other _____

ORTHOTIC RECOMMENDATION

UPPER LIMB			FLEX	EXT	ABD	ADD	ROTATION		AXIAL
							Int.	Ext.	LOAD
SEWHO	Shoulder								
EWHO	Humerus		▓						
	Elbow		▓						
	Forearm		▓				(Pron.)	(Sup.)	
WHO	Wrist				(RD)	(UD)			
HO	Hand								
	Fingers 2-5	MP			▓		▓		
		PIP			▓		▓		
		DIP			▓		▓		
	Thumb	CM			▓		(Opposition)		
		MP			▓				
		IP			▓		▓		

REMARKS:

_____   _____
Signature   Date

KEY: Use the following symbols to indicate desired control of designated function:

F = FREE   – *Free* motion.
A = ASSIST – Application of an external force for the purpose of increasing the range, velocity, or force of a motion.
R = RESIST – Application of an external force for the purpose of decreasing the velocity or force of a motion.
S = STOP   – Inclusion of a static unit to deter an undesired motion in one direction.
v = Variable – A unit that can be adjusted without making a structural change.
H = HOLD   – Elimination of all motion in prescribed plane (verify position).
L = LOCK   – Device includes an optional lock.

Fig. 1.2. Summary and Orthotic Recommendation—Right Upper Limb.

patients. As medical problems become more complex and orthotic technology becomes more sophisticated, clinics become more necessary not only for service but also for education of students who may attend as observers.

Other personnel may be required to meet special needs, for example, a

TECHNICAL ANALYSIS FORM   LOWER LIMB

Name_____ No._____ Age _____ Sex_____

Date of Onset_____ Cause_____ —

Occupation _____ Present Lower-Limb Equipment_____

Diagnosis_____
_____
_____

Ambulatory ☐   Non-Ambulatory ☐

MAJOR IMPAIRMENTS:

A. Skeletal
1. Bone and Joints: Normal ☐   Abnormal_____
2. Ligaments: Normal ☐   Abnormal ☐   Knee: AC ☐   PC ☐   MC ☐   LC ☐
                                              Ankle: MC ☐   LC ☐

3. Extremity Shortening: None ☐   Left ☐   Right ☐
    Amount of Discrepancy: A.S.S.-Heel_____   A.S.S.-MTP_____   MTP-Heel_____

B. Sensation: Normal ☐   Abnormal ☐
1. Anaesthesia ☐   Hypaesthesia ☐   Location:_____
    Protective Sensation: Retained ☐   Lost ☐
2. Pain ☐   Location:_____

C. Skin: Normal ☐   Abnormal: _____

D. Vascular: Normal ☐   Abnormal ☐   Right ☐   Left ☐

E. Balance: Normal ☐   Impaired ☐   Support:_____

F. Gait Deviations: _____
_____

G. Other Impairments: _____

─────────────────────── LEGEND ───────────────────────

= Direction of Translatory Motion

= Abnormal Degree of Rotary Motion   60°

= Fixed Position   30°   1 CM.

/\/\ = Fracture

Volitional Force (V)
N = Normal
G = Good
F = Fair
P = Poor
T = Trace
Z = Zero

Hypertonic Muscle (H)
N = Normal
M = Mild
Mo = Moderate
S = Severe

Proprioception (P)
N = Normal
I = Impaired
A = Absent

D = Local Distension or Enlargement

= Pseudarthrosis

= Absence of Segment

Fig. 1.3. Technical Analysis Form with legend—Lower Limb.

rehabilitation counselor and a social worker. A rehabilitation counselor may be needed to provide information relating to plans for vocational rehabilitation. The social worker can often assist as liaison between the clinic and paying agencies and explain the need for the orthosis and physical restoration program to the family as well as to the patient. Ideally, both of these

Summary of Functional Disability _____

_____

_____

_____

_____

_____

Treatment Objectives:

Prevent/Correct Deformity ☐　Improve Ambulation ☐
Reduce Axial Load　　　　 ☐　Fracture Treatment ☐
Protect Joint　　　　　　 ☐　Other_____

ORTHOTIC RECOMMENDATION

LOWER LIMB			FLEX	EXT	ABD	ADD	ROTATION Int.	ROTATION Ext.	AXIAL LOAD
HKAO	Hip								
KAO	Thigh								
	Knee								
AFO	Leg								
	Ankle		(Dorsi)	(Plantar)					
		Subtalar					(Inver.)	(Ever.)	
FO Foot		Midtarsal							
		Met.-phal.							

REMARKS:

_____
Signature

_____
Date

KEY: Use the following symbols to indicate desired control of designated function:

F = FREE — *Free* motion.
A = ASSIST — Application of an external force for the purpose of increasing the range, velocity, or force of a motion.
R = RESIST — Application of an external force for the purpose of decreasing the velocity or force of a motion.
S = STOP — Inclusion of a static unit to deter an undesired motion in one direction.
v = Variable — A unit that can be adjusted without making a structural change.
H = HOLD — Elimination of all motion in prescribed plane (verify position).
L = LOCK — Device includes an optional lock.

Fig. 1.4. Summary and Orthotic Recommendation—Lower Limb.

individuals should have some training and experience in orthotics and the biomechanical principles involved.

Indications for Orthoses

We have said that it is important to identify the primary purposes of an orthotic appliance. In this respect, all orthoses are prescribed for one or more of the following:

TECHNICAL ANALYSIS FORM   SPINE

Name_____ No._____ Age____Sex____Weight_____Height_____

Diagnosis_____ Occupation_____

Present Orthotic Equipment_____
_____

Ambulatory☐   Non Ambulatory☐   Wheelchair☐

Standing Balance: Normal ☐   Impaired ☐   Walking Aid_____

Sitting Position: Stable☐   Unstable☐   Reclined ☐   Upright ☐

Sitting Tolerance: Normal☐   Limited ☐

MAJOR IMPAIRMENTS

A. Structural: No Impairment ☐

   1. Bone: Osteoporosis ☐   Fracture☐   Level_____

             Other_____

   2. Disc Space: (Describe)_____
             _____

   3. Alignment: Scoliosis☐   Kyphosis☐   Lordosis ☐

B. Sensory: No Impairment☐

   1. Anesthesia☐   Location_____

   2. Pain☐   Location_____

C. Upper Limb: No Impairment ☐

   1. Amputation☐ _____

   2. Other_____

D. Lower Limb: No Impairment ☐

   1. Limb Shortening: Right☐   Left☐   Amount_____

   2. Hip Contracture ☐   Ankylosis☐   Flexion☐   Degree_____

      Adduction☐   Degree_____;   Abduction☐   Degree_____;

      Extension☐   Degree_____

   3. Major Motor Loss☐   Location _____

   4. Sensation: Anesthesia ☐   Location_____;

      Hypesthesia☐   Location _____

      Pain☐   Location _____

E. Associated Impairments:_____
_____

Fig. 1.5. Technical Analysis Form with legend—Spine.

1. Relief of pain by limiting motion or weight bearing.
2. Immobilization and protection of weak, painful, or healing musculoskeletal segments.
3. Reduction of axial load.
4. Prevention and correction of deformity.
5. Improvement of function.

Summary of Functional Disability:_____
_____
_____

Treatment Objectives:

        Spinal Alignment ☐   Motion Control ☐
        Axial Unloading ☐   Other _____

ORTHOTIC RECOMMENDATION

| SPINE | FLEX | EXT | LATERAL FLEXION | | ROTATION | | AXIAL LOAD |
			R	L	R	L	
CTLSO Cervical							
TLSO Thoracic							
LSO Lumbar							
(Lumbo sacral							
SIO Sacroiliac							

REMARKS:

KEY: Use the following symbols to indicate desired control of designated function:

F = FREE – Free motion
A = ASSIST – Application of an external force for the purpose of increasing the range, velocity, or force of a motion.
R = RESIST – Application of an external force for the purpose of decreasing the velocity or force of a motion.
S = STOP – Inclusion of a static unit to deter an undesired motion in one direction.
v = Variable – A unit that can be adjusted without making a structural change.
H = HOLD – Elimination of all motion in prescribed plane: specify position, e.g. in degrees or (+) (-).
L = LOCK – Device includes an optional lock.

Signature _____

Date _____

Fig. 1.6. Summary and Orthotic Recommendation—Spine.

In many instances these goals overlap. However, in prescribing and designing orthoses, the clinic team must always keep primary purposes in mind, and the patient and his family must be constantly reminded of them. The orthosis may be rejected otherwise, because the patient may walk better without it. Orthoses, in other words, are not always for improvement of function, and this may need particular emphasis in certain situations.

Relief of Pain by Limiting Motion or Weight Bearing

Musculoskeletal pain may be the result of stretch of a muscle, ligament, or tendon or of irritation of the synovial membrane. It may be due to abnormal motion in a joint, muscle, or ligament. Joint pain may be caused by inflammation with resulting swelling and distension. Pain may be induced even by minimal motion, or only at the extremes of motion or upon actual stretching. Compression or traction of neural structures, as in cervical spondylosis with encroachment on cervical roots, may bring on pain. Relief of pain caused by any of the above factors requires determination of motions to be avoided, of where stress or weight bearing should be allowed, and of what muscles may be contracted safely and usefully. If a part is to be fixed, the position of fixation may be of paramount importance. For example, in a patient with lumbar disc disease the position of comfort may be one of slight flexion. The orthosis should be constructed to meet this requirement; for example, there may be some allowance for a certain amount of flexion, as in the Williams flexor back brace.[2] The opposite may also be true; flexion may be painful or contraindicated, as in osteoporosis of the spine with incipient compression fractures of one or more vertebrae. In this case a Taylor back brace may be prescribed.[3]

Another example of orthosis to relieve pain is the cervical collar; it limits motion that may be painful and can be adjusted to redistribute the weight of the head according to the most comfortable position for the patient. Limitation or complete avoidance of motion reduces pain, as in Fig. 1.7, which illustrates the various positions that may be prescribed.

Pain may also be diminished by changing the axis of weight bearing, especially in the lower limb. By observing the gait, we may note eversion or inversion of the ankle or the lateral or medial thrust of the knee. From the side view, hyperextension or flexion of the knee or excess flexion of the hip, or abnormal positions of the ankle, can be noted. Based on these observations, the shoes may then be wedged or straps may be used on the lower limb orthosis to guide joint loading.

In acute musculoskeletal conditions or where pain is produced by overuse, fatigue, or stretch, pain may be relieved by immobilization. Thus, resting splints are commonly used for the wrist in rheumatoid arthritis, or a supporting sling for the shoulder is used in a patient with painful stretch of the glenohumeral joint following a stroke. An example of this is illustrated in Fig. 1.8.

Immobilization and Protection of Weak or Painful Musculoskeletal Segments

Perhaps the commonest use for an orthosis is to immobilize a body segment. This has its most obvious application in fracture bracing where

---

[2] See Fig. 6.12.
[3] See Fig. 6.15.

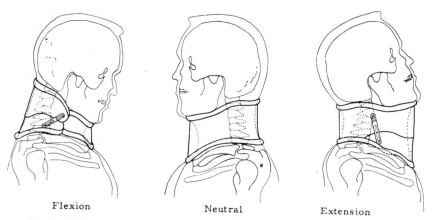

Flexion   Neutral   Extension

Fig. 1.7. Neck may be splinted in flexion, extension, or neutral position.

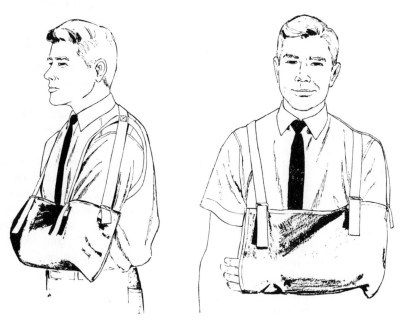

Fig. 1.8. Gaylord upper limb sling.

prevention of stress during fracture healing is required. Chapter 10 reviews fracture bracing, and Sarmiento (9), a pioneer in this field since 1963, in 1974 summarized his experience. Other indications include minimizing joint damage and pain from repeated trauma and painful synovitis in rheumatoid arthritis. Although joint support may be regarded as an example of bracing to prevent arthritic deformity, the primary purpose is joint protection. Unless this is realized, the secondary goal of avoiding deformity will not be achieved. The design utilized may be quite different from that used specifically to improve function in the painless or asymptomatic joint. Temporary subsidence of symptoms should not be an indication for discarding the orthosis since its protective function in an arthritic joint or hemophiliac joint is prophylactic. Effective wear will be achieved only if the patient understands that orthoses are for protective function, not just to relieve pain.

Resting orthoses are generally of simple design and made of relatively light materials, except in the case of weight-relieving apparatus for the lower limbs. Since the introduction of light thermoplastic materials, it has been much easier to achieve compliance with device wearing than previously, when all resting splints were made of plaster of Paris. Unlike many other arthritic devices, they are relatively inexpensive, as many can be supplied from stock sizes.

A newly developing area in orthotics relating to the goals of immobilization and protection of the musculoskeletal system as well as prevention of deformities has been the provision of adapted seating for the disabled. It has been recognized, particularly in children, that little can be accomplished in rehabilitating a severely handicapped person unless he can be maintained in an effective seating position.

An excellent discussion of this by Motloch (6) points out how physically impaired persons confined to chairs must re-educate the weight-bearing areas to function in an unfavorable environment. Skin in the buttock area is basically a temperature control device mechanically protecting the underlying tissues and serving as a bacterial barrier. As buttock skin becomes primarily a weight-bearing surface for the entire body, problems often develop in disabled patients. With prolonged seating, impaired circulation and poor ventilation with an increase in humidity produce conditions in which bacteria flourish. These undesirable skin conditions may exist for up to 10 to 15 hours per day, day after day for years. Skin ischemia, pressure sores, and infections follow, resulting in tissue damage to the area and misery for the patient. Therefore, a need has arisen to fit and fabricate special seats for the physically disabled to prevent these problems.

The principle of providing seating that will ensure comfort and prevent complications such as joint deformities and pressure sores is somewhat dependent on the disability. In cerebral palsy patients such seats will ensure positions that improve posture and inhibit untoward reflexes. One may need to give particular attention to head control so that the subject can relax from an abnormal uncontrollable posture and achieve a position or feeling of comfort and security. This type of seating often takes very careful study, including temporary mock-up-type seating. In cases of severe muscular dystrophy and other paralytic conditions where spinal deformities are produced basically by uncontrolled forces of gravity and muscle imbalance, it is particularly important to maintain normal lumbar lordosis and as the limb muscles become progressively more involved to provide not only trunk but also often head, arm, and leg support. Another special type of seating is required for the patients with sensory loss over the buttock area. This demands studies of pressure tolerance of tissue in order to obtain a seat that will minimize skin pressures over the longest possible time.

Although many different approaches, from custom-molded foam seating to motorized rollers, have been tried, prevention of skin breakdown continues to be a complex problem. Even the best custom seating does not always provide a satisfactory answer, but it is often very helpful.

Reduction of Axial Load

Reduction of the weight borne along the long axis of the limb or the trunk is listed as a separate purpose on the technical analysis forms discussed earlier. Actually, this feature of the orthosis may serve several purposes. For example, although ischial weight-bearing braces which unload the lower limb were useful for relief of pain in the knee or hip, a specially designed brace, such as that used in Legg-Perthes disease, serves to protect the hip from forces leading to femoral head deformity (7). Reduction of axial loading in the lower limb is sought to reduce pain and to prevent deformity or to reduce mobility.

The Milwaukee brace (2) is another example of an orthosis to reduce axial loading. This orthosis attempts to prevent axial gravitational forces from increasing the scoliotic deformity by stimulating the wearer to keep the spine in optimal alignment. Reduction of the axial loading forces of gravity is also a notable feature of the halo apparatus now commonly used to maintain reduction after cervical spinal fractures (see Chapter 5).

Prevention and Correction of Deformities

Prevention of deformity has its most common application in orthotics for children. In the growing child, deformity results either from lack of properly balanced muscle forces around the joint or from other intrinsic or extrinsic forces imposed on developing skeletal parts. "Biologic plasticity" in response to such unbalanced forces leads to abnormal development. Unfortunately, once the skeletal deformity is fixed, rarely will an orthosis correct it. Furthermore, incorrectly applied forces from poorly designed orthoses can even create deformities, as reported in some cases of induced leg deformity by Lusskin (5).

Prevention or correction of deformity in a child by an orthosis requires constant supervision and instruction to the family. This may be achieved in a children's orthotic clinic where well-organized follow-up reviews of braces are practiced. The patient and his family can generally be assured that the use of the orthosis is usually necessary only during the growth period. Muscle transplants and joint stabilizations at the conclusion of growth may allow the brace to be discarded. However, satisfactory surgical correction is usually only possible with the help of bracing to minimize the degree of deformity remaining at full growth.

Dynamic orthoses which apply forces with elastic bands or springs are commonly used to prevent or correct deformity in both children and adults. As they stimulate muscle activity and motion, they are more effective than passive devices in paralytic conditions. Passive or resting orthoses that do not cause the patient to actively exercise must frequently be removed so that the joint can be put through an optimal range of motion.

Designing an effective and acceptable orthosis to prevent deformity and improve function is particularly challenging in the upper limbs. Here, even the most basic functions require a considerable range of motion and versatility. Cosmesis and interference with sensory function may also be problems, particularly in hand bracing. In general, splints for correction or prevention of deformity in upper limbs must be lightweight and easily applied and removed or they will not be utilized. Unfortunately, the ideal orthosis for many upper limb problems has not yet been designed. For example, there is no good functional orthosis for the hemiplegic, or even hemiparetic, upper limb following strokes or head injuries.

Deformities develop in such a creeping, subtle manner that prevention must be considered at the first threat to musculoskeletal integrity. The common conditions that may produce deformities or contractures without suitable orthotic protection are:

1. Muscle imbalance around a joint, whether from upper or lower motor neuron paralysis or muscle disease.
2. Muscle disease or other paralytic conditions leading to unopposed gravitational forces.
3. Progressive fibrous tissue diseases, such as Dupuytren's contracture.
4. Lesions leading to reactive scarring, such as local trauma, burns, or inflammation involving joint structures or muscles.
5. Arthritis, especially of the shoulders, elbows, and knees, leading to pain-induced inhibition of muscular action.
6. A disrupted blood supply to a muscle or limb, such as Volkmann's ischemic contracture.
7. Any painful state of bone, joint, or muscle where inhibition of muscle contraction occurs.

Once a deformity or a contracture has developed and tissue extensibility and normal gliding planes have been lost, force will be required to extend contracted fibers. The longer the condition has existed, the less the chances for recovery of normal physiologic function. Therefore, orthoses for correction should be prescribed early and are far more complex than those for prevention.

Any stretching force may lead to further tissue tears with accompanying reactive scarring and, so, forces must be kept within levels of tissue tolerance. Furthermore, if the stretching force induces undue pain, the patient will actively contract the muscles to fight the force imposed by the brace. Stretching splints are perhaps most effective at night, when the patient is relaxed. Nevertheless, continued stretching may cause pain which may awaken the patient and negate the value of traction. If this occurs, night braces to prevent or correct deformities may have to be worn intermittently, and the patient may be specifically advised concerning wearing times.

A brace to correct a deformity should be constructed to apply an optimal degree of pressure for a long period: months as opposed to weeks. This principle has been applied for many years in different deformities by progressive wedging of plaster casts. An orthosis that will allow some joint motion and thereby preserve active use and muscle strength has definite advantages over a plaster cast. This can be accomplished with a hinge joint with adjustable dial lock which can force the joint into a progressively more extended position. If braces are applied for this purpose to limbs, support should be close to the joints around the contracture to prevent incipient subluxation of the distal segments. The lever arm should be as long as possible for comfortable stretching.

In preventing or correcting a deformity with orthotic devices, what constitutes adequate joint mobility depends on the patient's potential for full recovery. If return to normal is expected, full range of motion should be sought. However, less mobility may be preferred, if as a result of the disease process a considerable permanent loss of strength or control is expected. Not only does this avoid treatment directed towards a purposeless goal, but also some contractures are valuable sources of functional stability. Useful contractures, for example, are the mild finger flexion deformities in the hands of a C-6 quadriplegic patient. Here, tightness in the extrinsic finger muscles allows active wrist extension to flex the fingers and improve grasp. Even severe finger flexion deformities in such a patient may prove useful by allowing him to have a hook grasp if regular grasp cannot be achieved. In such patients, the therapeutic objective in deformity control may be to preserve the useful component of contracture while avoiding further deformities which would reduce function.

The most effective way to reduce any deformity or contracture is to have a normal physiologic force, that is, an active muscle contraction, counteracting the deformity. Unfortunately, this is not always possible in paralytic states, but in nonparalytic conditions such as arthritis any method that can be developed to induce the patient to contract muscles and counteract the progressive loss of joint mobility should be tried.

Lately, there have been developed small, electronic monitoring devices attached to orthoses that inform the patient when he is slipping into a undesirable position such as excess joint flexion (12). One such device, termed "a knee load monitor," has been developed at the Krusen Rehabilitation Engineering Center.[4] In such a device, if pressure is applied for too long in one position an alarm sounds; to turn off the alarm, the patient must

---

[4] Moss Rehabilitation Hospital, Philadelphia, Pa.

contract the muscle that relieves the pressure. More sophisticated information systems have been incorporated into other devices, such as sensing electromyographic activity and giving the electronic signals to the patient either by sound or sight, or by both simultaneously.

We expect that in the next few years biofeedback systems to prevent and correct deformities will be developed in conjunction with many orthotic devices. The advantages of having normal physiologic internal forces opposing the deformity, as compared with mechanical external forces, are obvious.

Improvement of Function

Function is improved by virtually all orthoses by diminishing pain, relieving weight bearing, and preventing deformity. In many orthoses, nevertheless, the primary purpose is to improve function. Such types include all those devices that assist in ambulation, feeding, dressing, and other activities of daily living. An orthosis used to improve function may do so by stabilizing unstable limb segments, stopping or limiting undesired motions, or assisting desired weak motions. Many orthoses feature components that can apply active or passive forces such as springs, elastic bands, or active motions powered by electricity or compressed gas. Devices with neural stimulation of muscle contraction by electricity, such as the electrically assisted drop-foot brace, also fall into this category (11).

Although not strictly classed as orthoses, but rather as the "etcetera" portion of the title of this book, all apparatus such as wheelchairs, respirators, environmental control apparatus, driving aids, etc. may be considered as functional orthoses. Progress in biomedical engineering is leading to more functional types of such instruments and, hence, improved function.

When we consider only those devices that are attached to the body, certain limitations are obvious, particularly in the upper limb. If the device applies external forces, it is only effective in the relaxed limb; if it pulls against simultaneously active antagonistic muscles, skin pressures may greatly exceed tissue tolerance. Speed of action of the dynamic device must also be within physiologic ranges. If it is too slow, the patient will be impatient with the delay and will reject the device. Consequently, dynamic functional orthoses for the upper limb are seldom of value in cases of central nervous system motor disorders. The uncontrollable muscle activity brought on by spasticity, reflex posturing, and primitive motor patterns produces antagonistic muscle action at undesirable times. With rare exceptions, therefore, spring-driven devices or motorized devices are only appropriate for cases with loss of motor units or lower motor neuron disorders (1).

Unwanted and uncontrollable motions such as those occurring in athetoid cerebral palsy are particularly difficult to check with functional orthoses. Some of these can be controlled with weighted cuffs at the wrists or friction-controlling devices, usually with limited success. Unfortunately, our present approach to this type of central nervous system problem is merely trial and error. A great need exists for better orthotic devices to control involuntary movement disorders.

In the upper extremity, another great limitation of functional orthoses is sensory impairment. Although with just visual direction one can place and use the hand, the entire task must be performed within the line of sight. Lack of proprioception or intrinsic feedback makes it impossible to accomplish smooth movements. Each task must be slowly and laboriously accomplished step by step, the appliance being readjusted to each new position required. Therefore, patients with lack of sensation will restrict their use of dynamic or powered orthoses only to simple situations, such as feeding, where another aid will not quite perform the same function or will be less acceptable from the self-care standpoint.

The problem of prescribing functional orthoses for the lower limb is not so much to provide joint immobility or overcome sensory loss as it is to provide strong durable materials to control the large gravitational and muscular forces. Ability to effectively restrict or alter joint motions without intolerably heavy materials must also be considered. Providing a motorized system of control to facilitate walking has not yet been achieved in a functional orthosis with any practical success, although some systems have been developed to control gait in spastic patients by electrical stimulation. The problem is the large amount of power required from the motor to overcome the forces of gravity and inertia in the lower limbs. In our present state of knowledge, the motor and control systems are too heavy and awkward. Furthermore, durability of component is a problem. Such orthoses must take considerable strain, and parts must move many hundreds of times daily if they are to assist walking. The problem is simpler in children, and perhaps we may one day be able to provide a system for storage of energy low in weight and high in output. We may also develop a miniaturized, noiseless motor that will be cosmetically acceptable and functional.

Any application of an orthosis to improve function in an adult is likely to be permanent. Therefore, providing such orthoses requires special care in evaluation to be sure that the appliance will improve function and correct the biomechanical deficiencies without adding problems outweighing the desirable effects.

Functional orthoses are the most difficult and challenging type of appliances to design and prescribe. If such an appliance is uncomfortable, fails to significantly improve function, or is not reasonably cosmetic, it may one day be rejected. Ease of application is also essential. Unless the patient can don and doff the orthosis easily himself, or with minimal assistance, he may become frustrated and discard it. Nevertheless, some orthoses, by improving function, may be an aid to motivation during rehabilitation. A typical example is the flexor-hinge tenodesis orthosis used in quadriplegic patients. Certain orthoses may also aid in building up the strength in the trunk and upper limb muscles so that eventually if the patient decides not to wear his orthosis, his progress toward independent living has been accelerated.

Training is the key to effective motor substitution with functional orthoses. This is especially true if the wearer has to control a switch activating a motor. Unfortunately, none of our available orthotic techniques match the versatility of the human nervous system. Patients will have to adapt to certain restrictions in motor patterns and control mechanisms in almost all functional orthoses. Thus, many functional orthoses require psychological readiness and a natural adaptability; unfortunately, such traits are too often lacking. In poorly motivated patients, the need for psychological and social assessment prior to prescribing such orthoses becomes very apparent.

Failure to keep patients on a training program until the device operates effectively may lead to a high percentage of discarded functional aids. Only when the activities to be performed are achieved with reasonable speed and accuracy can training be discontinued. Both training and performance checkouts should be carried through by conscientious and competent physical or occupational therapists.

Principles of Orthotic Applications

Adequate surface area for comfortable pressure distribution with accurate contouring is one of the basic principles of design applicable to all orthoses. The desired function of the brace will determine the amount of surface needed for comfort. If a joint is to be mobilized, the orthosis should employ the longest lever practicable with the widest possible pressure distribution to give maximum comfort and wearability. Where accurate contouring is difficult, it is desirable to work from cast models. This is particularly true in the lower limb, where there are much greater forces involved than in the upper. It should be remembered that a change of position may cause redistribution of pressure points to which the apparatus must be adapted, particularly in the case of trunk supports. For that reason, corsets often seem more adaptable to many patients than do rigid metal braces.

Comfort in an orthosis is not only determined by surface area but also by joint positioning. For example, a knee joint positioned below the anatomical knee joint will cause considerable calf band pressure when the knee is flexed, as in sitting. A joint that is too high will loosen the calf band when the patient is sitting but tighten it on standing. Single-axis joints in both the lower and the upper limbs, therefore, require careful review. Joint design and placement in a brace should be as close to the anatomical features of the encircled joint as possible. For example, dual-axis joints at the knee, although they increase the cost, may be necessary in some situations where knee mobility is very desirable.

Pain and limb constriction produced by orthoses are unfortunately rather common. The part to be fitted must be examined closely. Tender areas of skin over muscle or bone should be marked. Painful nodules of rheumatoid arthritis, skin erosions, and bony prominences must also be noted and avoided since pressure over them will be painful. The course of nerves and blood vessels should be outlined with a skin pencil, if necessary, to avoid localized compression. Supporting bands around the thigh and calf or in the arm may have to be relocated or reshaped to accommodate local lesions. The possibility of a constructing band of a brace causing distal edema must also be considered, particularly in patients for whom this is a problem from previous history. It may be necessary in some instances for the patient to wear an elastic supporting stocking or other garment under the brace to prevent such a problem from occurring. Edema presents a particularly difficult problem in the newer type of total-contact contoured plastic braces, such as the plastic ankle-foot orthosis. It may be impossible to adjust the device to accommodate for variations in the swelling.

It is important in all types of bracing that the wearer be able to don and doff his own appliance whenever possible. The brace should conserve the time and energy of the patient, thereby encouraging activity, not increasing his energy consumption. Closing devices should be simple. Velcro, for example, is much easier to use than buckles and straps and is much less damaging to overlying clothing. The patient should practice donning and doffing of the appliance under the supervision of his therapist and, if any additional assistive aids are needed, these can then be provided.

For maintenance, orthoses should be as simple and durable as possible since frequent visits to a repair shop may result in less than adequate utilization. Patients should be taught simple maintenance of their braces, such as cleaning the leather and oiling the joints if necessary. Most braces will be immersed in water periodically and so should be constructed to withstand it. Marks of bending tools or unnecessary holes in the metal or leather should be avoided since these are potentially weak points. Final adjustments frequently require moving leather or plastic bands and redrilling uprights. A good orthotist will add support to these weak points if such adjustments must be made. Some useful advice as to maintenance was given by Deaver (3) in the first edition of *Orthotics Etcetera*:

1. Open all locks every week and, with a hairpin or fine wire, remove the lint which collects in the joints.
2. Place a drop of machine oil in each joint every week.
3. Keep leather parts in good repair. Have tears repaired at once. Perspiration stains of leather cannot be completely removed, but washing the leather in lukewarm water with a good saddle soap will help preserve it.
4. Keep the heels and soles of the shoes in good condition so that no part of the brace touches the floor while walking.
5. When the brace has been removed, prop it carefully against the wall or lay it on the floor or table in good alignment. Handle braces with care and avoid injuring them.

6. Examine the skin every night for pressure marks; no metal should rub against any part of the body.
7. Before applying, inspect braces for (a) parts wearing out, (b) loose or missing screws or bolts, and (c) the condition of the straps or buckles.

Cost, unfortunately, is a serious problem with orthotic appliances. If it means the difference between activity or inactivity, it should be secondary to function and comfort. With a view to saving the patient money, we should anticipate the likely progress of the disease or condition. Thus, a patient may be fitted with a temporary adjustable type of brace, and only when he returns home should a permanent one be ordered. During the training period, for example, he may be able to switch from an above-knee type of orthosis to one below the knee. Cost control is of considerable concern to the suppliers of orthoses. The high cost of appliances has been partly due to the orthotic tradition of fabricating all separate components for the brace, although this is rapidly changing. Prefabrication of parts has been steadily increasing since World War II. This has markedly improved orthotic quality since orthotists can devote time and skill to fitting and patient management rather than to spending hours on metal work. In the future, we may see major advances in more modular designs for orthoses, just as we have for prostheses. At present, we still have a multitude of component parts for orthoses, very few of which are interchangeable—if certain parts wear out, a whole new brace may be required. By standardizing the different shapes or sizes, much in the same way that children's "Tinker Toys" are standardized for different designs, the goal of reducing cost and lessening the reliance on custom-made components will be achieved.

Finally, another possibility for cost control is more central fabrication. Facilities with multiple components for orthotic devices are being developed in major geographic distribution centers. In small local facilities, orthotists send the measurements made directly on patients to the central fabrication center. In return they receive a completed orthosis that needs only to be fitted and perhaps slightly modified to the needs of the individual patient. A much smaller inventory of fabrication equipment, parts, and supplies need to be carried by the smaller local facilities. This saves money, and there is minimal delay from measurement to fitting because of the large volume of the central fabrication facility (8).

REFERENCES

1. AMERICAN ACADEMY OF ORTHOPAEDIC SURGEONS. *Atlas of Orthotics*. C. V. Mosby Co., St. Louis, 1975.
2. BLOUNT, W. P., AND MOE, J. H. *The Milwaukee Brace*. Williams & Wilkins Co., Baltimore, 1973.
3. DEAVER, G. G. Lower limb bracing. In *Orthotics Etcetera*, edited by S. Licht. Elizabeth Licht, New Haven, 1966.

4. HARRIS, E. E. A new orthotics terminology. *Orthotics Prosthet.*, *27:* 6–10, 1973.
5. LUSSKIN, R. The influence of errors in bracing upon deformity of the lower extremity. *Arch. Phys. Med. Rehabil.*, *47:* 293–298, 1966.
6. MOTLOCH, W. M. Seating for the physically impaired. *Orthotics Prosthet.*, *32:* 11–21, 1977.
7. TACHDJIAN, M. O., AND JOVETT, T. O. Trilateral socket hip abduction orthosis for the treatment of Legg-Perthes Disease. *Orthotics Prosthet.*, *22:* 49–62, 1968.
8. THRANHARDT, T. Delivery of prosthetics and orthotic services: current status and future needs. *Orthotics Prosthet.*, *31:* 43–46, 1977.
9. SARMIENTO, A. Fracture bracing. *Clin. Orthop.*, *102:* 152–159, 1974.
10. STANIC, U., et al. Multichannel electrical stimulation for correction of hemiplegic gait. *Scand. J. Rehabil. Med.*, *10:* 75–92, 1978.
11. WATERS, R. L., McNEAL, D. R., AND TASTO, J. Experimental correction of foot drop by electrical stimulation of the peroneal nerve. *J. Bone Joint Surg. (Am.)*, *57:* 1047–1054, 1975.
12. WOOLRIDGE, C., LEIPER, C., AND OGSTON, D. Biofeedback training of knee joint position of the cerebral palsied child. *Physiotherapy (Canada)*, *28:* 138–143, 1976.

2

Mechanics of Orthotics

EDWIN M. SMITH, M.D.
ROBERT C. JUVINALL, M.S., M.E.

Orthotic devices traditionally are applied to the body for one or more of the following reasons: (a) to support or immobilize a body part; (b) to correct or prevent deformity; and (c) to assist or restore function (8, 13). There is a common denominator, however, in the way that these objectives are achieved. In each instance the device creates its effect through application of forces.

The forces applied by the device in turn affect movement about skeletal joints. Some devices restrict movement or eliminate it altogether. Others control the path of joint movement and still others act to cause movement.

The reason for altering movement about a joint may simply be that the joint is diseased and must be protected. More commonly, devices are applied to counteract abnormal forces that have developed about or within the joint itself and are causing the movement to be abnormal. This disturbance in forces may be the result of imbalance, weakness, or absence of muscle contraction, or it may occur when tissues serving to constrain joint movement are damaged so that the geometry of the joint is altered.

Thus, the rational use of orthotic devices must be based on an understanding of how internal force systems are deranged and on the way external forces can be applied to correct the derangement. An orthosis must be viewed as combining with body parts to form a mechanical system that obeys mechanical laws and achieves mechanical effects. This chapter, therefore, is concerned with forces; what they are, how they produce different types of motion, how they act in various mechanical systems, and what their effects are on materials and body parts themselves.

Motion

To understand the effects of forces in producing motion, it is necessary first to know the characteristics of motion. All movement can be broken down into one or a combination of two forms: rotation and translation.

Rotation is angular motion relative to a fixed line or axis, and translation is motion without change in angular orientation, usually in a straight line.

Any movement whatever of a rigid body can be expressed as the vector sum of six possible motion components, or motion in six possible degrees of freedom. These consist of translation (displacement) along any three arbitrary but mutually perpendicular axes and rotation about the same three axes. Consider, for example, the aircraft pictured in Fig. 2.1. The plane can translate along the X, Y, and Z axes, and it can also rotate about these axes. In the human body, each joint is capable of providing one or more of the six possible movements. For example, the metacarpophalangeal (MCP) joint permits rotation about the flexion-extension and abduction-adduction axes and, to a slight extent, the longitudinal axis. Although translational movement also is possible at this joint, it is negligible.

Sometimes it is necessary to apply a brace to a skeletal joint without restricting movement of the joint. One way this can be accomplished is through the use of an analog brace, that is, one in which the axes of rotation coincide with those of the anatomical joint. An analog brace, therefore, must be able to duplicate the degrees of freedom inherent in the joint.

Forces

The relative condition of rest or motion of an object is changed by the action of forces on the object. Forces exert their effect by pull (tension) or push (compression), and they are described according to their magnitude, direction, and point of application. Conventionally, an arrow is used to represent a force, because the arrow can indicate each of these parameters.

A basic principle of force systems is that the vector summation of all forces acting on an object must equal zero if the object is to be in a state of equilibrium. Another fundamental characteristic is that whenever a force is applied to an object by a second object, there is an equal and opposite force

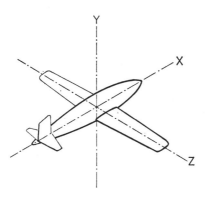

Fig. 2.1. Coordinate system of an airplane.

applied by the second to the first object. This is the action-reaction principle of Newton.

Two or more forces which intersect can be combined into a resultant vector, and likewise a single force can arbitrarily be broken down into two or more component vectors. In either instance, the combined effect of the multiple forces is the same as the individual effect of the resultant force.

To determine the component of a force acting in the direction of a given axis, the force is projected onto that axis. For example, Fig. 2.2 shows a force F of arbitrary orientation resolved into three mutually perpendicular components, F_x, F_y, and F_z, by being projected onto axes x, y, and z. The action of the resultant force F is identical to that of the three component forces acting together.

Application of these principles is illustrated by Fig. 2.18, which shows the first dorsal interosseous muscle acting at the MCP joint. The tension in the tendon is resolved into three mutually perpendicular components tending to translate the finger volarly along the y axis, radially along the z axis, and proximally along the x axis. However, in the normal MCP joint, counteracting internal forces are developed which prevent more than minimal displacement in any of these directions.

TORQUE

The first dorsal interosseus also attempts to rotate the finger about each of the three axes, and in this it succeeds when not opposed by other muscles or structures. The strength of the rotating tendency about any axis is the product of the force component in a plane perpendicular to the axis times the perpendicular distance from the force component to the axis. This distance is the moment arm, and the strength of the rotating tendency is the torque, or the moment, acting about the axis.

Thus, the tendon force (FDI) also creates torques T_x, T_y, and T_z about the three MCP axes (Fig. 2.3). T_y is the greatest of the three torques; hence, radial deviation by the first dorsal interosseus is stronger than either flexion or longitudinal rotation at the MCP joint. [In reality, the movements of

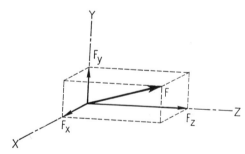

Fig. 2.2. Resolution of a force (F) into its components.

longitudinal rotation and deviation are linked together by the action of passive joint restraints (12).]

The concept of torque is vital to an understanding of the action of any muscle on a joint. The effectiveness of the muscle depends as much on its distance from the axis of rotation as it does on its strength of contraction. Thus, it is possible for a relatively weak muscle to have a much greater effect on a joint than its tension-generating capacity would indicate. For example, the abdominal muscles are powerful flexors of the spine largely because of their long moment arms. Conversely, if the moment arm of a muscle is shortened, the effect is the same as weakening the muscle itself. One reason patellectomy causes reduction in strength of knee extension by the quadriceps is that the perpendicular distance between patellar ligament and knee axis of rotation is shortened. The process of testing muscle strength clinically is really one of assessing torque produced by the muscle.

The principles of torque are equally valid, of course, for an external force applied by an orthotic device. The greater the perpendicular distance from the skeletal axis to the line of action of the force, the greater the torque generated by the device about that axis. For example, orthoses that power elbow flexion generate more torque when a given actuating force is placed farther from the elbow axis.

The gain in torque, however, must be purchased with reduced angular excursion of the part being moved. This is so because for a given expenditure of input energy, there can be no change in total work output (torque times angular displacement), despite variation in torque.

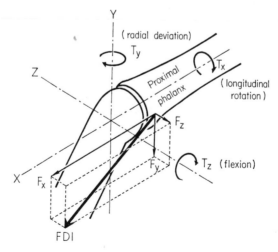

Fig. 2.3. Forces and torques produced at the metacarpophalangeal (*MCP*) joint by the first dorsal interosseous muscle (*FDI*).

EQUILIBRIUM OF TORQUES

In the example of torque produced by the first dorsal interosseus, the muscle was seen to exert translational forces without causing significant translational movement. Displacement is prevented by equal and opposite forces developed within the joint structure. If there is no translation, the first condition of static equilibrium is met.

Joint rotation can still occur, however, unless the second condition of static equilibrium is also met, namely, that the vector sum of all torques acting on an object must be zero. To prevent rotation of the MCP joint, other muscles or structures must generate opposing torques when the first dorsal interosseus contracts.

Thus, for an object to remain at rest there must be no unbalanced force along any axis and no unbalanced moment about any axis. If the requirements for static equilibrium are satisfied with respect to any three mutually perpendicular directions, they are automatically satisfied with respect to all other directions. If balance is lost, motion in the direction of unbalance will be initiated, thereby creating a dynamic system.

FREE-BODY ANALYSIS OF STATIC EQUILIBRIUM

One of the difficulties in studying force systems within the body is the problem of measuring directly the tension generated by individual muscles. However, values can often be estimated indirectly through the technique of free-body analysis of systems in static equilibrium (3). This technique, which is invaluable in the study of deformity (17), is useful also in determining force requirements of orthotic systems designed to counteract the deformity.

Free-body analysis is based on the principle that characteristics of static equilibrium apply not only to a complete body but also to any segment of it isolated by an imaginary cutting plane. Thus, the effect on a single skeletal joint of forces acting on multiple joints can be calculated, as can the internal forces and moments at various points between the joints.

As an example, consider a simplified analysis of forces acting during weight bearing about a knee (22) with a 25° flexion contracture. In Fig. 2.4a, the entire limb is shown as a free body in static equilibrium during a portion of the stance phase. Body weight (W) acts downward from the center of gravity, while an equal and opposite force (W) is applied to the foot by the floor. To determine the strength of quadriceps contraction needed to keep the knee from buckling, the femur alone may be considered as a free body (Fig. 2.4b). Equilibrium of this member requires that the summation of moments of all forces about the knee axis be zero. If the patellar ligament lies 1½ inches in front of the instantaneous axis of the knee (dimension a) and if the weight line passes 3 inches posterior to the axis (dimension 2a) during the portion of the stance phase depicted, then the quadriceps must contract with tension (Q) twice body weight to preserve equilibrium. If weight of the body (minus the leg below the knee) is 150 pounds, 450 inch-pounds of extension torque or 300 pounds of quadriceps tension are required to keep the flexed knee from buckling (Fig. 2.4*b*). When the weight line is so located, the same amount of torque must be developed by a long leg brace used in these circumstances to prevent flexion of a flail knee.

Free-body analysis also permits calculation of the bone-compressive force (*C*), applied in this example to the articulating surfaces. Based on the assumption that no muscles other than the quadriceps are contracting, and that the angle of the quadriceps tendon is as shown, then horizontal and vertical forces are in equilibrium if the bone compressive force (*C*) is equal to approximately 2.9 *W*, or 435 pounds. This solution can be derived by constructing the force polygon illustrated in Fig. 2.4*b*. Thus, in the presence of painful disease of the flexed knee joint, bone-compressive forces can be reduced a sizable amount by straightening the knee or by using a brace to substitute for quadriceps function.

For the sake of completeness, the analysis can be extended below the femur to the compression and extension forces acting on the tibia (Fig. 2.4*c*). These forces are of the same magnitude, but in the opposite direction, as those acting on the femur.

Beam Loading

When forces are applied to a rigid beam, they become distributed within the beam in a predictable manner. If the applied forces are not colinear with the reacting forces, two types of load are created within the beam:

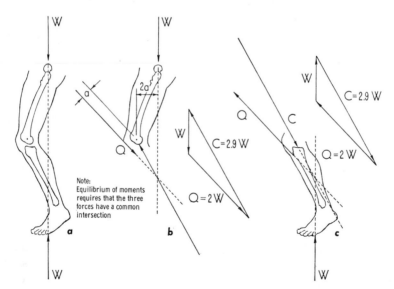

Fig. 2.4. Leg as a free body in static equilibrium. *a*, femur and tibia in equilibrium; *b*, equilibrium of forces on femur; *c*, equilibrium of forces on tibia. *W*, body weight; *Q*, quadriceps tension; *C*, bone-compressive force.

bending moments and transverse shear forces. Because of their importance in orthotics, each will be considered in some detail.

BENDING MOMENTS IN BEAMS

It can be shown that the bending tendency due to forces acting on a beam varies in different parts of the beam. Fig. 2.5*a* depicts a beam with a load at the center supported by reacting forces at either end. In this illustration a clockwise moment acting to bend the beam at the center is caused by the left reaction and is equal to 10 pounds times 12 inches. To satisfy equilibrium of moments at the center, there must be an equal counterclockwise torque of 10 pounds times 12 inches produced by the right reaction.

In Fig. 2.5*b*, a segment of the beam is isolated by an imaginary cutting plane. The magnitude of the moment acting to bend the beam in a clockwise direction at this particular plane is equal to 10 pounds times 8 inches, or 80 inch-pounds. This is balanced by a counterclockwise, or negative, torque of 80 inch-pounds. This is produced by the 20-pound downward force acting on a 4-inch moment arm (80 inch-pounds) minus the 10-pound upward force acting on a 16-inch moment arm (160 inch-pounds).

If the imaginary cutting plane were moved progressively along the beam, the magnitude of the bending moment would vary from zero at the ends to maximum under the middle load (see bending-moment diagram, Fig. 2.5*a*).

By applying the same principles, it can be shown that when the location of the load is shifted, reaction forces of different magnitudes are required for equilibrium. Fig. 2.5*c* shows the load shifted 4 inches to the left and increased to 30 pounds to preserve the original bending moment of 120 inch-pounds at the center. In this case, a bending moment of 160 inch-pounds exists in the plane of the load. As will be seen, the effects of shifting loads

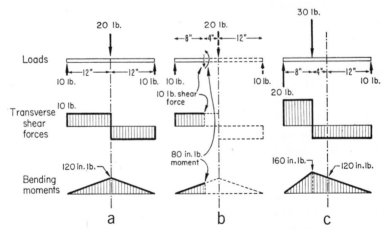

Fig. 2.5. Shear forces and bending moments resulting from beam loading. *a*, load at beam center; *b*, effect on plane 4 inches to left of center load; *c*, off-center load selected to produce same effect at center as in *a*.

on a beam have importance in bracing when the required torque is fixed by the internal characteristics of the body part.

Although a beam is generally thought of as a rigid member, the same principles apply if a joint is inserted, provided there are sufficient restrictions to rotation for the joint to transmit a bending moment. In the body, skeletal joints can be considered as beams and as subject to principles governing beam loading.

BENDING MOMENTS AS APPLIED IN ORTHOTICS

One of the more common braces used in medicine is the type applying force at three points. Such braces generally are used to cause or restrict rotation of joints through creation of bending moments. A "middle" force is located at or near the joint affected and is directed more or less opposite to the two "end" forces. Several features of three-point braces deserve consideration.

Since the bending moment is proportional to the length of the moment arm, the effectiveness of a three-point brace is strongly influenced by the location of the forces relative to the skeletal joint axis. The farther the end forces are from the joint, the greater will be their moment arms and the smaller will be their magnitudes needed to produce a given torque at the joint. If the end forces can be thus reduced, the middle force will be correspondingly diminished. This is so because the sum of the end and middle forces must equal zero if equilibrium is to exist. Similarly, if the middle force is moved away from the joint toward one end, the required corrective torque can be provided only if the middle force and the end force toward which it is moved are increased (Fig. 2.5c). Finally, if multiple joints (as in the spine) are spanned, the bending moment will be greatest at the particular joint closest to the middle force. Thus, for a three-point brace to provide a corrective torque with the least possible pressure, the middle force should be located directly over the affected joint, and the end forces as far away as practical.

A good example of a brace applying bending moments is the common drop-foot brace (Fig. 2.6). This device with its spring-loaded ankle applies three points of pressure: (a) on the metatarsal heads by means of the sole of the shoe; (b) on the dorsum of the ankle by means of the proximal shoe lace; and (c) on the upper calf through the calf band. The bending moment required at the ankle is determined by the internal characteristics of the wearer's lower limb. The forces producing this moment can be minimized by keeping the dorsal application directed as close to the flexion-extension axis of the ankle as possible and the calf and sole applications as far away as possible. In practice, other considerations such as anatomical factors limit the length of the moment arms.

While the brace is applying forces to a body part, it is at the same time receiving equal and opposite forces from the body part (action-reaction

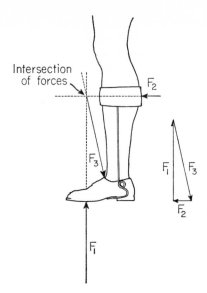

Fig. 2.6. Equilibrium of forces (*F*) applied by a drop-foot brace.

principle). Thus the brace serves as a beam and is also subjected to bending moments. In the drop-foot brace, the shoe must resist this bending as the rest of the brace does. The moment is greatest at the point of stirrup attachment and least at the metatarsal head area. A shank that is too flexible can negate the effect of the brace, just as can the use of elastic shoe laces on the dorsum.

Up to this point, only the effect of loading a beam in a single plane has been considered. If forces in two different planes are applied, a more complex reaction occurs. In general, bending moments are developed in two or more planes also, creating a twisting action or torsion within the beam.

This principle can be shown by introducing a 90° bend into the beam illustrated in Fig. 2.5*a*. In this situation, the three points of pressure are no longer in the same plane, even though they remain parallel (Fig. 2.7). The forces still balance, but the moments about the *x* and *y* axes do not. The correction of this imbalance requires the introduction of torques T_x and T_y as shown.

This situation makes a subtle appearance in orthotics when a brace applying side loads undergoes a bend as, for example, during flexion of a long leg brace with a valgus dial. When the knee is extended, the three points of pressure necessary for valgus correction all act in the same plane, creating a bending moment in the leg which is maximum at the knee (Fig. 2.8*a*). With flexion, however, the mechanics of the brace are as shown in Fig. 2.8*b*. To establish equilibrium of moments about the *x* axis, a torque (T_x) equal to $12F_1$ is necessary, and about the *y* axis a torque (T_y) of $12F_2$ must exist.

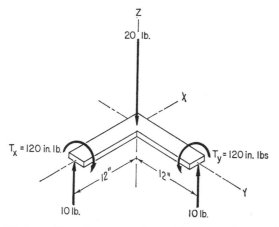

Fig. 2.7. Equilibrium of bending moments and forces on beam with 90° bend. *T*, torque.

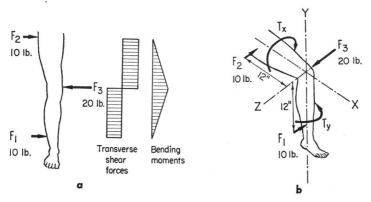

Fig. 2.8. Beam loading produced by brace for correction of *genu valgum. a,* leg loaded as a straight beam; *b,* leg loaded as a beam with 90° bend. *T*, torque.

If there is no provision for T_x during flexion, the brace will rotate about the *x* axis until the net value of F_1 becomes zero, and if there is no T_y, the brace will rotate about *y* until the net of F_2 is zero. If neither countertorque is provided, the net values of both F_1 and F_2 will become zero, and to satisfy equilibrium of forces the corrective force F_3 will also be lost. This situation prevails even though both uprights make positive contact with the leg. Rotation will occur about each axis until pressure of the upright on the medial aspect of the thigh and lower leg equal those on the lateral aspect, resulting in a net correction force of zero.

In practice, T_y is provided in part by attaching the brace to the foot through the shoe, but T_x usually remains minimal because of inadequate torsional attachment of brace to thigh. Without T_x, F_1 would become zero leaving only F_2 to counteract corrective force F_3. Thus, valgus correction tends to be considerably reduced whenever the brace is not completely extended.

TRANSVERSE SHEAR FORCES IN BEAMS

As previously indicated, when opposing forces which are not colinear are applied in the same plane to a beam, they produce not only bending moments but also transverse shear forces within the beam. The shear forces act to displace one segment of the beam relative to another along the plane of action of the forces. If the beam thus loaded is cut transversely, the cut ends will displace. The magnitude of the shear forces at any one point in the beam is equal to the sum of all forces on either side of the cutting plane (Fig. 2.5).

It follows that braces employing three points of pressure create shear forces as well as bending moments. For example, a posterior splint used to stretch a flexion contracture of the knee also develops forces acting to displace the tibia on the femur. If the lower strap of the knee pad is fastened more tightly than the upper strap, the shear forces act to subluxate the tibia posteriorly (Fig. 2.9), and if the upper strap is the tightest, the tibia tends to be displaced anteriorly (Fig. 2.9*b*). It is possible, however, to retain the extension torque while eliminating the brace-induced shear force at the knee. This can be done by tightening the upper strap so that it exerts the same force as the posterior thigh contact and the lower strap the same force as the calf contact (Fig. 2.9*c*). Because forces within the knee may tend to subluxate the tibia posteriorly as the knee is stretched, it is often preferable to lessen this tendency by tightening the upper strap only.

Occasionally, it is desirable to apply shear forces to a joint without causing associated bending moments. This can be done by utilizing four points of pressure instead of three. For example, a long leg brace is sometimes used

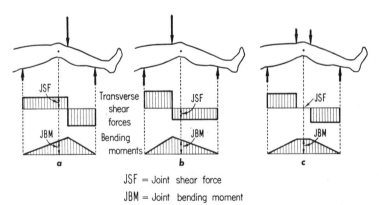

JSF = Joint shear force

JBM = Joint bending moment

Fig. 2.9. Effect of anterior strap placement on stretching a knee flexion contracture with a splint. *a*, strap placed distal to axis; *b*, strap placed proximal to axis; *c*, straps placed to eliminate brace-induced shear force on joint.

to control anteroposterior instability at the knee while still permitting free flexion-extension. To prevent the femur in Fig. 2.10 from displacing anteriorly, it would be necessary to tighten the upper strap of the knee pad and make the calf band shallower than the lower thigh band. In doing this, torques F_1a and F_2b would be developed acting to rotate the brace at the knee. These would be balanced by opposing torques F_3c and F_4d, utilizing forces developed at the upper posterior thigh band and anterior shoe respectively. The shear forces at the knee would not be neutralized, however, because forces F_1 and F_2 adjacent to the knee are smaller than forces F_3 and F_4 distant from the knee. The magnitude of the shear force is equal to $F_2 - F_4$, which is also equal to $F_1 - F_3$.

Alignment of Device and Skeletal Axes

When considering the effects of applying a brace to a body part, it is often assumed that if there is a joint in each, their axes coincide. In practice, however, the axes do not always coincide, either by design or by accident. When they do not, new sets of forces which may not be desirable are introduced during portions of the joint excursion. These new forces in general are antagonistic to the desired force and tend to cause binding and sliding of the brace on the body part.

For the customary brace with a single axis, the best attainable alignment may be limited by normal shifting of the skeletal axis with joint motion. The knee axis, for example, shifts several centimeters between extremes of flexion and extension (9), so that small amounts of binding between brace and leg are inherent in single-axis long leg braces allowing knee movement.

More often than not, however, misalignment is the result of failure to locate the brace axis on the skeletal axis. In general, the location of the skeletal axis of a hinge joint can be estimated by finding the tubercles of the proximal bone. It is from the tubercles that the collateral ligaments arise,

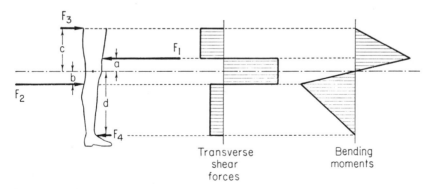

Fig. 2.10. Force system producing shear forces without bending moment at the knee.

and it is about the approximate origins of these ligaments that the distal bone tends to rotate.

There are two ways in which the skeletal and devices axes may fail to be colinear. They may fail to be parallel, or they may be parallel but displaced from each other. To illustrate these two types of misalignment, consider the knee as a simple hinged joint with a long leg brace attached (Fig. 2.11). It is assumed that the ankle joint (A) of the brace is rigidly positioned by a metal stirrup attached to the shoe and that about the knee the brace has four contact points: anterior thigh, anterior tibia, posterior thigh and posterior calf. Proximally, the brace is constrained by anterior and posterior thigh contacts. If the brace axis is coincident with the axis of the knee, the pressure exerted by the various contact points should remain essentially unchanged during extension (Fig. 2.11a) and flexion (Fig. 2.11b).[1]

AXES PARALLEL BUT DISPLACED

If the axes of the knee and brace are parallel but displaced, binding forces are created in the plane of movement. In the following examples, it is assumed that the brace is fitted with the knee in extension so that the binding occurs as the knee flexes.

The first example involves displacement of the brace axis posterior to the knee axis (Fig. 2.12). To visualize the consequences of this type of displacement, a pin can be imagined as passing through the brace and thigh at point T. As the knee flexes, the knee and brace axes are forced closer together. This creates extra pressure on the posterior calf and thigh bands and serves to resist flexion (Fig. 2.12b). Since there is no pin at T, the force on the posterior bands can be reduced by sliding the brace proximally and shifting the top posteriorly on the thigh. The net effect of posterior displacement of the brace axis is to cause some degree of all of these actions during knee flexion. If the brace axis is located anterior to the knee axis, the effects are just the opposite.

When the brace axis is misaligned proximally, the effects can be pictured by again imagining a pin through T (Fig. 2.13a). During flexion in this situation, pressure is developed on the posterior thigh and anterior leg (Fig. 2.13b). Because the brace is not fixed at T, the top tends to shift distally and posteriorly on the thigh. If the brace axis is placed too low, the reverse effects are created.

As previously indicated, this analysis assumes that the brace is fitted to the extended knee. If the knee is flexed 90° during fitting, the binding and sliding would occur during extension, and forces resulting from each type of misalignment would be reversed. Fitting of the brace with the knee partially flexed would cause resistance to the extremes of both extension and flexion, but to a lesser degree.

---

[1] With changes in knee position, there may be corresponding changes in soft tissue position, so that altered bulk beneath the contact points may affect the contact pressures.

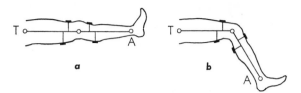

Fig. 2.11. Long-leg brace aligned with knee axis. *T,* proximal end of bace; *A,* ankle joint.

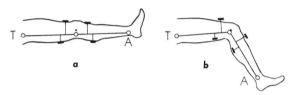

Fig. 2.12. Brace axis located posterior to knee axis (brace fitted in extension). *T,* proximal end of brace; *A,* ankle.

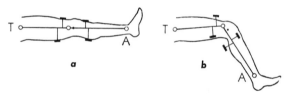

Fig. 2.13. Brace axis located superior to knee axis (brace fitted in extension). *T,* proximal end of brace; *A,* ankle.

It should be pointed out that other factors can also influence binding. The length of the various moment arms, closeness of fit at each contact point, tissue compressibility, stiffness of the brace, and shift of skeletal axes all can play roles.

AXES NONPARALLEL

The second type of joint misalignment occurs when the axes of a brace and hinged skeletal joint are not parallel but intersecting. There are two ways in which parallelism may be lost. Using the long leg brace again as an example, the brace and its axis may be rotated internally or externally relative to the knee axis (Fig. 2.14*a*), or the brace axis may be tilted in the medial or lateral plane, placing it, in effect, in the varus or valgus position relative to the knee axis (Fig. 2.15*a*). In both instances the result of the misalignment is that the knee attempts to flex and extend in one plane and the brace in another.

In the circumstance where the brace axis is internally or externally rotated (Fig. 2.14*b*), flexion of the brace fitted in extension causes progressively large side loads to develop (Fig. 2.14c) which act to resist the flexion. These side loads occur on the inside (or outside) of the ankle and thigh together with an opposing force on the outside (or inside) of the knee in a different plane. Although the forces are balanced, their moments are not in equilibrium (Fig. 2.8b) and thus tend to twist the leg in the brace, and the brace on the leg, until the axes are parallel. As a consequence, this type of misalignment tends to be self-correcting. The extent of correction depends on how readily the brace can rotate axially on the body part. The foot is often the limiting factor, as it constrains internal or external rotation of the shoe and the attached brace.

When parallelism is lost because the brace axis is tilted relative to the skeletal axis, for example, set into varus or valgus, side loads (Figs. 2.8, 2.15b) again create twisting torques between brace and body part. In this

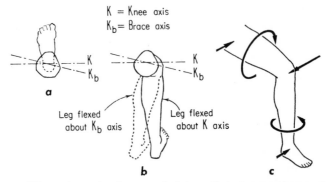

Fig. 2.14. Effect of rotating brace axis internally to knee axis. a, relation of axes (looking down from top, knee extended); b, leg position when flexed about skeletal and brace axes, respectively (looking down from top); c, side loads and resulting twisting moments applied to leg as a free body in equilibrium (see Fig. 2.10b).

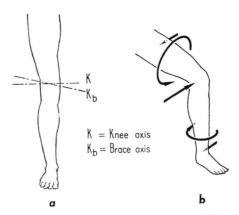

Fig. 2.15. Effect of tilting brace axis into valgus relative to knee axis. a, relation of axes; b, side loads with resultant twisting moments.

case, however, it is not possible to eliminate binding by rotating the brace on the leg.

Thus, both types of parallelism loss can be detected by checking for changing side loads and axial rotation as the joint goes through its range of motion. In the first type, the misalignment can be corrected by rotating the brace axially on the body part, but in the second type it cannot.

Intentional Use of Nonparallel Axes

In joints or joint complexes with multiple axes, bracing is sometimes used to prevent rotation about undesired axes. In this situation, the single axis of the brace is made nonparallel with the undesired axes, and through creation of side loads the brace forces the skeletal parts to move in the desired path. A short leg brace, for example, may be used on an ankle with a varus deformity to confine ankle excursion to a more normal arc. The effectiveness of a brace in such a situation will depend on how closely the brace axis parallels the desired axis and on how well the corrective forces constrain the skeletal links to rotate on that axis. In practice, it is sometimes necessary to overcorrect with the brace to compensate for tissue compression and shear and the inability of the device to induce skeletal motion identical to its own.

Intentional Use of Displaced Axes

Little value is obtained, as a rule, from deliberately displacing the axis of an analog brace. The resultant sliding or binding action is seldom beneficial. When a brace is a weight-bearing structure, however, axis displacement can sometimes be put to advantage by controlling the location of the axis relative to the brace's weight-bearing line. In the functional free-hinge knee brace, the axis of this partially weight-bearing device is placed posterior to the weight-bearing line (1). In this way, an extension torque is created which contributes significantly to the stability of the knee during weight bearing.

When a device spans multiple joints and is not an analog of the body part to which it is attached, displacement of the device axes generally is not important. For example, the balanced forearm orthosis does not require axes colinear with the elbow and shoulder joints, even though it spans these structures by attaching to the forearm and the trunk (through the wheelchair). Because multiple links are involved in both the device and the upper extremity, movement of one need not coincide with movement of the other. The important requirement of such a system is that the device provide the degrees of freedom and excursion desired for the body parts affected.

Force-related Behavior of Materials

The forces applied by orthotic devices must be transmitted through both the external "hardware" and internal tissues. The response of these materials to loads can influence not only the force balances which prevail, but the effectiveness of the device itself. Four types of force-related behavior characteristics govern the response of materials to loads: friction, elasticity, viscosity, and inertia. Nearly all aspects of the passive response of a given substance to force can be described according to one or more of these characteristics.

Forces associated with a particular response are commonly given the same name as the behavior characteristics. For example, forces developed in a spring are often called elastic forces. It should be remembered, however, that a description of a force is not dependent on its source, but need include only magnitude, direction, and point of application.

Friction

Common usage of the term friction refers to the dry or "Coulomb" type of friction, as distinguished from viscosity. Dry friction involves development of a force which opposes motion or a tendency toward motion between two mating surfaces (Fig. 2.16a). The coefficient of static friction between the two surfaces is the ratio of the force necessary to induce relative motion between the surfaces to the force acting perpendicular to the surfaces. Once motion is established, friction force usually decreases; thus, the coefficient of dynamic friction is generally less. It tends to remain constant, however, for all values of velocity other than zero (Fig. 2.16a). In normal skeletal joints, friction tends to be negligible and to have little influence on joint motion (7, 24).

Elasticity

Elasticity is the property of an object or material which permits it to resist deformation and to return completely to its original size and shape when the deforming force is removed (Fig. 2.17a). Elastic behavior implies a time-dependent normally linear relationship between force and deformation (displacement) and is measured by the slope of the force-displacement curve (Fig. 2.17b). The slope, in turn, is dependent on the elastic properties of the material and on the size and shape of the specimen tested. The basic elastic property of a material is described by its "modulus of elasticity," the ratio of force per unit area (stress) to stretch per unit length (strain).

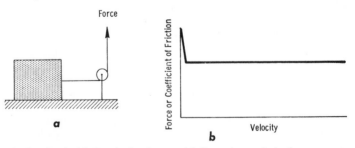

Fig. 2.16. Coulomb friction behavior. a, friction element; b, force necessary to maintain constant sliding velocity as a function of velocity.

Although the relationship between force and displacement is usually linear, it is not always so. The spring in Fig. 2.18a with unequal spacing between its coils exemplifies nonlinear elastic behavior. Under load, the bottom coil closes and no longer contributes to the deflection. The spring thus becomes stiffer. If the spring is wound with a continuously increasing pitch, it becomes progressively stiffer when compressed, as is shown by the curve in Fig. 2.18b. Human connective tissue (20) shows this characteristic of stiffness increasing with load.

Viscosity

Viscosity was described by Newton as "the lack of slipperiness of the parts of the liquid." It is actually a form of friction which is dependent on the velocity of movement between portions of a material. It is exemplified by a piston moving through a viscous liquid, as in a dashpot (Fig. 2.19a).

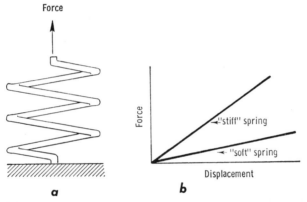

Fig. 2.17. Linear elastic behavior. a, linear elastic element (spring); b, force necessary to maintain constant displacement as a function of displacement.

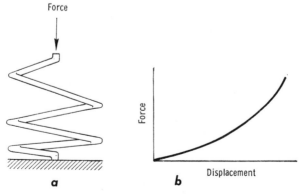

Fig. 2.18. Nonlinear elastic behavior. a, nonlinear elastic element (spring); b, force necessary to maintain constant displacement as a function of displacement.

Whereas an elastic substance tends to return to a position of zero displacement, a viscous substance tends to return to a state of zero velocity (the first time-derivative of displacement). The force-velocity relationship of viscous materials typically is linear, as shown in Fig. 2.19b, although nonlinear relationships have been described for some materials, such as synovial fluid (2).

Inertia

All bodies possess mass, and inherent in mass is inertia, the resistance to acceleration of the mass (Fig. 2.20). Thus, inertial behavior is characteristic of all matter. Inertial force is equal to mass times acceleration (the second time-derivative of displacement). In orthotics, inertial forces are relatively unimportant because of the limited accelerations and masses involved.

Comparison of Elasticity, Viscosity, and Inertia

Before examining combinations of these basic behavioral characteristics, the simplicity and similarity of relationships governing linear elasticity, viscosity, and inertia should be considered. Elastic forces are proportional to displacement and tend to restore zero displacement. Viscous forces are

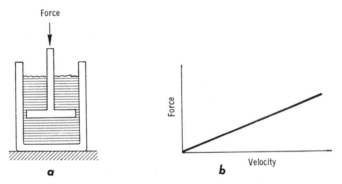

Fig. 2.19. Viscous behavior. a, viscous element (dashpot); b, force necessary to maintain constant velocity as a function of velocity.

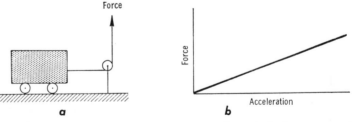

Fig. 2.20. Inertial behavior. a, inertial element (mass); b, force necessary to maintain constant acceleration as a function of acceleration.

proportional to velocity and tend to restore zero velocity. Inertial forces are proportional to acceleration and tend to restore zero acceleration. Elastic forces are totally independent of velocity and acceleration, viscous forces are totally independent of displacement and acceleration, and inertial forces are totally independent of displacement and velocity. As previously mentioned, velocity is the first time-derivative of displacement, while acceleration is the first time-derivative of velocity, or the second time-derivative of displacement.

RHEOLOGY

Rheology is the science that deals with the deformation or flow of matter in relation to its frictional, elastic, viscous, and inertial response to stress (15). In most examples of material deformation, however, acceleration is negligible, so that inertial behavior is usually of minor importance. Because the design and function of orthotic devices in part depends on rheologic properties of body tissues, this science will be considered further.

If a constant continuous force is applied to a spring in parallel with a dashpot (Fig. 2.21*a*), the spring will elongate gradually. The initial rate of elongation will depend on the viscosity of the dashpot fluid; however, the subsequent rate will decrease as increasing elastic resistance builds up (Fig. 2.21*b*). As the elastic resistance approaches the applied force, the velocity— and hence viscous resistance—approaches zero. On removal of the load, the elastic forces act to restore the initial position. This type of response is sometimes termed anelastic behavior.

In contrast, a constant force applied to a spring in series with a dashpot (Fig. 2.22*a*) produces a quite different effect. The spring will immediately elongate fully, and with the passage of time further displacement will occur as the piston moves in the dashpot (Fig. 2.22*b*). Release of the force will

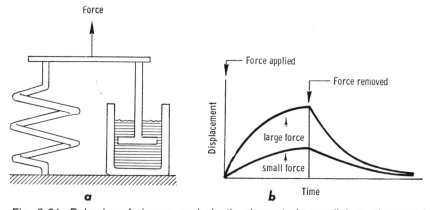

Fig. 2.21. Behavior of viscous and elastic elements in parallel. *a,* elements in parallel; *b,* displacement as a function of time for different constant forces.

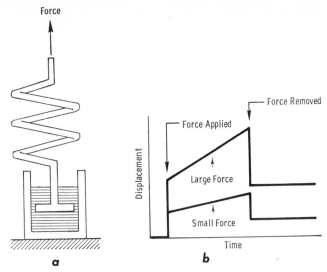

Fig. 2.22. Behavior of viscous and elastic elements in series. a, elements in series; b, displacement as a function of time for different constant forces.

result in immediate restoration of the initial spring length but no restoration of dashpot length. Permanent deformation of the system will have resulted.

A third common type of material behavior is represented by a friction element connected in parallel with a dashpot (Fig. 2.23a). A constant force too small to overcome the static friction of the system causes no movement, but if it exceeds the static friction force, that is, the yield point of the system, the weight slides at a constant velocity determined by the viscosity. (If there were no viscous element in the system, the weight would accelerate continuously). As shown in Fig. 2.23b, the force required for a given velocity is the sum of that required to overcome friction (Fig. 2.16b) and viscosity (Fig. 2.19b). Once the force is removed, there is no recovery of original length (Fig. 2.23c). This model illustrates idealized plastic deformation of a material. No deformation occurs until a yield point is exceeded, and then irreversible deformation develops.

A related combination is the spring fastened in series with a friction element (Fig. 2.24a). If a constant force is applied which is inadequate to overcome friction, the spring elongates but no permanent deformation occurs. A larger force exceeding the yield point causes the weight to move with increasing velocity as long as the force is applied (Fig. 2.24b). Upon removal of the force, the spring shortens and the block stops. Since permanent deformation occurs, this system represents another form of plastic change.

Of course, any combination of elements is possible. To describe the rheologic properties of body tissues requires models which are more complex, as will be seen.

A term not previously mentioned, but sometimes encountered in rheologic descriptions, is "creep." It refers to the total time-dependent phase of deformation, regardless of whether the change is permanent. Its common use is in connection with materials having slow rates of deformation.

Rheologic Properties of Joint-Constraining Tissues

The direction and extent of passive movement of a joint are determined by the characteristics of tissues constraining the joint. The tissues involved include bone, cartilage, muscle, connective tissue, skin, and even blood

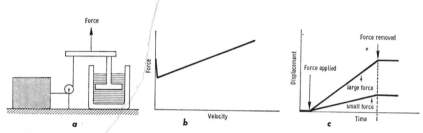

Fig. 2.23. Behavior of viscous and Coulomb friction elements in parallel. *a,* elements in parallel; *b,* force necessary to maintain constant sliding velocity as a function of velocity; *c,* displacement as a function of time for different constant forces.

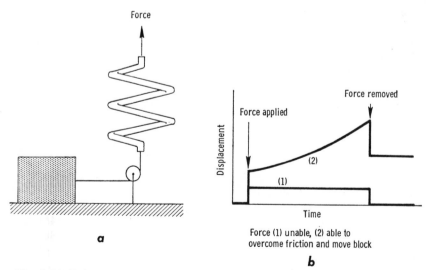

Fig. 2.24. Behavior of elastic and friction elements in series. *a,* elements in series; *b,* displacement as a function of time for different constant forces.

vessels and nerves. With the exception of contracting muscle, these structures are passive in the sense that they generate no mechanical energy, even though they are able to store such energy. The forces applied by orthotic devices are in large part reacted by these tissues, and to this extent the tissue properties influence device function.

If gravity were eliminated, a relaxed joint with its minimal Coulomb friction would come to rest consistently at the same general angle. For example, when a person is submerged in water so that buoyant forces substantially counteract gravity, the relaxed elbow comes to rest in flexion of about 75°, the wrist flexes about 10°, and the metacarpophalangeal (MP) and proximal interphalangeal (PIP) joints each flex about 45°. This is because in these positions, and only in these positions, there is equilibrium of all the torques that arise from the elastic forces about the joint. As the joint is moved in either direction, equilibrium is lost, and there is a net increase in elastic torque generated by relaxed muscles and other soft tissues acting to restore the joint to its position of equilibrium. The magnitude of these torques acting on the elbow of an average person is shown in Fig. 2.25.

Elastic forces become quite critical in the use of devices such as the balanced forearm orthosis (16). Precise control of the overall balance with this device is necessary in part to counteract tissue elasticity which might otherwise restrict movement of the severely weakened upper extremity.

That these elastic forces are not negligible can also be affirmed by anyone wearing a splint which holds a normal part in other than its resting position, as for example a cock-up splint with hand platform holding the wrist and fingers in extension.

Johns and Wright (6) have determined that in the midrange of wrist motion of an anesthetized cat, the capsule contributes 47% of the restoring torque, relaxed muscle and associated tendons 51%, and skin 2%. At the extremes of joint motion, the relative contribution of each tissue is unknown,

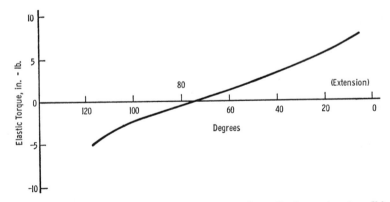

Fig. 2.25. Elastic torque acting in midrange of elbow flexion-extension. [Modified from Smith and Juvinall (16).]

but it is likely that further motion is restrained primarily by connective tissue, cartilage, and bone. Since connective tissue is the most yielding of these, and often the most deformed by forces applied by orthotic devices, its response to stress will be examined in more detail. Studies of pathologic connective tissue are limited, but considerable work has been done to define the properties of normal connective tissue.

Fig. 2.26 depicts a stress-strain curve obtained *in vitro* from human tendon. This curve, which approximates the response of connective tissue in general, shows a nonlinear time-dependent relation between stress and strain (20). As the applied load is increased, the material becomes progressively stiffer, *i.e.*, shows progressively less gain in strain (23). The total elongation that can occur before moist tendon ruptures has been reported variously as between 5 and 10% of the initial length *in vitro* (4, 21).

The slope of the stress-strain curve is affected also by the rate at which the force is applied (Fig. 2.26) (20), indicating that connective tissue possesses viscous as well as elastic properties. The viscoelastic nature is further evidenced by the response of connective tissue when a constant force is applied. Application of a weight to an anchored ligament or tendon causes a rapid initial elongation followed by additional slow stretching, *i.e.*, creep, of the tissue over a period of time, even though the force remains unchanged (Fig. 2.32) (11, 18). The amount of creep which occurs is related both to the magnitude of forces (Fig. 2.27) and to the temperature (Fig. 2.28) (11).

The relaxation characteristics of connective tissue following removal of large forces are incompletely understood. Two phases of recovery have been observed: an initial rapid phase followed by a secondary prolonged phase (11). The instantaneous phase is pure elastic recovery, while the prolonged phase is viscoelastic. An important question still unresolved is whether the prolonged recovery phase is ultimately complete if the applied force has been large but not in excess of the tensile strength. Thus, it is not known whether normal connective tissue has plastic properties and can undergo

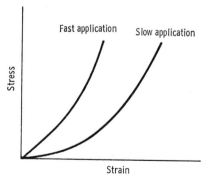

Fig. 2.26. Stress-strain relationship of human tendon for different rates of force application. [Modified from Van Brocklin and Ellis (20).]

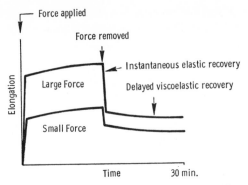

Fig. 2.27. Tendon elongation as a function of time for different constant loads; temperature constant. [Modified from LaBan (11).]

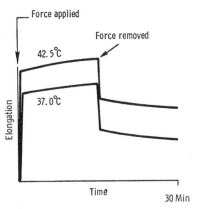

Fig. 2.28. Tendon elongation as a function of time for different temperatures; load constant. [Modified from LaBan (11).]

permanent elongation when stretched by a force that does not actually tear the fibers.

A tentative model employing viscous and elastic elements to explain the behavior of connective tissue as now understood is illustrated in Fig. 2.29. This model assumes complete recovery of initial length. A more precise model must await further experimental data, particularly on the recovery phase following force removal.

The response to compression of skin and subcutaneous tissues is in many ways similar to that of stretching connective tissue, even though such additional materials as skin, fat, and compartmentalized fluids are involved. Compression studies (5) of the human earlobe show that it, too, becomes progressively stiffer as the applied force is increased. Creep also occurs during tissue compression (Fig. 2.30b), with the magnitude being a function of pressure. Similarly, recovery passes through an instantaneous and delayed phase. The creep phenomenon and the delayed recovery reflect the visco-elastic nature of tissue response to compression, and these characteristics can again be represented by a rheologic model such as that depicted in Fig. 2.31 (5).

Adverse Effects of Pressure

In some instances it is the adverse effects of pressure on tissue which limit the total force that a device can be allowed to exert. The most important adverse effects result from the action of compressive and shear forces on subcutaneous and deeper tissues and from frictional forces on skin.

When force is applied to a surface, the amount of compression occurring in underlying structures is a function of pressure, that is, force applied per unit area. It is well recognized that a force concentrated in a small area is potentially much more harmful to tissue than the same force distributed over a large area.

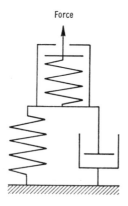

Fig. 2.29. Simplified mechanical analog model of connective tissue. [Modified from Final Report, Univ. Mich. Orth. Res. Proj. (19).]

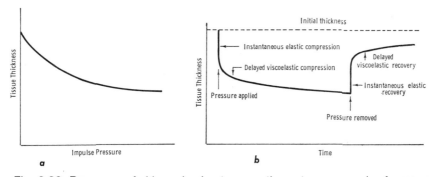

Fig. 2.30. Response of skin and subcutaneous tissue to compressive forces. a, tissue thickness as a function of impulse pressure, impulse time constant; b, tissue thickness as a function of time, pressure constant. [Modified from Hickman (5).]

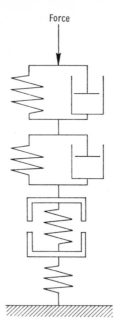

Fig. 2.31. Simplified mechanical analog model of skin and subcutaneous tissue. [Modified from Hickman *et al.* (5).]

The effects of pressure are also influenced by the compressibility of tissues between brace and bone. Compressibility, in turn, is related to the rheologic characteristics of the tissues and to their thicknesses. In Fig. 2.32*a*, compressed tissues are represented arbitrarily by springs located between bone and the contoured plate of a brace. Because the contour matches that of the bone, pressure distribution tends to be uniform. If, however, the plate is flat rather than contoured (Fig. 2.32*b*), the tissue directly over the bone is compressed more than the tissue at the periphery, resulting in unequal distribution. The thinner the layer of intervening tissue, the stiffer the equivalent springs and the more nonuniform the pressure distribution. Thus, tissues over bony prominences are the most vulnerable to the adverse effects of pressure, particularly when such prominences are superficial.

The harmful effects of pressure result largely from interference with blood flow, particularly at the capillary level. Kosiak (10) has shown that the amount of pressure causing damage is related inversely to the duration of application. He required 12 hours to produce ischemic ulceration in a dog when using a pressure of 150 mm Hg, but only 2 hours with a pressure of 500 mm Hg. The large pressures have the added disadvantage of causing venous thrombosis, with the persistence of and even the spread of ischemia after the pressure has been removed.

Sensory warning usually prevents true ischemic necrosis, but when the orthotic device is over an anesthetic area or the patient is unconscious, pressure ulceration can result. When sensory awareness is intact, a major deterrent to the use of a brace is often the pain associated with excessive localized pressure, even though the pressure may not be great enough to damage the tissue irreversibly. Pressure discomfort is probably the most frequent complaint the orthotist hears. Hence, it is important to consider ways to reduce pressure without compromising function.

Pressure effects can be minimized by reducing the total force or by increasing the area over which the force acts. A practical means of reducing total force without sacrificing effectiveness is to make the link distance between points of application as long as practical. In this way less force is required to achieve a given corrective torque.

Increasing the area of force application is important particularly over bony prominences. For the increased area to be fully effective, the brace should be contoured to distribute the pressure as uniformly as possible over the surface of the prominence.

Edges of orthotic devices are also a common site of pressure concentration, particularly when the device is not properly aligned or fitted. If the edge is

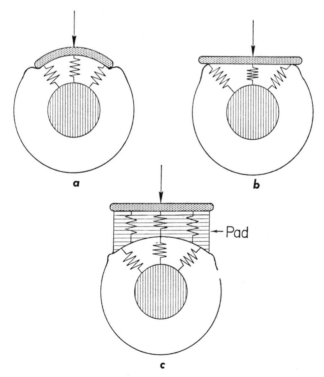

Fig. 2.32. Compression of tissue between bone and a rigid plate; tissue represented by springs. a, compression by a contoured plate; b, compression by a flat plate; c, compression by a padded plate.

at all sharp, the local pressures can be surprisingly high. A force of only 3 pounds acting on an edge that measures 2 inches × 0.05 inches creates an average edge pressure of 30 pounds per square inch. Rounding, contouring, or padding the edges increases the area of force application and reduces the pressure correspondingly.

The use of padding is most effective over bony prominences and along edges of braces. It decreases the stiffness of materials between bone and brace and, hence, increases the uniformity of pressure distribution (Fig. 3.1c). It should be remembered, however, that even though the padding distributes some of the concentrated force to adjacent areas, much of it still remains over the "high spots" where compression is the greatest. Thus, contour fitting is important, even with well-padded braces.

ADVERSE EFFECTS OF SHEAR

In addition to the damaging compressive forces, there can be equally damaging shear forces (14). Sliding movements of the brace can be transmitted to underlying tissue planes where attachments between interfaces provide less resistance to movement than does friction at the skin surface. Such displacement in subcutaneous tissue is the normal accompaniment of body movement and ordinarily causes no harm. However, excessive shear forces applied for too long a period are potentially damaging. Blood vessels are subject to kinking and stretching as they cross the shear plane, particularly when they are relatively fixed to underlying structures. The consequent impairment of blood flow can add to and extend ischemia resulting from pressure.

There are also occasions when resistance to shear movement is less at the surface or in superficial layers of skin than in underlying tissues. This can occur when the skin is relatively bound down to rigid deeper structures, or when the limits of shear movement in underlying tissues are exceeded. As a consequence, shear forces acting on superficial portions of the skin may cause abrasions to form as progressive layers are rubbed off by the brace.

To counteract the harmful effects of shear forces, several things can be done. Movement between brace and body can be minimized by aligning and fitting the brace properly, and pressure points can be selected in areas where there is sufficient skin mobility to prevent damage to underlying tissues. When these steps are inadequate, friction can be reduced between skin and brace so that movement occurring at this interface is less abrasive and less productive of shear forces between the varius layers of skin.

In selecting low-friction materials for braces, the interaction of the material with the skin must also be considered. For example, smooth materials applied forcefully to the skin can create an unsuspectedly high friction because of their "suction effect." As the material is pressed against the skin, air is forced out of the irregularities on the skin's surface. This can form a partial vacuum which is sealed by the moisture normally present, and the effect is much as if the skin were composed of multitudes of tiny suction cups. Since moisture tends also to soften the skin, it is not surprising that abrasions may form when smooth surfaces rub over damp skin.

Thus, if reduced friction is desired at the skin-brace interface, the surface covering of the brace should not only have a low coefficient of friction but also a surface texture minimizing vacuum seal formation. Leather and many fabrics fit this category. Smooth plastic or metal surfaces adjacent to skin are generally less desirable if abrasions are a factor. When such surfaces are necessary, interposition of clothing may be helpful because the coefficient of friction between clothing and brace, or between layers of clothing, tends to be less than that between clothing and skin. The adverse effects of moisture can usually be minimized by selecting absorbent materials and by constructing the brace to allow maximum ventilation of the skin.

REFERENCES

1. ANDERSON, M. H. Biochemical considerations in the design of a functional long leg brace. *Ortho. Prosthet. Appl. J., 18:* 273, 1964.
2. BARNETT, C. H., DAVIES, D. V., AND MACCONNAILL, M. A. Synovial Joints, Their Structure and Mechanics. Springfield, Ill., 1961.
3. DEMPSTER, W. T. Free-body diagrams as an approach to the mechanics of human posture and motion. *In Biomechanical Studies of the Musculo-Skeletal Systems,* edited by T. Evans. Charles C Thomas, Springfield, Ill., 1961.
4. ELLIS, D. G. Personal communication, 1965.
5. HICKMAN, K. E., LINDAN, O., CORELL, R. W., RESWICK, J. B., AND SCANLAN, R. H. Rheological behavior of tissues subjected to external pressure. *Proc. San Diego Symp. Biomed. Engl., 3:* 133, 1963.
6. JOHNS, R. J., AND WRIGHT, V. Relative importance of various tissues in joint stiffness. J. Appl. Physiol., 17: 824, 1962.
7. JONES, E. S. Joint lubrication. *Lancet, 1:* 1043, 1936.
8. JORDAN, H. H. Orthopedic Appliances. ed. 2. Charles C Thomas, Springfield, Ill., 1963.
9. KLOPSTEG, P. E., AND WILSON, P. D. *Human Limbs and Their Substitutes.* McGraw-Hill, New York, 1954.
10. KOSIAK, M. Etiology and pathology of ischemic ulcers. *Arch. Phys. Med. Rehabil., 40:* 62, 1959.
11. LABAN, M. M. Collagen tissue: implications of its response to stress *in vitro. Arch. Phys. Med. Rehabil., 43:* 461, 1962.
12. LANDSMEER, J. M. F. Anatomical and functional investigations on the articulation of the human fingers. *Acta Anat. (Basel), 25 (Suppl. 24):* 1955.
13. NANGLE, E. J. *Instruments and Apparatus in Orthopaedic Surgery.* Blackwell Scientific Publications, Oxford, 1951.
14. REICHEL, S. M. Shearing force as a factor in decubitus ulcers in paraplegics. *J. A. M. A., 166:* 762, 1958.
15. REINER, M. The flow of matter. *Sci. Am., 201:* 122, 1959.
16. SMITH, E. M., AND JUVINALL, R. C. Theory of "feeder" mechanics. *Am. J. Phys. Med., 42:* 113, 1963.
17. SMITH, E. M., JUVINALL, R. C., BENDER, L. F., AND PEARSON, J. R. Role of the finger flexors in rheumatoid deformities of the metacarpophalangeal joints. *Arthritis Rheum., 7:* 467, 1965.
18. SMITH, J. W. The elastic properties of the anterior cruciate ligament of the rabbit. *J. Anat., 88:* 369, 1954.

19. University of Michigan Orthetics Research Project. Final Report. Ann Arbor, Mich., 1964.
20. VAN BROCKLIN, J. D., AND ELLIS, D. G. A study of the mechanical behavior of toe extensor tendons under applied stress. *Arch. Phys. Med. Rehabil., 46:* 369, 1965.
21. WALKER, L. B., HARRIS, E. H., AND BENEDICT, J. V. Stress-strain relationship in human cadaveric plantaris tendon; a preliminary study. *Med. Electron. Biol. Eng., 2:* 31, 1965.
22. WILLIAMS, M., AND LISSNER, H. R. *Biomechanics of Human Motion.* W. B. Saunders, Philadelphia, 1962.
23. WRIGHT, D. G., AND RENNELS, D. C. A study of the elastic properties of plantar fascia. *J. Bone Joint Surg. (Am.), 46:* 482, 1964.
24. WRIGHT, V., AND JOHNS, R. J. Physical factors concerned with the stiffness of normal and diseased joints. *Bull. Johns Hopkins Hosp., 108:* 215, 1960.

3

Materials for Orthotics[1]

JOHN B. REDFORD, M.D.
SIDNEY LICHT, M.D.

A wide variety of materials are now available for orthotic appliances. With space age technology, new ones are constantly being introduced. These new materials have opened up new possibilities for better design, stronger support, increased durability, and improved cosmetic appearance in orthotics. However, traditional materials such as steel and leather are still widely used. Very obviously, there is no ideal material that will serve all orthotic problems, as completely different properties are needed for different clinical situations, or even for parts of the same device.

This chapter is not intended as a detailed elaboration and description of all orthotic materials in use today. Knowledge of these materials is a fundamental part of the training of orthotists. Postgraduate prosthetic and orthotic education schools have manuals giving details of construction of orthotic devices and materials to be used (14). The orthotic team will rely on the orthotist, for the most part, in selecting materials. However, for those interested in more detail, there is a guide available in the *Annual Book of ASTM Standards*, published by the American Society for Testing and Materials (ASTM). This guide includes specifications and recommended practices that can be applied to orthotics (1). Valuable information on properties and treatments of different materials used in orthotics is available from various manufacturers, such as steel, aluminum, and other metal companies. Information about properties of plastics is available from various chemical companies and manufacturers of orthotic devices. For a complete American list of suppliers of materials and equipment used in orthotics, the reader should consult the product index of the yearbook provided by the American Orthotic and Prosthetic Association.

Metals for Orthotics[1]

The metals most suitable for orthotic appliances are steel and aluminum alloys. Magnesium and titanium alloys are mentioned but at present have

---

[1] Reprinted with permission from S. J. Rosenberg (15).

little or no use in conventional orthoses. An alloy is a substance that has metallic properties and is composed with two or more chemical elements, of which at least one is an elemental metal. Properties of importance in orthotic appliances are strength, weight, resistance to deformation, fatigue, wear and corrosion, ease of working, and fabrication and cost.

The strength of metal is measured conventionally by the tensile test. In such a test, a sample of uniform cross-section is subjected to a constantly increasing tensile force until fracture occurs. When an external load is applied to the ends of the bar, the change in length that occurs is called elongation. Stress is generally defined as the load per unit cross-section of material. When the values of stress are then plotted against the corresponding values of strain (total elongation divided by gage length), a stress-strain curve is obtained.

In this curve for heat-treated steel (see Fig. 3.1), the portion from the origin to the proportional limit (P. L.) is a straight line. Thus, within this range of stress (elastic range), strain is proportional to stress (and *vice versa*). Furthermore, when the stress is removed, the corresponding strain disappears. However, if the metal is stressed above this value, some permanent deformation will remain after complete removal of the load. The slope of the straight line below the proportional limit that is obtained by dividing any stress by the corresponding strain is termed the modulus of elasticity, *i.e.*, the physical measure of the amount of stress necessary to cause a given strain. For instance, in the example shown, a stress of 30,000 pounds per square inch (psi) causes a strain of 0.001 inch per inch. Conversely, if a strain of 0.001 inch per inch exists, this indicates that the material has a modulus of elasticity equal to 30,000,000 psi.[2]

Soft steels exhibit a "yield point," that is, a sudden drop of stress accompanied by a markedly increased strain. Heat-treated steels, however, as indicated in Fig. 3.1, do not have a "yield point." For such steels and many nonferrous alloys, a "yield strength" is taken that corresponds to some definite value of strain, in this case 0.002 inches per inch, or 0.2%. When a steel does exhibit a yield point, this usually corresponds very closely to its yield strength.

The maximum stress attained by the specimen is the tensile strength. Once this value is obtained during testing, the stress begins to drop while the strain increases; nicking occurs, followed by fracture. The strength of metals, in a very general fashion, can be deduced from their hardness, as these two properties parallel each other.

In orthotic applications, the compressive yield and tensile strength are important. For all practical purposes, the compressive strength, both yield and maximum, may be assumed to be equivalent to the corresponding tensile properties. Another important factor in use of metals is shear strain. When an external load is applied obliquely, the change in the object is an

---

[2] International System of Units may be used: 1 psi = 6900 Newton per square meter.

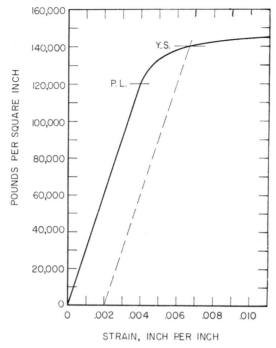

Fig. 3.1. Typical stress-strain curve for a heat-treated steel. Observe that strain is proportional to stress up to the proportional limit (P. L.). No permanent deformation remains after release of stress if stress does not exceed this value. Y.S., yield strength (see text).

angular deformity, and this change is called shear strain. Obviously, shear strength is also of importance in orthotic design. The shear strength of metals may be assumed to be about 55% of their tensile strength.

The densities (weights are proportional to the densities) of the four base metals of interest are listed in Table 3.1.

The various alloys based on these metals will have slightly different densities, depending on the alloy elements, but generally the values will not be too far from those given above. As a rough measure, it may be assumed that magnesium alloys are one-quarter as heavy as steel, aluminum alloys one-third as heavy, and titanium alloys 3/5 as heavy. Obviously, these values become important when strength is considered on a strength-weight basis.

The modulus of elasticity of the four metals of interest is roughly as follows:

Iron   29,000,000 psi
Titanium   17,000,000 psi
Aluminum   10,000,000 psi
Magnesium   6,500.000 psi

TABLE 3.1. *Four Base Metals: Their Density*

Metal	Density	
	lb/in^3	g/cm^3
Iron	0.2845	7.874
Titanium	0.1628	4.507
Aluminum	0.0975	2.699
Magnesium	0.0628	1.738

These values are not changed significantly either by alloying or by heat treatment. The practical significance of these figures is that elastic deformation (the strain or elongation under equal stresses) of the four metals varies inversely as their modulus of elasticity.

In many orthotic applications, such as in the upright of a lower extremity orthosis, the deformation under bending stresses is very important. For equal volumes and shapes of a member, it is evident that under the same load, the deformation of aluminum will be 3 times as great as that of iron. However, if the members are compared on the basis of equal weight, and the additional volume is used to increase the thickness of the member, the deformation (under equal load) of aluminum will be less than that of iron. This is because the resistance to bending is proportional to the square of the thickness. Thus, where resistance to bending or stiffness is important, proper design with light metals can result in superior rigidity. Proper design may require the usage of hollow sections or ribbing for stiffness.

When a metal is used in a long column, the danger of failure by buckling exists even though the calculated compressive strength may be more than adequate. The resistance to buckling (stiffness) may be increased by distributing the area so that it is farther from the center of the cross-section. Thus, a tube will be stiffer than a solid rod of equal cross-sectional area, though there are limits beyond which this principle may not be applied in orthotics.

Metals often fail under repeated or fluctuating stresses at values far below their tensile strength or even yield strength. Such failures are caused by a phenomenon termed metal fatigue. Fatigue fracture entails a rather complex process of propagation of cracks through the material. It usually originates at some discontinuity called points-of-stress concentration, such as a notch, a sharp change in section, a gouge, a scratch, or even a surface inclusion in the metal. The susceptibility to fatigue failure can be materially reduced by eliminating all locations of stress concentration, or at least by minimizing their harmful effects by proper design and workmanship. It is particularly important that welds be finished so that they blend smoothly into the joined metals. Therefore, design and workmanship cannot be overemphasized. Fatigue fracture is probably the most prevalent form of failure of orthotic devices (12).

A brittle fracture, in contrast to a fatigue fracture, is sudden failure of material under stress. Conditions such as sharp edges, extreme stiffening, or other unusual configurations may alter the performance of metals so as to produce brittle fractures. A discontinuity such as a hole in the upright of a brace may cause significant local buildup of stress or stress concentration. A suddenly applied load will produce failure and a brittle fracture. Obviously, this kind of sudden failure may be very dangerous for a patient wearing an orthotic device, as a brittle fracture in a key part of the orthosis can lead to injury.

STEEL

Steel is an iron-base alloy, malleable in some temperature range as initially cast, containing alloying elements. Steels can be divided into *carbon steels*, which owe their properties to the carbon additions, and *alloy steels*, which owe theirs both to carbon and alloy additions. The alloy steels can be further divided into low alloy and high alloy, depending on the proportion of the alloy mixed with the iron. Stainless steel, which should be more accurately termed corrosion-resistant steel is a subclass of alloy steel.

The elements commonly found in steel are carbon, manganese, phosphorus, sulfur, and silicon. Of these, carbon is the most significant, imparting strength and the ability to be hardened to a soft steel condition. Manganese and silicon are essentially cleansing agents used to deoxidize the steel during the melting operation while phosphorus and sulfur are undesirable impurities. Many types of steel exist with extremely varied properties, for example, tensile strength may vary from less than 50,000 to more than 500,000 psi. The AISI-SAE (The American Iron Steel Institute-Society of Automotive Engineers) system of identification of steel assigns 4-digit numbers to steels. The first two digits indicate the type of steel, the last two digits indicate the carbon content. Straight carbon steels are indicated by the first two digits, 10. For alloy steel, the first digit identifies the type, and the second digit indicates the approximate percent of alloy (see examples below).

Carbon Steels

At a low concentration of carbon (0.05 to 0.1%), steels are very ductile and have a low yield strength. An increase in proportion of carbon, therefore, increases yield strength and decreases ductility. Heat treatment at a given level of carbon also increases yield strength and decreases ductility. The actual yield strength of carbon steel may vary from 30,000 to 125,000 psi, depending on carbon content and heat treatment. High-carbon steels, such as AISI 1090, which has a carbon content of 0.9%, are frequently used, for example, in springs.

Alloy Steels

Low alloy steels have features that place them between the carbon steels and the high alloy steels; they are rarely used in orthotics. High alloy steels, on the other hand, can be obtained with extremely high strength-to-weight ratios. If corrosion is not a problem, they can be used for structures subject to large repetitive loads, such as brace joints, but are more expensive and difficult to fabricate than more common steels.

Stainless Steels

Stainless steels or corrosion-resistant steels all contain chromium; the minimum amount is 12%. Addition of this element imparts to the steel the ability to form a very thin, adherent oxide film that protects the base metal from attack. To assist the formation and maintenance of this film, the stainless steels are "passivated" by treatment in a dilute solution of nitric acid. Periodic cleaning of stainless steel with 20% nitric acid is good housekeeping.

The stainless steels that contain only chromium as a major alloying element fall into two categories: martensitic and ferritic. The martensitic steels can be hardened by heat treatment; the ferritic steels cannot. The martensitic steels are the only ones used in orthopedic appliances. Although they possess good corrosion resistance, this property is almost completely dependent on proper heat treatment and surface finishing. The addition of nickel to high-chromium steels effects a radical change in their properties. These steels become soft, ductile, and nonmagnetic and cannot be hardened by heat treatment, but can be hardened by mechanical deformation (cold working). Although there are many varieties in this group, they are all referred to generically as "18-8" because they all contain chromium and nickel in approximately this ratio. As a group, these steels are very corrosion resistant, easily worked and formed, and readily welded. AISI type 302 (18% Cr, 9% Ni, 9.20% C Max.) stainless steel and type 304 are almost the same in composition and are widely used for orthoses.

The major advantage of steel in orthotics is its low cost, abundance, and ease or working. Steel is fatigue resistant and combines high strength with high rigidity or ductility, depending on the alloy used. Steel is widely used in prefabricated joints, metal uprights, metal bands and cuffs, springs, and bearings. The main disadvantage is its weight and the need for expensive alloys to prevent corrosion. As more parts become prefabricated of stainless steel for modular orthoses, chrome plating of steel is becoming less widely used in orthotics.

ALUMINUM

Aluminum is useful in orthotics, particularly in its alloy form because of its corrosion resistance and high strength. Aluminum alloys may be divided into two broad groups: *non-heat-treatable* and *heat-treatable*. The strength of the first group depends on the hardening effects of certain alloying elements, usually enhanced by various degrees of cold working. In the second group, the hardening effects of the alloying elements is enhanced essentially by heat treatment.

Although the system of designation of alloys is complex, as a general guide, when the alloy designation is followed by the letter "O," the alloy is in the annealed condition or temper. When followed by the letter "H," the alloy has been strain hardened. The letter "T" indicates that the alloy has been heat treated. Typical alloys where strength is not important include the 1100 alloy containing 99% aluminum (the rest chiefly silicon and iron), which has excellent workability. Another useful alloy is 3003 (1 to 1½% Mn, 0.6% Si, 0.7% Fe). The tensile strength for these alloys range from 13,000 to 24,000 psi for 1100 and from 16,000 to 29,000 psi for 3003.

Useful heat-treatable alloys for orthotics are 2024 and 6061. Although these can be used in the annealed condition, advantage should be taken of the strength potentials that can be developed by heat treatment. Typical tensile strengths are 68,000 to 72,000 psi for 2024 and 35,000 to 45,000 for 6061.

Although the corrosion resistance of aluminum gives it definite advantages over steel, it still can be damaged by alkalis and acids, which may remove the protective aluminum oxide coating. Aluminum can be coated with protective film by subjecting it to electrolytic action or anodizing. This gives it a very attractive and corrosion-resistant surface, which is greatly appreciated in orthotics.

The main benefit of aluminum in orthotics is its high strength-to-weight ratio. Thus, it is used whenever light weight is a major consideration, as in upper limb orthoses. Unfortunately, although its static loading strength is good, aluminum has a lower endurance limit under repeated dynamic loading condition than does steel. Endurance limit is defined as the greatest repetitive stress which a material can stand without failure. Therefore, if loading conditions are known to be great and highly repetitive, as in an adult full lower limb brace [knee-ankle-foot orthosis (KAFO)], steel is superior to aluminum. Proper selection of steel for the orthosis will permit it to be repeatedly stressed almost indefinitely, whereas an aluminum alloy cannot stand repeated loading at high levels of tensile stress.

TITANIUM AND MAGNESIUM

Titanium alloys have some attractive properties, such as strength comparable to steel, but with only 60% the density. They are also more resistant to corrosion than aluminum alloys or steel so that they should have more applications in orthotics. Unfortunately, at the moment, titanium alloys have very limited use because of limited availability and high cost.

Magnesium alloys, by virtue of their very light weight, may have some possibilities for use in orthotic appliances. They are particularly useful where bulk instead of strength is the important requirement. Magnesium is still lighter than aluminum and its modulus of elasticity even lower. Such alloys are also resistant to corrosion and are amenable to welding and brazing.

Leather for Orthotics

Leather can be defined as the hide or skin of an animal, or any portion of such skin, when tanned, tawed, or otherwise dressed for use. Skins of many animals can be used for leather, but basically in orthotics the most commonly used are cattle hides.

Most animal skins originate in the packing house where the food animal is flayed. The animal skin includes epidermis, hair, and glands, along with adherent flesh, fat, and blood vessels. By tanning, these are eliminated. To reduce the high (65%) moisture content of fresh hide, the skin is cured by applying sodium chloride to its flesh side or by immersing the skin in a brine solution. When the moisture content is lowered sufficiently, bacteria and enzymes cease to act on the skin. This is an indispensible step toward preservation.

At the tannery, the cured hides are sorted and trimmed and then soaked in water to clear debris and salt from them. The skins are then depilated with a saturated lime solution to which sulfur compounds or amines have been added. The swollen and highly alkaline hide is bated to reduce the alkalinity of the surfaces and to some extent the swelling. During the bating, acid or acid salt and enzymes are added to digest the unwanted remnants of hair roots and nonfibrous materials. From this point, processing varies according to the type of tannage to be used. Since orthotic leather may frequently contact human skin, vegetable tanning is preferred over chemical. When great strength is sought, the hide may be treated with chromium compounds or other minerals, but skin contact must be avoided with "chrome" leathers (13).

For vegetable tanning, the leather is treated with tannins extracted from the bark, wood, leaves, or fruits of the chestnut, oak, acacia, quebracho, and hemlock trees. Vegetable tanning requires weeks or months, longer than chrome tanning. After the tanning period, the leather is treated with conditioning materials, then bleached to produce the desired color and lubricated with various oils.

Leather to be mineral-tanned is pickled in a bath of acids and salt in water. For convenience, the same vat is used successively for bating and pickling as a continuous process. The chrome-tanned stock is split or shaved to a uniform thickness and then dyed or lubricated with an oil emulsion called fatliquor.

Leather can retain a molded shape permanently. It has tensile properties equalled by no other comparable material of the same weight. Few other flexible materials are more puncture resistant. Leather can be cut, skived, split, perforated, and cemented. It can be sewed, dyed, and buffed. Generally, leather requires minimal care: it can be cleaned with mild soap solution and oiled or waxed to maintain the natural softness.

In construction of footwear, no synthetic or other material offers factors of foot comfort comparable to leather. These factors include a) good thermal conductivity, b) capacity to absorb water from moist air surrounding the foot, c) ability to draw perspiration away from points of heavy sweating and redistribute it, and d) ability to stretch as the shoe becomes moist and thus prevent constriction of hot or sweaty feet (13).

According to the finish desired, pigment, resin, or aniline may be applied to leather. Colors generally available include cream, pearl, brown, black, and white. Leather is ironed by machine or hand to achieve a smooth finish.

The average size per side of leather is 22 to 24 square feet, and fine weights are most commonly used in orthotics. Leather is available in thicknesses from paper thin to ¼ inch or more. Thickness is expressed in the number of ounces per square foot. The following are the commonly used terms:

2–2½ ounces	extra light weight
2½–3 ounces	light weight
3½–4 ounces	medium weight
5–6 ounces	heavy weight
7–8 ounces	extra heavy weight.

Sole leather and other heavy leather are measured in "irons" using a special gage. One iron is equal to ¼₈ inch.

USE OF LEATHER IN ORTHOTICS

Most leather used in orthotic appliances is vegetable-tanned for texture and to prevent skin irritation. Chrome-tanned leather is used where there will be no skin contact and where great strength is required. Some of the most common uses for leather in orthotics are as covering for braces, straps, covering pelvic bands, and various types of molded applications, such as the girdle for Milwaukee braces. In orthotics the following are the principal applications followed by the usual type of leather:

Molded leather around a body part	Calfskin as rawhide
Brace covering	Vegetable-tanned calfskin
Strap, skirting, lining, covering	Vegetable-tanned cattlehide
Molded arch support	Vegetable-tanned cattlehide
Binding straps or lacing	Chrome-tanned cattlehide, rawhide
Cover for appliance	Chrome-tanned cattlehide, calfskin, or elk (a special cattlehide).

Among the many operations which leather undergoes in orthotics, perhaps the most common are cutting, skiving, sewing, and molding. Leather may be stamped out with a die or cut by a sharp knife. Skiving is shaving leather to make it less thick throughout or at the edge. Leather is molded by sponging the flesh side evenly with cold water until the grain side shows wet spots. It is kept damp and rolled for about 24 hours so that it can be stretched tight and smooth over a form until dry. Leather may be reinforced by lamination or impregnation with a plastic or other strengthener.

There are many unique terms used in relation to leather and footwear. A complete list of these terms can be found in Chapter 5 of the first edition of *Orthotics Etcetera* (13) by O'Flaherty. Some of the above material is modified from his original chapter while most of the terms related to leather can be found in a separate list at the end of Chapter 11 "Shoes and Their Modifications."

Rubber for Orthotics

The term rubber refers to a group of compounds both natural and synthetic that have elastic properties. The chemical industry classifies all these compounds as elastomers. Rubber, because of its tough resiliency and high shock-absorbing qualities, is capable of fulfilling a variety of functions in orthotics. There are so many varieties of rubber that can be produced by compounding that it is often possible to produce material which meets the exact requirement for a particular application (11). Rubber is generally divided into either solid forms and cellular or porous rubber.

Natural rubber has excellent elastic properties and good tear and abrasion resistance. It also has good resistance to cold and aging, but it is not very resistant to sunlight, water, or to most oils and solvents. Butyl rubber, which is the commonest synthetic rubber, has a greater resistance to water and aging and to heat and sunlight than does natural rubber. However, it does not have the resilience and wear resistance of natural rubber, and compression and permanent set characteristics are not quite as good. Polysulfide rubbers have a strong objectionable odor but have marked resistance to petroleum products, corrosive agents, oils, solvents, and greases. Polysulfide rubbers are usually used in gas caps and seals which are in contact with gasoline, oil thinners, etc. Neoprene has excellent resistance to wear and to oxidation and heat. As it has good resistance to oil and gasoline compounds, it is frequently used in the chemical and petroleum industry (5).

Table 3.2 gives examples of trade names of the various types of synthetic rubbers, with their chemical classification (5).

Cellular Rubbers

The ASTM (1) has divided cellular rubbers into three classes: sponge, expanded rubber, and latex foam. These, in turn, are divisible into either

TABLE 3.2. *Examples of Trade Names*[1]

Common name	Chemical designator	Trade name
Buna S. GR-S	Styrene-butadiene	Polysar Ameripol SBR Plioflex Naugopol
Buna N. GR-A	Butadiene acrylonitrile (NBR)	Butaprene Chemigum Hycar Nitrile Paracril
Neoprene GR-M Butyl GR-I	Chloroprene (CR) Isobutylene-isoprene	Neoprene Enjay Butyl Polysar Butyl
Silicone	Polysiloxane	Silastic Silicone
Polyurethane	Poluyurethane Diisocyanate	Adiprene Chemigum SL Elastothane Texin Vibrathane

[1] From a brochure from Stalwart Rubber Company—Stalwart Rubber Selector.

open-cell or closed-cell structure. In an open-cell structure, fluids can flow through the holes; in a closed-cell structure, each void is a separate sealed hole. Three factors are involved in producing material of uniform density and cell structure in expanded materials that are synthetic: (1) size of individual cells, (2) ratio of cell space to total volume, and (3) continuity or discontinuity of the cells. All foam materials, including nonelastomeric materials, are classified according to these criteria.

Open-cell structures are inherently softer than the closed-cell structures of similar material. However, they do absorb moisture like a sponge. The open-cell structure does allow ventilation, although this factor is minimized when foam rubber is glued to a solid orthotic component such as metal or rigid plastic. As closed-cell structures are firmer and offer better support and do not absorb perspiration, they are usually preferred in orthotics.

A unique type of foam material is silicone polymer. This polymer, when mixed with a cellulose and a blowing agent, produces a material that expands and cures at the same time. The foam that is produced may be shaped at a very low pressure. This has made it possible to pour a foam mixture inside a prosthetic socket and have it harden within 5 or 10 minutes to make a comfortable cushion between the end of the stump and the socket. Such expandable foams will probably find more use in the future in orthotics, just as they have in the ski industry, where they have been used for assuring optimal fit of ski boots.

USE OF RUBBER

Elastic deformation of rubber is acquired at relatively low force levels. Rubbers of various types can be utilized, for example, in padding for various assistive devices, seals in hydraulic mechanisms, and padding in body jackets and limb orthoses. Rubber can also be used for insulation and to protect from heat or skin irritation from some thermosetting resins.

In upper extremity orthoses, rubber can be used to stretch contractures, particularly of the fingers. In lower extremity orthoses, rubber twisters may be used to correct rotation deformities or rubber elastic straps to assist joint motion. Rubber is a much better elastic energy absorber than any metal or rigid plastic, so it is used in bumpers, shoe heels, and crutch tips. In cane and crutch tips, it not only absorbs shock but also provides skid resistance because of its large friction coefficient (7). This also makes it useful in many types of footwear.

If rubber is to be used in a particular orthosis, its properties can be described in detail by the manufacturer.

Care of Rubber

Some general rules apply to prolong the service life of rubber (5):
1. Rubber may be affected by heat, light, and air. This aging process is particularly notable in natural rubber. Therefore, to minimize the problem, rubber should be stored in a cool dark place and, if stocked in sheet form, folds should be eliminated.
2. Generally, vegetable, mineral, and animal oils cause deterioration of rubber. Oil should be removed by washing with soap and water or cleaning with solvents.
3. Rubber should not be exposed to high temperatures. This increases the aging process.
4. If rubber is used in conjunction with another material such as elastic webbing bandages, the fabrics should be thoroughly dried after washing and before storing.

Plastics for Orthotics

Plastics have truly revolutionized orthotic practice. The term plastic may be applied to any synthetic material that may be molded, extruded, laminated, or hardened into any desired form. There are over 30 major families of plastics. However, only those used in orthotics can be considered here. Plastics presently used have all characteristics required for ideal splinting material. Some of which, as proposed by Hershall and Scales (6), are 1) suitable for direct application to the patient or to an anatomical model, 2) easy to mold to desired form, 3) of little or no toxicity, 4) unaffected by fluids such as water, urine, oils, etc., 5) radiolucent, 6) easy to modify or manipulate without elaborate apparatus, 7) of quick setting or hardening time.

Plastics for orthotics may be grouped into two major types: *thermoplastics* and *thermosetting plastics.* Thermoplastics soften when heated and harden when cooled so they can be molded and remolded by heating. Thermosetting materials develop a permanent shape when heat and pressure are applied and maintain a memory. Therefore, they cannot be softened when reheated and be reshaped (5).

THERMOPLASTICS

Thermoplastics can be divided into low-temperature and high-temperature types. Those requiring no more than 80°C (180°F) to become workable may be termed low-temperature thermoplastics and may be shaped directly to the body. High-temperature thermoplastics, on the other hand, must be shaped over a model. They are much more resistant than low-temperature types to creep, that is, change in shape with continued stress and heat. Therefore, they are ideal for long-term use or permanent use in limb orthoses, body jacket, etc.

LOW-TEMPERATURE THERMOPLASTICS

Low-temperature thermoplastics cannot be used effectively in applications where high stress is anticipated, as in spasticity or in many lower extremity applications. Their principal use is in upper limb orthotics, where rapid provision of an assistive or protective orthosis is often desirable. As no cast is needed, these plastics hasten orthotic fittings and are so easy to use that most rehabilitation personnel can form devices over the body with minimal practice and equipment. The only equipment needed to use most of these materials is a supply of hot water, scissors, and a source of hot air, such as a heat gun or an oven.

Low-temperature thermoplastics are usually marketed in sheets, except for a few which come as rolls of plastic impregnated bandage (see Table 3.3). This bandage can be wrapped around the patient's limb or applied in overlapping layers. Less rigid materials require laminating several layers or ridging at stress points to provide adequate strength.

Cutting low-temperature thermoplastics with scissors or a sharp knife generally leaves a smooth edge. However, for some cuts, a saber or coping saw may be needed, and then the edges will need sanding. A pattern for a low-temperature thermoplastic orthosis can either be traced from a book or around the part on which it is to be fitted. A template or pattern may be made of paper and a trial fit made on the limb. This pattern can be used in cutting the plastic in order to conserve material.

In cutting splints from patterns, one may need to allow for shrinkage; various materials reduce in size when heated. If the pattern for molding the

TABLE 3.3. *Low-Temperature Thermoplastics*[1]*

Trade name(s)	Characteristics	Fabrication
Aliplast, Plastazote, surgical orthopedic splinting (SOS)	Closed cell foamed polyethylene sheets. Resilient. Plastazote, SOS: perforated and unperforated. Aliplast: unperforated only. Matte opaque white; Plastazote also in black and pink. Very light weight, various densities. Flexibility depends on density. Low flammability; flame causes melting.	Cut with knife or scissors. Heat only with hot air 110–140°C (220–280°F) in oven protected with talcum, Teflon, or brown paper. Shape on stockinette-protected patient. Reinforce with polyethylene strips. Setting and curing time 1–5 minutes. Self-adherent.
Aquaplast	Polyester sheets. Waxy hard smooth surface. Perforated and unperforated. Glossy opaque yellowish-white. Very rigid. Low flammability; flame causes melting.	Cut with scissors. Heat until transparent; 60°C (140°F) in pan protected with plastic net separator. Shape on patient whose skin has been lubricated with water, petroleum jelly, or soap to prevent Aquaplast from sticking to hair; extremely elastic when hot. Trim when hot. Setting time 10 minutes. Curing time 20 minutes. Self-adherent.
Bioplastics	Polyvinyl chloride sheets. Hard smooth surface. Shiny transparent pale blue. Very rigid, high-impact strength, difficult to reshape. Low flammability; flame causes charring.	Cut with coping or band saw when cool or with scissors when warm. Heat to 80–110°C (170–220°F). Shape on stockinette-protected patient. Scrape, sand, or buff edges. Setting and curing time 1–2 minutes. Not self-adherent.

TABLE 3.3—Continued

Trade name(s)[1]	Characteristics	Fabrication
Glassona	Cellulose acetate plastic bandage. Hard porous surface. Opaque white. Lightweight. Pliable, resists chipping and cracking, difficult to remold once set. Very toxic solvent activator; strong acids cause decomposition; strong alkalis cause swelling. Very flammable.	Moisten bandage in acetone. Wrap the stockinette-protected patient. Cut with scissors. Setting time 10–15 minutes. Curing time 24 hours. Self-adherent and adherent to other materials.
Hexcelite	Polycaprolactone bandage and splints. Hard, very porous mesh surface. Matte opaque white. Very rigid, difficult to reshape. Flammable.	Apply polypropylene or cotton stockinette over body part. Heat with hot water only 70–80°C (160–180°F). Wrap the part, discarding polyethylene separator. Fold edges to avoid roughness. If using splints, apply to limb. Cut with scissors or shears. Setting time 3–5 minutes. Curing time 15–20 minutes. Self-adherent.
Kay-Splint, Polyform	Polyester polycaprolactone sheets; Polyform also in preformed orthoses. Hard smooth surface, semiglossy, opaque; Kay-Splint; pink, unperforated; Polyform; white, perforated and unperforated. Flammable.	Heat to 65–75°C (150–170°F). Cut with scissors; stretches, but has minimal shrinkage. Shape on patient. Setting time 2–5 minutes. Curing time 24 hours. Self-adherent only if surface is dissolved with methylene chloride, toluene, or aromatic hydrocarbon solvent.

TABLE 3.3—*Continued*

Trade name(s)[1]	Characteristics	Fabrication
Lightcast	Fiberglass and acrylic resin bandage. Hard porous surface. Opaque yellowish-white. Pliable, resists chipping and cracking, difficult to remold once set. Not flammable when cured.	Apply polypropylene stockinette over body part. Wrap the part with bandage. Harden by ultraviolet radiation, 3200 to 4000 Angstrom units. Setting and curing time 3 minutes. Self-adherent.
Orthoplast, San-Splint	Synthetic rubber sheets. Hard smooth surface; perforated and unperforated. Semiglossy opaque; Orthoplast; white, San-Splint; pink, with grain on one side. Slightly rigid; dissolves in aromatic and chlorinated solvents, *e.g.*, carbon tetrachloride. Flammable.	Heat to 65–80°C (150–175°F); if heated in oven, use silicone release paper. Cut with scissors; minimal shrinkage; minimal elastic memory. Shape on patient. Setting time 10 minutes. Curing time 2 hours. Self-adherent.
Polysar	Synthetic rubber sheets and tubes. Hard smooth surface. Matte opaque pink. Very rigid. Flammable.	Heat to 70–80°C (160–180°F); if heated in oven, use separating material. Cut with shears. Shape on stockinette-protected patient. Setting and curing time 5–10 minutes. Self-adherent only if hot and dry.
Warm-N-Form	Polyvinyl chloride sheets and orthoses. Hard smooth surface. Transparent shiny amber on one side, gold knit fabric on other side. Very rigid. Flammable.	Cut with coping or band saw when cool or with scissors when hot; minimal stretchability, minimal memory, minimal shrinkage. Heat with dry heat only to 55–80°C (130–180°F). Shape on patient, fabric side next to skin. Setting and curing time 1–3 minutes. Not self-adherent.

[1] The most common trade name precedes alternate versions of the same material.
[2] Reprinted with permission from: J. Compton and E. Edelstein (3).

orthosis does not compensate for this, there may be an insufficient amount of plastic to form the orthosis, and fitting may be a problem. Return to the original fabricated shape after material is mechanically stressed is called elastic memory—a very desirable property in plastic orthoses. Low-temperature thermoplastics with good elastic memory may stretch a good deal when heated during molding but may return to the original dimension when cool. If the plastic orthosis is to be fitted correctly, dimensions must be carefully planned before heating.

Attaching straps can be done with ease to most low-temperature thermoplastics. Straps may be speed-riveted. Heat can bond the plastic to the strap material, or two layers of plastic can be bonded together to enclose the strap. To improve self-adherence, one may use a solvent to dissolve a thin portion of the surface and then press together the parts to be bonded. Several different types of low-temperature thermoplastics may be laminated together to improve rigidity or strength. For example, a trunk orthosis made of Plastazote or Aliplast can be reinforced with strips of Orthoplast or San-Splint.

Closed-cell foam polyethylene materials such as Plastazote differ from the other low-temperature plastics in that they require higher temperatures (110 to 140°C) for molding. However, as air convection cools their surfaces so rapidly that they can be formed safely on the skin, they can be grouped with low-temperature thermoplastics. Different types of closed-cell foam plastics are particularly useful for cushioning and lining orthoses made of more rigid materials. They are very useful in an area such as the neck, which is difficult to fit comfortably with rigid plastic orthoses (17). Foamed polyethylene has proved particularly helpful in fabrication of custom-made inner soles for foot deformities (see Chapter 11).

The polyethylene foams have several definite disadvantages even for temporary application. They compress and lose their springy quality under repeated pressures, as in shoes, and so must be frequently remade. As they are nonrigid and very friable, they have a short life expectancy. Although perforated, they permit very little air circulation, so that patients frequently complain of discomfort from heat and perspiration.

Table 3.2[1] summarizes pertinent information on the characteristics of the low-temperature thermoplastics currently available (3). Detailed instruction on their use can be secured from the manufacturers and suppliers who are listed in the *Modern Plastics Encyclopedia* (11). Two useful manuals for temporary orthoses using low-temperature thermoplastics have been written by Malick (9, 10).

HIGH-TEMPERATURE THERMOPLASTICS

The major types of high-temperature thermoplastics that are most widely used in orthotics are acrylic, polyethylene, polypropylene, polycarbonate, ABS (acnyonitrile-butadiene-styrene) and the group of vinyl polymers and copolymers which include polyvinyl chloride (PVC), polyvinyl alcohol

(PVA), and polyvinyl acetate. These are widely used in sheet form for the manufacture of permanent orthotic devices using vacuum-forming techniques.

Acrylics

The acrylic plastics are a family of thermoplastics mostly polymerized from methyl methacrylate monomers. The standard acrylics possess qualities—quite attractive in orthotics—of light weight, high transparency, good dimensional stability, and resistance to breakage. They are the most weather-resistant thermoplastics known and are available in a wide range of transparent, translucent, and opaque colors. Some properties of a well-known acrylic, cast methyl methacrylate, are specific gravity of 1.172 to 1.20, tensile strength of 8,000 to 11,000 psi, and compressive strength of 11,000 to 19,000 psi (5, 11).

The acrylic plastics are available in the form of sheets, rods, tubes, and molding powder. The cast sheets can be thermoformed over plaster of Paris molds by vacuum or air pressure with temperatures of 150 to 160°C (300 to 350°F).

Acrylic polymers are used at present in manufacturing lenses, dentures, and many self-help aids. Acrylic monomers are used as components in some adhesives, and acrylic dispersions are used in leather finishing. Textiles such as Acrilon and Orlon are made of acrylic fibers. In commercial use, acrylics are extensively used to substitute for glass in light fixtures, etc. and are widely used in outdoor signs.

Orthotic devices composed of acrylic plastic can be fabricated or modified by filing, drilling, sawing, routing, and buffing. Solvents such as acetone, methyl ketone, or methyl isobutyl ketone are used to weld acrylics or polish and finish cut edges. Adhesives used with acrylics may be monomeric cements, bodied adhesives containing thermoplastics, or thermosetting resins or solvents. Acrylics can be polished by an oxyhydrogen flame technique. Acrylics are unaffected by alkalis, nonoxidizing acids, or saltwater but are attacked by strong alcohols or solvents. They are combustible materials, and fire precautions must be observed in handling, storing, and using them.

Polyethylene

Polyethylene, while having one of the simplest structures of all polymers, can be produced with such varied properties that a simple descriptive statement is impossible. Polyethylene used in orthotics is a wax-like material possessing properties of toughness and flexibility with good dimensional stability. It has very good electrical resistance and cold-resistant properties. It is also light in weight, has no objectionable odor or taste, and is nontoxic. Although in very thin films it can be clear or translucent, additives usually make it white and opaque or colored. It is generally classified as being of low density, medium density, or high density. The higher the density, the greater the tear strength and impact strength but the higher the mold shrinkage. Low-density polyethylene has a specific gravity of 0.912 to 0.925 and a tensile strength of 600 to 2300 psi. Medium-density polyethylene has a specific gravity of 0.926 to 0.980 and a tensile strength of 1200 to 3500 psi. High-density polyethylene has a specific gravity of 0.941 to 0.965 and a tensile strength of 3100 to 5500 psi and a compressive strength of 3200 psi (5, 11).

Low-density polyethylene can be vacuum formed or hand formed on a plaster of Paris model after being softened in an air-circulating oven. After modeling, it can be machined with wood-working tools. For nonweight-bearing appliances such as hand or wrist supports, polyethylene makes a supporting device with more rigidity than many of the low-temperature thermoplastics.

High-density polyethylene (Ortholen, Vitrathene) is generally used where a more rigid weight-bearing support system is required. It has been used in a wide variety of situations, such as the production of spinal jackets, and as the main component of KAFO and ankle-foot orthoses (17). It is generally used as a heat-softened sheet which is vacuum formed over a plaster model. However, stock items such as cervical collars are available. One advantage of high-density polyethylene is that it can be bonded to closed-cell polyethylene sheets such as Plastazote so that it will be easy to line rigid orthoses.

High-density polyethylene requires a considerable amount of hand finishing and does not stand up to repeated heavy loading, as does polypropylene. It fatigues when subjected to repeated stresses and therefore should be mostly used where there is little repetitive motion, as in a body jacket. All types of polyethylene can be welded by the use of a plastic welding gun with hot gas and welding rod of ⅛-inch diameter. The polyethylenes are very resistant to alkalis but are affected by strong oxidizing agents such as nitric acid. A tendency to crack may increase when they are repeatedly exposed to active compounds such as alcohol, strong soaps, and hydrocarbons. Polyethylene orthoses should not be placed in front of an electric fire, on top of gas cookers, or any place where temperatures may reach 100°C or more. Although stabilizers are present in polyethylene plastics, they are still somewhat sensitive to ultraviolet light and must be protected from excessive exposure to sunlight. As with all plastics, polyethylene can burn, but its flammability is in no way a hazard, as it is very difficult to ignite.

Polypropylene

Polypropylene is a very rigid thermoplastic material with an extremely stable molecular structure. It is tough and odorless and has high-impact strength with good mechanical properties. It is one of the lightest thermoplastics, and shaping can be done very conveniently on vacuum-forming machines. Polypropylene can be tailored for different uses by controlling molecular weight and molecular weight distribution and by additives. It is sensitive to ultraviolet light and, because of this, ultraviolet absorbers or screening agents are available. It is also sensitive to strong oxidizing agents and extreme cold. Polypropylene has a specific gravity between 0.90 and 0.91, a tensile strength range from 2900 to 4500 psi, and a compressive strength range of 3700 to 8000 psi (11).

Polypropylene has unique flexing properties which enable it to stand several million repetitive flexes before showing signs of a failure. Therefore, it is very useful in orthotic hinge joints. In fact, it is becoming the most popular type of thermoplastic and is now widely used in all types of limb and spinal orthoses (17). It can be easily sawed and buffed with regular woodworking tools. Like polyethylene, it can be heat-welded but will withstand higher temperatures and can be placed in boiling water without losing its shape. It can easily be washed in soap and water and should be washed daily if used in an orthosis. As paint will not stick readily to polypropylene, several different colors are available. Polypropylene is nick and notch sensitive, particularly at low temperatures: its impact resistance decreases by a factor of 4 between 23°C (74°F) and 18°C (60°F).

Polypropylene is being widely used in preformed plastic orthoses, which can be fitted to individual needs. There are a number of stock items on the market such as polypropylene ankle-foot orthoses that can be modified to suit a particular patient. Preformed modules can be stocked in various sizes that can be assembled and modified depending on the need. The Boston system of modular spinal bracing uses polypropylene model prefabricated components (16) (see Chapter 7). Polypropylene is also widely used for custom fitting of vacuum-formed orthoses from plaster molds.

Polycarbonate

Polycarbonate is another high-temperature thermoplastic that has been introduced recently in orthotics, but so far it is less popular than polyethylene, polypropylene, and acrylics. It is also more expensive than the other thermoplastics. A variety called Lexan is an extremely strong thermoplastic material with a tensile strength of 9000 psi. It has very high-impact strength and is totally transparent, making it very desirable for fabrication of prosthetic sockets and orthotic items where it may be desirable to see underlying skin. Unlike many other thermoplastics, it can be steam sterilized (11).

Its main disadvantage is that it is hydroscopic so that any water absorbed from air results in bubble formation when the material is molded at vacuum-forming temperatures. Therefore, it must be dried and dehydrated by prolonged heating prior to molding. Because of its extreme strength and durability, it may be more utilized in modular orthotics in the future. Its present use is limited primarily to forming of prosthetic sockets.

ABS

ABS is a thermoplastic composed of three different monomers—acrylonitrile, butadiene, and styrene. Depending on the proportion of the components, a wide variety of properties can be achieved. ABS resins are generally tough and rigid and have good dimensional stability. They have hard surfaces, good chemical and weather resistance, and good resistance to staining by foodstuffs. The specific gravity is between 0.97 and 1.22, and the tensile strength is from 3000 to 8000 psi. Characteristic of ABS is its capability of formation in a ductile manner over a wide range of temperatures (11). It particularly is suitable in applications where extreme fatigue resistance is required as, for example, in chair seats and backs.

In orthotics, ABS is mainly used in the form of sheet material that can be thermoformed. Equipment made from ABS material can be drilled, sawed, etc. with conventional wood and metal-working tools. ABS can be repaired by heat or solvent welding. Thermoforming temperatures range from 275°F to 325°F. In applications such as modeling to body contours it must be thermoformed over a cast and is actually not very popular for this purpose. ABS is currently widely used for wheelchair seat inserts, self-help aids, and for other applications where extremely rugged properties are desirable.

Vinyl Polymers and Copolymers

PVC and other related compounds are probably the most commonly used materials in orthotics. Some forms of PVC have been listed with the low-temperature plastics (see Table 3.3) but other forms are used at high temperatures. By compounding PVC with plasticizers, lubricants, and fillers, a great range of properties are possible in the finished product. Compounds of PVC can provide a wide range of flexibility from extreme rigidity to great pliability (5).

PVC solutions are used for coating orthoses by dipping, spraying, or fluidized bed coating. These coatings are not affected by mineral or acid alcohols, greases, or aliphatic hydrocarbons, and they resist attack by weathering. Plastisols, which are PVC dispersions, are used in both molding and coating. Since very little skill or equipment is required for applying and processing plastisols, they offer good possibilities as covers for metal brace components and as substitutes for leather bands and cuffs. The metal is preheated to 150°C (300°F) and dipped in liquid plastisol, and then the excess is immediately dripped away. The coated metal is then cured in an oven for a short time at a higher temperature. In general, the higher the temperature, the greater the thickness: about 0.6 to 2 mm (0.025 to 0.08 inches) are the usual depth of coating (5).

Rigid PVC is a hard tough thermoplastic material that can be thermoformed with the vacuum forming or hand molding. The material can be modified with the use of standard metal and woodworking tools.

Copolymers of vinyl chloride and vinyl acetate are more flexible than PVC. They are odorless, tasteless, water-resistant, and flame-resistant. They also can be modified, depending on the addition of plasticizers, stabilizers, etc.

PVC and its related compounds have been used for prosthetic restoration, vinyl-coated fabrics, and seat covers on wheelchairs and padded parts. Some of the common commercial uses are wastepaper baskets, raincoats, weather stripping, heat-shrinkable tubing, vinyl shoe soles, and winter footwear.

The specific gravity of rigid PVC is 1.45, tensile strength is 5,000 to 9,000 psi, and compressive strength is 8,000 to 13,000 psi. For the flexible PVC, specific gravity is 1.3 to 1.7, and tensile strength is 1,000 to 3,500 psi (5).

PVC and its related compounds are not affected by weak acid or weak or strong alkalis, but strong acid has a bad effect. The vinyl compounds resist alcohols and aliphatic hydrocarbons and oils but are affected by ketones and esters and swell in aromatic hydrocarbons.

THERMOSETTING PLASTICS

The introduction of many new thermoplastics to orthotics in the past 10 years has caused a decline in the use of thermosetting plastic materials. These are somewhat more difficult to use than thermoplastics and generally cause more body irritation or allergic reaction.

Polyesters

Polyester resins are especially useful for laminating purposes in orthotics (5). The gel time of the resins can be controlled, and the resins can be cured with low or contact pressure at room temperatures. When reinforced with fibers such as nylon, dacron, and cotton, the strength and impact resistance is good; if glass fibers are used, the laminates exhibit excellent strength-to-weight ratios, comparable to steel. Typical values of polyester resins reinforced with glass cloth are specific gravity of 1.5 to 2.1, tensile strength of 18,000 to 55,000 psi, and compressive strength of 25,000 to 60,000 psi. Rigidity of the laminates can be varied, depending on the individual need from very stiff to very flexible.

Polyester laminates have an advantage over the thermoplastics, as they can be readily pigmented to approximate skin color and can be given a high gloss or dull finish. When cured, the polyester-cured resins are chemically stable with no odor. The heat produced during the curing stage of the polyester resin prohibits fabricating laminates next to the skin, so they must be formed over a cast. Although skin toxicity from the cured material is unusual, if there is any doubt, a skin patch test should be made.

The polyester laminates can be drilled, sanded, buffed, or riveted by regular metal-woodworking tools. They do not absorb moisture and can be kept clean by washing with soap and water.

Typical applications in orthotics are hand orthoses, body jackets, and sockets for ischial weight-bearing and patellar tendon-bearing lower extremity orthoses.

Rivets are generally used for attaching straps. Reactive glues which depend on a catalytic action to join the two materials with an interlayer of thermosetting resin are used as adhesives for polyester laminates. Dissimilar materials such as leather and rubber can be glued to polyester laminates by elastomeric adhesives based on natural or synthetic rubber.

Polyester resins are affected by sunlight and generally are not affected by organic solvents or weak acids, although they may be attacked by strong acids and alkalis.

Epoxies

Epoxy resins are compounds or mixtures of compounds containing one or more epoxide group per molecule, or a combination of epoxide and secondary hydroxide groups. Epoxy resins formulated for laminating are noted for their high tensile, compressive, and flexural strength, high-impact resistance, and superior bonding strength. They have good chemical resistance and excellent resistance to weathering (11). Like polyester resins, they can be reinforced with various materials such as glass, cloth, glass mat, nylon, and dacron and can be formed over contoured shapes at low or contact pressure. They are generally used over plaster molds and require a separator or release agent to prevent adhesion of the resin to the mold.

Epoxy resins are excellent as adhesives. It is probably in this form that they are most widely used in orthotics today. This is because when used in fabricating orthoses, they are more expensive than polyester resins and more inconvenient to use than the thermoplastics. Furthermore, they are difficult to handle, as they can cause skin, eye, or respiratory tract irritation during the curing process. Persons fabricating with the resins must work in a well-ventilated room and protect hands and arms by wearing rubber gloves or protective ointments.

Slight color change takes place in epoxies exposed to sunlight. They are not affected by weak acids or alkalis or organic solvents but are slightly affected by strong acids and alkalis.

Polyurethane Foam

Polyurethane foams are widely used plastics that meet certain special orthotic needs, primarily as cosmetic covers and pads for orthoses or other devices. They can be bonded not only to other plastics but also to metal or plywood.

Rigid Urethane foam offers an alternative for plaster of Paris casts (2). It has the advantage of being much lighter, waterproof, and quickly applied. In addition, it is more easily penetrable by x-rays.

Rigid polyurethane is used in a two-component system of resin and hardener that can be either hand-mixed or mixed with a high-speed mixer. It must be poured 30 seconds after mixing and will set in 5 to 10 minutes. It requires 30 minutes to reach full strength.

The density of the foam may be controlled between 2 and 10 pounds per cubic foot, depending on the formulation of components. Applications in orthotics and prosthetics include the fabrication of temporary casts and shaped cosmetic covers for orthoses and prostheses.

Flexible Polyurethane Foam is an elastomer that has wide use in padding in orthotics and in pads and cushions for wheelchairs and seats. Its density can be widely varied according to the pressures to which it will be subjected. A discussion of polyurethane foam mattresses and pads is given in Chapter 14, "Beds for Patients."

OTHER PLASTICS

There are a number of classes of plastics that have been used in orthotics in the past, such as polyamide (nylon), and cellulosic plastics, such as cellulose acetate, cellulose acetate butyrate, and ethyl cellulose. At the present time, nylon in orthotics is almost entirely confined to its use in textiles. Cellulose body jackets may still be seen occasionally, but cellulosic plastics are, in general, not as easy to use as the new high-temperature thermoplastics. Therefore, these have largely replaced cellulosic plastics in popularity.

While this section has been a survey of the general types of plastics available for orthotic use, more specific information can be found on each of these plastics by consulting the manufacturers listed in the yearbook of the American Orthotic and Prosthetic Association or at the end of other chapters in the book. New plastic materials are constantly under development, and we can probably expect new developments in the field, particularly in the use of plastic combinations with very high tensile strength, such as boron-coated tungsten filaments with epoxy resins that have been used in the space program. Extreme stiffness is also possible with graphite fibers laminated with epoxy, and these are less expensive than boron plastic combinations (12).

Fabrics for Orthotics

Most braces rely on a rigidity in at least one part, but they usually also incorporate some nonrigid substance to protect the skin and to permit selective yield, or to aid in fastening or snug fit. Such soft materials as leather or rubber may be excellent for support, but for fastening or for less rigid support, primarily in corsets, girdles, belts, and stockings, fabrics are necessary. Most textiles or fabrics are woven or knitted from threads or yarn, but a few are molded with pressure, heat, or chemicals.

Woven fabrics are made of yarn. Yarn may be made of single strand, but it is almost always a collection of fibers or filaments which have been twisted into yarn or thread for strength or flexibility. The constituent fibers may be of animal, vegetable, or mineral origin. Of these, the most important in orthotics are the vegetable, and the most common of these is cotton in one of its many forms.

The most important component of vegetable fibers is cellulose and, of animal fibers, protein. The mineral fibers are asbestos, ceramic, glass, and metal. Vegetable fibers are classified according to the type of plant from which they are derived. Bast fibers are made from the bast or inner bark of the stems of dicotyledons (flax or linen); leaf fibers are made from the longitudinal bundles of leaves of monocotyledons (sisal). The prime example of fiber made from seed hair or floss is cotton. The flower of the cotton plant develops a seed pod or boll which bursts open at maturity to display fibers or fluff.

When the ripe cotton fluff is picked, the seeds are removed from the lint in a gin. The cotton is cleaned, carded, drawn, and combed into slivers and twisted into yarn. The size of the cotton yarn is the count or number of 840-yard hanks in a pound. Mercerized cotton is a stronger cotton produced by immersing it in a solution of caustic soda and holding the cotton at its original length. It develops a luster and makes a stronger fabric which is widely used in orthotic applications.

The two principal animal fibers are wool and silk. Wool fibers grow in groups of 5 to 80 hairs in the skin of the lamb or sheep, which is shorn once or twice a year. The raw wool is scoured in warm water with detergent. When dried, it is spun into wool or worsted yarn. Wool is thick and full; worsted is fine, firm, and smooth.

When the silkworm prepares to change from a chrysalis to a moth, it spins a silken fiber around itself to form a cocoon of a continuous fiber, which may be a mile long. Usually, two cocoons are unwound, and their filaments are twisted into silk thread measured in deniers. A denier of yarn is the weight in grams of 9,000 meters of the thread.

PROPERTIES OF FIBERS

The important properties of fibers for fabrics, especially with reference to orthotic garments, are: tensile strength, weight per surface unit (specific gravity), elongation, elastic recovery, wet strength (rayon becomes weaker in water, cotton becomes stronger), stiffness, effect of heat, and smoothness.

MANUFACTURE OF FABRICS

There are five methods of making fabrics from yarn: interlocking (felt), braiding, netting (lace), knitting, and weaving. Of these, weaving is perhaps the most important, but interlocking is of interest because of the frequency in which felt and wadding are used for padding in orthotics. Fibers of wool tend to coil and entangle permanently. When pressure and heat are added to this natural process, felt results. Felt is a warm resilient fabric which may be made in many thicknesses. It does not fray, and it permits the passage of air, but its tensile strength is relatively low.

Woven fabrics are made by interlacing two or more sets of yarn at right angles. The longitudinal thread is called the warp and the transverse thread the weft. By varying the pattern of interlacing, many types of weaving may be achieved. The principal varieties of weaving are plain and twill. In plain weaves, the weft intertwines alternately above and below successive strands of warp. Twill is a closely woven fabric with diagonal ridges; it is heavier and sturdier than comparable plain weaves.

Woven fabrics are mainly used for straps and geometric designs. However, when a fabric must be tailored to a complex three-dimensional shape, such as a stump sock or a custom-made elastic stocking, knitting is more suitable. Complex knitting machines are available that can custom fit a garment of almost any shape or dimension required to cover a limb or body part.

Manufactured fibers may be made from naturally occurring basic materials or from synthesized products. When a fiber is made from a naturally occurring cellulose, it is called regenerated cellulose. Such material is most easily derived from wood. Wood cellulose, when treated with alkalis and sulfides, converts into a viscous alkaline solution. This, when injected into an acid bath, coagulates into long filaments called rayon.

Synthetic fibers are composed of long molecules joined end to end. These molecules link into a very long chain which is physically, as well as chemically, a long filament. Such a simple long molecule is called a monomer; several long molecules of different length joined together form a polymer. Caruthers was the first developer of a synthetic filament formed from a polymeric amide. He called this nylon. Fabric made of nylon is perhaps still the most widely used synthetic fabric, but many more are now available on the market. It would be impossible to discuss all of these in detail, but typical examples, including trade names (in parentheses) have been classed by Cook (4) as follows:

1. Polymides (Nylon)
2. Polyester (Dacron)
3. Polyvinyls
   Polyacrylonitrile (Orlon)
   PVC (Avisco)
   Polyvinylidene chloride (Saran)
   PVA (Mewlon)
   Polyfluorocarbon (Teflon)
   Polyvinylidene dinitrile (Darvan)
4. Polyolephines
   Polyethylene (Proloft)
   Polypropylene (Herculon)
5. Polyurethane
   Spandex (Lycra)

The Federal Trade Commission has given synthetic fibers the following generic names: acetate, acrylic, azlon, modacrylic, nylon, nytril, olefin, polyester, rayon, saran, spandex, vinyl, and vinyon.

In the previous edition of *Orthotics Etcetera*, Licht listed in alphabetical order most of the fibers and fabrics that are used in the manufacture of orthotic devices, including details about the use of the individual types of fabrics (8). If still further detail on these synthetic fabrics is desired, it is possible to find the information in the *Modern Plastics Encyclopedia* (11).

REFERENCES

1. AMERICAN SOCIETY FOR TESTING AND MATERIALS. *Annual Book of ASTM Standards.* Philadelphia (revision issued annually), 1978.
2. BLOMER, A., FISCHER, K., BERG, H., AICHINGER, R., AND ALBRECHT, F. Development and application of a new polyurethane plastic support bandage. *Arch. Orthop. Unfall-chir., 85:* 1, 1976.
3. COMPTON, J., AND EDELSTEIN, J. E. New plastics for forming directly on the patient. *Prosthet. Orthot. Int., 2:* 43, 1978.
4. COOK, J. C. *Handbook of Textile Fibers.* Third edition. Merrow, Watford, England, 1964.
5. HAMPTON, F. Rubber and plastics for orthotics. In *Orthotics Etcetera*, edited by S. Licht. Elizabeth Licht, New Haven, 1966.
6. HERSHALL, W., AND SCALES, J. T. Plastic splints and appliances in orthopedic surgery. *J. Bone Joint Surg. (Br.), 30:* 298, 1948.
7. KENNAWAY, A. On the reduction of slip of rubber crutch tips on wet pavement, snow and ice. *Bull. Prosthet. Res., 10–14:* 130–144, 1970.
8. LICHT, S. *Fabrics for orthotics.* In *Orthotics Etcetera*, edited by S. Licht. Elizabeth Licht, New Haven, 1966.
9. MALICK, M. H. *Manual on Dynamic Hand Splinting with Thermoplastic Materials.* Harmarville Rehabilitation Center, Pittsburgh, 1974.
10. MALICK, M. H. *Manual on Static Hand Splinting—New Materials and Techniques.* Harmarville Rehabilitation Center, Pittsburgh, 1974.
11. *Modern Plastics Encyclopedia.* McGraw-Hill, New York, 1977.
12. MURPHY, E. F., AND BURSTEIN, A. H. Physical properties of materials including solid mechanics. In *Atlas of Orthotics.* C. V. Mosby, St. Louis, 1975.
13. O'FLAHERTY, F. Leather for orthotics. In *Orthotics Etcetera*, edited by S. Licht. Elizabeth Licht, New Haven, 1966.
14. PROSTHETIC ORTHOTIC CENTER, NORTHWESTERN UNIVERSITY MEDICAL SCHOOL. *Spinal Orthotics for Orthotists (Manual for Orthotics 701) and Lower Extremity and Spinal Orthotics for Physicians, Surgeons, and Therapists (Manual for Orthotics 722 and 723).* Northwestern University Medical School, Chicago, Ill. Undated.
15. ROSENBERG, S. J. Metals for orthotics. In *Orthotics Etcetera*, edited by S. Licht. Elizabeth Licht, New Haven, 1966.
16. WATTS, H. G., HALL, J. E., AND STANISH, W. The Boston brace system for the treatment of low thoracic and lumbar scoliosis by the use of a girdle without superstructure. *Clin. Orthop., 126:* 87, 1977.
17. YATES, G. Molded plastics in bracing. *Clin. Orthop., 102:* 46, 1974.

4

Corsets and Soft Supports

V. NANDA KUMAR, M.D.
SIDNEY LICHT, M.D.

Almost since the time of recorded history, women interested in high fashion have worn garments in an attempt to modify the shape of the human figure. The narrowest circumference of the trunk is the waist, and at times, the waistline has been so constricted by corsets that the abdominal viscera, and possibly health, have been compromised. Andreas Vesalius condemned the tight corset in the middle of the 16th Century and, in 1793, Samuel Soemmering of Berlin also write against it in *Ubedie Wirkung der Schnurbruste*. It was not until the 20th Century that the corset was prescribed for other than cosmetic reasons. During the first half of this century, corsets were medically prescribed for back pain, ptosed abdominal organs, hernia, and paralysis. Since the decline in the number of cases of poliomyelitis, back pain has become the chief indication (12).

A corset is an encircling garment with stiffening reinforcement which attempts to contain soft tissue under pressure at a desired elevation, to compress bony and other tissues to restrict or prevent motion, or to support the muscles and other soft tissues.

The word corset is probably a derivative of the Latin 'corpus', meaning body. The American Orthotic and Prosthetic Association has described a corset as a soft spinal orthosis having vertical or horizontal reinforcements (metal stays), but not both.

Materials

The soft support is made of fabric woven from natural fiber, synthetic fiber, or a combination of the two, sometimes with the addition of rubber, fiberglass, or metal. Cotton is used most often, plain or treated, as in canvas or duck. Cotton is soft and absorbent, can be made shrink resistant, and is easily laundered. It resists high temperatures and, unlike rayon, it is strong when wet. Of the synthetic materials, the most popular for soft supports are dacron, rayon, and spandex. Some fibers are elastic; they may be stretched considerably and yet return to their original length. Other fibers are relatively nonelastic. When a fabric is woven with elastic fibers, it can be made to stretch one way only, two ways, or more. Most corsets utilize one-way stretch.

Corsets for the torso (human trunk) are usually stiffened with longitudinal strips of material. Until the 18th century, the strip was made of wood or metal. In the 19th century, whalebone became very popular since it was highly flexible, light in weight, and fairly strong. In the 20th century, steel and other tensile materials replaced the bone.

Reinforcements are still called bones, and the process of fitting them into corsets is called boning. Bones are classified according to width, thickness, and strength. Steel bones come in many lengths (from 3 to 25 inches), with a tensile strength of about 200,000 psi and a Rockwell hardness of 15 N. The rigid steels are usually inserted into long narrow pockets called bone casings, which are free at one end so that they may be removed when the garment is laundered. Other metal parts of quality garments are usually made of nickel-plated brass and include buckles, eyelets, hooks, and zippers.

Corsets are made by sewing together pieces of pattern-cut fabric. The corset is open at the front, side, or back and secured to the human frame by buckled straps, Velcro fasteners, clasps, hooks and eyes, laces or elastic fabric. There are two schools of thought on the advisability of using lace for closing. One group believes that if there is one lace between the top and bottom of the garment, there will be a tendency for the laced portion below to spread and accommodate the greatest tension, which is usually where the support is needed. It is considered that this objection is overruled if there are many separate lace segments, with about three pairs of eyelets to the unit in a series of many (Fig. 4.1). Many orthotists favor tape and buckle for maximum control, or Velcro. Most of the corsets come in different sizes and are convenient for ordering stock models. The custom fit corset, to fill a medical prescription, is made by large manufacturers, and even these manufacturers have developed a system for sizing stock models that can be altered by an orthotist.

Fitting

Good measurement is essential for a proper fitting of the corset. After sections of the corset have been cut and trimmed to proper size, they are sewn together, measured again, and fitted with steel reinforcements. The completed corset must be tried on the patient. The patient must feel comfortable after all fasteners have been secured to the farthest maximum position for daily wear. The corset must be centered on the body. The fitter should observe the garment in place to ascertain position, levels, creases, and areas of unwanted excessive pressure. The patient should be measured and fitted in a sitting as well as standing position to determine the length of

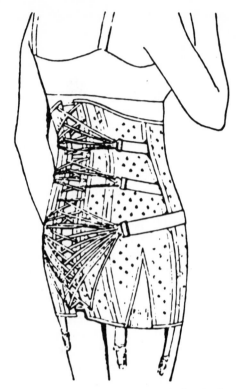

Fig. 4.1. Showing separate lace segments (lumbodorsal orthosis).

the front bones and to avoid their touching the lower ribs or coming well over them if they are prominent. Care is taken with the obese patient not to make the front so high that flesh is forced up in a seated position. This measurement is critical in specifying the corset length down for proper fit of the groin. The physician should prescribe the height at the back of the corset when he wishes stiff or rigid steels for added support. In general, the higher the lesion, the higher the top edge of the corset.

In the custom-made garment, riding out of place is at a minimum. Not only are the curves placed physiologically appropriate for the individual, but a measurement is taken from the waist down over the buttocks to where the lower limbs join and a gripped shape is cut into the corset.

Stock garments may have a tendency to ride too high or too low. If the garment is form fitting on a torso with well-marked curves, the shape of the garment will probably keep it in place. Otherwise, shoulder straps may be used to anchor the garment (Fig. 4.2). In general, certain variations in soft supports are best suited for specific body contours and shapes.

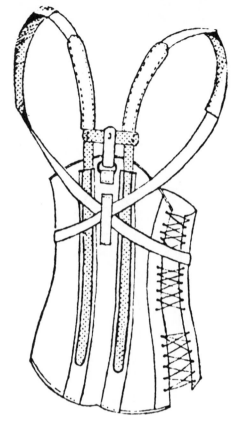

Fig. 4.2. A laced corset with shoulder straps.

Thorax

For fractured ribs or any other condition for which maximum mobilization of the ribs is desired for an ambulatory patient, a rib belt may be applied. The rib belt should be at least 8 inches wide to provide a wide spread of pressure and to prevent bruising of the skin. It may be made of an elastic fabric, joined in front or in back with tapes or velcro. It may be made of foam material, with shoulder straps, and with tapes and buckles which permit maximum tightening.

Abdomen

Soft supports are used to support and elevate abdominal muscles and viscera, to distribute the gravitational pull on the back, and to aid in diaphragmatic breathing (Fig. 4.3). With improved appearance, there is frequently an improved outlook on life.

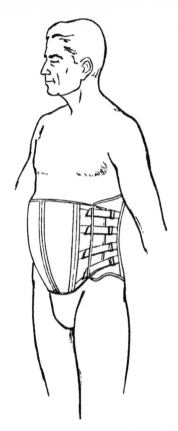

Fig. 4.3. A corset for pendulous abdomen.

The abdominal viscera are suspended, along with the omentum, from the anterior aspect of the spine. The abdominal muscles, in health, are among the strongest in the body per unit of volume. When they become weak (from disease, trauma, surgery, or multiple pregnancies), the weight of the viscera tends further to separate weakened muscle fibers, and the abdominal wall continues to sag even more. This is also true in quadriplegia where abdominal muscles are paralyzed. To support relaxed tissues, the "Hoke" corset is used with good results. This corset extends in the upper part close to the nipples, and the lower part of the garment should be parallel to the inguinal ligament but should not be folded when the patient is sitting.

An abdominal hernia is often held back with a pad placed against the hernial sac. The pads may be made of foam rubber covered with felt and velcro for easy adjustment of position. Controllable inguinal hernia is managed by: (a) a separate device encircling the greater trochanters with the bones placed diagonally and perineal straps attached thereto; the egg shaped pad is set on velcro so that it is movable to satisfactorily cover the hernia; (b) an addition may be secured to the belt front for a corrective garment to achieve the same end.

Back

Corsets are prescribed frequently for low back pain. A corset should be long enough in front to lift and support the abdomen, but instead of fitting the curves of the back snugly as was once recommended, it should be straight to reduce the lumbosacral angle (lumbar lordosis). The garment should be long enough posteriorly to grip the buttocks. A tight fit over the iliac crests is the most important factor.

Corsets for Low Back Pain

Perhaps the chief indication for corsets is low back pain. They should be prescribed and checked by the physician to validate their efficacy. Lumbosacral corset (flexible LSO), lumbosacral belt (flexible LSO), and sacroiliac belt (flexible SIO) are commonly used in practice (3, 11). Mechanisms of back pain and types of supports are discussed and illustrated more completely in the chapters on spinal bracing.

Lumbosacral Corset (Flexible LSO)

The biomechanical features of the LSO corset include anterior and lateral trunk containment to assist the abdominal musculature in elevating intracavity pressure. Depending on vertical stays, three-point pressure systems are applied that tend to restrict spinal motions.

Design and Fabrication. This orthosis is essentially a cloth garment that wraps around the torso and hips and is adjustable in circumference by means of side, front, or back laces or hooks. Anteriorly, the superior border is ½ inch below the xiphoid process or above the lower ribs, and the inferior border is ½ to 1 inch above the symphysis pubis. Posteriorly, the superior border is just below the apex of the gluteal bulge for men and the gluteal fold for women (1). The corset is usually a stock garment but should snugly fit all body contours. Wrinkles, failure to maintain position, and discomfort require tucks or alterations for a proper fit. If a stock garment cannot be used, a custom corset should be fabricated based on a pattern derived from careful measurement of the individual patient. Additions that may be necessary include posterior rigid or semirigid steels, posterior pads or shingles, extra-abdominal reinforcements, and a thoracic extension with shoulder straps. Posterior steels can be shaped so as to flatten (not maintain) lumbar lordosis.

Lumbosacral belt: (Flexible LSO)

The LSO belt, although not as effective in restricting motion, like the LSO corset does biomechanically assist in alleviating intra-abdominal pressure and may be useful in the obese to support a pendulous abdomen.

Additions that may be necessary include posterior rigid or semirigid steels, posterior sacral pads, and extra-abdominal reinforcements.

Design and Fabrication. A cloth garment that wraps around the pelvis and lower abdomen and is adjustable in circumference by means of side, front, or back laces, hooks, or Velcro. Anteriorly and posteriorly, the superior border is at the iliac crest level. Anteriorly, the inferior border is ½ to 1 inch above the symphysis pubis and, posteriorly, it extends to the apex of the gluteal bulge (15). For cosmetic reasons, the superior border may rise to just above waist level, and the inferior border may descend to the gluteal fold, thus reducing bulging. This orthosis is prefabricated and may require tucks or alterations for a comfortable fit.

Sacroiliac Belt (Flexible SIO)

This type of orthosis partially stabilizes sacroiliac joints and the symphysis pubis. This is a fabricated belt, 2 to 4 inches wide, which encircles the pelvis between the iliac crest and the trochanters. It is mainly used in postpartum and post-traumatic separations of the sacroiliac joints and symphysis pubis. It can be used in other causes of back pain, but does *not* significantly immobilize the sacroiliac joints. It most likely relieves pain by relieving strain on tense muscles, ligaments, or tendons and prevents sudden stressful movements of the spine.

Wearing Corsets for Back Pain

It is a common experience that back pain is relieved in some patients with a tight-fitting belt or girdle. When this occurs, the relief of pain may be due not to approximating "separated" bones or closing the gap in a sacroiliac joint, but to relieve strain from tense muscles, tendons, or ligaments, or by merely restricting the activity of the small joints in the spine.

The length of time a corset or belt should be worn will depend upon medical indications. Corsets, like back braces, are worn when the patient is up and about—walking, sitting, or otherwise active. In acute low back pain secondary to disk disease, we usually ask the patient to wear the support for 24 hours a day. This permits a comfortable night of sleep, not interrupted by the pain of trunk movement, which the unsupported back may experience. In some patients, it may be necessary to release the binder to permit sleep. If properly supportive and comfortably fitted, a corset may be worn till the acute symptoms are overcome. Corsets or back braces are not substitutes for good abdominal and back muscles. Exercises for these muscles should be prescribed along with the use of these supports.

Posture Correction

Corsets may also be prescribed to regulate posture, to promote or reduce lumbar lordosis or a dorsal kyphosis secondary to this position of the lumbar spine. If the corset is used to immobilize the spine, more work will be required of the gluteus maximus and other hip muscles when the patient bends; this is especially important in patients who have either weakness of the muscles that control the hips or painful conditions such as osteoarthritis. Corsets may be made as rigid as desired by the addition of more rigid stays or bones and by their placement. For the patient who needs only light support, light and flexible stays may be used. Position and molding of the stays determine the position of the back. When the corset stays are straight and the corset fits snugly, the lumbar lordosis will flatten; in other words, the lower back will be pulled into the corset. Conversely, if we markedly increase the curve in the stays when molding them, we can produce an increased lumbar spine extension and an increased flexion in the dorsal spine. This can further increase the extension at the cervical spine to achieve postural balance. Thus, we may be able to influence the spinal curvature considerably by the manner in which we mold the stays.

Corsets for Support of Limb Joints

"Corsets" are also available for the support of joints, such as knee, ankle, and wrist. Only the hinged knee support (KO) will be considered. Biomechanically, this orthosis provides mediolateral stabilization. Control of flexion or extension depends on stop or lock used at knee, and that cannot be effectively applied in this orthosis. The material used is one-way stretch elastic with two hinged bars on each side, enclosed in cowhide leather casing. Hinged bars are nickel-plated brass with a nylon washer to prevent friction. Encircling leather straps top and bottom help to stabilize the position of the hinge. An additional feature of front lacing may be added for ease of application and adjustment when swelling is a factor (Fig. 4.4). Actually, it is more likely that the hinged knee corset and other soft joint supports produce increased stability by increasing patients' sensory awareness of the joint position than by use of any mechanical stabilization.

Soft Supports for Limbs

Soft supports for the limbs may be indicated for disorders of the veins or lymphatics, or for orthostatic hypotension. Anatomically, such supports may be divided into four categories: below the knee, full-length lower limb, waist-high garment or leotard, and arm supports.

Each support is available with different pressure variances. The usual pressure of an elastic stocking is equal to 30 to 40 mm Hg, but they may be ordered for higher pressures. The supports are usually flesh colored, but on special demand, different colors are available. The lower limb supports should be closed at the toe so that more pressure may be exerted distally, and less proximally on the limb. Reduction of edema is assisted as the pressure variance built into the stockings furnishes a milking action when the wearer walks in them, or in the arm support when the patient performs isometric contractions.

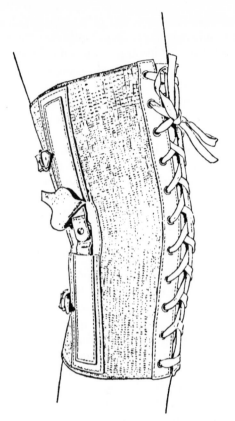

Fig. 4.4. Laced hinge knee support (KO).

Indications for Compression Supports

1. Edemas (14). All edemas of the lower limbs which cannot be cured definitely by active treatment must be compressed by compression stockings.

　　a. Venous edemas. Almost all edemas of primary varices are excluded from these indications. These include: postthrombotic syndrome sequelae of phlebitis of the deep veins of the lower limbs (13); high venous compression, as in compression of iliac veins; intra-abdominal compression by an inoperable inflammatory or malignant tumor; ligature of the inferior venae cava to prevent pulmonary embolism recurring after phlebitis of the lower limb.

　　b. Lymphatic edemas (10). Lymphatic edemas are due to atresia, obstruction, or removal of the lymphatic vessels without apparent venous dilatations. These include: congenital lymphedema which appears at birth or only a few years after; acquired lymphedema—

postoperative upper extremities following mastectomy (2, 18), or following radical groin disection.

2. Venous Diseases (17). Most venous diseases are accompanied by edema of the lower extremities as a secondary symptom. These include: chronic venous insufficiency; varices of pregnancy; varicose veins after sclerotherapy; and after stripping operation of varicose veins.

3. Orthostatic Hypotension. The waist-high garment is particularly useful for this problem, as it provides improved venous return throughout the entire lower body segment (6).

4. Post-burn healing (see following section on burns).

Precautions in Using Compression Supports (4)

1. Insufficient Compression. Edemas which are not already reduced to some degree by drugs or physical treatment should not be fitted with a compression stocking. The purpose of a compression stocking is not primarily to treat edema, but to maintain the limb free of edema or with minimal degree of edema.

2. Excessive Compression. Generally in peripheral arterial disease, it may increase danger of gangrene and compression supports should not be used.

3. Skin Disorders. Skin disorders such as moist dermatoses and cutaneous infections like furuncles, erysipelas, and abscesses are complete contraindications.

4. Difficulties in Donning. The patient who cannot put on his stockings by himself needs somebody else to help. Make sure that a second person is available to put on stockings before prescribing. Examples of conditions where such caution is needed include organic brain syndrome, hemiplegia, and paraplegia.

Prescription of the Compression Supports

Wearing limb supports regularly requires a certain degree of intelligence on the part of a patient, expressed by a cooperative attitude in order to obtain the best possible results. It also requires a detailed motivation of the doctor for his decision and reasonably good explanation for the patient about the possible benefits. Because they like to be elegant, many female patients are apprehensive about wearing compression stockings. The doctor should take time to explain the absolute necessity and therapeutic benefits, assuring the patient about the availability of numerous colors and sizes that would improve the esthetic value.

A good support must meet the following criteria.

For strong compression it must have maximum compression at the distal part, becoming less and less as it is followed proximally.

The pressure should be at least between 30 to 40 mm Hg for good therapeutic benefits.

The texture must be airy and porous in order to avoid possible allergies.

Timing of the Prescription

Four timings may be considered.

Immediate Prescription. In disorders which do not require previous treatment, stockings can be prescribed on first visit. The wearing of the stocking can of course be associated with other treatments. These conditions include varices of pregnancy, chronic venous insufficiency, venous malformations, and orthostatic hypotension.

At the End of Treatment. After physical treatments, supports are needed to maintain favorable results obtained from such therapy as intermittent pneumatic compression or an elastic bandage which are not very efficient in maintaining compression. In venous or lymphatic edemas, decrease of edema is easily verified by a good measurement of the leg or arm circumferences. If the circumference of the limb does not diminish any longer from one day to the next, the support may be prescribed based on the smallest measurements. Those varicose or post-thrombotic ulcers that precariously cicatrise with areas of white scarring require regular wearing of limb supports to prevent relapses.

Additional Treatment. Stockings are needed to improve the result obtained by another therapeutic method. For example, sclerotherapy of varicose veins, particularly the big caliber ones, will require the addition of compression after injection to avoid superficial periphlebitic reactions and obtain the best cosmetic results. Another use is following stripping of the saphenous veins which can cause secondary hemorrhages on the track of the stripped vein. Moreover, risk of deep postoperative thrombosis exists. Powerful compression of the whole lower limb will be achieved best by a compression stocking on the operating table.

During Treatment. The limb compression dressing is used for treatment of leg ulcers due to chronic venous insufficiency. The essential measure for cicatrization of an ulcer is ambulatory elastocompression. Bandages are commonly used. Their compression is reinforced by rubber sponges; sometimes an Unna's boot is applied. The Unna's boot is made up of zinc oxide gelatin nonstretchable pliable adhesive mold applied to the leg. It sets up a pumping action which is generated by the movements of the ankle. It is effective in reducing the edema due to chronic venous insufficiency in lower limbs. The application requires special technique, so the mold does not contract with the shrinking leg and must be reapplied to take up the slack. The boot must often be left on the leg for several weeks, which may be objectionable to patients (8). The compression support has all the advantages of the mobile bandage without any of the disadvantages. It may be taken off at night, which allows the exudates to dry. As the compression value is determined by the doctor, the daily activities of the patient do not interfere with treatment.

Measurements for the Prescription

Since it is desirable for the stocking to fit the limb contour as accurately as possible, measurements are taken with encircling tapes at intervals of 2 inches from the foot to the knee or above (Fig. 4.10). Similar measurements for supports can be made for the upper extremities. Only custom-made supports are really effective in controlling severe edema. Other elastic stockings or supports, although much less expensive, can only be used for mild edema or as a preventative measure.

Soft Supports in Burns

Contractures and hypertrophic scars are the two most frustrating sequelae of thermal injury. Extensive studies conducted at the Shriner's Burn Institute in Galveston, Texas, have indicated that more than 80% of patients who have suffered second and third degree burns will develop hypertrophic scarring throughout the burn areas after new skin and grafts have healed (Fig. 4.5). If no attempt is made to control the development of scar hypertrophy, crippling disfigurement is likely to occur due to severe contractures and the unchecked formation of thickened, knobby, red scar tissue. In normal burn-wound healing, there is a great increase in vascularity to form the granulation tissue which the body uses to restore the damaged skin site. Studies by Linares et al. (7) indicate that the granulation tissue shows an increase of fibroblasts.

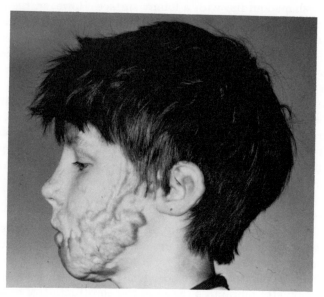

Fig. 4.5. Hypertrophic scarring following second degree burns. Courtesy of Jobst Institute, Inc.

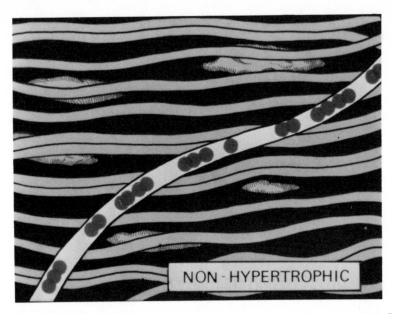

Fig. 4.6. Microscopic appearance of nonhypertrophic scar (diagrammatic). Courtesy of Jobst Institute, Inc.

In the development of normal skin dermis, fibroblasts appear to be irregular in shape and flat with a lumpy surface. However, the fibroblasts which develop within the reticular layer of a hypertrophic scar are spider-shaped with nodular rounded body (Figs. 4.4–4.7). These fibroblasts produce an excessive number of collagen fibers which entwine with each other to produce whorl-like patterns. In addition to the irregular shape of the nodules, a hypertrophic scar will synthesize collagen at more than four times the rate of normal skin. It is this pileup of collagen-filled nodules which gives rise to the thickened rigid hypertrophic scar which later can cause contractures. It has been known for some years that the application of controlled consistent pressure to the surface of an immature hypertrophic scar will, in time, reduce the scar and leave a smooth, pliable skin surface (Fig. 4.8). Research studies suggest that the application of pressure decreases the rapid blood flow through the vascular bed, thereby preventing an uncontrolled proliferation of fibroblasts and the excessive collagen buildup characteristic of hypertrophic scar(5). Initially, pressure dressings and elastic wraps were tried, but these materials slipped, bunched up, constricted, or came loose.

In 1960, Jobst Institute in Toledo, Ohio, developed a special Dacron spandex Bobbinette fabric to be used in the construction of custom-fitted pressure gradient garments. The Bobbinette fabric was unique in that it was porous, not occlusive. Its elastic weave was especially designed to

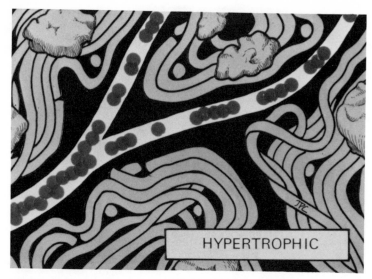

Fig. 4.7. Microscopic appearance of hypertrophic scar (diagrammatic). Courtesy of Jobst Institute, Inc.

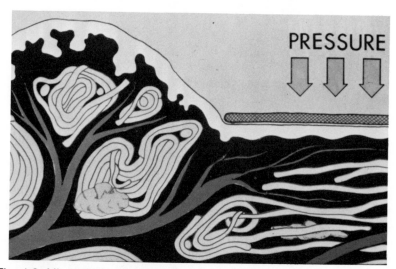

Fig. 4.8. Microscopic appearance of immature scar under consistent pressure (diagrammatic). Courtesy of Jobst Institute, Inc.

provide tridimensional control by employing unidirectional tension threads wrapped with prestressed fibers permitting maximum pressure effectiveness. Garments constructed from this new fabric, when accurately measured, fit, and consistently worn by the burn patient, provide and usually maintain adequate pressure to prevent hypertrophic scar formation (Figs. 4.9 and

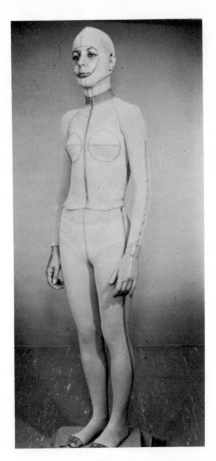

Fig. 4.9. Jobst body garment.

4.10). The multidirectional stretch of the fabric also allows any normal movement of the body. The garments are custom made and tailored for each patient, providing a gradient pressure on the burn scar area which just exceeds the interstitial pressure within the healing tissue. This early continuous pressure prevents hypertrophic scar formation and can diminish and control immature hypertrophic scarring for up to 6 months post burn (9).

Timing. The measurement and fitting of pressure gradient garments may begin as soon as the open areas of newly healed scar tissue are reduced to the size of a quarter (Fig. 4.11). The garments can then be made to apply pressure directly over the burn areas, including an entire body extremity. The healed areas should be measured and garments ordered as early as possible, leaving large unhealed areas for measurement at a later date.

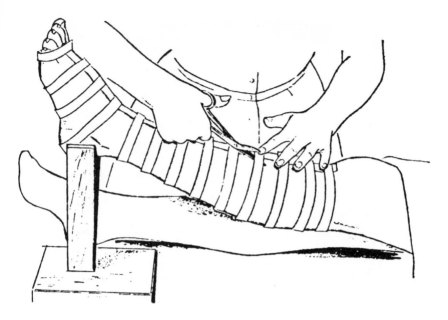

Fig. 4.10. Technique of measuring for garment.

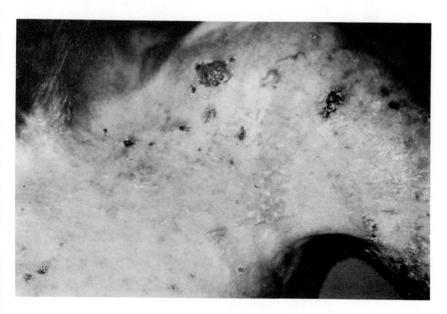

Fig. 4.11. Newly healed scar ready for Jobst garment.

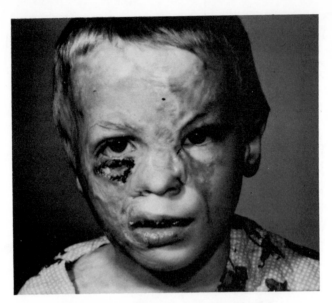

Fig. 4.12. Facial scar ready for garment.

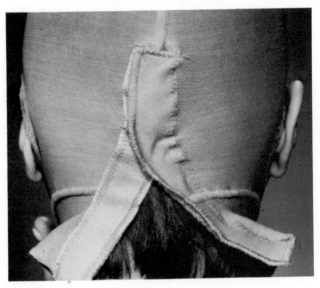

Fig. 4.13. Garment fitting (posterior view).

Of all of the body parts, the face is the most difficult area in which to achieve adequate pressure (Figs. 4.12–4.14). Because of underlying bone structure, the forehead and mandible line are the only areas where sufficient pressure is guaranteed.

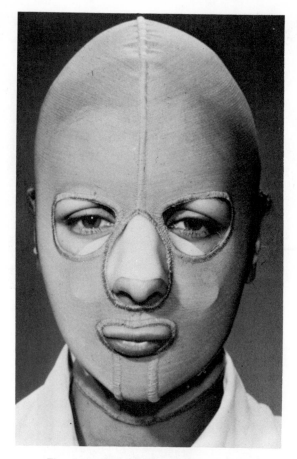

Fig. 4.14. Fitting of face (nose spared).

If the soft areas around the mouth, nose, and chin are a part of these extensively damaged areas, additional materials, such as molded low-temperature plastic or a high-density foam, such as Spenco padding (Fig. 4.15), would have to be inserted under the mask to guarantee consistent adequate pressure to all burn areas. When moderate anterior neck burns are present, a soft neck (16) support can be used to prevent cervical contractures and, at the same time, apply pressure (Fig. 4.16).

Whenever possible, efforts should be made to measure a patient for garments before hospital discharge. If body weight increases more than 15 pounds, remeasuring is necessary. The garments should be carefully hand washed, rinsed, and then squeezed gently or rolled into a Turkish towel to remove excessive moisture. They should then be hung up to dry. They should never be put in a dryer, as excessive heat will damage the elasticity quickly. With proper care, Jobst garments have an average life of 3 months.

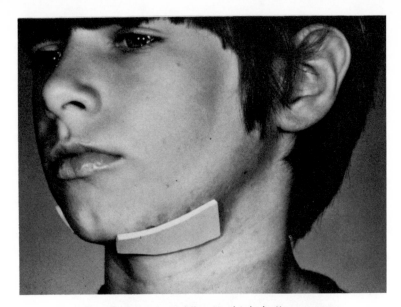

Fig. 4.15. Spenco padding to obtain better pressure.

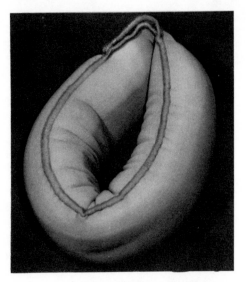

Fig. 4.16. Soft collar for neck burns.

Daily washing is not only important to the life and usefulness of the garment, but is also essential to prevent any infection underneath the garment. Petroleum-based lotions are discouraged because they can damage the elasticity of the fabric. To be fully effective, pressure gradient garments should be worn until the scar tissue is mature. Depending on the patient, this process could take from 9 to 14 months.

REFERENCES

1. BERGER, N., AND LUSSKIN, R. Orthotic Components and Systems, In *Atlas of Orthotics*, Ch. 19, pp. 334–372. C. V. Mosby & Co., St. Louis, Mo., 1975.
2. BRITTON, R. C., AND NELSON, P. A. Post mastectomy lymphedema of the arm. *J. A. M. A., 180* (2): 92, 1962.
3. HARRIS, E. E. A new orthotics terminology. *Orthotics Prosthet., 27* (2): 6–19, 1973.
4. HUSNI, F. A., AND GOYETTE, E. M. Elastic compression of the lower limbs: merits and hazards. *Am. Heart J., 82* (1): 132, 1971.
5. LARSON, D. L., ET AL. Techniques for decreasing scar formation and contractures in the burned patient. *J. Trauma, 2* (10): 807–823, 1971.
6. LEVIN, J. M., RAVENNA, P., AND WEISS, M. Idiopathic orthostatic hypotension. *Arch. Intern. Med., 114* (1): 145, 1964.
7. LINARES, H. A., KISCHER, C. W., DOBRKOVSKY, M., AND LARSON, D. L. On the origin of the hypertrophic scar. *J. Trauma, 13:* 70, 1973.
8. LIPPMAN, H. I., AND BRIERE, J. P. Physical basis of external supports in chronic venous insufficiency. *Arch. Phys. Med. Rehabil., 52:* 555–559, 1971.
9. MANI, M. M., ROBINSON, D. W., MASTERS, F. W., AND KETCHUM, L. D. Burn update-management of scars and contractures. *J. Kans. Med. Soc.,* 118–120, 1978.
10. NELSON, P. A. Recent advances in treatment of lymphedema of the extremities. *Geriatrics, 21* (4): 162, 1966.
11. NORTON, P. L., AND BROWN, T. The immobilizing efficiency of back braces. *J. Bone Joint Surgery, 39A:* 111, 1957.
12. PERRY, J. The use of external support in the treatment of low back pain. *J. Bone Joint Surgery, 52A:* 1440–1442, 1972.
13. SCHIRGER, A., AND KAVANAUGH, G. J. Swelling of legs in the aged. *Geriatrics, 21* (5): 123, 1966.
14. SIGG, K. Compression with pressure bandages and elastic stockings for prophylaxis and therapy of venous disorders of the leg. *Fortschr. Med.,* (15), 601–606, 1963.
15. Spinal Orthotics, New York Post Graduate Medical School, Prosthetics and Orthotics, New York, 1973.
16. WILLIS, B. A., LARSON, D. L., AND ABSTON, S. Positioning and splinting the burned patient. *Heart Lung, 2:* 5, 696–700, 1973.
17. WOOD, J. E. The Veins. Little, Brown & Co., Boston, Mass., 1965.
18. ZEISSLER, R. G. B., AND NELSON, P. A. Post mastectomy lymphedema: late results of treatment in 385 patients. *Arch. Phys. Med. Rehabil., 53:* 159, 1972.

5

Cervical Orthoses

JAMES D. HARRIS, D.O.

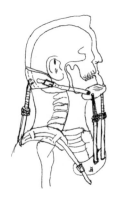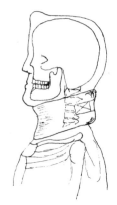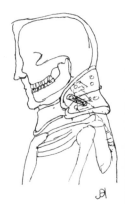

Fig. 5.1. Extension; neutral; flexion.

Bracing of the neck for pain and other problems is centuries old (Fig. 5.1). Documentation of the first cervical orthosis is difficult, and its uses have been varied, but through the centuries the materials have changed from natural fiber to man-made metals, plastics, and fabrics with further refinement in combination usage. Recently, quantified documentation in the literature concerning the indications and limitations of different types of cervical orthoses has assisted the physician in his choice of the best-suited orthoses. This chapter is dedicated to classification and quantification of the advantages and disadvantages of the different types of cervical orthoses.

A cervical orthosis is a device applied to the exterior of the body which influences neck motion by assisting, resisting, blocking, or unloading part of the head weight.

The cervical orthoses are used to treat many diseases and injuries of the neck, ranging from muscle guarding to serious bony instability. Common cervical orthotic goals are:

1. Bony stabilization with maintenance of alignment.

2. Muscle relaxation with analgesia.
3. Deformity prevention.
   a. Skeletal.
   b. Soft tissue contracture (*i.e.*, third degree neck burns, torticollis).
4. Skeletal distraction to decrease neural compression.
5. Motion limitation for soft tissue healing.
6. Motion amplification to facilitate range of motion.
7. Partial unloading of the weight of the head.

The *patient* who wears the cervical orthosis and his family should be educated as to the need and goal of the orthotic device. Common areas of concern are:

1. Patient and family *acceptance of the need* of the external "artificial" support system, which is highly visible and may affect the patient's self-image.
2. *Independent* application of the orthosis is desirable but may be a problem for a person with limited hand function or lack of antigravity strength in the upper extremity.
3. Willingness to *care for* and *maintain* and not abuse the orthosis.
4. *Secondary motivation* for wearing the device: "A sign of disability" in "whiplash" litigation, "need for compensation," or "need for special consideration."
5. *Cost* for the custom-made cervical orthosis may need explanation, justification, and communication prior to fabrication.

The cervical region is difficult to brace due to its special anatomic and functional demands, which are primarily motion and protection. The cervical area is the most mobile segment of the entire spine. This *mobility* is essential for adequate positioning and focusing of the major sensory receptors located in the skull (sight, smell, taste, hearing, and balance), and any immobilization may affect all of these functions. The musculoskeletal structures in the neck protect not only the entire neurological pathways of the caudal body but also the blood supply to the head and passageways for nutrition and respiration.

Mobility of the cervical spine is greatly increased in the very young, with dislocation and relocation injury being more common. Rigidity of the cervical spine in the elderly with decreased vascular supply to the head region must be considered, as well as the age-related general curvature changes, prior to prescribing the cervical orthosis.

The cervical spine has both a static structural support system as well as a dynamic mobile mechanism, which can be drastically changed by disease or injury. The cervical spine compensates for the lower vertebral curvatures and gravitational forces by alignment stability and strives to maintain optimal position of the head for sensory input.

The specific systemic diseases may have unique complications affecting the cervical spine:

1. *Rheumatoid arthritis*—synovial joint pathology, particularly at the atlantoaxial articulation, characterized by decreased ligamentous stability and odontoid pathology.
2. *Rheumatoid spondylitis*—connective tissue autoimmune pathology with ultimate spinal rigidity and ankylosis.
3. *Duchenne muscular dystrophy*—lack of muscle support and head control to defy gravitational forces.
4. *Parkinson's disease*—lack of synergistic neurological control with neck rigidity and postural changes.
5. *Cerebral palsy*—lack of volitional fine motor coordination, which may necessitate head positioning to help control tonic neck reflexes. The athetoid cerebral palsy patient creates tremendous repetitive abnormal forces on the cervical spine which increase wear and breakdown of the joint surfaces.
6. *Congenital cervical anomalies*—fusion or partial vertebral absence changes the stress pattern of breakdown, buildup, and replacement that is continually taking place.

Cailliet (3) nicely stated that abnormal stresses on normal structures or normal stresses on abnormal structures lead to functional loss.

Traumatic injury to the cervical spine can be devastating in altering the mechanisms for static support and mobility. Understanding the nature, sequence, and effect of trauma on the cervical spine is essential in prescribing the most suitable orthotic device. A cervical spine radiograph is only one aspect of the neck evaluation. The subjective and objective neurological findings, as well as the musculoskeletal palpatory assessment of the cervical structures in combination with the history and laboratory findings, are all part of the decision-making process for the treatment.

The effects of different types of trauma on the cervical spine need to be considered, and these are grouped as follows:

Repetitive stresses—a history of abnormal posturing and occupational stresses may be significant.

Acceleration forces—these focus primarily at the C-4 vertebral area from the hyperextension type of injury (12).

Deceleration forces—these focus on the C-5-6 vertebral area from the hyperflexion type of injury (3).

Other cervical anatomical areas need special consideration which are as follows.

The C-7, T-1 area is a transitional zone between the highly mobile cervical spine and the more rigid thoracic spine and, so, is often subject to injury. It is associated with the lower roots of the brachial plexus, which are primarily involved with hand function.

Odontoid and atlas fractures may be missed on early nonstressed radiographic examination but, when stressed, can be fatal. Serial radiograph examinations may be indicated of the C-1, C-2 area in the patients complaining of upper cervical pain, or with a history of head trauma, especially if there was loss of consciousness.

Anatomical Structure

A discussion of cervical orthoses requires a brief description of the anatomy and kinesiology of the cervical spine. The cervical spine is an aggregate of superimposed "functional units" (3). The seven cervical vertebrae form the normal adult cervical lordotic posture. The "functional unit" as described by Cailliet (3) is two adjacent vertebrae separated by an intervertebral disc. This unit can be conceptually divided into an anterior and posterior portion. The *anterior* portion is the weight-bearing vertebral body with the cushioning intervertebral disc, which is relatively insensitive as far as pain sensation is concerned. The *posterior* portion consists of the lamina, facets, and transverse and spinous processes. This posterior portion is nonweight-bearing and relatively sensitive as far as pain sensation is concerned. The processes serve as the site of muscle attachment. Both the anterior and posterior portions of the functional unit are heavily guyed by ligamentous structures.

The cervical spine is unique in that the upper articulation, the atlanto-occipital areas, have encapsulated synovial joints. The superior atlantal joint surface has bilateral elongated cups with a sagittally oriented joint motion, which receives the two occipital condyles. The backward, extension motion of the head is greater (25°), and the forward, flexion motion is less (10°). The joint capsule is lax and lies close to the first cervical nerve root and the vertebral artery. Hyperextension of the head upon the cervical spine can cause compression of the neural vascular bundle (vertebral arteries and C-1), especially if there are exostoses present. This explains some of the complaints of "dizziness" in older persons upon looking up.

The atlantoaxial articulation is complex; the atlas has no body or disc and is designed primarily for rotation about the odontoid of the axis. Four synovial joints lie between the atlas and axis: two lateral and two medial. The odontoid is held in close approximation to the atlas ring by the transverse ligament of the atlas. Fifty percent of the total neck rotation occurs between C-1 and C-2.

The vertebral arteries transit up through the foramen in the transverse processes of C-6 through C-1 to supply the brain stem.

The cervical intervertebral discs are wedge shaped, the anterior being two to three times thicker than the posterior margin. The resulting curve is partially reversed by the wedge-shaped vertebral bodies C-3 through C-7. In normal adults cervical lordosis is a result of the cervical disc and body curves. The cervical body end plates are curved. The superior surface is concave with an increased margin in the posterior lateral area which makes up the lateral intervertebral joint (hemiarthrosis intervertebralis lateralis of von Luschka). The inferior surface of the vertebral body is concave in the saggital plane but is convex in the coronal plane. The wedged cervical disc has a rocker effect on flexion and extension; thus, it has a multifocal axis.

There is a total of five joints in the cervical "functional unit": the vertebral body, the pair of articular facets, and the pair of lateral interbody joints of von Luschka.

Ligamentous Support

Neck ligaments are resilient enough to control extremes of motion and lax enough to permit a great range of motion. Mechanically, the head is a heavy eccentrically balanced globe on a relatively narrow elastic mobile support. Stability of the atlantoaxial joint is dependent upon the ligamentous structure and muscular support. Function of the various ligaments are as follows: the anterior longitudinal ligament re-enforces the disc annulus anteriorly, and the posterior longitudinal ligament is a double-layered ligament and re-enforces the posterior aspect of the disc and laterally re-enforces the facet capsules. The ligamentum flavum encompasses the posterior arch (laminar area) and also helps to re-enforce the facet capsule. The interspinous ligaments help check hyperflexion. The ligamentum nuchae is the fan-shaped extension of the interspinous ligament checking the atlantoaxial hyperflexion.

Musculature and Kinesiology

The beauty of the synchronization of the prime movers, stabilizers, agonists, and antagonists is well demonstrated in the large number of cervical muscles. Cailliet (3) divides the neck musculature into two major functional groups: head (capital) flexors and extensors and neck (cervical) spine flexors and extensors. The *head flexors* are predominantly the short recti and longus capitis. The *head extensors* are the four short muscles: posterior rectus capitis (minor and major), obliquus capitis superior and inferior, and two long muscles, splenius capitis and splenius cervicis.

The *sternocleidomastoid* muscles are bilaterally paired, forming a "V" anteriorly. They are the prime movers of flexion of the cervical spine when contracting bilaterally in unison. Unilateral contraction contributes to lateral bending and rotation to the opposite side. When the head is stabilized, this muscle will assist in respiration by elevating the rib cage.

Scaleni are three in number which are bilaterally symmetrical muscles (anterior, middle, and posterior). They are prime movers for lateral bending and assist in flexion of the spine.

Longus Colli assists with flexion and lateral bending of the cervical spine.

Longus Capitis assists with flexion and lateral bending of the head and cervical spine.

Rectus Capitis muscles are of two types: anterior, which are an assistive head flexor, and lateralis, which are assistive in lateral head bending.

Intertransversarii—unilateral action causes lateral bending and bilateral contraction causes extension of the spine.

Interspinalis are prime movers for extension of the spine.

Rotatores—unilateral contraction causes rotation of the spine to the opposite side; bilateral contraction causes extension of the spine.

Multifidus—unilateral contraction causes lateral bending and rotation to opposite side; bilateral contraction causes extension of the spine.

Semispinalis cervicis—unilateral contraction causes lateral flexion and rotation to the opposite side; bilateral contraction causes extension of the spine.

Semispinalis capitis—unilateral contraction causes lateral bending of the head and cervical spine; bilateral contraction causes head and neck extension.

Iliocostalis cervicis—unilateral contraction causes lateral bending and rotation to the same side; bilateral contraction causes extension of the cervical spine.

Longissimus cervicis—unilateral contraction causes lateral bending and rotation to the same side; bilateral contraction causes cervical spine extension.

Spinalis cervicis—unilateral contraction causes lateral bending of the cervical spine; bilateral contraction causes extension of the cervical spine.

Splenius cervicis—unilateral contraction causes lateral bending and rotation to the same side; bilateral contraction causes extension of the cervical spine.

Splenius capitis—unilateral contraction causes rotation to the same side and lateral bending of the head and cervical spine; bilateral contraction causes extension of the head and cervical spine.

Suboccipital muscles (rectus capitis posterior major, rectus capitis posterior minor, obliquus capitis superior, obliquus capitis inferior)—unilateral contraction causes lateral bending and rotation of the head to the same side; bilateral contraction causes extension of the head. This group of muscles is frequently involved in tension and post-deceleration neck trauma.

Pain-sensitive Tissues in the Cervical Spine Area

The dura mater is a pain-sensitive tissue and is innervated by the recurrent spinal meningeal nerve. The articular facets and joint capsules are pain sensitive through the medial portion of the posterior primary division of the spinal nerve. The posterior longitudinal ligament and the capsule structures of the lateral intervertebral joints receive their nerve supply from the recurrent spinal meningeal nerve (sinuvertebral), which contains somatic sensory and efferent sympathetic nerves. Here is where we see a close association with the somatic and visceral innervation. The spinal nerve root is a pain-sensitive tissue, and there are three commonly acceptable mechanisms of irritation: dural sheath tension, dorsal sensory root involvement, and sensory fibers of the motor root (3). Stretching the nerve and its dural sheath causes impaired vascular supply, which may be the cause of "nerve pain." "Pain is the cry of a nerve deprived of its blood supply," according to Sir Henry Head, which is in agreement with A. T. Still's quote, "The rule of the artery is supreme." In summary, the pain-sensitive tissues of the cervical areas are: anterior and posterior longitudinal ligaments, nerve roots, articular capsules and facets, and supportive musculature. This excludes the cervical intervertebral disc, which is aneural and avascular in the adult. We must not overlook "central pain" as the etiological factor of neck pain.

Nomenclature of Cervical Orthoses

Standardization of the nomenclature that is logical with minimal usage of eponyms is a goal of this chapter.

Cervical orthoses can be categorized into two general types: *skin* contact (soft tissue devices) and *bony* contact (skeletal devices).

Skin contact cervical orthoses are of six basic designs which are named according to the regional anatomy that is involved:

1. Cervical Orthoses (CO)
2. Head Cervical Orthoses (HCO)
3. HCO, custom-molded.
4. HCO, poster type.
5. Head Cervical Thoracic Orthoses (HCTO)
6. Head Cervical Thoracic Lumbar Orthoses (HCTLO)
7. Head Cervical Thoracic Lumbar Sacral Orthosis (HCTLSO)

Bony contact cervical orthoses are of six basic designs which are of two major types:

1. Halo type.
   a. Halo bed.
   b. Halo vest, skull cervical thoracic orthoses (SCTO).
   c. Halo jacket, skull cervical thoracic lumbar orthoses (SCTLO).
   d. Halo pelvic hoop, skull cervical thoracic lumbar pelvic orthoses (SCTLPO).
   e. Halo femoral pin, countertraction.
2. Tong type.

Skin Contact Cervical Orthoses

In a review of cervical orthotic fitting, Fisher (8) found that fitting of cervical orthoses by the traditional method of subjective "approval" response, even by a certified orthotist, produced increased pressure (105 mm Hg pressure at chin and occiput pad). When a pressure device was used, the average pressure was 25 mm Hg. The capillary pressure of human skin is 30 mm Hg: sustained pressure above this will cause ischemia which will lead to pain and may lead to necrosis if prolonged. Fisher's study (8) indicated that cervical immobilization gained with pressures greater than 30 mm Hg was not significantly greater than fitting with pressures at 25 mm Hg. Therefore, he suggested that the fitting orthotist should be using a pressure sensor to obtain the best possible fit within tolerable pressure limits. This would increase the patient's comfort and reduce the likelihood of loosening his own device, which decreases its effectiveness.

The common problem of fitting a cervical orthosis that has not been resolved is fitting in one position but losing this fit when the anatomical and gravitational forces are changed by assuming a different position, that is, supine to sitting or standing.

I. Cervical Orthoses (CO)

The orthopedic type of collars are divided into soft and rigid types (Fig. 5.2).

Soft Cervical Collar. This type of cervical orthosis typically is made of foam rubber covered with cotton stockinette, which fastens with Velcro behind the neck (Fig. 5.2A). It also has been made of many different materials, such as towels, felt, newspaper, leather and inflatable, (Fig. 5.2B), and the elastic Jobst Cervical Garments (Fig. 5.2C). The cervical orthosis (soft type) is usually considered comfortable by most wearers but is the least effective appliance in limiting all motions of the head and neck in the study of Johnson et al. (13). He also reported that it was comfortable and may serve as a reminder to the patient to restrict motion and provide sufficient support for some symptomatic treatment. He measured the effects of the soft cervical collar and showed that the gross cervical flexion-extension was restricted to 26% of normal motion. Colachis and Strohm (4) found that the use of the soft collar did not restrict neck flexion and only slightly restricted extension. Jones (14) used cineradiographic techniques and further agreed that the soft collar afforded little immobilization. He did relate that the height of the collar was directly proportional to the fixation of the upper cervical spine through restriction of head motion. He concluded that the motion of the head must be prevented if immobilization of the cervical spine is desired. Furthermore, Hartman et al. (11) found that the soft cervical collar restricted flexion-extension and lateral bending up to 5 to 10% by motion picture studies, but there was no evidence of restriction seen on cineradiographic evaluation.

An *inflatable neck support* has been described by Taylor (23) (Fig. 5.2B) which was introduced as a supplemental soft collar and cervical traction device. There have been wrap around as well as bivalved types on the market, but no published data as to their effectiveness is readily available.

The *Jobst Cervical Garment* is designed to control hypertrophic scar formation and help prevent contracture in the cervical area by continuous splinting and pressure until the scar tissue matures (an average of 6 to 12 months) (Fig. 5.2C). Larson (18) has recommended a minimum of 20 mm Hg pressure and has used this in combination with molded plastic inserts and more rigid cervical orthoses to prevent the catastrophic neck flexion hypertrophic scar contractures.

Hard Cervical Collar (Thomas, Mayo, Wire-frame types) (Fig. 5.3). The studies of Hartman *et al.* (11) have shown that the adjustable Thomas collar (Fig. 5.3A) restricted flexion-extension motion by 75%. Half of the remaining motion occurred between the occiput and atlas; the rest of the motion was seen between C-2 and C-7 in diminishing amounts. Lateral bending was also restricted by 75%, and the remaining motion was distributed between C-2 and C-7, as analyzed by cineradiographic technique. Cervical rotation was restricted by 50%, and the majority of the motion took place between C-1 and C-2.

The *wire frame collar* (Fig. 5.3B) is rigid and more difficult to fit, but it allows better skin ventilation of the neck and does not cover the tracheal area. There needs to be more quantitative comparative research done to document the effectiveness of the wire frame type of rigid cervical orthosis.

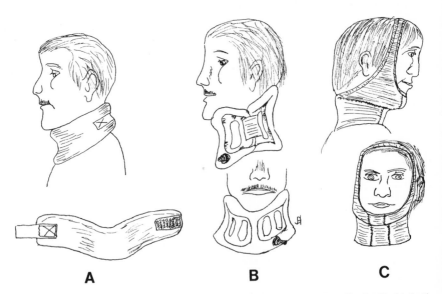

Fig. 5.2. Soft cervical orthosis. *A*, soft collar; *B*, inflatable collar; *C*, elastic (Jobst).

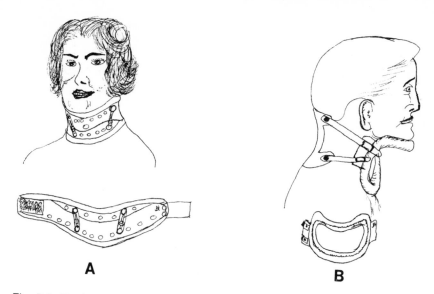

Fig. 5.3. Hard cervical orthosis. *A*, Thomas or Mayo collar; *B*, wire frame collar.

II. Head Cervical Orthoses (HCO)

These include *chin piece collar, Queen Anne collar, double-support collar,* and *molded collar with chin and occipital support* (Fig. 5.4). These types of cervical orthoses, all made of firm plastic, give more neck control than the previously mentioned cervical orthoses by restricting more head motion.

Colachis (4) showed that the *chin piece collar* (Fig. 5.4*A*) was more effective in limiting flexion of the cervical spine when compared to the soft and Queen Anne type of cervical orthosis (Fig. 5.4*B*). It restricts atlantooc-cipital and atlantoaxial flexion without limiting extension. On the other hand, the *Queen Anne type* is more effective in limiting cervical extension when compared to the soft and chin piece type of cervical orthoses, but it has little effect on limiting atlantoaxial extension.

The studies of Fisher *et al.* (9) showed that the *polyethylene plastic collar* with chin and occipital pieces (Camp Manufacturing Co.) provided the best sagittal immobilization of C-1, C-2, and atlantooccipital areas in a comparative study with the sternal-occipital-mandibular immobilizer (SOMI) and four-poster cervical orthosis. However, it is less effective in restricting overall cervical motion when compared to the SOMI and four-poster cervical orthosis. Since forward movement of the head is not restricted, complete cervical immobilization is impossible with these orthoses. Forward movement of the head does produce flexion in the middle and lower cervical

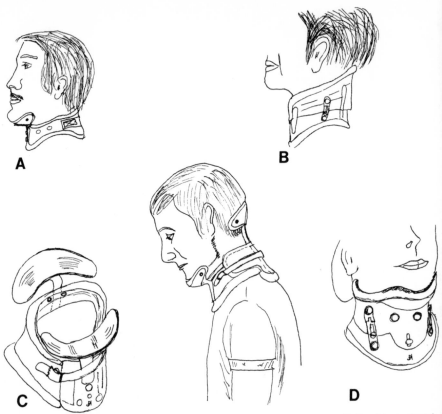

Fig. 5.4. Head cervical orthosis. *A*, chin piece; *B*, Queen Anne; *C*, Double support (Camp)-Chin-Occiput; *D*, molded.

segments. Therefore, if immobilization of the cervical spine is desired, forward motion of the head must be prevented.

III. HCO (Custom-molded)

Custom-molded Type (Philadelphia or Plastazote Collar) (Fig. 5.5). The *polyethylene foam two piece cervical orthosis* comes in three sizes and three heights and is heat malleable. The studies of Johnson *et al.* (13) showed that this custom-molded HCO restricts gross flexion and extension of the cervical spine to 29% of the normal motion but is less effective in controlling rotation and side bending when compared to the four-poster orthosis.

The studies of Fisher *et al.* (9) demonstrated that the custom-molded HCO is as effective in immobilizing the cervical spine as the SOMI is for

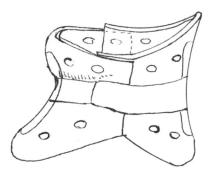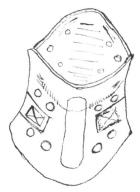

Fig. 5.5. Head cervical orthosis, custom-molded type. Philadelphia or plastazote collar.

restricting extension and the four-poster is in restricting flexion. This type of orthosis is bivalved and has lateral Velcro fasteners which make it ideal for fitting the bedridden patient, as it is easily applied and removed.

IV. HCO (Poster)

Poster Type (four-poster, Victoria-type) (Fig. 5.6). The *four-poster cervical orthosis* controls the head through padded mandibular and occipital supports which are attached to the thoracic and chest plates by two rigid adjustable uprights anteriorly and posteriorly. Bilateral flexible leather straps connect the mandibular and occipital supports.

The study of Johnson *et al.* (13) shows that the total cervical flexion-extension was restricted to 21% of normal, that rotation was restricted to 27% of normal, and that lateral bending was least restricted, that is, only 46% of normal when the four-poster HCO was used. The study of Fisher *et al.* (9) found the four-poster more effective in restricting extension of the cervical spine when comparing it to the SOMI. The study of Hartman *et al.* (11) showed that the four-poster type of HCO was 80 to 85% effective in limiting flexion-extension and lateral bending but was only 60% effective in restricting the rotation of the cervical spine. Berger (1) reported that control of motion can be increased by adding rigid side bar attachments between the chin and occipital pads. He also related that a thoracic extension could be added to provide increased support and rotational support. However, he cautioned that this increased trunk support may impart undesirable trunk motion to the head and neck.

V. Head Cervical Thoracic Orthoses (HCTO)

This includes *SOMI, Wilson, Guilford, and rigid APRO* (Anterior-posterior rotational orthosis) (Fig. 5.7).

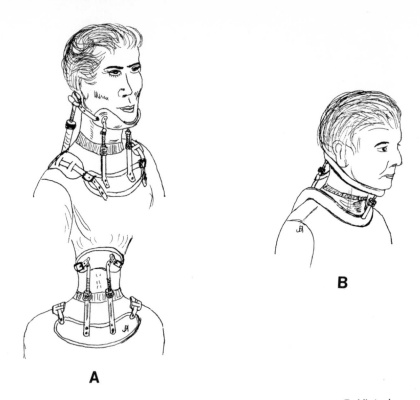

Fig. 5.6. Head cervical orthosis, poster type. *A*, four-poster; *B*, Victoria.

SOMI Type of HCTO is sensibly named according to its attachment points (sternal-occipital-mandibular immobilizer) (Fig. 5.7*A*). Modified usage of the basic SOMI loses the meaning of its name, such as the headband modification or the SOMI superstructure attached to a thoracic-lumbar-sacral-orthosis (TLSO) as described by Lund *et al.* (19) or the modification by Wilson. The study of Fisher *et al.* (9) showed that the unmodified SOMI is the best orthosis in limiting cervical spine flexion when compared to the four-poster and custom-molded Philadelphia type HCO.

The SOMI is easy to fit on the supine patient, and the occipital piece can be easily removed from the supine patient.

The *new SOMI headband* (3B 101-60) is designed as an auxiliary support to be used when the mandibular support is removed for eating, shaving, etc. (Fig. 5.7*B*). The headband is made of thin flexible plastic which attaches bilaterally in the back via snaps to the occipital pad. The headband encircles the cranium and has a Velcro closure. Quantitative effectiveness studies need to be published in reference to this modification. Lund's presentation

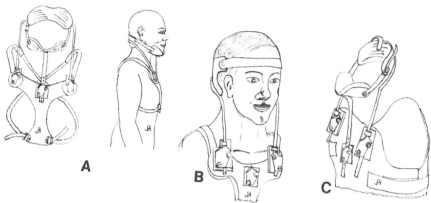

Fig. 5.7. HCTO. *A*, SOMI; *B*, SOMI head band; *C*, SOMI mounted on a bivalved TLSO.

(19) of the SOMI suprastructure on a bivalved TLSO (Fig. 5.7*C*) gives the advantages as:

1. Easy and safe donning and doffing of the device, which enable better hygiene and soft tissue checks.
2. Light weight.
3. Less encumbrance of the patient when compared to the halo.

Wilson's evaluation (24) presented with the need of a new noninvasive halo orthosis for immobilization of the cervical spine (Fig. 5.8). He described his modified SOMI as a total motion control device. The Wilson type of HCTO allows the chin to be free for talking and chewing and that there is no undesirable force applied over the temporomandibular articulation. His opinion is that his brace is "almost the treatment of choice whenever rigid immobilization of the cervical spine is indicated."

The *Wilson type of HCTO* is a modified SOMI (Fig. 5.8). The occipital pad has been removed, and the uprights are extended to attach to the posterior opening of a split-ring Sansplint headpiece which encircles the forehead and temples and most of the occipital area. There is a second set of adjustable uprights which attach from the temple portion of the headpiece and attach caudally to the occipital rods that go posterior from the SOMI chest plate.

Comparative studies are needed to document the advantages of this orthosis and to show how much immobilization can be attained.

HCTO, four-poster type (Fig. 5.9), is similar to the four-poster HCO but is more rigid due to a larger thoracic surface area combined with the metal connections between the occipital and mandibular pads and the axillary straps between the sternal and thoracic plates.

The study of Johnson *et al.* (13) shows restriction of total cervical flexion

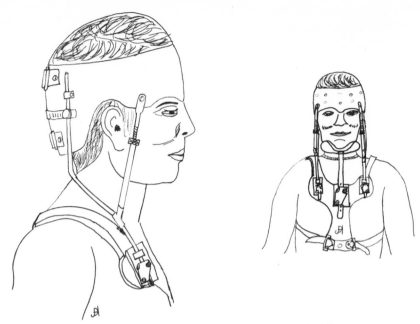

Fig. 5.8. HCTO. Wilson modification of SOMI.

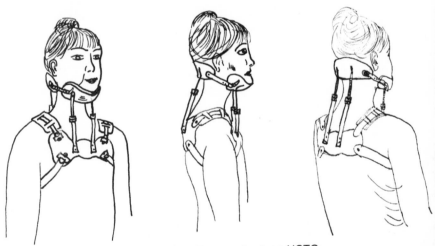

Fig. 5.9. HCTO. Four-poster type HCTO.

to 13% of normal motion, as compared with 28% for the SOMI. Although the SOMI restricts flexion better in the upper and middle cervical region, the HCTO four-poster type is more effective in controlling extension, and it allows only 18% of normal cervical rotation. Both the SOMI and the four-poster HCTO were not good inhibitors of lateral bending.

Guilford type of HCTO (Fig. 5.10) is unique in that the chin piece has bilateral posterior metal projections which lock into channels of the occipital piece. This provides a rigid ring head support. The studies of Hartman *et al.* (11) showed that the Guilford type of two-poster HCTO restricts all motion by 90 to 95%. This device is superior in its ability to immobilize the head and neck when compared to the soft cervical collar, the rigid plastic Thomas type of collar, the four-poster HCO, and the long two-poster HCTLO (see below).

Rigid APRO (anterior-posterior-rotational-orthosis) *and HCTO* (Fig. 5.11) appear to be a combination of the SOMI chest plate and the four-poster superstructure with the addition of a posterior SOMI chest plate. The effect of this new orthosis needs more quantitative comparative study and documentation in the literature.

VI. Head Cervical Thoracic Lumbar Orthoses (HCTLO)

These include the *Florida two-poster type cervical brace*, the *cervical attachment for the Jewett brace*, and the *Dennison-Boldrey supportive cervical immobilizer.*

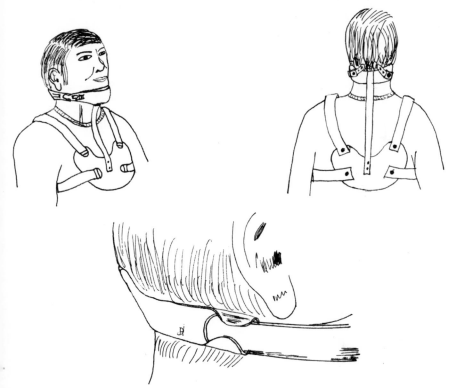

Fig. 5.10. HCTO. Guilford type of HCTO.

The Florida two-poster cervical HCTLO (Fig. 5.12) gives the advantages of good trunk stabilization, but the occipital and mandibular portions are not rigidly connected, using only leather straps. The study of Hartman *et al.* (11) reported restriction of normal cervical motion: flexion and extension 90 to 95%, lateral bending 90%, and rotation 90% of normal. Hartman felt that some rotation occurs as the chin slides on the chin piece and found the Florida two-poster cervical HCTLO less effective in restricting cervical motion when compared to the Guilford two-poster HCTO (11).

Cervical attachment to the Jewett back brace (Fig. 5.13) is an orthosis that attempts to gain stability through increasing the area of attachment. The ease of orthotic application, which has been characteristic of the Jewett,

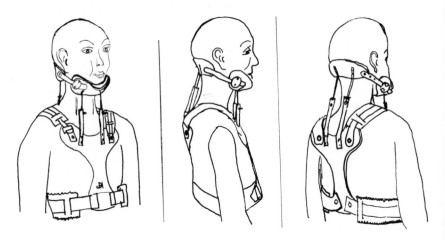

Fig. 5.11. HCTO. Rigid APRO HCTO.

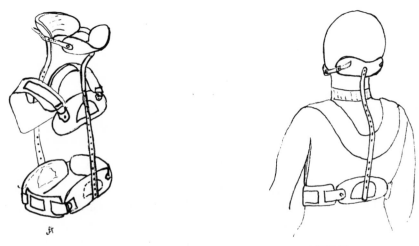

Fig. 5.12. HCTLO. Two-poster, Florida-type HCTLO.

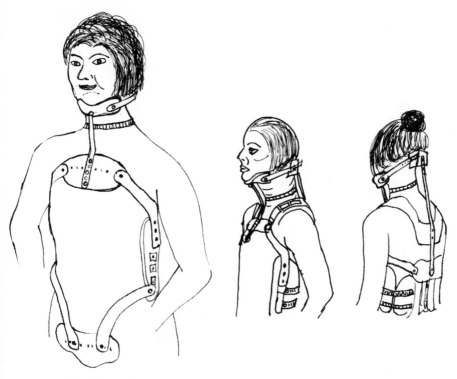

Fig. 5.13. HCTLO. Cervical attachment to Jewett back orthosis.

is diminished with the attachment of the posterior occipital structure. There needs to be more published data as to the effectiveness of this new adaption of the Jewett back brace.

Boldrey supportive cervical immobilizer (Fig. 5.14) was first reported by Boldrey in 1945 (2) as a different way of immobilizing the head to avoid mandibular pad problems. "The usual cast or splint is built up beneath or around the chin to such a degree that eating is severely interfered with; if the jaw is permitted movement, then there is likewise movement of the cervical spine." The Boldrey cervical immobilizer is constructed with an aluminum cup, molded to the occipital-and-suboccipital region, which projects laterally and anteriorly partially encircling the ear. This cup is attached to a steel upright bar which is attached caudally to a padded thoracic plate and lumbar band. The supra-auricular portion of the head cup is attached to a broad webbing strap that encircles the frontal area of the skull to hold the head firmly in the cup and decrease flexion-extension motion. The infra-auricular projection of the head cup has a ball-and-socket joint which allows the attachment of a contoured aluminum prong that is fitted to the maxilla and infrazygomatic region to the nasolabial fold. This prevents rotation and

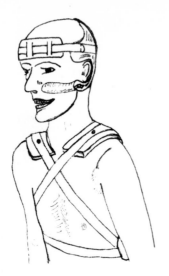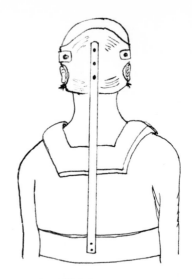

Fig. 5.14. HCTLO. Boldrey type of HCTLO.

further impedes flexion and extension. This concept of cervical immobilization needs further comparative quantitation.

VII. Head Cervical Thoracic Lumbar Sacral Orthoses (HCTLSO)

Stryker cervical immobilizer HCTLSO was designed to fit the following requirements according to Kerr (16) (Fig. 5.15):

1. Provide secure immobilization with traction of the cervical spine up to 30 pounds applied by skeletal tongs or head halter.
2. Enable patient transportation with ease and safety.
3. Permit cervical spine x-ray examination in the brace without interference in either anteroposterior (AP) or lateral projections.
4. Permit lumbar puncture and myelogram without difficulty.
5. Adjust to any adult body shape and to older children.
6. Apply and remove with ease (lightweight and reasonably comfortable).

Bony Contact Cervical Orthoses

There are two major categories: *halo and tong type* (Fig. 5.16).

The Halo Orthosis

The *halo* is a means of skeletal skull fixation which gives a three-dimensional control method applying forces through the head and neck. It was introduced in the early 1960's and has become very popular. The advantages of the halo skeletal traction are:

A. Rigid fixation with improved rate of fracture union.

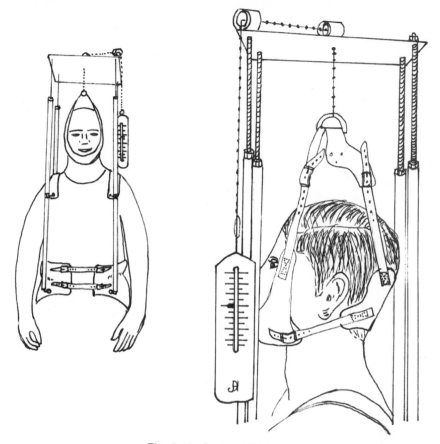

Fig. 5.15. Stryker HCTLSO.

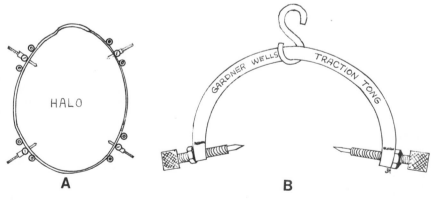

Fig. 5.16. Bony contact CO. *A*, halo; *B*, Gardner Wells tongs.

B. Increased force application without the problems of skin necrosis.
C. Close tolerance, three-dimensional rigid adjustment.
D. Versatile countertraction in fixation which can allow early mobility from the bed.

The five most common types of cervical bony contact orthoses are: *halo bed, SCTO halo vest, SCTLO halo body jacket, SCTLPO halo hoop,* and *halo femoral pin traction.*

The disadvantages of the halo skeletal fixation are:

A. Special technical skills required in application and adjustment. There is a smaller margin for error due to the increased forces and rigid fixation.
B. Prolonged usage slows down the rehabilitation process by prohibiting the use of the head and neck and trunk movements which are essential for balance and some activities-of-daily-living (ADL) skills.
C. Local pin site infection, slippage, and central migration of the pin necessitates close observation and maintenance.
D. Soft tissue necrosis under the vest or cast countertraction setup.
E. Loss of alignment, with some neurological root loss when reduction is lost in transferring the bed countertraction to a jacket or vest countertraction according to the method of Kelly (15).

Stauffer (21) has provided a general table for usage of the halo apparatus and its removal. "Eight weeks of immobilization in the reduced position allows sufficient callous bone healing and fibrous ankylosing to remove the halo apparatus and replace it with a Dennison cervical type of brace for an additional 4 to 6 weeks. During this period the patient may safely be treated with a soft collar while he is recovering in bed, but should also use the Dennison brace when he is in the upright position ambulating or in the wheelchair" (20).

Tong or Caliper Type (Gardiner Wells or Crutchfield) Used with an Orthosis

Tongs are traditionally used with the frame or bed type of traction, but they have been used in conjunction with a body jacket or a pelvic girdle countertraction unit. The traction through a cervical head halter is limited due to the ischemic skin necrosis process.

Use of Halos or Tongs. We must individualize the orthotic needs for each patient but avoid the pitfalls of prolonged halo traction stabilization. Using only radiographic evidence of calcification as the only indication of when to remove the halo traction orthosis can be too conservative. In the rehabilitation process, the quadriplegic patient needs mobility of his trunk, head, and neck to do and learn his activities-of-daily-living skills (ADL). The time following injury is a critical psychological period of adjustment and reorganization. It is important to speed up the rehabilitation process so that the patient can have goal attainment and see progress, not just be left in a halo traction unit until there is a dense bony callus formation.

Summary

The goal of this chapter has been to review the cervical anatomy and function, categorize cervical orthoses, and compare their relative effectiveness in limiting motion.

The majority of studies reported on in this chapter were done on normal subjects and not on patients with disease or unstable cervical spines. Therefore, the findings should be applied with caution and clinical judgment to each individual patient.

REFERENCES

1. BERGER, N., AND LUSSKIN, R. Orthotic components and systems, cervical orthoses. In *Atlas of Orthotics*, pp. 361–363. C. V. Mosby Co., St. Louis, 1975.
2. BOLDREY, E. Supportive immobilization of the cervical spine. *Surg. Gynecol. Obstet., 80:* 107–108, 1945.
3. CAILLIET, R. *Neck and Arm Pain.* F. A. Davis Co., Philadelphia, 1964.
4. COLACHIS, S. C., JR., AND STROHM, B. R. Radiographic studies of cervical spine motion in normal subjects: flexion and hyperextension. *Arch. Phys. Med. Rehabil., 46:* 753–760, 1965.
5. COLACHIS, S. C., JR., STROHM, B. R., AND GANTER, E. L. Cervical spine motion in normal women: radiographic study of effect of cervical collars. *Arch. Phys. Med. Rehabil., 54:* 161–169, 1973.
6. CRABBE, W. Bracing the neck. In *Orthotics Etcetera*, edited by Sidney Licht, ed. 2, pp. 148–151. Elizabeth Licht, New Haven, 1966.
7. DEWALD, R. L. Halo traction systems. In *Atlas of Orthotics*, chap. 24, pp. 407–417. C. V. Mosby Co., St. Louis, 1975.
8. FISHER, S. V. Proper fitting of cervical orthoses. *Arch. Phys. Med. Rehabil., 59:* 505–507, 1978.
9. FISHER, S. V., BOWAR, J. F., AWARD, E. A., AND GULLICKSON, G., JR. Cervical Orthoses effect on cervical spine motion: roentgenographic and goniometric method of study. *Arch. Phys. Med. Rehabil., 58:* 109–115, 1977.
10. HARRIS, E. E. A new orthotics terminology. *Orthotics Prosthet., 27 (2):* 6–19, 1973.
11. HARTMAN, J. T., PALUMBO, F., AND HILL, B. J. Cineradiography of braced normal cervical spine: comparative study of five commonly used cervical orthoses. *Clin. Orthop., 109:* 97–102, 1975.
12. JACKSON, R. *The Cervical Syndrome*, ed. 3. Charles C Thomas, Springfield, Ill., 1966.
13. JOHNSON, R. M., HART, D. L., SIMMONS, E. F., RAMSBY, G. R., AND SOUTHWICK, W. O. Cervical orthoses: a study comparing their effectiveness in restricting cervical motion in normal subjects. *J. Bone Joint Surg., 59:* 332–339, 1977.
14. JONES, M. D. Cineradiographic studies of collar immobilized cervical spine. *J. Neurosurg., 17:* 633–637, 1960.
15. KELLY, E. G. Loss of Reduction of Fracture Dislocation of the Cervical Spine after Placement in Halo Body Jacket for Immobilization. *Abstract from ASIA Meeting,* University of Pittsburgh, Pittsburgh, Pa., 1979.
16. KERR, F. W. L. A brace for the management of fracture dislocation of the cervical spine: traction, immobilization, and myelography. *J. Neurosurg. 30:* 97–101, 1969.
17. KOTTKE, F. J., AND MUNDALE, M. O. Range of mobility of cervical spine. *Arch. Phys. Med. Rehabil., 40:* 379–382, 1959.
18. LARSON, D. L. *The Prevention and Correction of Burn Scar Contracture and Hypertrophy.*

Schriners Burns Publication. Institute of the University of Texas Medical Branch, Galveston, Texas.

19. LUND, S., DRALLE, A., AND LEHMANN, J. Orthotic management of high thoracic, low cervical fractures. *Orthotics Prosthet., 32:* 11–14, 1978.

20. SHERK, H. H. Atlantoaxial instability and acquired basilar invagination in rheumatoid arthritis. *Orthop. Clin. North Am., 4:* 1978.

21. STAUFFER, E. S. Orthotics for spinal cord injuries. *Clin. Orthop. Related Res., 102:* 1974.

22. STEINDLER, A. *Kinesiology of the Human Body.* Charles C Thomas, Springfield, Ill., 1955.

23. TAYLOR, A. N. An inflatable neck support. *Clin. Orthop., 81:* 87, 1971.

24. WILSON, C. L. A new non-invasive halo orthosis for immobilization of the cervical spine. *Orthotics Prosthet., 32:* 16–19, 1978.

6

Spinal Orthotics for Pain and Instability

DONALD B. LUCAS, M.D.

Nicolas Andry (1658–1742), who is credited with originating the word "orthopédie" from the Greek *orthos* (straight) and *paidos* (child), described corsets that assisted in spinal support in his treatise published in 1741. Spinal braces have been in abundant use for the past 200 years and are prescribed for a variety of disorders of the trunk. In all probability, spinal bracing predated Andry and is, in one form or another, nearly as old as civilization.

Lorenz Heister (1683–1758) is often given credit for the introduction of the spinal brace which was called the "iron cross." This rather crude apparatus consisted of a single posterior upright with a crossbar at the level of the shoulders. A simple ring served for support of the head, and straps were attached to the shoulders; an abdominal strap held the appliance to the lower portion of the trunk. A similar type of apparatus was designed by Levacher about 1764. The vertical posterior bar was extended over the head to form a curved arc to which a snugly fitting cap that gripped the head was attached. This design was later altered slightly and became known as the "jury-mast."

Since the introduction of spinal braces, new ones have periodically made their appearance, and older versions have been modified so that there now exists a host of appliances of similar design but with different names in different regions of the country. Some modifications have been accomplished to improve the fit and some to take advantage of new materials. Most, however, have stemmed from the designer's attempt to improve the treatment or control of disorders as concepts of their pathomechanics have changed. These concepts are based on contemporary understanding of normal functional anatomy and spinal mechanics, as well as of pain mechanisms, but unfortunately our knowledge is always incomplete, and spinal appliances have of necessity developed for the most part on an empirical basis.

The objectives of spinal orthotics are (a) control of pain, (b) protection from further injury, (c) assistance for muscle weakness, and (d) prevention and correction of deformity. Bracing for a given patient usually includes more than one objective since the factors are usually interrelated. Other considerations in the application of a brace are its effect on gait, energy expenditure required during walking, and its acceptability to the patient.

Spinal appliances are divided into two groups: (a) corrective and (b) supportive or immobilizing. They may be considered according to the region of the body as trochanteric, sacroiliac, lumbosacral, thoracolumbar, and cervical. In general, they are classified as flexible, semirigid, and rigid. Nearly all are constructed of a combination of cloth, leather, metal, plastic, and rubber. They include belts, corsets, braces, jackets, and plaster casts.

Before considering individual appliances, it would be helpful to review some of the pertinent anatomy of the spine and trunk, as well as the biomechanics and function of the spine and the mechanisms of pain in this region. For review of the embryology and gross anatomy of the spine, the previous edition of *Orthotics Etcetera* may be consulted, and the reference section contains a number of excellent reviews (6, 7, 11, 16, 17, 31, 38, 41, 51, 59, 61, 64, 65, 69, 72, 74).

Biomechanics of the Spine

The spinal column serves as a sustaining rod for the maintenance of an upright position of the body and as such is subjected to innumerable forces of different types, for example, compression, shearing, tension, bending, and twisting (Fig. 6.1, *A–E*). The column possesses an intrinsic as well as an extrinsic stability. The former is due to its disc and ligamentous support while the latter is related to the muscle support. The intrinsic stability is the result of the pressure within the discs, which tends to push the vertebral bodies apart (53, 63), and the resistance provided by the ligaments, which

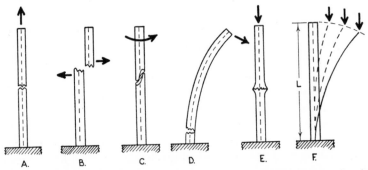

Fig. 6.1. Schematic drawing of elastic rods to show failure as a result of various forces. *A*, distraction; *B*, shear; *C*, twisting; *D*, bending; *E*, compression; *F*, critical load (a condition in which the rod buckles without permanent deformation as a result of a specific load, P_{cr}, applied at the top).

tends to force the bodies together. It has been shown that the ligamentous spine (the spine devoid of musculature) may be considered to be a modified elastic rod, and as such obeys the physical laws which apply to elastic rods (Fig. 6.1F) (72). It has been shown further that the critical load value (P_{cr} in Fig. 6.1) for the ligamentous spine, which is fixed at the base and free at the top, is approximately 4.5 pounds (2.0 kg). At that load, the upright spine buckles. It is apparent that the extrinsic support provided by the trunk musculature is responsible for the ability of the spinal column to withstand the great loads to which it is subjected.

The spine, which is composed of alternating rigid and elastic elements, possesses a considerable degree of flexibility that is primarily due to the intervertebral discs. The amount of flexibility depends on the material characteristics, size, and shape of the disc, but also on the restraint offered by the intervertebral ligaments. It can be said that the flexibility between two vertebrae varies directly with the square of the vertical height of the disc and indirectly with the square of the horizontal diameter of that body. Because of the proportionally greater height of the lumbar disc, the range of intervertebral motion is somewhat greater in the lumbar region, but because of the greater horizontal diameter the flexibility is less than in the thoracic region.

The discs are of prime importance for the flexibility and motion of the spinal column. Normally, they may be considered to act as universal joints, permitting motion in four directions between vertebral bodies: (1) translational motion in the long axis of the spine occurring because of compressibility of the disc, (2) rotatory motion about a perpendicular axis, (3) forward-backward bending, and (4) lateral bending.

The centers of the axes of motion pass close to or within the nucleus pulposus, so that for most practical purposes the nucleus may be considered the center of motion. Experimentally, however, it has been found that the axis of motion changes its position somewhat with changes in the arc of motion. For example, during full extension of the spine the axis passes through the disc immediately behind the nucleus; during full flexion it passes immediately in front of the nucleus. This change of position is progressive throughout movement and is compatible with a hypothesis that the vertebral bodies normally rock over the nucleus (32, 50).

The nucleus pulposus is well suited for this function. Because of its high water content and plastic nature, it functions according to the laws of hydrodynamics (9, 27, 35, 37, 55). The tension of the elastic anulus fibrosus and of the intervertebral ligaments keeps the nucleus under pressure even when the disc is not bearing weight. Forces are transmitted across the disc partly by the nucleus and partly by the anulus. Because of the semiliquid center of the disc, these transmitted forces are uniformly distributed to the intervertebral surfaces of the bodies of the vertebrae in a wide range of movement. Only when the angulation is sufficient to displace all the liquid medium from one portion of the central "cavity" and when apposition of the vertebrae occurs does the distribution become unequal.

The range of motion between adjacent vertebrae is guided and controlled by both the ligamentous structures and the posterior articulations.

In the thoracic region, the articulations form part of the surface of a cone and are aligned close to the coronal plane. This arrangement allows for flexion and axial rotation, but extension is limited.

In the lumbar region, the articulations are aligned closer to the parasagittal plane. The facets have cylindrical surfaces, with the upper surface concave and the lower convex. This arrangement allows for flexion, extension, and lateral motion. There is only slight axial rotation in the lumbar part of the spine, except at the lumbosacral level, where the facets tend more toward the coronal plane (Fig. 6.2).

The combined intrinsic and extrinsic support of the spinal column enables it to withstand the great forces to which it may be subjected. At the same time, the great number of articulations and interposed intervertebral discs give the column considerable mobility and allow its action as a modified elastic rod. A number of biomechanical experiments have been carried out to determine the strengths of the discs and vertebral bodies. By placing two vertebral bodies with their intervening discs in a material-testing compression machine or by subjecting them to sudden dynamic forces, considerable information has been obtained.

Compression tests have shown that the disc behaves as an elastic body only up to a maximum total pressure of 1,400 pounds (636 kg) [this was in specimens from young adults—in specimens from older persons, the elastic limit was approximately 350 pounds (160 kg) (8, 28)]. Beyond this amount, the disc is rapidly deformed by very little additional pressure. These tests

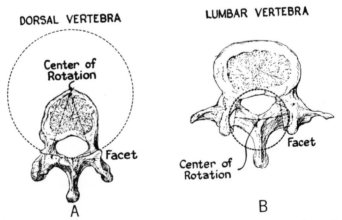

Fig. 6.2. Drawings to show determination of center of rotation of vertebrae based on alignment of facets. *A*, thoracic; *B*, lumbar.

have also shown that the vertebral body possesses certain elastic qualities similar to those of the disc (20).

Compression forces have been imposed up to the point of failure of a particular segment of the spine being studied (12, 14, 57, 62). This failure is characterized by an audible crack followed by leakage of sanguineous fluid from one of the vertebrae (usually the superior), through the vascular foramen, and, occasionally, at some point along the attachment of the peripheral fibers of the anulus to the vertebral bodies. The evidence of failure is often difficult to visualize either upon gross examination or roentgenographically. It may consist of compression of a few spicules of bone, cracks in the end-plate or, sometimes, collapse of the plate. It has been shown that this failure occurs in specimens from young persons at a compressive load of 1,000 to 1,300 pounds (454 to 590 kg). When specimens from older persons were studied, the critical load was much less, even as little as 300 pounds (136 kg).

It is noteworthy that when the anulus is intact, its elastic limits cannot be exceeded without vertebral fracture. The end-plate is most susceptible to fracture as a result of the forces exerted on the spine, and this structure generally gives way first. It may fracture centrally or peripherally, or a fissure may appear across the entire plate. The central type of fracture is most apt to occur when the disc is normal and when the resistance of the vertebral body is greater than the pressure generated in the nucleus. This type of end-plate failure would explain the origin of the so-called Schmorl's nodes in young persons. The other two types of end-plate fracture occur when various degrees of disc degeneration are present, which leads to an abnormal distribution of forces across the disc space.

The vertebral body itself is the next most susceptible portion of the segment under study and usually collapses before herniation of the nucleus occurs through the anulus (60). Even when well-developed defects of the anulus are present, end-plate or vertebral fractures are more likely to occur than disc herniation. Furthermore, in experiments with use of discography and x-rays of the specimen, it has been possible to demonstrate that new fissures developed in the anulus without disc herniation, even though the forces applied were always sufficient to fracture the vertebra (49). It has also been shown experimentally in dogs that a single violent trauma will cause fracture of the vertebra more often than disc herniation (24, 25, 44). This would agree well with the opinion that trauma *per se* seldom causes disc herniation. Inorganic as well as organic materials generally are able to withstand stresses during a short period more readily than stresses exerted for longer periods of time. It has been shown that an approximately equal number of end-plate fractures occurred when a static force of 620 kilograms was exerted, as when dynamic stresses of 1,200 kilograms were applied.

The question often arises as to how the lumbar vertebrae and discs are able to withstand the forces to which they are apparently subjected during normal activities. It can be readily shown from a static diagram that when an individual bends forward to lift a heavy weight, a large axial force is transmitted along the spine. This force results from the contraction of the erector spinae muscles acting through a very short lever arm. The ratio of the proximal to the distal lever arm is approximately 10 to 1. This means that if a weight of 200 pounds (91 kg) is lifted, an axial force of 2,000 pounds (910 kg) is transmitted along the vertebral bodies to the lumbosacral joint (Fig. 6.3) (6, 52).

One possible explanation for the ability of the spine to withstand such forces is to consider the spine as a segmental elastic column supported by the paraspinal muscles and attached to the sides of and within two chambers, the abdominal and thoracic cavities, which are separated by the diaphragm. The first cavity is filled with a combination of solids and liquid, while the second is filled largely with air. The action of the trunk musculature converts these chambers into rigid-walled cylinders of air and semisolids capable of transmitting forces generated in loading the spine and thereby relieving the spine itself (5).

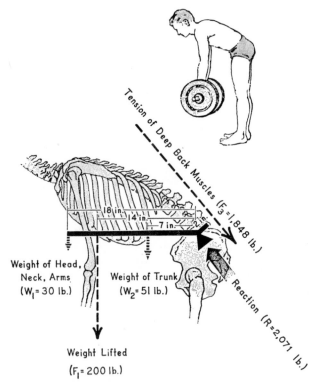

Fig. 6.3. Calculated static forces on lower lumbar part of spine when a 200-pound weight is lifted. [Reproduced with permission from: J. M. Morris *et al.* (52)].

This hypothesis was studied by Morris *et al.* (52), who were able to show that during the act of lifting, the action of the intercostal muscles and the muscles of the shoulder girdle rendered the thoracic cage quite rigid. An increase in intrathoracic pressure resulted, converting the thoracic cage and the spine into a solid sturdy unit capable of transmitting large forces. By contraction of the diaphragm, which is attached to the lower margin of the thorax and overlaps the abdominal viscera and the muscles of the abdominal wall (especially the transversus abdominis), the abdominal contents were compressed into a semirigid mass, thereby making the abdominal cavity a semirigid cylinder. The force of weights lifted by the arms is thus transmitted to the spinal column by the muscles of the shoulder girdle, principally the trapezius, and then on to the abdominal cylinder and the pelvis, partly through the spinal column and partly through the rigid rib cage and abdomen. The larger the weight lifted, the greater the activity of the trunk and chest and abdominal musculature was found to be. Also, a concomitant increase in intracavitary pressures resulted. The calculated force on the lumbosacral disc during the lifting of any load was found to be 30% less because of the cavitary pressures, and the load on the lower thoracic portion of the spine was about 50% less than it would have been without support by the trunk. Thus, when 200 pounds (91 kg) is lifted, instead of approximately 2,000 pounds (910 kg) of force being transmitted along the spine, only about 1,500 pounds (681 kg) is actually transmitted (Fig. 6.4). It is interesting to note that when a tight corset was worn about the abdomen, an increase in the intra-abdominal and intrathoracic pressures resulted from tightening of the corset. At the same time, during the act of lifting there was a decrease in the activities of the thoracic and abdominal muscles, indicating that the effect of the muscles can be replaced by an external pressure appliance.

In a further study by Nachemson and Morris (56), intradiscal pressures were measured *in vivo*. A needle with a pressure-sensitive polyethylene membrane at its tip was inserted into the disc under study. Intradiscal pressures of 10 to 15 kilograms/sq cm were found in normal discs with subjects in the sitting position. There was approximately 30% less pressure during standing and about 50% less in the reclining position. From this it can be seen that the lower lumbar discs of adults have to support total loads of as much as 100 to 175 kilograms when the subjects are seated. For the standing position, total loads of between 90 and 120 kilograms were calculated from the pressure values obtained. When an inflated corset was worn during the experiment, the pressure in the examined discs decreased by about 25%. This last experiment demonstrates quite well how an increase of the intrathoracic and intra-abdominal pressures decreases the superincumbent load on the disc, an important consideration in view of the fact that the behavior of the spine in the living subject depends on the integrity of the intervertebral disc.

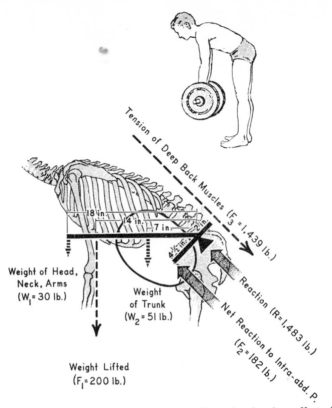

Fig. 6.4. Same as in Fig. 6.3, with consideration of reduction effected by intra-abdominal pressure. [Reproduced with permission from: J. M. Morris *et al.* (52)].

Pain Mechanisms

Disc degeneration is no doubt the basic factor in the production of pain in the majority of patients with low back pain problems. Friberg, in studying this problem roentgenographically, noted: (1) instability, or displacement, of the upper vertebra on the lower; (2) disc narrowing; and (3) osteophytes in one-half of all adults examined for complaints of back pain (18, 19).

Changes in the disc due to degeneration begin at about 20 years of age and increase progressively throughout life (12, 13, 45, 57). Initially, progressive fibrosis is observed in association with increasing cellular degeneration, central fissuring, and cavitation, as well as focal deposition of calcium salts. The cartilage plates become thinner, and the anulus shows swelling of the layers, with areas of mucinous degeneration between them which stain dark blue with hematoxylin. These areas give rise to concentric fissures which enlarge and coalesce increasingly with age. The fibrous structure becomes increasingly homogenized or hyalinized and may become fragmented. Radial fissures occur, especially posteriorly on the lower lumbar discs. These fissures begin centrally and may extend through the anulus, causing bulging; they disturb the function of the disc more than the other regressive changes. Fibrous tissue with vascularization may be seen at the borders of the anulus after trauma. Areas of brown pigmentation may be seen in the region of fissure, presumably from hemosiderin deposits. In the nucleus, the water content decreases with age. In the newborn it is 90%, whereas in persons in their 70's it is only 75%.

In attempting to explain the relatively early degeneration of the disc, several factors must be taken into account. The pertinent degenerative changes in the nucleus and anulus are similar to the early changes seen in many other mesenchymal tissues, for example, articular cartilage, tendons, and loose connective tissue (6, 33, 70). There is no conclusive evidence that heavy physical labor is the direct cause of disc change since nearly the same incidence of disc degeneration is seen in sedentary workers as in heavy laborers. However, if it is considered that these partly physiological changes not only become more frequent as age advances but are also found more often in the lower lumbar discs than in any other, the assumption cannot be avoided that mechanical forces in some way play a part in degeneration of the disc and the decreased resistance of the anulus to rupture.

The effect of mechanical stresses has been pointed out by Brown and his group, who demonstrated that both anulus and nucleus of the disc are better able to withstand compressive or single dynamic forces than the end-plate or the adjacent vertebra (8). On the other hand, in a fatigue test in which a disc and adjacent vertebrae were studied, a horizontal tear occurred through the anulus after only 1,000 cycles of flexion and extension when a 15-pound load was applied at 1,100 cycles per minute.

Pressure is also a factor to be considered since the radial fissures are first seen and are most pronounced in the portion of the disc on the concave side of the spinal curve, i.e., posteriorly in the lumbar region and anteriorly in the thoracic region. It is also worth noting that when Lindblom (47) fixed rats' tails in a position in which they were bent at an acute angle, he induced radial ruptures of the anulus in the portion of the disc along the concave surface.

There is some evidence that hereditary factors may play a part. It is a common observation that in dogs of the chondrodystrophy type (dachshund, Pekingese, and French bull), disc degeneration is much more pronounced than in dogs of other breeds (30).

When some of the more basic elements of disc degeneration are more closely studied and the sequence of events is outlined, the relationship between lumbosacral pain and disc degeneration becomes more apparent. While regressive changes begin in the nucleus, no ruptures occur in the anulus unless the nucleus shows advanced structural changes. The nucleus is described as a three-dimensional lattice gel system composed of interlacing collagen fibers coated by the chondroitin sulfuric acid/protein complex which gives the nucleus its marked hydrophilia. The efficient functioning of the disc depends largely on the elasticity of the nucleus, which is in turn related to its water-binding capacity (68). There are two possible physico-chemical bases for this water retention: (1) osmosis; or (2) imbibition pressure exerted by the protein/polysaccharide gel. That osmosis is relatively unimportant is shown by the fact that the water content of the nucleus remains almost the same when it is placed in liquids of different tonicity. Therefore, it is virtually certain that the hydration of the nucleus is due to the imbibition pressure of the gel (10). It is interesting to note that a gel with a saturation of 1% will have an imbibition pressure of 5,000 atmospheres (that is, this amount of force is necessary to separate the water in the solid phase). This characteristic of gels provides a powerful and adaptable force to meet the functional needs of the disc.

In the process of disc degeneration, the amount of collagen within the nucleus increases in relation to the amount of mucopolysaccharide; the collagen protein occupies a larger number of polar groups of the polysaccharide in the ground substance, and a smaller number will therefore be available for water binding. The effects of this are first to decrease the strength of water binding within the nucleus and later to decrease the actual amount of water. Studies by Hendry (27) have shown that the degenerated nucleus is markedly less hydrophilic than the normal nucleus. When the material of the degenerated nucleus is subjected even to low pressures, it will lose much more water than normally.

The importance of this is seen when the effects are considered. Normally, the stress through the vertebral bodies can be regarded as being resolved into two components: (1) a force balanced by the imbibition pressure of the nucleus and wholly contributed by the nucleus itself, and (2) a remaining force transmitted by the anulus. Hirsch (28, 29) has reported that if the nucleus loses part of its ability to produce an even distribution of pressure, the anulus is not capable of meeting even physiologic demands upon it. Such a reduction of the imbibition pressure of the nucleus has three effects. First, a greater proportion of the total strain is borne by the anulus. This aspect has also been studied by Nachemson (53), who calculated, by means of measuring intradiscal pressures in normal and degenerated discs in cadaver spines, that if the nucleus is degenerated, the stress on the anulus is four times as great as in the normal disc. He has also calculated that the weight-bearing capacity of the normal disc is 50% greater than that of the degenerated disc. Second, the characteristic of the stress on the anulus may change from alternating tension and compression to unrelieved compression. The collagen fibers of the anulus are adapted to withstand tensile forces, but they degenerate when subjected to compression. Third, under certain conditions of prolonged relaxation, the nucleus will imbibe fluid, only to be unable to retain it when stress is reapplied. This will cause a sudden loss of fluid and a rapid redistribution of hydrostatic pressure, which cannot be dissipated rapidly through the avascular disc. This forceful expulsion of fluid from the nucleus into existing small fissures and cracks within the anulus tends to enlarge the fissures and separate the layers of the anulus. When it is recalled that the elastic properties of the anulus depend on the sheets of fibers oriented perpendicularly to each other, it is reasonable to assume that the physical separation of these sheets would allow for increased motion of one upon the other and possibly allow more compression and bulging of the anulus. This in turn would permit increased motion of one vertebra on another and lead to the clinical condition of instability.

As intervertebral disc degeneration progresses, fibrosis of the nucleus and fibrous proliferation in the anulus (partially due to ingrowth of granulation tissue through fissures) transforms the disc space into a fibrous ankylosis between the two vertebrae. At this time, which is usually 5 to 10 years after the onset of degeneration, there is little danger of nuclear herniation. Pain, if it has been present, usually subsides and often largely disappears (30). This concept agrees with the clinical observation that while disc degeneration proceeds on into old age, the peak incidence of disc herniation and acutely painful back episodes occurs in the 30- to 50-year age group.

Whether or not mechanical derangement of the disc occurs in a particular patient presumably depends on the age and activity of the patient at the time of degeneration, on the speed and extent of collagen deposition in the nucleus, on the relation of anular damage and fibrosis to hydrostatic effects, and perhaps on unknown biochemical factors.

It may be that the difference between normal aging and that seen in degenerative disc disease lies in the relative speeds of the mucopolysaccharide loss and collagen deposition. In normal aging it is presumed that a slow orderly mucopolysaccharide loss with simultaneous collagen replacement would allow progressive physiologic dehydration to occur without damage to the anulus and without the appearance of hydrostatic effects characteristic of degenerative disc disorders.

While it is recognized that disc degeneration and low back pain are closely related, the exact pain mechanism is not clearly understood.

It has been shown that degeneration of the disc leads to an alteration in the intrinsic stability of the spine which, as described above, results from the tension of the binding ligaments opposed by the turgor, or imbibition pressure, of the nucleus. With the combination of loss of turgor (desiccation) of the nucleus and the fissuring, separation of the layers, and settling of the anulus, the tension of the spinal ligaments is markedly decreased. These factors give rise to an abnormal amount of movement between contiguous vertebrae (46). In extension the upper vertebra is displaced posteriorly, and in flexion it may be displaced anteriorly. Instability is said to exist when the amount of motion exceeds the normal limit of 3 millimeters of displacement in either direction. This condition is most frequently seen at the L-4/L-5 disc (next most frequently at the L-5/S-1 disc) and is the first sign of disc degeneration which is detectable roentgenologically. With increasing degeneration, the disc space is narrowed, and bulging of the anulus elevates the periosteum at the edges of the vertebral body. Beneath this elevated periosteum, new bone forms, *i.e.,* osteophytes, or spurs. This excessive mobility of the unstable spine may cause pain by the undue stress placed upon the surrounding structures, especially the ligaments and the anulus.

Narrowing of the disc tends to cause posterior displacement of the center of motion of the involved segments. In severe degeneration, the axes of motion may even pass through the posterior articulations. The abnormal motion thus imposed on these posterior facet joints leads to degenerative changes of various degrees (23), *e.g.,* fibrillation and pitting of the cartilage, fibrosis, and fractures of the articular surfaces. These changes may result in bony impingement of an articular process against the laminae of adjacent vertebrae, or even subluxation of one process on another. Pain may be associated with motion within the degenerated facet articulations, with capsular stretching, with bony impingement, or, occasionally, with entrapment and squeezing of redundant synovia between the articular surfaces. The last condition is believed to be the basis (at least in some cases) for the so-called "catch" in the back.

Another mechanism by which pain is produced is suggested by Hirsch and Schajowicz (29, 34). They were able to reproduce back pain in patients by injecting saline into the degenerated disc. If procaine was used, pain did not occur. They believe that the pain was due to distention of the anulus, causing tension in the posterior ligament at its junction with the anulus. They have also suggested that pain may arise from irritation of the vascular granulation tissue which grows into anular fissures from the periphery. In another experiment, they injected a hypertonic solution of saline (11%) into lumbar synovial joints. The severe, fairly localized pain which immediately resulted gradually spread to the sacroiliac, gluteal, and trochanteric regions. When the same solution was injected into the fourth and fifth discs, an extremely severe deep pain occurred, identical to a "lumbago." The patients could not locate the site, and the deep ache was felt across the low back. Less severe, fairly localized pain also resulted from injections into the ligamentum flavum, interspinous and supraspinous ligaments, and dorsal fascia.

In all these conditions, the existing pain is usually of the deep type and may be associated with visceral symptoms. Radiation may occur across the back or down the thigh. This radiation does not correspond with the classic dermatome or with the distribution of sensory nerves in the region, but follows a more or less constant reproducible sclerotomic pattern characteristic of "deep pain," as described by both Kellgren and Feinstein and coworkers (15, 41, 42).

Finally, low back pain with or without sciatica may arise from irritation of the spinal nerves in the intervertebral foramen. Such irritation occurs most commonly in the lower two lumbar and the first sacral nerves. Presumably, it may be caused by herniated nuclear material, posterior anulus bulge, osteophytes, and/or hypertrophic ligamentum flavum (3, 4, 21, 26, 36, 39, 43, 48, 59).

The cause of sciatic pain or low back pain in cases of nerve root compression is difficult to elucidate. Certainly, compression alone is not the answer. When pressure is exerted on a nerve, the first fibers to be blocked are the large myelinated fibers that transmit touch and proprioception, as well as the motor impulses. This block occurs, for example, when the leg "goes to sleep" as a result of pressure on the sciatic nerve during sitting. The pain fibers (especially the smaller amyelinated fibers that transmit deep pain) are affected later.

In sciatica, however, pain is one of the first symptoms. Some mechanism must therefore be assumed to lower the threshold of pain fibers. Perhaps the precipitating factors are the edema and inflammation of the nerve root found in conditions of intermittent compression and irritation associated with intermittent disc bulging. Nerve stretching and ischemia may play a role in the cause of pain.

In addition to the pain resulting from the degenerative disc process, back pain is frequently associated with neoplasm, acute trauma, inflammatory processes, osteoporosis, and metabolic bone disorders. The pain mechanisms in these instances do not differ from those operating in other parts of the body afflicted with these disorders. Stress of any kind will aggravate the pain, and bracing is usually employed to restrict motion and relieve superincumbent weight.

An additional condition associated with pain is faulty posture (40). This may be superimposed upon an already existing painful condition, with resulting aggravation of the pre-existing condition, or it may be a primary source of pain. In the latter case, the pain is probably secondary to stretching of the ligaments. Many patients seem to tolerate faulty posture extremely well until a degenerative disc process arises in conjunction with it, when the added stress usually gives rise to back pain.

In spite of the foregoing discussion, Nachemson (54) has recently reviewed what is known about the lumbar disc and concludes that the answer to how it causes back pain still is not clear. There remain many cases of chronic low back pain where no pathological, mechanical, or other presumed physical derangement in the area can explain the symptoms. These cases, for want of better terminology, may be said to suffer from "tension myositis"— a situation analogous to other psychosomatic disorders such as peptic ulcer, spastic colitis, noncardiac chest wall pain, and tension headaches (66). The term, unfortunately, is not completely accurate, although tension implies the psychosomatic overtones. The term "myositis," defined as a specific inflammation of the muscle, is not exactly accurate, but perhaps is comparable to the term colitis in the phrase "spastic colitis," where there is no definite inflammation of the colon. The actual origin of pain in this condition remains speculative, but it is suspected to be a local disorder of the contractile state of the muscle—only occasionally is it widespread enough to be perceived by the patient as muscle spasm (66). A common characteristic of all of the patients with this complaint is one or more of the following personality features: compulsive striving for success, a tendency toward chronic worry and depression, and somatization of emotional distress through complaints in other body systems (67).

Spinal Appliances: General Considerations

EFFECT OF SPINAL ORTHOSES ON GAIT AND ENERGY EXPENDITURE DURING WALKING

While spinal appliances may be necessary in order to achieve objectives in the treatment of spinal disorders, the use of appliances may create additional problems. Usually, the disadvantages are far outweighed by the advantages; nevertheless, the physician should be aware of them so that they may be kept to a minimum. Aside from the inconveniences and relative confinement imposed by the brace, the major disadvantages are impairments which can occur with respect to gait and energy expenditure.

During normal level walking, the pelvis rotates approximately 10° about the vertical axis with each step. The shoulder girdle rotates an equal amount but 180° out of phase with the pelvis. The amount of rotation varies directly with the length of stride. Arm swing is in the opposite direction to leg swing and apparently serves as a passive pendulum counterbalance. Since the shoulders and pelvis rotate in opposite directions, there is a neutral point in the spine where no rotation occurs. With use of steel pins placed in the spinous processes, Gregersen and Lucas (22) were able to establish that, in the several individuals tested, the neutral point was at the level of the seventh thoracic vertebra.

In experiments in which the spine was immobilized by a posterior plaster shell which eliminated axial rotation of the pelvis and shoulders, Chapman and Ralston (71) found an average increase of 10% in the oxygen consumption of 7 young adult subjects during level walking at a comfortable speed. This is of some significance to the patient who wears a full-length spinal orthosis.

A patient wearing an appliance that restricts axial rotation of the spine usually has to shorten the stride during level walking to conform to the restrictions imposed by the orthosis, thereby eliminating discomforts at the skin/orthosis interface. In addition, a slower pace is usually adopted, which serves to lessen the increased energy requirement and improve balance. These limitations imposed by rigid bracing are the reason that flexible appliances are generally more popular.

The problem of energy expenditure becomes a major consideration to the patient with muscular dystrophy or to one who has muscle weakness resulting from poliomyelitis. It is of importance also to the debilitated, elderly, or otherwise weakened person.

One additional effect of the use of a spinal appliance is the tendency for spinal motion to be increased in the spinal segments adjacent to the ends of the appliance. This was demonstrated by Norton and Brown (58), who were able to show increased lumbosacral motion during trunk flexion when a long spinal orthosis extending only to the upper part of the pelvis was worn, this motion being a compensation for decreased motion of the thoracolumbar region. A corresponding increase in thoracic or thoracolumbar motion occurs in patients wearing short spinal braces. This increased motion and strain may be a cause of pain, particularly if degenerative processes are present, and should be especially taken into account in prescribing an appliance that does not follow the contour of the back for the patient who has restricted motion resulting from advanced degenerative changes. If the orthosis tends to flatten the lumbar part of the spine, the thoracic part must be extended to maintain balance. Such extension often results in significant localized thoracic pain and negates the effectiveness of the appliance. When the focus of the pain is at the lumbosacral level, the immobilized proximal segments provide an effective lever to increase the stress at the lumbosacral joint during motion of the trunk.

It follows that in order to limit motion at any point in the spine, the brace must extend well beyond that point. This is particularly true when a brace is prescribed for the lumbosacral joint when motion is the cause of pain. Norton and Brown found that in such cases the brace had to extend well down onto the pelvis and grip it firmly in order to eliminate lumbosacral motion.

In a study by Waters and Morris (73) of the electrical activity in the back muscles, the rigid lumbosacral orthosis (LSO) (like the chairback or Knight orthosis in Fig. 6.5) and the lumbosacral corset either decreased or had no effect on the electrical activity recorded from deep back muscles in standing subjects. Muscle activity was also unaltered when the subject walked at his usual speed. However, while wearing the rigid orthosis and walking at a fast

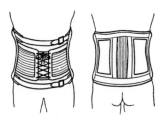

Fig. 6.5. Knight brace.

pace, subjects showed an increase in electrical activity when they were compared under the same condition without spinal support. On the other hand, subjects wearing a corset and walking at the same fast pace did not show such an increased electrical activity.

Although these studies were on healthy subjects, we can probably assume that spinal orthoses do not exert their effects by specifically reducing the involuntary activity of the back muscles.

Basic Types of Spinal Appliances

Each physician has his preference among the spinal appliances in common use today; the total number available is far too great to describe or enumerate here. For a relatively complete listing, the reader is referred to the standard atlases (1, 2).

In order to simplify the problem of selection of a spinal appliance, the list of orthoses to be described here has been reduced to the minimum which is necessary for the treatment of the majority of disorders commonly seen. Braces used in the treatment of scoliosis have been excluded since they are described in Chapter 7.

The appliances to be discussed are: (1) trochanteric belts; (2) sacroiliac and lumbosacral belts; (3) corsets; (4) rigid braces (chairback and dorsolumbar); (5) hyperextension braces; and (6) jackets.

With the single exception of the hyperextension brace, all the appliances rely at least in part on abdominal compression to accomplish their purpose. It has been pointed out earlier that an increase of intra-abdominal pressure partially relieves the spine of weight from superincumbent structures. In addition the increase in intra-abdominal pressure provided by the appliance tends to straighten the lordotic lumbar curve and simultaneously to decrease the intervertebral joint motion.

There is considerable indirect evidence to support the contention that abdominal compression provided by spinal appliances is the major factor in the relief from back pain. It is more than coincidental that many women rely on the use of an elastic girdle to control fatigue backache. Heavy laborers frequently wear wide leather belts while working or, in some countries, tightly wrapped sashes. Abdominal strengthening exercises, used in the treatment of low back pain, probably owe their success, in part at least, to improved abdominal compression.

There are those who argue that relief from pain through abdominal compression is brought about by the decrease in lumbar lordosis. There is no question that this is a factor; however, it is probably not the major one since it has been frequently observed that pain relief often follows application of an abdominal support without a concomitant change in lumbar lordosis.

Although gross trunk motion is reduced by both rigid and flexible orthoses, the exact degree of motion control between vertebrae has had to be measured using biomechanical principles. Undoubtedly, part of the effectiveness of spinal orthoses lies in inhibiting voluntary motion. The sensation of wearing a corset or brace serves as a reminder to the patient not to make certain movements that increase his symptoms.

Unfortunately, this useful function also has a negative effect. The patient may become psychologically and physically dependent on wearing the orthosis, and if isometric exercises are not performed along with orthotic wear, the trunk muscles—so essential in spinal support—become weakened. Whether or not to prescribe an orthosis for back pain, therefore, should be very carefully considered, particularly if emotional factors seem to play a major role in perpetuating the back pain (67).

Non-rigid Orthoses
TROCHANTERIC BELT ORTHOSES

The trochanteric belt (Fig. 6.6A) is a belt made of canvas, leather, or other heavy material, usually 2 or 3 inches wide, which encircles the pelvis between the trochanters and the iliac crests. It is fastened in front and may be equipped with perineal straps to prevent it from riding upward. It is used frequently to provide a barrel-hoop type of support for pelvic fractures during the healing period. It may also be helpful in improving the gait of patients with long-standing congenital dislocation of the hip. The tightly worn belt possibly serves to restrict the upward movement of the femoral heads during weight-bearing.

This orthosis is frequently prescribed for pain felt in the region of the

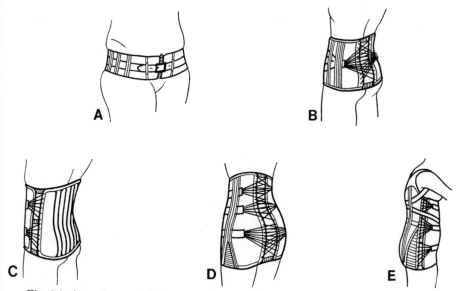

Fig. 6.6. *A*, trochanteric belt; *B*, sacroiliac belt; *C*, lumbosacral belt; *D*, lumbosacral corset; *E*, thoracolumbar corset.

sacroiliac joints or posterior superior spines of the ilium, as well as for conditions of rheumatoid arthritis involving the sacroiliac joints. Except in the case of the rheumatoid patient, the origin of this type of pain is often obscure. The orthosis is also prescribed for so-called instability of one or both joints, a condition which, in the author's experience, is rare except after severe trauma. Pain felt in this region is more commonly due to lumbosacral disorders and should be treated accordingly.

SACROILIAC ORTHOSES (SIOs) AND LUMBAR SACRAL ORTHOSES (LSOs)

The SIOs (Fig. 6.6B) and LSOs (Fig 6.6C) are similar in design and function. The distinction between them is based on width. They were discussed earlier in Chapter 4 and may be termed belts or corsets, depending on patient preference—men seem to prefer the term "belt." They are obtainable as stock items in most orthotic facilities and require fitting by an experienced orthotist or corsetier. They are made of a heavy cotton cloth such as coutil or duck and are usually reinforced with lightweight stays. Posterior steels may be added on either side of the spine to increase rigidity and allow counterpressure to be applied evenly over the back. Frequently, these supports come equipped with a sacral pad to provide better contact over the sacrum and give the patient a feeling of pressure over this region, with resulting sense of security.

The sacroiliac belt orthosis (SIO), which is worn at the level of the sacroiliac joint, varies in width from 4 to 6 inches and usually fastens with snaps in the front. The anterior portion contributes considerably to the support of the spine through its compressive action on the abdomen. Compressive force is obtained by means of adjustable side or back laces which allow for the desired amount of tension through single or double pulls. Perineal straps may be necessary to prevent the brace from sliding upward.

Belt-type LSOs range in width from 8 to 16 inches. Extra paraspinal steel inserts are provided if additional stiffness is desired.

SIOs and LSOs are prescribed for low back pain associated with degenerative disc disorders, postural fatigue, acute flexion injuries, and other conditions for which abdominal compression is felt to be a factor in the relief of pain. They do not provide enough immobilization to be suitable for use after most surgical spinal procedures, but they are sufficiently restrictive to relieve pain where excessive motion is an aggravating factor.

CORSETS

Corsets differ from belts in their basic design. In addition to supplying abdominal compression, they extend down over the buttocks and upper thighs to provide a more acceptable contour. Hose supporters can be added for convenience and aid in holding the garment at the proper level. Corsets are obtainable at corset and orthotic facilities; they must be fitted very carefully by an experienced corsetier to ensure an accurate fit, as determined by the superior border. Three types of corsets are available: sacroiliac (Fig. 6.6*B*), lumbosacral (Fig. 6.6*D*), and thoracolumbar (Fig. 6.6*E*).

Corsets may lace at the back, side, or front. The back and side lacing models have self-adjusting laces which provide for a variable amount of pressure on the abdomen by means of either two or three pullstraps. Elastic inserts are used to prevent binding and to ensure better fit. When desired, contoured steel uprights may be inserted paraspinally to increase the rigidity of the appliance and to provide a better distribution of counterpressure for abdominal compression.

The thoracolumbar corset extends well over the scapulae and is equipped with shoulder straps that are supposed to maintain thoracic extension. The paraspinal steel uprights, as well as additional stays, are important in providing the necessary rigidity usually required by this appliance.

Corsets are made from several different fabrics, including cotton, nylon, and rayon. Because corsets tend to be uncomfortable in hot climates, mesh fabrics may be utilized if necessary. Some loss of support may then occur.

The shorter corsets are prescribed for lumbar and lumbosacral disorders, including degenerative disc disorders, postural fatigue, acute flexion injuries, osteoarthritis, osteoporosis, and other painful conditions. The longer, full-length corsets are helpful for control of pain in generalized osteoporosis, metastatic malignancy, myeloma, and osteoarthritis of the midthoracic and lower thoracic parts of the spine. The shoulder straps must be pulled reasonably tight to support the thoracic spine. This may cause some local discomfort from axillary pressure, and care must be exercised to avoid venous obstruction here.

The corset, adequately reinforced with stays and paraspinal steels, is nearly as rigid as a back brace, and women usually prefer it to a rigid brace. As a practical point, it may be noted that people who are moderately obese commonly derive far more relief of pain from the use of corsets than do thin people. This may be due to the greater ease with which abdominal pressure can be applied in heavier patients without causing painful pressure over bony prominences.

A modified full-length corset with extra steels laterally, as well as paraspinally, is useful in treating children with trunk weakness. The corset has enough strength when applied snugly to hold the trunk upright, even in the presence of rather severe involvement of the erector spinae and abdominal muscles, such as is seen following poliomyelitis or in muscular dystrophy. There may be some restriction of chest excursion, but diaphragm breathing is aided by the abdominal support.

Abdominal supports with special lacing are available for prenatal patients. These should be worn with care so that undue abdominal pressure is avoided. As a general rule, the obstetrician should be consulted before such a garment is prescribed.

Other conditions benefited by corsets are abdominal hernia and pendulous abdomen. Naturally, definitive correction of the disorder is preferable whenever possible, followed later by an abdominal muscle-strengthening program.

Rigid Orthoses

Rigid appliances, including corsets with paraspinal steel supports, provide an efficient means of obtaining abdominal compression with an anterior force and, at the same time, distributing the counterforce over an extensive area. If the appliance is properly fitted, the posterior corset steels will follow the contour of the spine and paraspinal muscles, providing a broad area of contact, while the apron in front will contact as large an abdominal area as possible. The net effect is to surround and compress the entire abdomen, pelvis, and lower back.

The pressure generated in the abdomen is distributed equally against its walls, including the spine. If lordosis is to be reduced, it is best accomplished slowly, with gradual straightening of the paraspinal uprights. Any patient so treated should carry out concomitant abdominal strengthening exercises in order to avoid weakening the abdominal muscles. While the orthosis passively corrects the lordosis through the pressure mechanism, the abdominal muscles use a combination of this and the levers afforded by the ribs and pelvis to actively correct the lordosis.

The rigid back orthosis most commonly used is the lumbar or LSO type. Frequently termed the chairback brace, it probably has more variations than any other single type of orthosis. Basically, it is a short spinal brace consisting of a pelvic band, which is located at a level between the greater trochanter and the iliac crest, and a thoracic band, which is located 1 inch inferior to the angle of the scapula; these bands are joined by two posterior and two lateral metal uprights with an apron or corset front. This brace acts in the same manner as the lumbosacral corset or belt, even though it differs in design. Anterior pressure is exerted by the apron or corset front, and posterior counterpressure is supplied by the metal frame.

In most instances, the posterior uprights are contoured to fit the normal curve of the spine so that a smooth even pressure is applied to the back (an equally well-distributed anterior pressure is furnished by the conforming apron). When the orthosis is applied to reduce lumbar lordosis, the posterior uprights are straightened, and anterior pressure supplied by the apron or corset front draws the spine back against the uprights.

Because of its lateral uprights, the short metal LSO is considerably more rigid than the corset. Some flexibility may be secured, however, if the posterior uprights of the brace are made from flexible steel and the lateral uprights are omitted. Additional rigidity in the metal LSO is obtained by the use of double pelvic bands, one below and one above the iliac crest, in order to gain a better purchase on the pelvis. The greatest rigidity is achieved by the addition of anterior rigid uprights. In this case, a hinge must be placed in the back of the brace for application and removal of the appliance.

The physician is naturally dependent on the orthotist in his locality for custom construction of the rigid brace. Brace makers tend to specialize in the construction of certain types of braces, which means that the physician may have to utilize the services of several orthotists to obtain a wide selection.

Typical of short spinal braces are the commonly used Knight and Brackett braces (Figs. 6.5, and 6.7A). The Williams brace (Fig. 6.7B) is a specialized short spinal brace which allows free flexion but limits extension and utilizes a lever action to gain additional flattening of the lumbar part of the spine.

The MacAusland brace (Fig. 6.8A) has clock-spring posterior uprights

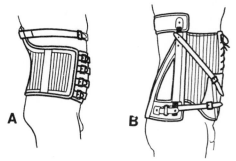

Fig. 6.7. A, Brackett brace; B, Williams brace.

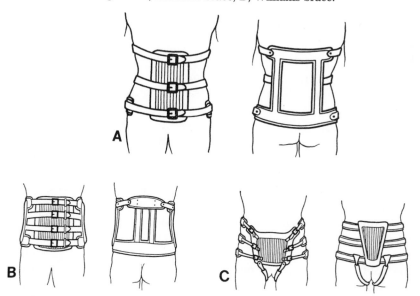

Fig. 6.8. A, MacAusland brace; B, Wilcox, or Lipscomb, brace; C, Osgood, or Goldthwait, brace.

and no lateral uprights, an arrangement which allows some flexibility while at the same time providing abdominal pressure.

The Wilcox, or Lipscomb, brace (Fig. 6.8B) employs a movable joint where the lateral uprights join the pelvic band, permitting some mobility. This adds to the comfort of the wearer and provides for easier fitting and adjustment.

The Osgood, or Goldthwait, brace (Fig. 6.8C) is one of the shortest orthoses and also one of the most effective in providing lower abdominal pressure and pelvic arch support without significantly limiting lumbar motion. It is more properly referred to as an SIO whereas the other braces mentioned are LSOs. The Osgood brace has its corollary in the sacroiliac belts and corset. Because of its hoop effect, it is prescribed for the treatment of pelvic fractures and when immobilization of the sacroiliac joints is to be attempted. It is effective in some cases of lumbosacral arthralgia because of its efficient lower abdominal pressure pad, which is instrumental in increasing intra-abdominal pressure and thereby relieving some of the load on the lower lumbar segments. All rigid short spinal orthoses or LSOs are useful in contouring the lumbar part of the spine and in providing abdominal compression, measures which have been clinically observed to be associated with reduction of pain symptoms. Immobilization of the lumbosacral spine by these braces is more difficult. Complete immobilization is impossible unless the brace is worn so tightly that the lower part of the back is converted into a rigid column. In this case, the flattening of the lumbar part of the spine reduces axial rotation to a minimum and almost eliminates further flexion. Extension is possible only as far as the anteriocompressive force permits.

THORACOLUMBAR ORTHOSES

The long spinal orthosis is the corollary of the full-length corset and is called a thoracolumbar brace or, using the new terminology, a thoracolumbosacral orthosis (TLSO). Generally, this device is designed to fix the lumbar spine to the pelvis to provide a base and then to hold the thoracic part to the rigid paraspinal uprights, in varying amounts of extension. The prototype of the TLSO is the Taylor brace (Fig. 6.9A), which consists of a wide-fitted pelvic band extending forward to the midaxillary lines, with two long posterior paraspinal uprights extending to the shoulders. The uprights are joined by a short transverse bar in the midthoracic region; straps pass from the uprights over the shoulders and under the axillae to this transverse bar. A full-length abdominal apron attached by straps and buckles completes the orthosis.

The holding action exerted on the thoracic part of the spine is achieved in the Magnuson (Fig. 6.9B) and Arnold (Fig. 6.10A) braces by means of a fairly rigid, long transverse dorsal band which extends forward under the axillae and curves upward to terminate in padded ends which exert pressure

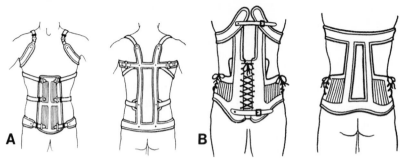

Fig. 6.9. *A*, Taylor brace; *B*, Magnuson brace.

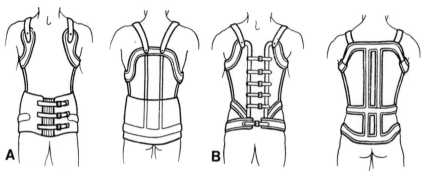

Fig. 6.10. *A*, Arnold brace; *B*, Steindler brace.

bilaterally in the infraclavicular region. Additional longitudinal rigidity is obtained by the use of lateral uprights (Bennett brace) or anterior uprights (Magnuson brace). The most rigid of all is the Steindler brace (Fig. 6.10*B*), which employs a double pelvic band for pelvic stability, as well as anterior, posterior, and lateral uprights and infraclavicular pressure pads combined with shoulder straps.

From the foregoing, it is obvious that varying degrees of rigidity can be built into the long spinal brace, the required amount of rigidity being dictated by the needs of the patient. When moderate assistance to maintain extension is the objective, the less rigid appliances are adequate and are probably better tolerated by the patient.

The Arnold brace can be worn comfortably and is useful in treating patients with osteoporosis, degenerative joint disease, rheumatoid spondylitis, and moderate muscle weakness. The Taylor brace provides slightly more rigidity because the straps serve to pull the shoulders back, but they also make the brace less comfortable. This orthosis is effective when used after vertebral-body compression fractures and in the treatment of patients with severe round back secondary to epiphysitis, spondylitis, or marked weakness of the trunk. While it is also prescribed for support and immobilization after surgical treatment of the thoracic part of the spine, it probably does not effectively immobilize the upper third of the thoracic segment unless a cervical extension piece is added.

When maximum immobilization is required, the Steindler brace will serve most effectively, particularly in limiting axial rotation.

Naturally, the more confining the brace, the more bulky and uncomfortable it becomes. For this reason, the physician will usually prescribe the simplest orthosis possible to obtain his objectives. In general, the full-length corset and brace are interchangeable, and both can be modified to provide varying amounts of rigidity. As a rule, women prefer corsets for esthetic reasons, and men prefer rigid orthoses, possibly because they seem more masculine. This is an artificial distinction but, nevertheless, a realistic one from the standpoint of the patient's acceptance.

ANTERIOR HYPEREXTENSION ORTHOSES

The full-length anterior hyperextension orthosis (Fig. 6.11) is probably the only appliance which relies solely on the "three-point-pressure" principle to achieve its purpose. First described by Hoadley in 1895, this brace has been modified and popularized by Griswold, Jewett, Baker, and Graham and Bradford. Basically, it consists of a modified rectangular metal frame which is applied anteriorly so that the ends exert pressure over the pubis and manubrium while counterpressure is being maintained over the midback by means of a modified strap which attaches to the sides of the frame. Additional pelvic and thoracic straps may be added to hold the brace in place. Pads are incorporated to distribute the pressure more evenly over the manubrium and sternum.

While this orthosis may be used whenever hyperextension is desired, it is usually recommended as an efficient aid to permit ambulation during treatment of compression fractures of the vertebral bodies. It is rather uncomfortable since the corrective forces are applied over a small area.

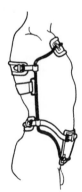

Fig. 6.11. Anterior hyperextension brace.

Also, the hyperextension extends into the lumbar part of the spine and may give rise to postural back pain of considerable degree. The greatest virtue of the brace is its lightweight construction. When it is prescribed and used only as a protective device to prevent excessive flexion, it can be applied with less than ordinary pressure so that it then meets with considerably greater approval from the patient.

MOLDED SPINAL ORTHOSES

Molded jackets are frequently prescribed for spinal support (Fig. 6.12). They are constructed from plaster of Paris, leather, or plastic. Because they fit the contours of the body accurately, they distribute pressures evenly over the widest possible area of the body surface and thereby contribute to the comfort of the patient. This distribution of pressures becomes of paramount importance when the pressures to be applied are great; skin breakdown can become a problem, especially when the skin and underlying tissues are inordinately tender, as in the chronically ill or debilitated patient.

Since the materials used in the construction of molded jackets vary from rigid to semirigid, these jackets provide varying amounts of support. A surprising amount of rigidity, however, is supplied by even a flexible leather jacket which has been carefully molded and snugly laced. In principle, the orthosis is a large modified tube and derives its rigidity from this shape; the larger the cross-section, the greater the rigidity afforded. In the final analysis, of course, corsets and braces are also modified tubes which vary in rigidity according to the completeness of their walls and the materials used in their construction.

The simplest jacket—the easiest for the physician to construct—is the plaster of Paris molded support. It is molded directly onto the patient, who is placed in the desired position, often standing with a head-halter support.

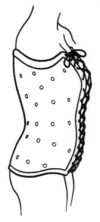

Fig. 6.12. Molded jacket.

The usual plaster cast is then constructed, trimmed, split down the front, and removed. After it has dried thoroughly, the edges are finished with adhesive tape to ensure smoothness, and the jacket is applied to the patient and held with two encircling webbing straps which can be taped in position. If a more permanent finish is desired, the jacket can be trimmed in leather and laced in front.

A new concept in spinal orthotics is the modular polypropylene spinal brace. The modules can be manufactured in standard sizes and then modified according to needs of individual patients. At present, this concept has been primarily applied to cases of spinal deformity, as described in Chapter 7, but its application in cases of back pain appears to be promising.

Most other types of molded orthoses require a positive mold which is made by the orthotist from a plaster cast often supplied by the physician. Corrections can be incorporated into the original cast and enlarged in the positive mold for inclusion in the final orthosis, but once the latter is completed, it seldom allows for the additional correction or adjustment possible in the belt, corset, or brace.

One type of molded orthosis can be formed directly on the patient. It is made of closed cell polyethylene foam sheets (Plastazote, Aliplast—see Chapter 3) which can be heated at a temperature low enough not to burn the patient when it is molded over the body contour. The surface of the material is soft and comfortable, but the material itself is bulky and rigid. Generally, to provide more rigidity, these orthoses are reinforced with strips of thin polyethylene (Orthoplast, Sansplint) which when heated will adhere to the surface of the jacket. These jackets are easy to apply even in a wheelchair; they are wrapped around the trunk and attached across a front opening by Velcro strap closure.

The main advantage of these jackets is the short time it takes to provide them, and they can be corrected or adjusted by reheating the low temperature thermoplastic material. However, they are not very durable and, although vented, may cause excessive heat. Patients also complain that they are very bulky under clothing.

Jackets are especially useful in providing spinal support for the aged, debilitated, or very weak patients. Patients with advanced metastatic tumor involvement of the spine, multiple myeloma, or severe osteoporosis benefit from the support and pain control afforded by jackets. However, they are often required in patients for whom standard types of orthoses are impossible to apply with any degree of comfort because of severe deformities resulting from multiple congenital anomalies or neglected spinal disorders. Further discussion of molded trunk orthoses is covered in Chapter 7.

Summary

This chapter is a review of the various devices used for supporting the spine in patients with back pain and instability. For proper utilization of these orthoses, physicians and those in allied health programs should understand what a back support can or cannot do. These types of orthoses will restrict but not prevent motion in the thoracic lumbar regions. The function of these orthoses basically is to create abdominal compression which converts the abdominal contents into a semirigid cylinder capable of transmitting stresses to the trunk through the abdomen, rather than having all of the force loading the spine. With few exceptions, the use of such restrictive back supports in treating back disorders should be only a temporary measure. The goal should be restoration of physiologic forces which support the spine through the intrinsic action of the individual's trunk musculature rather than through some type of external appliance (1).

REFERENCES

1. AMERICAN ACADEMY OF ORTHOPEDIC SURGERY. *Atlas of Orthotics.* St. Louis, C. V. Mosby, 1975.
2. AMERICAN ACADEMY OF ORTHOPAEDIC SURGEONS. *Orthopaedic Appliances Atlas. Braces, Splints, Shoe Alterations; a Consideration of Aids Employed in the Practice of Orthopaedic Surgery,* Vol. 1. Ann Arbor, Mich., Edwards, 1952.
3. BARR, J. S. Protruded discs and painful backs. *J. Bone Joint Surg., 33B:* 3, 1951.
4. BARR, J. S. Ruptured intervertebral disc and sciatic pain. *J. Bone Joint Surg., 29:* 429, 1947.
5. BARTELINK, D. L. The role of abdominal pressure in relieving the pressure on the lumbar intervertebral discs. *J. Bone Joint Surg., 39B:* 718, 1957.
6. BRADFORD, F. K., AND SPURLING, R. G. *The Intervertebral Disc, with Special Reference to Rupture of the Annulus Fibrosus with Herniation of the Nucleus Pulposus,* ed. 2. Springfield, Ill., Charles C Thomas, 1945.
7. BRODIN, H. Paths of nutrition in articular cartilage and intervertebral discs. *Acta Orthop. Scand., 24:* 177, 1955.
8. BROWN, T., HANSEN, R. J., AND YORRA, A. J. Some mechanical tests on the lumbosacral spine with particular reference to the intervertebral discs: a preliminary report. *J. Bone Joint Surg., 39A:* 1135, 1957.
9. BUSH, H. D., HORTON, W. G., SMARE, D. L., AND NAYLOR, A. Fluid content of the nucleus pulposus as a factor in the disk syndrome. *Brit. Med. J., 2:* 81, 1956.
10. CHARNLEY, J. The imbibition of fluid as a cause of herniation of the nucleus pulposus. *Lancet, 1:* 124, 1952.
11. COVENTRY, M. B., GHORMLEY, R. K., AND KERNOHAN, J. W. The intervertebral disc: its microscopic anatomy and pathology. I. Anatomy, development, and physiology. *J. Bone Joint Surg., 27:* 105, 1945.
12. COVENTRY, M. B. The intervertebral disc: its microscopic anatomy and pathology. II. Changes in the intervertebral disc concomitant with age. *J. Bone Joint Surg., 27:* 233, 1945.
13. COVENTRY, M. B. The intervertebral disc: its microscopic anatomy and pathology. III. Pathological changes in the intervertebral disc. *J. Bone Joint Surg., 27:* 460, 1945.
14. EVANS, F. G., AND LISSNER, H. R. Strength of intervertebral discs. *J. Bone Joint Surg., 36A:* 185, 1954.
15. FEINSTEIN, B., LANGTON, J. N. K., JAMESON, R. M., AND SCHILLER, F. Experiments on pain referred from deep somatic tissues. *J. Bone Joint Surg., 36A:* 981, 1954.
16. FERGUSON, W. R. Some observations on the circulation in foetal and infant spines. *J. Bone Joint Surg., 32A:* 640, 1950.
17. FLOYD, W. F., AND SILVER, P. H. S. Electromyographic study of patterns of activity of the anterior abdominal wall muscles in man. *J. Anat., 84:* 132, 1950.

18. FRIBERG, S. Anatomical studies on lumbar disc degeneration. *Acta Orthop. Scand., 17:* 224, 1947.

19. FRIBERG, S. Lumbar disc degeneration in problem of lumbago sciatica. *Bull. Hosp. Joint Dis., 15:* 1, 1954.

20. FRIBERG, S., AND HIRSCH, C. Anatomical and clinical studies on lumbar disc degeneration. *Acta Orthop. Scand., 19:* 222, 1949.

21. GHORMLEY, M. An etiologic study of backache and sciatic pain. *Proc. Mayo Clin., 26:* 457, 1951.

22. GREGERSEN, G. G., AND LUCAS, D. B. An *in vivo* study of axial rotation of the human thoracolumbar spine. *J. Bone Joint Surg., 49A:* 267, 1967.

23. HADLEY, L. A. Apophyseal subluxation disturbances in and about the intervertebral foramen causing back pain. *J. Bone Joint Surg., 18:* 428, 1936.

24. HANSEN, H-J. A pathologic-anatomical interpretation of disc degeneration in dogs. *Acta Orthop. Scand., 20:* 280, 1951.

25. HANSEN, H. J., AND OLSSON, S.E. The effect of a single violent trauma on the spine of the dog. *Acta Orthop. Scand., 24:* 1, 1954.

26. HARRIS, R. I., AND MACNAB. I. Structural changes in the lumbar intervertebral discs: their relationship to low back pain and sciatica. *J. Bone Joint Surg., 36B:* 304, 1954.

27. HENDRY, N. G. C. The hydration of the nucleus pulposus and its relation to the intervertebral disc derangement. *J. Bone Joint Surg., 40B:* 132, 1958.

28. HIRSCH, C. The reaction of intervertebral discs to compression forces. *J. Bone Joint Surg., 37A:* 1188, 1955.

29. HIRSCH, C. Studies on the mechanism of low back pain. *Acta Orthop. Scand., 20:* 261, 1951.

30. HIRSCH, C. Studies on the pathology of low back pain. *J. Bone Joint Surg., 41B:* 237, 1959.

31. HIRSCH, C., INGELMARK, B-E., AND MILLER, M. The anatomical basis for low back pain. Studies on the presence of sensory nerve endings in ligamentous, capsular and intervertebral disc structures in the human lumbar spine. *Acta Orthop. Scand., 33:* 1, 1963.

32. HIRSCH, C., AND NACHEMSON, A. New observations on the mechanical behavior of lumbar discs. *Acta Orthop. Scand., 23:* 254, 1954.

33. HIRSCH, C., PAULSON, S., SYLVÉN, B., AND SNELLMAN, O. Biophysical and physiological investigations on cartilage and other mesenchymal tissues. VI. Characteristics of human nuclei pulposi during aging. *Acta Orthop. Scand., 22:* 175, 1953.

34. HIRSCH, C., AND SCHAJOWICZ, F. Studies on structural changes in the lumbar annulus fibrosus. *Acta Orthop. Scand., 22:* 184, 1953.

35. HORTON, W. G. Further observations on the elastic mechanism of the intervertebral disc. *J. Bone Joint Surg., 40B:* 552, 1958.

36. HYNDMAN, O. R. Pathologic intervertebral disk and its consequences. A contribution to the cause and treatment of chronic pain low in the back and to the subject of herniating intervertebral disk. *Arch. Surg., 53:* 247, 1946.

37. INMAN, V. T. AND SAUNDERS, J. B. DE C. M. Anatomicophysiological aspects of injuries to the intervertebral disc. *J. Bone Joint Surg., 29:* 461, 1947.

38. JOPLIN, R. J. The intervertebral disc: embryology, anatomy, physiology, and pathology. *Surg. Gynecol. Obstet., 61:* 591, 1935.

39. KALLIO, K. E. Experiences with the problem of low back pain and sciatica. *Am. Acad. Orthop. Surg. Instruct. Course Lect., 14:* 23, 1957.

40. KEEGAN, J. J. Alterations of the lumbar curve related to posture and seating. *J. Bone Joint Surg., 35A:* 589, 1953.

41. KELLGREN, J. H. Observations on referred pain arising from muscle. *Clin. Sci., 3:* 175, 1938.

42. KELLGREN, J. H. On the distribution of pain arising from deep somatic structures, with charts of segmental pain areas. *Clin. Sci., 4:* 35, 1939.

43. KEY, J. A. Intervertebral disk lesions and low-back and leg pain. Introduction. The

intervertebral disk: anatomy, physiology, and pathology. *Am. Acad. Orthop. Surg. Instruct. Course Lect., 11:* 99, 101, 1954.

44. KELLGREN, J. H., AND FORD, L. T. Experimental intervertebral-disc lesions. *J. Bone Joint Surg., 30A:* 621, 1948.

45. KEYES, D. C., AND COMPERE, E. L. The normal and pathological physiology of the nucleus pulposus of the intervertebral disc. *J. Bone Joint Surg., 14:* 897, 1932.

46. KNUTSSON, F. The instability associated with disk degeneration in the lumbar spine. *Acta Radiol., 25:* 593, 1944.

47. LINDBLOM, K. Experimental ruptures of intervertebral discs in rats' tails: a preliminary report. *J. Bone Joint Surg., 34A:* 123, 1952.

48. LINDBLOM, K., AND HULTQVIST, G. Absorption of protruded disc tissue. *J. Bone Joint Surg., 32A:* 557, 1950.

49. LINDBOM, A. The roentgenographic appearance of injuries to the intervertebral discs. *Acta Radiol., 45:* 129, 1956.

50. MORGAN, F. P., AND KING, T. Primary instability of lumbar vertebrae as a common cause of low back pain. *J. Bone Joint Surg., 39B:* 6, 1957.

51. MORRIS, J. M., BENNER, G., AND LUCAS, D. B. An electromyographic study of the intrinsic muscles of the back in man. *J. Anat., 96:* 509, 1962.

52. MORRIS, J. M., LUCAS, D. B., AND BRESLER, B. Role of the trunk in stability of the spine. *J. Bone Joint Surg., 43A:* 327, 1961.

53. NACHEMSON, A. Measurement of intradiscal pressure. *Acta Orthop. Scand., 28:* 269, 1959.

54. NACHEMSON, A. L. The lumbar spine, an orthopedic challenge. *Spine 1:* 59, 1976.

55. NACHEMSON, A. Some mechanical properties of the lumbar intervertebral discs. *Bull. Hosp. Joint Dis., 23:* 130, 1962.

56. NACHEMSON, A., AND MORRIS, J. M. *In vivo* measurements of intradiscal pressure: discometry, a method for the determination of pressure in the lower lumbar discs. *J. Bone Joint Surg., 46A:* 1077, 1964.

57. NAYLOR, A. Changes in the human intervertebral disc with age. *Proc. R. Soc. Med., 51:* 573, 1958.

58. NORTON, P. L., AND BROWN, T. The immobilizing efficiency of back braces: their effect on the posture and motion of the lumbosacral spine. *J. Bone Joint Surg., 39A:* 111, 1957.

59. O'CONNELL, J. E. A. Protrusions of the lumbar intervertebral discs: a clinical review based on five hundred cases treated by excision of the protrusion. *J. Bone Joint Surg., 33B:* 8, 1951.

60. OLIN, H. A. The intervertebral disc: involvement in vertebral fractures and in spinal pathology. Report of fifty-six cases. *Am. J. Roentgenol., 42:* 235, 1939.

61. PEDERSEN, H. C., CONRAD, F. J. B., AND GARDNER, E. The anatomy of lumbosacral posterior rami and meningeal branches of spinal nerves (sinu-vertebral nerves), with an experimental study of their functions. *J. Bone Joint Surg., 38A:* 377, 1956.

62. PEREY, O. Fracture of the vertebral end-plate in the lumbar spine: an experimental biomechanical investigation. *Acta Orthop. Scand. 1* (Suppl. 25): 1957.

63. PETTER, C. K. Methods of measuring the pressure of the intervertebral disc. *J. Bone Joint Surg., 5:* 365, 1933.

64. PRADER, A. Die Entwicklung der Zwischenwirbelscheibe beim menschlichen Keimling. *Acta Anat., 3:* 115, 1947.

65. ROOFE, P. G. Innervation of annulus fibrosus and posterior longitudinal ligament: fourth and fifth lumbar level. *Arch. Neurol. Psychiatr., 44:* 100, 1940.

66. SARNO, J. E. Chronic back pain and psychic conflict. *Scand. J. Rehabil. Med., 8:* 143–153, 1978.

67. SARNO, J. E. Exercise for back pain. *Scand. J. Rehabil. Med.* (Suppl.), *1:* 1970.

68. SAUNDERS, J. B. DE C. M., AND INMAN, V. T. Pathology of the intervertebral disc. *Arch. Surg., 40:* 389, 1940.

69. SINCLAIR, D. C., FEINDEL, W. H., WEDDELL, G., AND FALCONER, M. A. The intervertebral

ligaments as a source of segmental pain. *J. Bone Joint Surg., 30B:* 515, 1948.

70. SYLVÉN, B., PAULSON, S., HIRSCH, C., AND SNELLMAN, O. Biophysical and physiological investigations on cartilage and other mesenchymal tissues. II. The ultrastructure of bovine and human nuclei pulposi. *J. Bone Joint Surg., 33A:* 333, 1951.

71. UNIVERSITY OF CALIFORNIA (SAN FRANCISCO AND BERKELEY). Biomechanics Laboratory. Effect of Immobilization of the Back and Arms on Energy Expenditure during Level Walking, by M. W. Chapman and H. J. Ralston. Technical Report no. 52. San Francisco and Berkeley, The Laboratory, June 1964.

72. UNIVERSITY OF CALIFORNIA (SAN FRANCISCO AND BERKELEY). Biomechanics Laboratory. Stability of the Ligamentous Spine, by D. B. Lucas and B. Bresler. Technical Report no. 40. San Francisco and Berkeley, The Laboratory, January 1961.

73. WATERS, R. L., AND MORRIS, J. M. Effects of spinal supports on the electrical activity of muscles of the trunk. *J. Bone Joint Surg., 52A:* 51, 1970.

74. WIBERG, G. Back pain in relation to the nerve supply of the intervertebral disc. *Acta Orthop. Scand., 19:* 211, 1949.

7

Orthotics for Spinal Deformity

MARC A. ASHER, M.D.
WALLACE H. WHITNEY, C.O.

Spinal deformities have been recognized since antiquity. However, only in this century has significant progress been made in the understanding and treatment of these problems.

Spinal deformities include scoliosis, hyper- and hypokyphosis, and hyper- and hypolordosis. These deformities may be the result of many different disease processes, including congenital vertebral anomalies, neuromuscular disease, neurofibromatosis, metabolic connective tissue disorders, trauma, infection, and spondylolisthesis. For the largest diagnostic category, idiopathic scoliosis, the etiology is unknown.

Some spinal deformities may progress (32) and, if sufficiently severe, may cause pulmonocardiac failure, pain, trunk imbalance, paralysis, or psychological maladjustment (9, 10, 59, 63). Increased longevity has made these problems more apparent. Fortunately, the natural history of these disease processes is now understood well enough to allow rational management recommendations. Treatment includes enlightened follow-up, a spinal orthosis, or surgery. Intermittent traction, manipulation, and physical therapy alone have not been shown to be effective.

Approximately 5 per 1000 newborns may eventually require treatment for spinal deformity. In the U. S., over 3 million babies are born each year. Thus, approximately 15,000 new spinal deformity cases who will eventually require treatment are born annually. For the majority, orthotic treatment will be definitive. For many, one or more replacement orthoses may be required. The magnitude of the problem is apparent.

Spinal Orthotic Deformity Development

Historically, spinal deformity orthotic development has occurred in three eras. These are the pre-Milwaukee brace, Milwaukee brace, and post-Milwaukee brace eras.

The pre-Milwaukee brace era dates from the middle ages. It includes an assortment of metal and leather corsets and body jackets. Most were underarm, and virtually all appeared to be based on the principle of passive correction maintained by total or three-point fixation. An exception appears to have been the brace of Spitzy (75), in which a neck ring with pointed submandibular spikes was used to stimulate dynamic correction. There does not appear to have been any scientific study of these braces. In addition to these removable orthoses, serial localizer plaster of Paris jackets were developed in the early part of the 20th century.

The Milwaukee brace era began in 1945, when Drs. Walter P. Blount and Albert Schmidt began the development of a brace as an alternative to plaster cast immobilization following spine fusion. Subsequent development has been extensively documentated (11–20, 49, 52). Since 1949, this brace has been used for the nonoperative treatment of scoliosis. By the late 1960's, the Milwaukee brace with numerous refinements had become virtually the only orthosis used for the nonoperative treatment of scoliosis.

There were two major problems with the Milwaukee brace. One was mandibular malocclusion resulting in bite deformity secondary to the chin piece (44). This was solved by lowering the chin piece and by the introduction of the throat mold in 1969. The second problem, patient noncompliance with brace wear, remains a small but significant problem.

The post-Milwaukee brace era began in the late 1960's, when experimentation with underarm (topless) total-contact orthosis was renewed. This development was made possible by the introduction of molded thermoplastics (93). These materials allow more precise molding and fitting and stimulated the application of prefabrication concepts to spine deformity orthotics. The effectiveness of these orthoses has been sparsely documented, and apparently no biomechanical studies have been done. The Milwaukee brace, still in widespread use, remains the standard for comparison.

Basic Science of Spine Deformity Orthotics

A spinal deformity orthosis is primarily intended to partially correct or prevent progression of spine deformity during completion of growth and maturation of the spine. In addition, it may be used for immobilization following surgery, to relieve pain in the older patient, or to improve sitting balance in the patient with severe neuromuscular disease. To better accomplish these goals, it is desirable to understand the basic principles of spine growth and development, spine morphology, and spine mechanics.

SPINE GROWTH AND DEVELOPMENT (4, 77, 78, 91)

From birth to age 3 years, and again during adolescence, the human spine undergoes periods of accelerated growth (77, 78). During adolescence, the spine grows approximately 12 to 13 cm (4). It is during this period that spinal deformity is most likely to develop and progress. This is especially true for idiopathic scoliosis. As a corrective device, the spinal deformity orthosis is only effective when the patient is actively growing. Parameters used to determine remaining growth include the plotting of longitudinal growth, the development of secondary sexual characteristics, onset of menses in females, skeletal age determination (estimation) by hand-wrist x-ray, iliac epiphyseal excursion and closure, and vertebral ring apophyseal closure. For growth estimation, skeletal age is more reliable than chronological age. The iliac epiphysis is a much less accurate parameter of true age, but it is frequently used because it is readily available.

For girls, the adolescent growth spurt starts at approximately 10 years 9 months of age. This is before the appearance of pubic hair and well before the appearance of the iliac epiphysis. The growth spurt peaks at approximately 12 years of age. Menses begins at about 12 years 6 months of age, usually before the iliac epiphysis appears. Ideally, detection, documentation of progression, and bracing should take place before the menarche.

For boys, a growth spurt begins at about 12 years 6 months of age; this is after the appearance of pubic hair. The growth spurt peaks at about 14 years of age, still before the appearance of the iliac epiphysis.

The majority of spine growth is complete for females at 15 years 6 months and for boys at 17 years 6 months of age. At this time, the iliac epiphysis has completed its excursion. Complete cessation of spine growth, however, occurs later, at about 17 years for girls and 19 to 20 years for boys (4). Complete closure of the vertebral ring apophysis is the best sign of complete cessation of spine growth.

SPINAL DEFORMITY MORPHOLOGY AND QUANTITATION

For descriptive purposes, the body in stance is divided into three orientation planes: these are the horizontal, sagittal, and frontal planes. By definition, they are perpendicular to each other and originate from the center of gravity of the body (76, 85).

Spinal deformity may occur in any one or several combinations of the three planes. Scoliosis, the most common and extensively studied spine deformity, is primarily a frontal plane deformity. In 1966, the Scoliosis Research Society adopted the Cobb measurement (Fig. 7.1) (29) and developed a glossary of terminology related to spine deformity (53). This glossary was updated in 1978 and has greatly assisted communication in this field.

Idiopathic scoliosis usually appears as one of the six basic curve patterns (Fig. 7.2). Similar curve patterns may be seen with scoliosis of known etiology. In addition, neuromuscular scoliosis often results in a long C curve, and congenital scoliosis may cause cervicothoracic or lumbosacral junction deformities.

Horizontal plane deformity always accompanies structural frontal plane deformity. The vertebral bodies rotate toward the convexity of the curve and result in pedicle asymmetry on x-ray (Fig. 7.3). This asymmetry can be

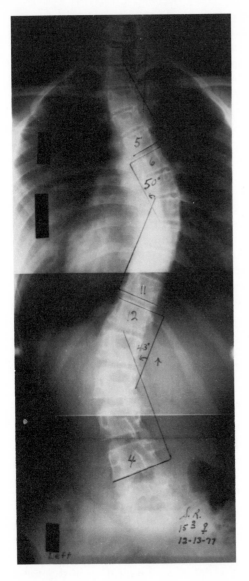

Fig. 7.1. Anteroposterior x-ray demonstrating the Cobb technique of curve measurement. End vertebrae are identified as those maximally tilted into the concavity of the curve. The curve angle is at the intersection of lines drawn parallel to the upper cortical plate of the cephalid vertebra and the lower cortical plate of the caudad vertebra. Except for large curves, these lines do not usually cross on the x-ray film. Therefore, the angle is measured at the intersection of lines drawn perpendicular to the end vertebral lines. This is a supplemental or identical angle.

quantitated (61, 64). Horizontal deformity is apparent clinically as a paravertebral prominence on the convex side and a paravertebral depression on the concave side. This deformity is particularly apparent with forward bending.

In the sagittal plane, the human spine normally has some posterior curvature (kyphosis) in the thoracic spine and anterior curvature (lordosis) in the cervical and lumbar spine. The Cobb technique has been adopted to

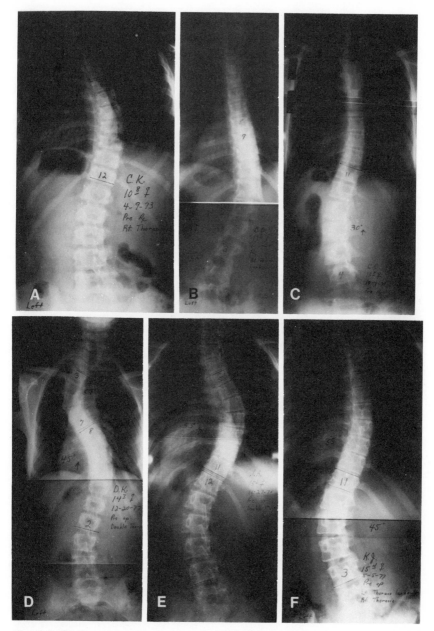

Fig. 7.2. Basic curve patterns seen in idiopathic scoliosis; *A*, right thoracic with apex T2-11; *B*, right thoracolumbar with apex at T12 or L1; *C*, left lumbar with apex L2-L4; *D*, double thoracic; *E*, right thoracic, left lumbar; *F*, left thoracolumbar, right thoracic.

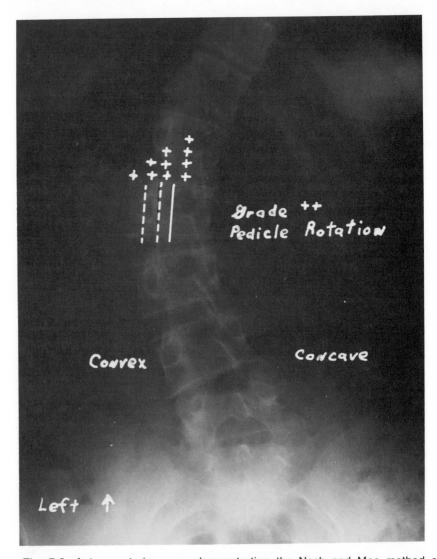

Fig. 7.3. Anteroposterior x-ray demonstrating the Nash and Moe method of grading vertebral rotation by measuring convex pedicle migration. The convex one-half of the vertebral body is divided into three equal segments. +, migration within first segment; + +, migration within second segment; + + +, migration within third segment; + + + +, migration past the midline.

quantitate these curves (Fig. 7.4). Normal values for cervical and lumbar lordosis are unknown, but for thoracic kyphosis the normal appears to be between 20 and 40 degrees (90). Sacral inclination should be about 45 degrees.

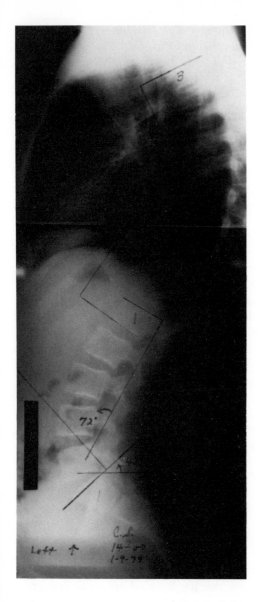

Fig. 7.4. X-ray showing the Cobb technique of curve measurement adopted for lateral plane quantitation.

SPINE BIOMECHANICS

The chest cage, abdominal cavity, and numerous extrinsic and intrinsic muscles attach to, provide support for, and influence the motion of the spine. Stripped of these attachments, the spine has been described as a semiflexible rod consisting of a sequence of rigid bodies (vertebrae) connected by deformable elements (ligaments). The vertebrae are further divided into the anterior (body) and the posterior (lamina, spinous process, pars interarticularis, facets, and transverse process) elements connected by pedicles. The bodies gain height by epiphyseal growth on their superior and inferior borders.

This structure allows mobility in any of the three body planes. These motions may be coupled, that is, one motion occurring simultaneously with another motion. For instance, with physiologic lateral bending of the upper spine, there is normally horizontal plane rotation of the vertebral body toward the concavity of the curve (84).

Without its soft tissue and rib attachments, the spine will support only about 2 kg before buckling laterally (8, 45). Adding the rib cage increases the stability by a factor of 3 (5). Experimental studies of scoliotic deformities suggest that transsection of the costal vertebral ligaments most nearly duplicates the clinical deformity (48). These studies demonstrate consistent but variable coupling of frontal plane curvature and horizontal vertebral body rotation toward the convexity of the curve.

With the exceptions of congenital vertebral anomaly and postirradiation scoliosis, spinal deformity apparently initially develops in the deformable ligaments (71). Eventually, the deformity results in slowing of vertebral epiphyseal growth on the concave side and wedging of the vertebral body. This is thought to be an example of the Heuter-Volkmann law, which states that pathological pressure on the epiphysis results in decreased growth whereas decreased pressure results in accelerated growth.

Mechanical properties of the ligaments are important in the development and treatment of spinal deformities. Mechanically, the ligaments behave in a viscoelastic manner, that is, the deformity or strain will depend on the deforming force (stress) and the time over which the stress is applied. Practical consequences of this are creep (increasing strain under constant stress) and relaxation (decreasing stress under constant strain) (86). Creep explains curve progression under the constant stress of gravity, and stress relaxation explains the need to frequently take up the slack in corrective orthotic pads.

Spine deformities are controlled by longitudinal and transverse forces. These forces may be applied actively by muscle contraction, or passively. Longitudinal forces are most effective in the treatment of large deformities. For frontal plane deformity (scoliosis), this has been estimated at 53 degrees or more (86). This is because they are being applied through relatively long lever arms. Longitudinal forces have very little corrective effect on rotation. Transverse forces are most effective on smaller curves, again, because they are acting through a longer lever arm. Combined longitudinal and transverse forces are more effective than either alone.

ORTHOTIC MATERIALS

Spinal deformity orthotics have traditionally been made from leather and metal, either steel or aluminum. During the 1960's, molded plastics were introduced (86). As it has become apparent that their properties most nearly meet the ideal requirements of orthotic material (56), the use of plastics has markedly expanded (50).

Plastics are classified as thermosetting or thermoplastic. Thermoplastics are the type most widely used in orthotics (50).

The low-temperature thermoplastics that are important in spine deformity are Orthoplast and K-Splint. The working temperature for these materials is approximately 140°F (60°C). In 1967, Orthoplast was introduced as a replacement material for the leather Milwaukee brace girdle. The main problem with Orthoplast has been lack of durability.

Expanded polyethylene foam (Plastazote) is a nonrigid thermoplastic with a working temperature ranging from 140–300°F (60–150°C), depending on the thickness of the material. Thick sheets have been utilized for the direct forming of supportive spinal jackets. Thin sheets may be used for lining. Other commonly used types of expanded polethylene foam are Aliplast, Alimed, and Pelite.

Rigid molded thermoplastics are now in common use for spinal orthotics. The working temperature is approximately 350–400°F (175–205°C), depending upon the material used. They are formed on positive molds of the patient. Polypropylene has excellent flexural strength characteristics and is currently widely used. Other rigid thermoplastics in common use are polyethylene and polycarbonate (Lexan). Polyethylene does not have the fatigue resistance of polypropylene. Polycarbonate is much more rigid and is more expensive.

Current Spinal Orthotics Practice

In 1975, a new nomenclature of orthotics was developed and published (2) (see Chapter 1). It is based on naming the joints crossed by the orthosis and the control desired for these joints (38). For the upper and lower extremities, this terminology seems to have been well accepted. This may be because extremity orthoses were already being referred to as short and long braces with few eponyms remaining in common usage. For the spine, this terminology has been less well accepted, apparently because the spine braces are still largely referred to by eponyms and not by a description of the brace. While making the transfer to a standard nomenclature, it will undoubtedly be necessary to retain the eponyms until the practice of spine deformity orthotics is more standardized. To be more specific, the prescription should, at this time, contain four items: diagnosis, generic nomenclature, eponum, and modifications.

Spinal deformity orthoses will be considered under the heading of: cervico-thoraco-lumbo-sacral orthoses (CTLSO); thoracolumbosacral orthoses (TLSO); and lumbosacral orthoses (LSO).

Cervico-thoraco-lumbo-sacral Orthoses (CTLSO)
MILWAUKEE BRACE (Fig. 7.5)

The Milwaukee brace is undoubtedly the most extensively analyzed and utilized spinal deformity orthosis. The principles involved have been borrowed to a greater or lesser extent by developers of subsequent orthoses.

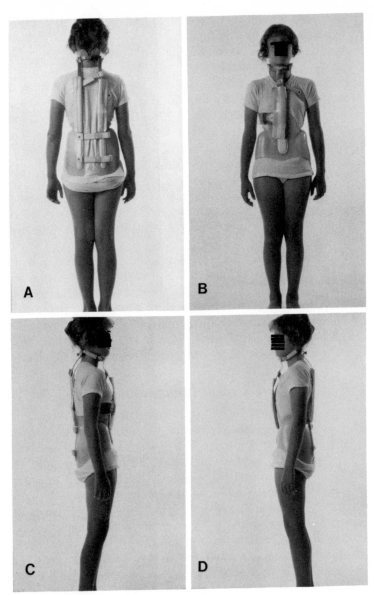

Fig. 7.5. Four views of a Milwaukee brace: *A*, posterior; *B*, anterior; *C*, right lateral; *D*, left lateral.

The basic Milwaukee brace consists of a pelvic girdle and superstructure. To this basic brace, corrective pads are added. The orthosis is constructed to provide as little unwanted restriction of the torso as possible. It is designed to develop and encourage both active and passive longitudinal forces and active and passive transverse forces. All indications are that the transverse forces predominate. The pelvic girdle is the foundation for the remainder of the brace. In principle, the brace controls the lower (caudad) portion of the spine, thereby gaining better control of the upper portion of the spine (33).

The pelvic girdle is formed on a modified positive plaster mold of the patient's pelvis. The developers cast the patient in an upright position without correction. Our preference is to cast the patient in a corrected position, utilizing longitudinal distraction and pelvic tilt in the standing frame (49). Specific modifications of the positive mold include deepening the indentation over the iliac crests, relief over the anterior iliac spines, flattening over the abdomen to encourage pelvic tilt, and continuation of the mold well down over the buttocks. This places the pelvis in a position of pelvic tilt with decreased lumbar lordosis. Only in patients with relative thoracic hypokyphosis should the pelvis tilt be less severe. Lack of proper pelvic tilt has been the most frequent serious construction deficiency in the Milwaukee brace. The girdle retains an abdominal apron which extends to just below the xiphoid process and just clears the lower ribs, thereby providing a compressive force on the abdomen. This produces a longitudinal corrective force on the spine by unloading the intervertebral discs (58). The girdle is opened and closed from the rear.

The original Milwaukee brace girdle was made from leather reinforced with Monel waist pieces. When thermoplastics became available, reuse of positive molds became feasible. With this came the realization that the girdle could be ordered and prefabricated on standard measurements. Some prefabricated girdles are available commercially. Over the years we have developed an inventory of 15 modified positive plaster models and approximately 90% of the time are able to prefabricate a girdle of the appropriate size.

Another advantage of the thermoplastic mold is the ease with which trochanteric extensions can be incorporated at the time of the trim. These extensions may be extremely helpful to balance the brace once corrective forces have been added above the pelvis.

The Milwaukee brace superstructure consists of three expandable metal uprights. The one placed anteriorly is made of aluminum to allow better visualization of the spine with x-rays. The two posterior uprights are of stainless steel. Superiorly, the uprights are attached to a stainless steel metal neck ring which is inclined approximately 20° anteriorly. The neck ring closes in back with a knurl nut. There are two occipital pads and one anterior throat mold attached to the neck ring. Originally, the latter was a mandibular pad and, combined, these pads were designed to provide constant passive longitudinal distractive force. This force, measured by dynamometers, in standing was 1.9 kg (35, 60) to 2.5 kg (30), with relatively more force on the mandibular pad than on the occipital pad. These forces increased to 5.1 kg in the supine sleeping position and 6.4 kg during lateral torso shift while standing (35). These changes indicate an increase in passive longitudinal distraction. These forces resulted in troublesome bite deformities. As a result, the neck ring was lowered and, in 1969, the mandibular pad was replaced with a throat mold. This lowered the passive distraction force to approximately 0.4 kg standing and 1.22 kg supine (55). These changes have eliminated mandibular deformities and do not appear to have affected the desired results obtained by wearing a Milwaukee brace. This observation is compatible with subsequent observations that passive longitudinal distraction force is less important than transverse corrective forces.

An assortment of pads may be added to the pelvic girdle superstructure (27). These are designed to provide transverse corrective forces. They will be discussed from caudad to cephalad.

The lumbar pad (Fig. 7.6) is designed to treat lumbar curves. It has undergone marked evolution since introduction of the brace. In fact, the lumbar pad, as we know it today, was not included in the original description of the brace. What has evolved is a delta-shaped polyethylene foam pad secured by opposing Velcro surfaces to the inside of the posterior portion of the girdle. The delta shape is necessary to avoid pressure on the lower ribs and the iliac crest, while at the same time delivering maximum pressure to the lumbar spine. The pad should contain radiopaque markers to allow x-ray confirmation of position. It should provide corrective force on the convex transverse processes of L2, 3, and 4. In this position, the pad provides a constant passive, transversely directed force which corrects both lateral curvature and horizontal plane rotation. The force can be increased by forceful active flexion of the lumbar spine, which further drives the convex side of the spinal column into the pad. It is necessary to have the girdle relief area posteriorly on the concave side in order to allow rotatory correction to occur.

The oval pad (Fig. 7.7) is designed for the treatment of thoracolumbar

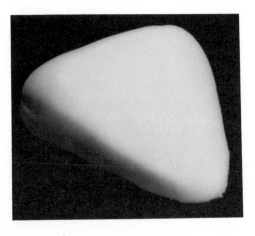

Fig. 7.6. Delta-shaped polyethylene foam lumbar pad added to the Milwaukee brace to treat lumbar curves.

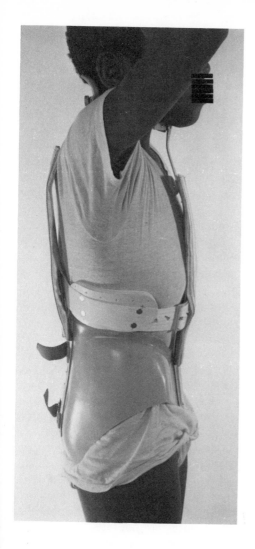

Fig. 7.7. View of a Milwaukee brace with the oval pad added for the treatment of a thoracolumbar curve.

curves. It is an Orthoplast or polyethylene-backed, Aliplast-faced pad suspended by 1 ½-inch wide Dacron straps from the anterior upright and the posterior upright on the convex side. It is used in conjunction with a lumbar pad and provides corrective force through the tenth and eleventh ribs, thereby providing symmetry to the thorax.

The "L" pad (Fig. 7.5C) is indicated for the treatment of mid and lower thoracic curves. It is an Orthoplast or polyethylene-backed, Aliplast-faced pad suspended by 1 ½-inch Dacron straps from the anterior upright and the posterior upright on the convex side. It should cover and control the inferior tip of the scapula and provide force through the ribs originating at the apex of the curve. If the standing lateral x-ray reveals a relative thoracic kyphosis, the medial border of the L pad should be placed under the posterior upright and an anterior outrigger should be included in order to clear the L pad support from the chest. If there is marked kyphosis, the Orthoplast pad is thickened, thereby putting more pressure on the ribs of the convex side. As the kyphosis and rib humps correct, additional thickness is added to the L pad under the upright, or the uprights are moved toward the thoracic cage as necessary to keep the L pad engaged on the thoracic hump. On the other hand, if there is relative thoracic lordosis, the L pad should provide little posterior pressure and thus be brought out from under the posterior upright. In addition, it should be elongated and the anterior outrigger shortened in order to move the horizontal vector from relative posterior to posterolateral (27, 92). It should not be moved directly laterally. In either case, the concave side posterior upright should clear the chest cage even during the thoracic arching exercise. This location of the posterior upright allows for the correction of the paravertebral depression (79).

Thoracic L pad pressures have been measured at 2.9 to 6.5 kg, and they are greater in curves over 40° (30). This pad produces the dominant transverse force which, if not checked, can overpower the other pads producing significant secondary curves (6).

Removal of the thoracic pad results in an increase in longitudinal distraction force of only 0.63 kg (60). In computer simulation studies, Andriacchi et al. (6) report that utilizing optimum known external Milwaukee brace forces, the optimum correction expected of a 43° right thoracic curve is 8.9°, or 21%. This is considerably less than the expected initial brace correction of 35% for thoracic curves (51). These observations suggest that the basic pelvic-girdle superstructure brace stimulates active corrective forces.

The costal margin pad (Fig. 7.8) is designed to improve the cosmetic deformity of the ribs. It may be an Orthoplast-backed, Aliplast-faced pad attached to a metal outrigger or an extension of a molded plastic girdle. The outrigger is attached to the anterior upright so that the pad provides pressure over the prominent anterior rib cage. It is located on the concave side of the thoracic curve and provides a counterrotation force.

The axillary sling (Fig. 7.5B) is sometimes used as a counterforce against the L pad. This sling helps balance the upper torso and provides longitudinal unloading. In our practice, the axillary sling is constructed like the lower half of a shoulder ring. It is a polyethylene or polypropylene C-shaped half-ring suspended by 1-inch wide Dacron straps from the anterior upright and the posterior upright on the convex side. Supplemental suspension to prevent excess axillary pressure is sometimes included to attach the half-ring to the pelvic girdle with an adjustable Dacron strap. The axillary C-shaped ring is sometimes discontinued after the patient has become acclimated to the brace and developed a righting reflex in order to bring the upper torso back in line against the displacement force of the L pad. The axillary C-shaped ring also helps elevate a depressed shoulder. On occasion,

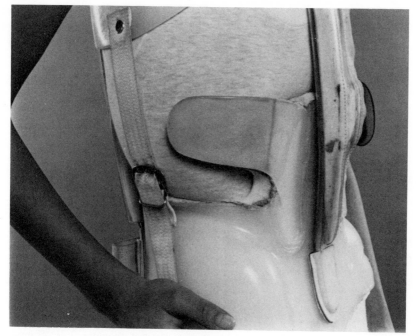

Fig. 7.8. View of a Milwaukee brace with a costal margin pad added.

we have used it to treat a mild upper thoracic curve, but have no proof of its efficiency.

The shoulder ring (Fig. 7.9, *A* and *B*) is also designed to treat some upper thoracic curves (apex above T6) when the shoulder is not elevated. It is made of polypropylene or polyethylene from a positive mold of the patient's shoulder. It is suspended by two Dacron straps, one anterior and one from the posterior far side upright, passing under the near side upright. The upper thoracic curve is the most difficult curve to treat and, therefore, this modification appears to provide less effective control than other pads. Fortunately, this curve pattern is not very common, but unfortunately is frequently overlooked unless 36-inch x-rays are utilized. Because the L pad for the midthoracic curve will tend to aggravate this upper thoracic curve, we must recognize this high curve and treat it effectively.

The trapezius pad may also be indicated for the treatment of the high thoracic curve, especially when it is associated with an elevated shoulder. This Orthoplast-backed, Aliplast-faced pad is contoured over the shoulder and attached to the uprights by Dacron webbing. The pull is directed inferiorly and medially.

For the treatment of kyphosis, Orthoplast-backed, Aliplast-faced pads are added to both posterior uprights and centered one vertebra below the apex. By increasing the thickness of the pads, progressive pressure can be devel-

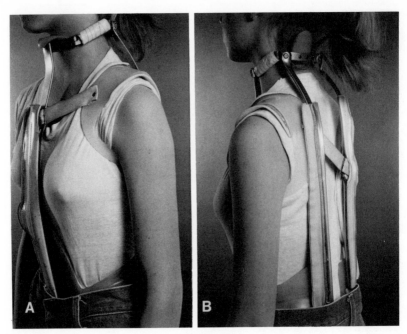

Fig. 7.9. Views of the Milwaukee brace showing the shoulder ring: *A*, anterior view; *B*, posterior view.

oped. In bracing for kyphosis, it is important to keep the throat mold well back into the neck, centering the head over the shoulders and trochanters in the lateral upright position. This increases the effectiveness of the kyphosis padding and is a point that must not be overlooked (Fig. 7.10, *A* and *B*) (66).

Some patients with thoracic hyperkyphosis have tight pectorals. These may be stretched by pectoral pads or shoulder slings. Pectoral pads are Orthoplast-backed, Aliplast-faced, and suspended from the anterior upright by metal outriggers which extend to the deltopectoral groove. They apply pressure to the anterior aspect of the shoulder. Shoulder slings are Orthoplast caps molded to the anterior deltoid surface and suspended by Dacron draw straps from outriggers on the posterior uprights.

With cervical scoliosis, it is occasionally necessary to add a superstructure to the cervical ring in order to control head position. This may apply pressure behind the mastoid or even extend up behind the ear toward the parietal area.

The Milwaukee brace prescription should indicate the deformity being braced, modifications of the brace girdle, and the specific pads to be added. In addition, leg-length discrepancy of greater than 1 cm, as indicated by the levels of the iliac crest on the standing x-ray, should usually be equalized by a shoe lift. We prefer to have the orthotist present when the prescription is

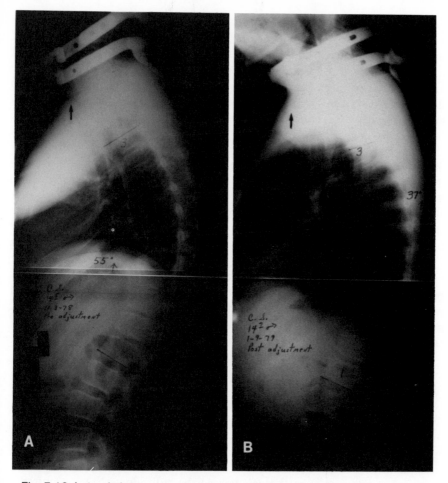

Fig. 7.10. Lateral plane x-rays showing the importance of the throat mold position while treating for kyphosis: *A*, preadjustment; *B*, postadjustment.

being written. He or she should have access to the x-rays during casting, preliminary fitting, and checkout.

Checkout Procedure

The patient is seen by the prescribing physician and the orthotist at or shortly after the time of brace pickup. This provides a checkout to be sure that the brace is properly prescribed, constructed, and fitted (24, 53). An upright, in brace x-ray is taken to ensure proper pad placement and curve correction.

In stance (Fig. 7.5, *A–D*), the anterior inferior trimline of the pelvic girdle must extend to the symphysis pubis and maintain a posture of posterior pelvic tilt. The anterior abdominal apron should extend superiorly to the xiphoid and the lower ribs. Posteriorly, the superior trim of the girdle and uprights should clear the lumbar spine. This allows for more correction of lumbar lordosis during pelvic tilt exercises. To accommodate sitting the anterior inferior edge should curve up over the thigh to allow 90° of hip flexion (Fig. 7.11, *A–C*). The posterior inferior trim line of the girdle should extend to within 2.5 cm of a firm seat. There should be a 4- to 5-cm gap between the edges of the girdle at its posterior closure. The uprights should then be checked to make certain that they clear the body, except for points of desired pressure, which are transmitted through pads. They are perpendicular to the girdle, and the posterior uprights are parallel to each other. The posterior uprights should pass just medial to the scapula. The neck ring should clear the neck laterally by about 1 to 1.5 cm on each side. The throat mold should be 1 cm inferior to the mandible and should clear the larynx by about 1 cm anteriorly when the gaze is level. For patients with a prominent larynx, a throat frame may be necessary (available from Fillauer Orthopedics, Inc.). The occipital pads should be placed inferior to (not behind) the occiput and bent posteriorly approximately 45° to a vertical reference line. With the patient sitting, the position of the neck ring should not change. If it does, the anterior and/or the posterior inferior trimlines of the pelvic girdle are probably too long.

The pads are then evaluated for proper placement. Residual skin blush or erythema upon brace removal will serve to identify the sites and intensity of pad pressure.

Proper alignment, pad placement, and deformity correction are confirmed by a standing x-ray (Fig. 7.12, *A* and *B*). In the case of scoliosis, an anterioposterior view is usually satisfactory. However, if the prebracing lateral x-ray has shown a deviation from normal in the sagittal plane, it is desirable to confirm correction of lumbar lordosis or thoracic hyperkyphosis and to ensure that thoracic hyperlordosis has not been produced. This requires a standing lateral x-ray in the brace. In scoliosis treatment, the standing anterioposterior x-ray of a patient in a well-fit orthosis can be expected to demonstrate an average correction of approximately 16% for an upper thoracic curve, 35% for a thoracic curve, and 43% for a lumbar curve (51).

The patient and family are then instructed in brace wear. It is recommended that a nonribbed cotton T-shirt which extends below the girdle be worn under the brace and changed frequently in order to keep the brace clean and dry and to protect the skin. Additional skin hygiene and skin toughening involves rubbing alcohol treatment of the skin. Salves and creams should not be used.

Initially, it is recommended that someone assist the patient in putting on the brace. In practice, most patients eventually become independent in brace application. A common problem in brace wearing is not applying the

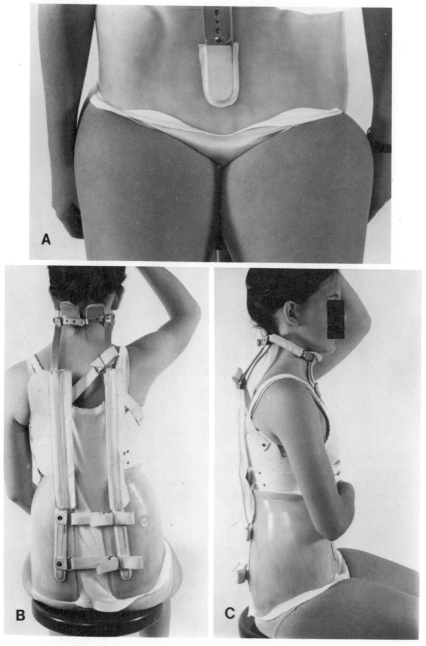

Fig. 7.11. Views of the Milwaukee brace showing: *A*, the anterior inferior trimline; *B*, the posterior inferior trim line; *C*, lateral view of the inferior trimlines, uprights, neck ring, throat mold, and occipital pads.

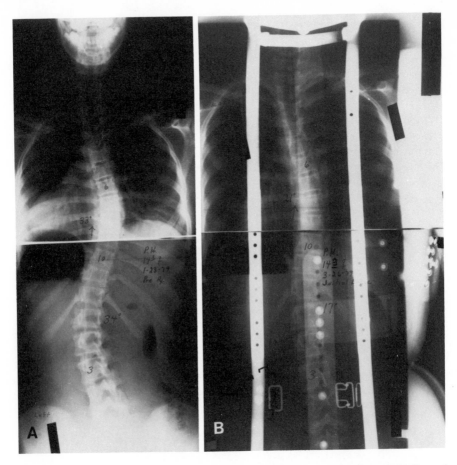

Fig. 7.12. *A*, anteroposterior x-ray showing a left thoracolumbar, right thoracic curve before treatment; *B*, anteroposterior x-ray of the same patient after being fitted in a Milwaukee brace, confirming proper pad placement, alignment, and deformity correction. (Delta pad marking staples and L pad rivets have been highlighted on x-ray.)

orthosis properly over the iliac crests. Also, the brace is often not tight enough, causing it to slide down over the iliac crest. The originators of the brace have indicated that no "break-in" time is necessary. We have tried this, but prefer a break-in time of 5 to 7 days to acclimate to full-time brace wear of 23 out of 24 hours.

The patients are instructed to wear the brace during physical education classes. They are requested not to participate in tackle football, hockey, wrestling, boxing, weight lifting (except for bench presses), springboard diving, trampoline, and highly flexible gymnastics. Otherwise, they are encouraged and expected to physically participate completely. In some situations we have allowed the patient to remove the brace during gym class, competitive sports, and other physical extracurricular activities. Out-of-brace swimming is encouraged, but the patient is instructed to remain in neck-deep water during this time.

Exercises

At or about the time of brace checkout, the patient is instructed by a trained physical therapist in an exercise program (14). This instruction includes both in- and out-of-brace exercises, and they should be done faithfully at least once daily, if not twice. Without these exercises, decreased trunk muscle activity could be expected to result in weakness (80). The exercises are designed to attain and maintain postural balance, curve correction, and muscle strength. They include pelvic tilt, lateral shift, and thoracic arching. Exercising in front of a mirror stimulates visual proprioceptive feedback and thereby reinforces exercise training (81). We emphasize that the thoracic arching maneuver is a means of correcting the rib deformity (79). In addition, breathing exercises are taught to improve chest expansion.

For patients with increased dorsal kyphosis, thoracic spine extension exercises are prescribed. We prefer an exercise with the patient out of the brace and resting on a bed or table in a prone position, with the hips bent 90° over the edge. This eliminates lumbar lordosis. The torso is then actively lifted, resulting in strong contraction of the spine extensors.

Follow-up

The first return visit should be in 1 to 2 months and thereafter at approximately 3-month intervals. The condition and fit of the brace, compliance of the patient to brace wear, and improvement of the curves are evaluated. A properly selected and fitted brace on a properly compliant patient will continue to improve the patient's curve for the first year or so that the brace is worn. The maximal improvement obtained is usually 17% for the upper thoracic curve, 38% for the thoracic curve, and 55% for the lumbar curve (51). Full-time wear is continued until the patient is skeletally mature (vertebral ring apophysis fused), or until stability of improvement has been proven. Spine stability is one of the most variable and difficult factors to assess and prove. We evaluate stability by comparing curve magnitude on in-brace and out-of-brace standing anterior-posterior (AP) or posterior-anterior (PA) x-rays (21). When do we start weaning the patient from the brace? After the patient has been out of the brace for 4 hours and there is not more than a 3°, or at most a 5°, loss in correction on a standing x-ray. This sequence is repeated at approximately 3-month intervals, increasing the out-of-brace time until the brace is worn at night only. This transition period requires approximately 1 year. This is one of the most difficult phases of the Milwaukee brace program, as there is tremendous pressure from the patient to hurry the weaning process. However, for optimal bracing results, proven stability is essential before weaning progresses.

Night wear continues for approximately 1 to 2 years while the patient's spine is stabilizing. The age at which spine stability occurs and curve progression ceases is most commonly between 17 and 19 years. It may be earlier or later. For optimum result, nighttime brace wear should continue until stabilization is proven. Continued nighttime wear under these circumstances is generally well accepted by the patient (21).

Results

The Milwaukee brace has reportedly been effective in the treatment of juvenile idiopathic scoliosis (42, 52), and at least several groups have independently documented its effectiveness in the treatment of idiopathic adolescent scolosis (34, 40, 47, 51, 64, 69). For idiopathic adolescent scoliosis, the average total brace time is approximately 3 years. At the completion of brace wearing, the improvement averages 10% for the upper thoracic curve, 24% for the thoracic curve, and 23% for the lumbar curve (51). Follow-up 5 years or more after the end of brace treatment reveals that on the average the curves have either returned to their pretreatment value (28) or improved 8% (47). Factors generally thought to favorably influence brace treatment are skeletal immaturity at the time of bracing, more flexible and less severe thoracic curves, compliant patients, and cooperative parents.

These results and the recent observation that 20% of growing patients with 20 to 30° curves observed a minimum of 2 years do not progress (68) have clarified bracing recommendations. Currently, spinal deformity bracing is primarily indicated for idiopathic scolosis patients with progressive curves, i.e. 10° progression for 15 to 20° curves and 5° progression for 20 to 30° curves, and for those whose curves are still small enough to be in the nonsurgical category at the end of treatment, roughly 30 to 45°. With increasing understanding of the natural history of idiopathic scoliosis, these recommendations remain subject to further refinement. Under ideal circumstances, lasting improvement may be obtained (Fig. 7.13, A–F).

Some surgeons continue to use the Milwaukee brace for its originally intended purpose, i.e., immobilization following surgical correction. By means of intervital wireless telemetry, Nachemson has demonstrated that their Milwaukee brace is as effective, if not more so, than the Risser cast in relieving pressure on the distraction rod. In supine patients, the Milwaukee brace relieved the force on the Harrington distraction rod by 2 to 4 kg, and in standing by 4 to 6 kg (60). These observations provide the only available direct evidence that the external forces developed by the brace effectively reach the spine.

Adolescent round back and Scheuermann's kyphosis reportedly respond

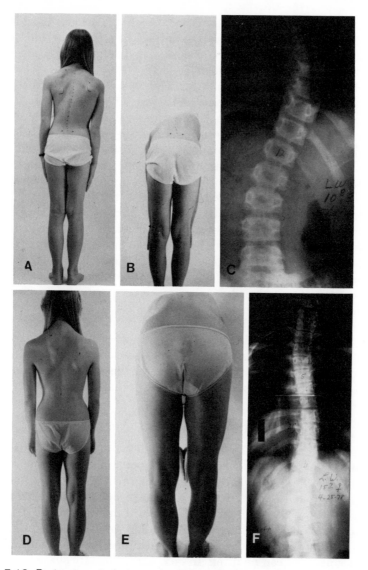

Fig. 7.13. Pretreatment photographs (*A* and *B*) of a 10-year 4-month-old female with right thoracic scoliosis measuring 40° (*C*). Current photographs (*D* and *E*) at age 15 years 7 months demonstrating satisfactory clinical correction. The curve now measures 21° (*F*). Her Milwaukee brace treatment continued for 55 months. (Fig. 7.13, *A–C*, also appeared in *J. Kans. Med. Soc., 76:* 287, 1975.)

favorably to Milwaukee brace treatment. Moe initiated this treatment in 1959, and Bradford *et al.* (22) have recently reported results of 75 patients, 28 boys and 47 girls, with Scheuermann's kyphosis who have completed brace treatment. The average age at initial treatment was 14 years 4 months, and the average wearing time was 34 months. Kyphosis improved from an average of 59° to 35°. Factors compromising correction included greater than 65° of kyphosis, iliac epiphyseal closure, and vertebral wedging of more than 10°.

The Milwaukee brace has been reported to be helpful in the treatment of congenital scoliosis when a hemivertebra is a small portion of a long flexible curve and to correct head tilt associated with a cervical thoracic curve (88). The brace has limited usefulness in preventing or retarding deformity progression in Marfan's syndrome (67). The brace has reportedly been effective in paralytic scoliosis, but only with extensive modification, including containment of the lower rib cage. These modifications significantly alter the basic structure of the Milwaukee brace (23).

There are a few other CTLSO's. The Lyonese brace used by Dr. Stagnara (54) in France restricts the chest cage and therefore is not recommended, either as a CTLSO or TLSO. We have no experience with the Orthodyne CTLSO developed by W. Keuhnegger (41); however, it does not appear to provide adequate pelvic control. The Boston brace (discussed below) with added superstructure is a CTLSO.

Thoracolumbosacral Orthoses (TLSO)

These orthoses in general can be divided into those that are prefabricated and those that are custom fabricated. While there are several prefabricated orthoses on the market, the dominant type at this time appears to be the Boston brace (Physical Support System, Inc.). Therefore, this will be most extensively discussed.

PREFABRICATED MOLDED PLASTIC TLSO

The Boston brace (36, 37, 81, 82) is illustrated in Fig. 7.14. The unique feature of the Boston brace is the prefabricated 3-mm-thick polypropylene rear-opening girdle. As the girdle is vacuum formed on a positive mold of a normal torso, areas of corrective pressure and relief are prebuilt into it. In addition, it features a systematized scheme of trimlines and pad placement to balance and correct frontal, sagittal, and horizontal plane deformity.

Twenty girdle sizes are available, and with these, approximately 95% of all scoliosis patients can be fitted. In fact, approximately 80% can be fitted with six of the sizes. Girdle fitting is aided by the 7-mm-thick polyethylene foam lining and the large iliac crest rolls of firmer polyethylene foam. This lining also increases the total contact of the girdle.

Modifications of the prefabricated girdle are at least partially guided by the development of a blueprint using a standing AP x-ray. The most important points in the x-ray blueprint are the perpendicular reference line, the degree of lateral pelvic tilt, and the location, size, and rotation of the scoliotic curve. From this information, the strategy for standard and modified trimlines and pad placement is developed. The anterior middle and thigh trim lines are kept as low as possible to still allow 90° of hip flexion for

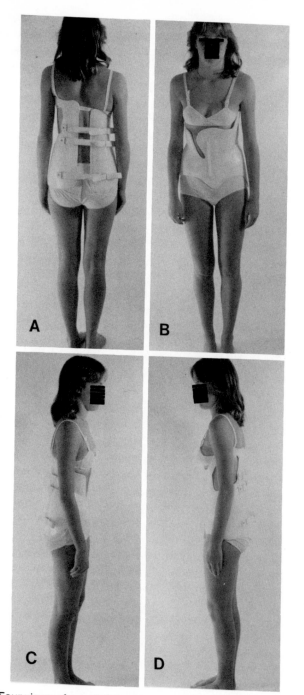

Fig. 7.14. Four views of a prefabricated polypropylene Boston brace; A, posterior; B, anterior; C, right lateral; D, left lateral.

sitting. Posterior trimlines just clear the seat of a hard chair by 1 or 2 cm. The lateral trimlines should pass about 1 cm above the trochanters unless trochanteric extension is desired to improve balance. This inferior extension is placed on the same side as the primary curve, that is, the one to which the most pressure is being applied. The width of the posterior opening should be the width of the largest lumbar vertebra. The posterior superior trimlines start at the level of T8 (inferior edge of the scapula) and sweep sharply to the top of the iliac crest pad. The superior anterior apron clears the edge of the ribs, and the xiphoid process then sweeps to the top of the iliac crest pad. Specialized trimlines may be necessary to control the rib cage, but exact trimlines for the treatment of the thoracic curve have yet to be established scientifically.

The key factor in treating the lumbar curve is the lumbar pad. Its location is similar to that described for the Milwaukee brace, that is, the pad clears the ribs above and the iliac crest below and is aimed at the transverse processes of L2, 3, and 4. In addition, anterior counterrotation pads are placed below and above the level of the lumbar pad on the same side and on the opposite side counterrotational posterior pressure points also above and below the level of the lumbar pad. This leaves a void on the concave side opposite the lumbar pad (Fig. 7.15). The pelvic tilt exercise further increases the derotational force on the lumbar spine.

The brace is fitted firmly and progressively tightened. This results in soft tissue atrophy and, as the brace is tightened, the posterior edges of the brace

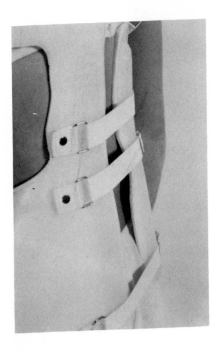

Fig. 7.15. Clinical photo showing the void on the concave side, opposite a left delta pad. This allows lumbar curve correction during active pelvic tilt.

come closer together. This causes the lumbar pad to become less effective. The position must be restored by filling the inside of the front of the brace with additional layers of polyethylene foam.

The Boston brace is designed primarily for the treatment of lumbar and thoracolumbar curves. For the treatment of thoracic curves with apex above T8, the developers of the Boston brace recommend addition of a Milwaukee brace superstructure and pads. This converts the Boston brace to a CTLSO. For the treatment of kyphosis, a floating anteriorly suspended apex pad has been substituted for the posterior upright pad of the Milwaukee brace.

The checkout and follow-up procedure is similar to that described for the Milwaukee brace. Both in-brace and out-of-brace exercises are emphasized. The brace wearer is urged to be physically active.

The developers report average improvement at the time of brace checkout of 54% for lumbar curves and 64% for thoracolumbar curves (82). Short-term results will soon be available on 60 patients who have been out of the brace for a minimum of 12 months. Without added superstructure, the curves showed a 3° (13%) improvement, and with the superstructure added, the average improvement was 2° (6%) (39). Thus, the results to date appear to be the same as those for the Milwaukee brace.

In summary, the most appealing aspects of the Boston brace girdle are its excellent control of the pelvis and lumbosacral junction, its correction of balance by the trochanter pad, and its cosmetic appearance. Prefabrication reduces expense and saves hours of orthotic construction time.

CUSTOM-FABRICATED MOLDED PLASTIC TLSO

One of the first post-Milwaukee brace era corrective body jackets was the front opening Orthoplast jacket developed at the Alfred I. DuPont Institute in Wilmington, Delaware (25, 26). It was fabricated directly on the patient while on a traction casting table, with full longitudinal traction as well as lateral corrective forces being applied. Improvement was documented by x-ray. Wearing time and wearing instructions were similar to those of the Milwaukee brace.

The DuPont Orthoplast jacket is the only body jacket for which intermediate results are available (26). They have recently reported on 48 patients with 63 curves. The average age when the patients were first braced was 11 years 10 months, and wearing continued for 59 months. At an average of 15 months following weaning, 55% of the curves were unchanged, 35% of the curves were improved more than 5°, and only 10% of the curves progressed more than 5°. The majority (73%) of the curves were less than 30° at the time of initial bracing. Thus, the patients were younger and had smaller curves than the series treated by Milwaukee bracing.

The major objection to the Orthoplast body jacket is that it restricts lung function; 18% on the average (25). In addition, it may result in permanent chest cage deformity. For these reasons, this orthosis has not gained widespread acceptance for the treatment of idiopathic scoliosis.

Essentially, all orthotic facilities dealing with spinal deformities are now custom-fabricating rigid molded plastic TLSO's for the treatment of idiopathic scoliosis. Among these are the front-opening orthosis (New York Orthopaedic) (94), the Prenyl jacket (65), and the Lexan jacket (31).

In general, it seems safe to conclude that for the treatment of lumbar and lumbosacral curves, custom-fabricated TLSO's have no advantage over the prefabricated Boston system, and when utilized for thoracic curve treatment, they suffer from all of the disadvantages of the Orthoplast jacket system.

The custom-fabricated TLSO has become useful in supporting the unstable spine of patients with neuromuscular disease. In addition, it has been helpful in the postoperative immobilization of patients with nonsensitive skin where access for care and cleaning is important. We prefer the side opening bivalved polypropylene TLSO (Fig. 7.16, *A–C*) and usually provide an anterior opening similar to that utilized in our postoperative plaster of Paris TLSO (Fig. 7.17). This is designed to provide minimum interference with respiration.

For some patients, casting on a frame is difficult. In these cases the negative cast may be obtained by overlapping sequentially placed anterior and posterior plaster of Paris shells.

SEATING ORTHOSES

Molded plastics have opened a new era of seating orthoses for the severely handicapped (92) (see Chapter 1). These are designed to promote upright seating and retard progression of scoliosis and kyphosis. They may be suspended from the wheelchair, allowing gravity correction of the curvature (73).

METAL TLSO'S

There are only a few metal orthoses in use that are designed to control spine deformities. These include the underarm orthosis of Dr. Ponte in Italy and the Kosair orthosis (a combined crutch-brace and Jewett hyperextension front) utilized by Dr. Leatherman in Louisville (43). We do not have experience with these. The Jewett hyperextension brace (see Chapter 6) has previously been shown to be ineffective in the treatment of juvenile kyphosis (46).

SOFT MATERIAL TLSO'S

For infants with scoliosis, the Kalibis harness may be utilized. It is designed to provide a 3-point corrective force system on the spine.

Lumbosacral Orthosis (LSO)

A modified Norton-Brown brace has been utilized for the treatment of excessive lumbar lordosis in the achondroplastic dwarf (74). Long-term

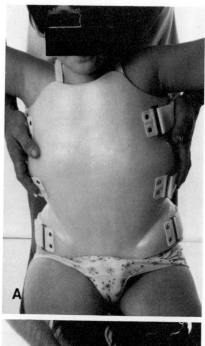

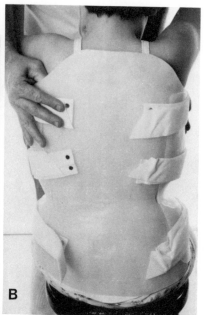

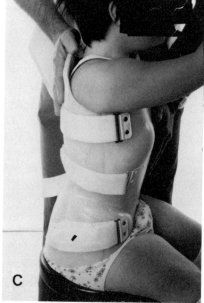

Fig. 7.16. Side-opening bivalved polypropylene thoracolumbosacral orthosis used for postoperative immobilization of neuromuscular patients: *A*, anterior; *B*, posterior; *C*, lateral.

results are not known. The same goal is obtainable with a Boston brace girdle.

Contraindications and Complications

Spinal deformity bracing is contraindicated in congenital scoliosis with an unsegmented bar, congenital kyphosis, classic neurofibromatosis, and acute

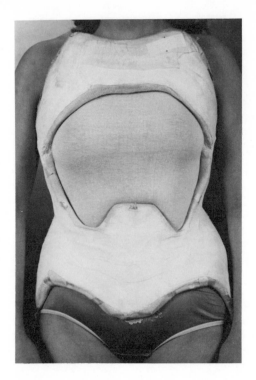

Fig. 7.17. Anterior opening recommended for custom thoracolumbosacral orthoses.

angle kyphosis secondary to myelomeningocele (89). In addition, hypokyphosis may be a contraindication (90).

There are many possible problems associated with spinal deformity bracing. These include: skin problems, nerve compression, wearing noncompliance, psychological disturbance, creation of secondary deformities such as chest cage constriction, overdevelopment of compensatory curves, restriction of pelvic ring growth, and fat thighs.

Skin problems may be related to pressure, the material used for the brace, or occlusion of the skin, especially in hot, humid climates. Pressure problems are related to an ill-fitted or outgrown brace. The most common site for pressure sores is the iliac crest (Fig. 7.18). The usual solution is localized relief either by bending out, cutting away, or by counterpadding. In some situations, it may be necessary to rebuild a portion of the brace. Impending or established pressure sores should be treated with temporary brace removal while alterations are made or sites protected from irritation by nonadherent Telfa. Adhesive dressings should not be used on pressure points under the brace.

The brace material can cause a chemical skin irritation or an allergic reaction. Any one or a combination of treatments may be necessary. The inner lining of the brace should be cleansed regularly using a moist cloth for leather and hypoallergenic soap and water for thermoplastics. Patients may

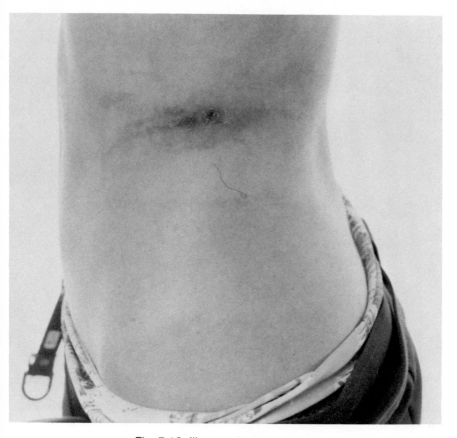

Fig. 7.18. Iliac crest pressure sore.

be allergic to detergents used to wash the undergarments. In such cases a change of the detergent or soap and multiple laundry rinses are recommended. In rare cases, it may be necessary to change the material lining the brace, cover the lining with moleskin, or even exchange the brace for one fabricated of a different material. Allergic skin rashes may be treated with a steroid cream.

Factors such as patient constitution or climate may result in excess perspiration, especially under the girdle or pads. Frequent T-shirt changes and brace ventilation with perforating holes usually solve the problem. When coupled with poor skin hygiene, skin maceration may be complicated by fungus infection (tinea). Compared to an allergic rash, tinea of the skin is less pruritic, is often scaly, and typically exhibits a raised "active" border (Fig. 7.19). The diagnosis is confirmed by fungus culture or microscopic visualization of mycelial filaments of fungi among skin scrapings suspended in potassium hydroxide. Treatment of funal infection consists of cleansings,

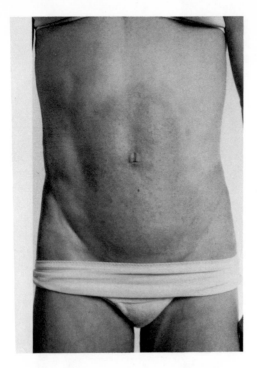

Fig. 7.19. Fungus infection coinciding with abdominal apron.

aeration, and topical antifungal agents such as sulfa salicylic acid ointment or miconazole cream.

Numbness along the anterior lateral aspect of the thigh indicates excessive pressure on the lateral femoral cutaneous nerve just medial to the anterior superior spine or on the lateral cutaneous branch of the iliohypogastric nerve. Treatment is by relief of the girdle in that area.

It has been widely assumed that a spinal deformity orthosis not extending above the neck (TLSO) would be more acceptable than one which extends above the neck (CTLSO). This has not been directly studied and remains to be proven.

It has been reported that several TLSO's have caused pulmonary constriction to a greater or lesser degrees (25, 54). However, the Milwaukee brace (CTLSO) does not appear to interfere significantly with pulmonary function (1, 62, 72).

Corrective force on the primary curve results in compensatory curves (6). At times, these compensatory curves may become more troublesome than the primary curves. For that reason, the compensatory curve should be protected by appropriate padding, and this problem will be avoided.

Restriction of pelvic ring growth does not appear to be a significant problem, and fat thighs can be expected to resolve soon after completion of brace wear (39, 83).

Noncompliance with brace wearing and psychological problems can be related but are not necessarily identical. For instance, some patients will not wear a spinal deformity brace but have no significant psychological problem. On the other hand, patients who wear the brace may develop significant psychological problems related to the brace.

The psychological aspects of spinal deformity bracing with the Milwaukee brace have been extensively studied (3, 7, 57, 70, 87). Factors thought to contribute to good wearing compliance are positive patient self-image, intelligence, cooperative parents, and a supportive home environment. The most effective adjustment mechanism appears to be denial (7). Adjustment and compliance problems are often related to preexisting conflicts. For most patients, it may actually be a character-building experience. However, some patients have varying degrees of difficulty adjusting to the brace. This is reflected by the fact that as many as 25% of patients are either partially or totally noncompliant to brace wear (51). For a few, the idea of brace wear is emotionally intolerable and, for these patients, bracing is contraindicated. A very small group of patients may become emotionally disturbed during the course of the brace treatment, and these patients should receive supportive therapeutic counseling.

Future Developments

It appears that the standard nomenclature for spinal deformity orthotics will become accepted and bracing practices standardized. Through research, a better understanding of the forces applied by the various spinal deformity orthoses and a better understanding of how to utilize these forces appear certain to develop. It seems likely that expanded utilization of prefabrication will occur.

Further study of spinal deformities should yield valuable information on such unknowns as prediction of curve progression, spinal stability, effectiveness of the various brace types, and better-defined bracing indications.

Alternative forms of treatment may be developed. Possibilities include paraspinal muscle stimulation either by implanted electrodes or surface electrodes, or biofeedback. As the pathogenesis and natural history of scoliosis and related spinal deformities are better understood, other treatment options may be developed. As always, change is inevitable.

Acknowledgment

The authors would like to thank Drs. Walter Blount, Milwaukee, Wisc., Wilton Bunch, Maywood, Ill., Hugh Watts, Philadelphia, Pa., and Robert Winter, Minneapolis, Minn. for providing invaluable assistance in the preparation of this chapter. We would also like to thank Janice Orrick, R.N., and Jan Brunks for major assistance in preparing the manuscript.

REFERENCES

1. ADLER, F. A., DEVINS, G., AND GUNN, W. Effect of Milwaukee brace on pulmonary function. Proceedings of SICOT Meeting, Jerusalem, 1972.
2. AMERICAN ACADEMY OF ORTHOPEDIC SURGEONS. *Atlas of Orthotics.* C. V. Mosby, Co., St. Louis, 1975.
3. ANDERSON, F., ASHER, M., CLARK, G., ORRICK, J., AND QUIASON, E. Adjustment of adolescent females to the treatment of idiopathic scoliosis. In preparation.
4. ANDERSON, M., HWANG, S-C., AND GREEN, W. T. Growth of the normal trunk in boys and girls during the second decade of life (related to age, maturity, and ossification of the iliac epiphysis). *J. Bone Joint Surg., 47A:* 1154–1164, 1965.
5. ANDRIACCHI, T., SCHULTZ, A., BELYTSCHKO, T., AND GALANTE, J. A model for studies of mechanical interactions between the human spine and rib cage. *J. Biomech., 7:* 497–507, 1974.
6. ANDRIACCHI, T. F., SCHULTZ, A. B., BELYTSCHKO, T. B., AND DeWALD, R. L. Milwaukee brace correction of idiopathic scoliosis. A biomechanical analysis and retrospective study. *J. Bone Joint Surg., 53:* 806–815, 1976.
7. APTAR, A., MOREN, G., MUNITZ, H., TYANO, B., MAOZ, B., AND WIJSENBEAK, H. The psychosocial sequelae of the Milwaukee brace in adolescent girls. From the Orthopaedic Department of Bailiason Medical Center and the Geha Psychiatric Hospital, Petah-Tiqua, Israel.
8. BELYTSCHKO, T. B., ANDRIACCHI, T. P., SCHULTZ, A. B., AND GALANTE, J. O. Analog studies of forces in the human spine: computational techniques. *J. Biomech., 6:* 361–371, 1973.
9. BENGTSSON, G., FALLSTROM, K., JANSSON, B., AND NACHEMSON, A. A psychological and psychiatric investigation of the adjustment of female scoliosis patients. *Acta Psychiatr. Scand., 50:* 50–59, 1974.
10. BJURE, J., AND NACHEMSON, A. Nontreated scoliosis. *Clin. Orthop., 93:* 44–52, 1973.
11. BLOUNT, W. P., SCHMIDT, A. C., KEEVER, E. D., AND LEONARD, E. T. The Milwaukee brace in the operative treatment of scoliosis. *J. Bone Joint Surg., 40A:* 511–525, 1958.
12. BLOUNT, W. P. Scoliosis and the Milwaukee brace. *Bull. Hosp. Joint Dis., 19:* 152, 1958.
13. BLOUNT, W. P. Bracing for scoliosis. *In Orthotics Etcetera,* B6 17-92, L617, p. 306, 1966.
14. BLOUNT, W. P., AND BOLINSKE, T. Physical therapy in the nonoperative treatment of scoliosis. *Phys. Ther. Rev., 47:* 919–925, 1967.
15. BLOUNT, W. P. Nonoperative treatment of scoliosis. In *Symposium of the Spine,* American Academy of Orthopaedic Surgeons, Cleveland, 1967, p. 188. C. V. Mosby Co., St. Louis, 1969.
16. BLOUNT, W. P. Use of the Milwaukee brace. *Orthop. Clin. North Am., 3:* 3–16, 1972.
17. BLOUNT, W. P., AND MOE, J. H. *The Milwaukee Brace.* Baltimore, Williams & Wilkins Company, 1973.
18. BLOUNT, W. P. Principles of treatment of scoliosis and round back with the Milwaukee brace. *Isr. J. Med. Sci., 9(6):* 745–750, 1973.
19. BLOUNT, W. P., AND MELLENCAMP, D. D. Scoliosis treatment—skeletal maturity evaluation. *Minn. Med., 56:* 382–390, 1973.
20. BLOUNT, W. P., AND BIDWELL, T. R. Milwaukee brace principles and fabrication. In *Atlas of Orthotics.* C. V. Mosby, St. Louis, 1975.
21. BLOUNT, W. P. Personal communication.
22. BRADFORD, D. S., MOE, J. H., MONTALO, F. T., AND WINTER, R. B. Scheuermann's kyphosis and round back deformity, results of Milwaukee brace treatments. *J. Bone Joint Surg., 56A:* 740–758, 1974.
23. BUNCH, W. H. The Milwaukee brace in paralytic scoliosis. *Clin. Orthop., 110:* 63–68, 1975.
24. BUNCH, W. H., AND KEAGY, R. D. *Principles of Orthotic Treatment.* C. V. Mosby Company, St. Louis, 1976.

25. BUNNELL, W. P., AND MACEWEN, G. D. Use of the Orthoplast jacket in the nonoperative treatment of scoliosis. Presented at the Tenth Annual Meeting of the Scoliosis Research Society, Louisville, Ky., September 11, 1975.
26. BUNNELL, W. P., MACEWEN, G. P., AND JAYAKUMAR, S. Plastic jackets in non-operative treatment of scoliosis. *J. Bone Joint Surg., 62A*: 31–38, 1980.
27. CARLSON, J. M. Fabrication of the Milwaukee superstructure and providing the appropriate corrective force system. AAOS Course: Orthotics for Spinal Deformities Advanced Workshop, Memphis, Tenn., June 12–16, 1978.
28. CARR, W., AND WINTER, R. Long term end results of Milwaukee brace. In preparation.
29. COBB, J. R. Outline for the study of scoliosis. *Instructional Course Lectures,* edited by J. W. Edwards, Ann Arbor, Michigan: American Academy of Orthopedic Surgeons, 1948.
30. COCHRANE, G. V. B., AND WAUGH, T. R. The external forces in correction of idiopathic scoliosis. *J. Bone Joint Surg., 51A*: 201, 1969 (Abstract).
31. COCKRELL, R., AND RISSER, J. Plastic body jacket in the treatment of scoliosis. Exhibit at the annual meeting of the American Academy of Orthopaedic Surgeons, Las Vegas, 1973.
32. COLLIS, D. K., AND PONSETI, I. V. Long-term followup of patients with idiopathic scoliosis not treated surgically. *J. Bone Joint Surg., 51A*: 425–445, 1969.
33. COTCH, M. D. Biomechanics of the thoracic spine. In *Atlas of Orthotics,* C. V. Mosby, St. Louis, 1975.
34. EDMONDSON, A. S., AND MORRIS, J. T. Followup study of Milwaukee brace treatment in patients with idiopathic scoliosis. *Clin. Orthop., 126*: 58–61, 1977.
35. GALANTE, J., SCHULTZ, A., DEWALD, R. L., AND RAY, R. D. Forces acting in the Milwaukee brace on patients undergoing treatment for idiopathic scoliosis. *J. Bone and Joint Surg., 52A*: 498–506, 1970.
36. HALL, J., AND MILLER, W. Prefabrication of Milwaukee braces. *J. Bone Joint Surg., 56A*: 1763, 1974.
37. HALL, J., MILLER, W., SHUMANN, W., AND STANISH, W. A refined concept in the orthotic management of scoliosis. *Orthotics Prosthet., 29*: 9–16, 1975.
38. HARRIS, E. E. A new orthotics terminology. *Orthotics Prosthet., 27*(2): 6–10, 1973.
39. JODOIN, A., HALL, J., WATTS, H., MICHAEL, L., RISEBOROUGH, E., AND MILLER, W. Treatment of idiopathic scoliosis by the Boston brace system: early results, in preparation.
40. KEISER, R. P., AND SHUFFLEBARGER, H. L. The Milwaukee brace in idiopathic scoliosis: evaluation of 123 completed cases. *Clin. Orthop., 118*: 19–24, 1976.
41. KUEHNEGGER, W. Research, design, and development of a CTLS (cervical-thoracic-lumbar-sacral) orthosis, Orthodyne, Inc. Report OD74-106, September 1974.
42. LARDONE, J., AND LEVINE, D. B. Milwaukee brace treatment in juvenile idiopathic scoliosis. *J. Bone Joint Surg., 55A*: 438, 1973.
43. LEATHERMAN, K. D., GAINES, R. W., BENSON, S., AND IBARRA, G. Kosair Scoliosis Orthosis. Informational material, Kosair Crippled Children's Hospital, Louisville, Kentucky, 1978.
44. LOGAN, W. R. The effect of the Milwaukee brace on developing dentition. In *Transactions of the British Society for the Study of Orthodontics,* pp. 1–8. London, 1962.
45. LUCAS, D. B., AND BRESLER, B. Stability of the ligamentous spine. Biomechanics Lab, University of California at Berkeley, Report #40, 1961.
46. McALLISTER, D. T., AND HARDY, J. H. Juvenile kyphosis; statistical survey and comparison of methods of treatment. *J. Bone Joint Surg., 53A*: 1323, 1973.
47. MELLENCAMP, D. D., BLOUNT, W. P., AND ANDERSON, A. J. Milwaukee brace treatment of idiopathic scoliosis. *Clin. Orthop., 127*: 47–57, 1977.
48. MICHELSSON, J. The development of spinal deformity in experimental scoliosis. *Acta Orthop. Scand., 81*(Suppl.), 1965.
49. MILWAUKEE BRACE, THE. A fabrication manual, Prosthetic-Orthotic Center, Northwestern University Medical School, Chicago, Ill., 1972.
50. MODERN PLASTICS ENCYCLOPEDIA. McGraw-Hill, New York, 1978.

51. MOE, J. H., AND KETTLESON, D. H. Idiopathic scoliosis. *J. Bone Joint Surg., 52A:* 1509–1533, 1970.
52. MOE, J. H. The Milwaukee brace in the treatment of scoliosis. *Clin. Orthop., 77:* 18–31, 1971.
53. MOE, J. H., WINTER, R. B., BRADFORD, D. S., AND LONSTEIN, J. E. *Scoliosis and Other Spinal Deformities.* Philadelphia, London, Toronto, W. B. Saunders, 1978.
54. MOE, J. H., *et al.* Ibid., citing STAGNARA, P. Lyon nonoperative treatment. Paper presented to the Scoliosis Research Society and the Group d'etude de la Scoliose. Lyon, France, September 25, 1973.
55. MULCAHY, T., GALANTE, J., DEWALD, R., SCHULTZ, H., AND HUNTER, J. C. A followup study of forces acting on the Milwaukee brace on patients undergoing treatment for idiopathic scoliosis. *Clin. Orthop., 93:* 53–68, 1973.
56. MURPHY, E. E., AND BURNSTEIN, A. H. Physical properties of materials including solid mechanics. In *Atlas of Orthotics,* St. Louis, 1975.
57. MYERS, B. A., FRIEDMAN, S. B., AND WEINER, I. B. Coping with a chronic disability: psychosocial observations of girls with scoliosis treated with the Milwaukee brace. *Am. J. Dis. Child., 120:* 175–181, 1970.
58. NACHEMSON, A., AND MORRIS, J. M. *In vivo* measurements of intradical pressure. *J. Bone Joint Surg., 46A:* 1077–1092, 1964.
59. NACHEMSON, A. A long-term followup study of nontreated scoliosis. *Acta. Orthop. Scandinav., 39:* 466–476, 1968.
60. NACHEMSON, A., AND ELFSTROM, G. Intravital wireless telemetry of axial forces in Harrington distraction rods in patients with idiopathic scoliosis. *J. Bone Joint Surg., 53A:* 445–465, 1971.
61. NASH, C. L., AND MOE, J. H. A study of vertebral rotation. *J. Bone Joint Surg., 51A:* 223–229, 1969.
62. NASH, C. L., VEGA, G. E., AND BROWN, R. Oxygen consumption studies in idiopathic adolescent scoliosis patients undergoing Milwaukee brace treatment. *J. Bone Joint Surg., 55A:* 439–440, 1973.
63. NILSONNE, U., AND LUNDGREN, K. D. Long-term prognosis in idiopathic scoliosis. *Acta Orthop. Scandinav., 39:* 456–465, 1968.
64. NORDWALL, A. Studies in idiopathic scoliosis relevant to etiology, conservative and operative treatment. *Acta Orthop. Scand. [Suppl.], 150:* 1–178, 1973.
65. PARK, J., HOUTKIN, S., GROSSMAN, J., AND LEVINE, D. B. A modified brace (Prenyl) for scoliosis. *Clin. Orthop., 126:* 67–73, 1977.
66. PAUL, S. W. Five years of nonoperative treatment of scoliosis and kyphosis. A followup study. *Orthotics Prosthet., 22:* 28, 1968.
67. ROBINS, P., MOE, J., AND WINTER, R. Scoliosis in Marfan's Syndrome. *J. Bone Joint Surg., 57A:* 358–368, 1975.
68. ROGALA, E., DRUMMOND, D., AND GURR, J. Scoliosis: incidence and natural history. *J. Bone Joint Surg., 60A:* 173–176, 1978.
69. SALANOVA, C. Les resultats lointains du corset de Milwaukee: les indications. *Acta Orthop. Belg., 43:* 606–615, 1977.
70. SCHATZINGER, L. A. H., NASH, C. L., JR., DROTAR, D. D., AND HALL, T. W. Emotional adjustment in scoliosis. *Clin. Orthop., 125:* 145–150, 1977.
71. SCHULTZ, A. B., LANOCCA, H., GALANTE, J. S., AND ANDRIACCHI, T. P. A study of geometrical relationships in scoliotic spines. *J. Biomech., 5:* 409–420, 1972.
72. SEVASTIKOGLOU, J. A., LINDERHOLM, H., AND LINDGREN, U. Effect of the Milwaukee brace on vital and ventilatory capacity of scoliotic patients. *Acta Orthop. Scand., 47:* 540–545, 1976.
73. SIEBENS, A. A., HOHT, J. P., ENGEL, W. E., AND SCRIBNER, N. Suspension of certain patients from their ribs. *Johns Hopkins Med. J., 130:* 26–36, 1972.

74. SIEBENS, A. A., HUNGERFORD, D. S., AND KIRBY, N. A. Curves of the achondroplastic spine: a new hypothesis. *Johns Hopkins Med. J., 142:* 205–210, 1978.
75. SPITZY, H. Scoliosis. In *Lehrbuch der Orthopadie,* edited by Lange and Lritz, Jena and Fischer, 1928. (cited by Moe et al. 1978).
76. STEINDLER, A. *Kinesiology of the Human Body.* Charles C Thomas, Springfield, Ill., 1955.
77. TANNER, J. M., WHITEHOUSE, R. H., AND TAKAISUE, M. Standards from birth to maturity for height, weight, height velocity, and weight velocity: British children, 1965. *Arch. Dis. Child., 41:* 454–471, 613–635, 1966.
78. TANNER, J. M. Some main features of normal growth in children. In *Scoliosis and Growth,* edited by P. A. Zorab. Churchill-Livingstone, London, 1971.
79. THULBOURNE, T., AND GILLESPIE, R. The rib hump in idiopathic scoliosis. Measurement, analysis, and response to treatment. *J. Bone Joint Surg., 58:* 64–71, 1976.
80. WATERS, R. L., AND MORRIS, J. M. Effect of the spinal support on the electrical activity of muscles of the trunk. *J. Bone Joint Surg., 52A:* 51–60, 1970.
81. WATTS, H. G. Manual for "Boston Brace System" Workshop, ed. 8. Boston, March 1979.
82. WATTS, H. G., HALL, J. E., AND STANISH, W. The Boston brace system for the treatment of low thoracic and lumbar scoliosis by the use of a girdle without superstructure. *Clin. Orthop., 126:* 87–92, 1977.
83. WATTS, H. Bracing in spinal deformities. *Orthop. Clin. North Am., 10:* 769–787, 1979.
84. WHITE, A. A. Analysis of the mechanics of the thoracic spine in man. An experimental study on autopsy specimens. *Acta Orthop. Scand. [Suppl.], 127:* 1969.
85. WHITE, A. A., PANJABI, M. M., AND BRAND, R. A system for defining position and motion of human body parts. *J. Med. Biol. Eng., 261:* 261–265, 1975.
86. WHITE, A. A., AND PANJABI, M. M. *Biomechanics of the Spine.* J. B. Lippincott Co., Philadelphia, 1978.
87. WICKERS, F., BUNCH, W., AND BARNETT, P. Psychological factors in failure to wear the Milwaukee Brace for treatment of idiopathic scoliosis. *Clin. Orthop., 26:* 62–66, 1977.
88. WINTER, R. B., MOE, J. H., AND EILERS, V. E. Congenital scoliosis: a study of 234 patient treated and untreated. *J. Bone Joint Surg., 50A:* 1–47, 1968.
89. WINTER, R. B., AND MOE, J. H. Orthotics for spinal deformity. *Clin. Orthop., 102:* 72–91, 1974.
90. WINTER, R. B., LOVELL, W. W., AND MOE, J. H. Excessive thoracic lordosis and loss of pulmonary function in patients with idiopathic scoliosis. *J. Bone Joint Surg., 57A:* 972–977, 1975.
91. WINTER, R. B. Scoliosis and spinal growth. *Orthop. Rev., 6:* 17–20, 1977.
92. WINTER, R. B., AND CARLSON, J. M. Modern orthotics for spinal deformities. *Clin. Orthop., 120:* 74–86, 1977.
93. YATES, G. Molded plastics in bracing. *Clin. Orthop., 102:* 46–57, 1974.
94. ZAMOSKY, I. New concepts in the corrective bracing of scoliosis, kyphosis, and lordosis. *Orthotics Prosthet., 32:* 3–10, 1978.

8

Upper Limb Orthotics

CHARLES LONG, M.D.

The purpose of this chapter is to discuss the structural and functional aspects of upper limb orthotics and provide the clinician with an illustrated text to which he may refer when confronted with a specific clinical problem. It also provides a background of facts and explanations for the student.

Uses of Upper Limb Orthoses

Upper limb orthoses are used to *substitute* for absent motor power, to *assist* weak segments, to *support* segments which require positioning or immobilization, to provide *traction,* to enforce specific, directional *control* or for the *attachment* of devices.

Substitution for Absent Motor Power. The deficit of motor power to drive a segment through its normal range of motion with sufficient force is a common indication for an upper limb orthosis. The method of substituting power varies from the use of rubber bands to electronically programmed carbon dioxide actuators. It is quite common in hand orthoses for the segment to have adequate muscle strength for one direction but not for the opposite direction. In such an instance, the patient is expected to use his own motor power for the controllable direction, and a substitute, usually elastic, for the return motion. The use of elastics for the production of motion against gravity and resistance requires strong antagonists (better than good-minus) to the substituted motion.

Assistance of Weak Segments. In a significant number of patients there is some motor power but not enough intensity or amplitude. Orthoses can be used to apply external power assistance to the weakened segment through the required range with the power increment needed. There is an important difference between this category and the preceding one of "substitution." When complete substitution is desired for a certain motion, we need only replace the lost motors with devices powerful enough to replace their function completely; however, when partial function persists in a segment, we must decide whether it is better to override the ramining, limited power completely, or to allow the patient to use his residual function. We decide by determining whether it would be detrimental to the patient if his remaining muscles would be destined to atrophy by overriding. The decision will depend upon the further recovery expected. If more recovery in the segment is not anticipated, overriding by external power is indicated and acceptable. If recovery is anticipated or even a possibility, the external power should not completely override the function of the recovering muscles but permit them to act at their safe limit in assisting control.

Adjustable external power sources are used to assist residual muscle function *without complete overriding*. These sources include springs and rubber bands, the tensions of which are adjusted to allow motion through a full range only when the patient uses his residual power to initiate and complete motion. There is no motion of the segment unless the patient uses his own residual power. Such elastic systems can allow the patient continued use and strengthening of his muscles, or at least prevent further atrophy of disuse.

Certain types of external power give more *complete override* of the intrinsic muscles of a segment. Complete override is a characteristic of nonelastic external power sources. These include the McKibben, carbon dioxide-powered, artificial muscle and the direct-current torque motors. Most cable systems which use distant, uninvolved muscles to drive a weakened segment are also used to override control (67). With all these devices, the patient cannot time or grade his residual segmental motor activity to operate in concert with external power properly.

There is no good method which allows the patient to assist the driving of a splint with his own muscles which assures powerful control of the segment. As mentioned above, the very method of balancing external elastic power and the residual function to produce motion precludes the production of a motion which can operate against resistance. The system, including residual motor power and external power, is set so that its total strength in full operation would grade fair—just enough to complete range of motion against gravity. As a by-product of their action, all elastics provide resistance during the active contraction of antagonistic muscles. However, the provision of resistive exercise is not a primary indication for an upper limb orthosis.

To Support Segments Requiring Positioning and Immobilization. Orthoses are often used for static positioning of a segment, either full or part-time. It is sometimes desirable to rest a group of muscles, tendon sheaths or joints for some periods of the day but allow their full use at other times. Removable splints are best suited for such instances. When full-time immobilization is desired, we may use a cast or a removable splint.

For the treatment of contracture we may use static splints for support or immobilization or traction splints. Such splints may be used during the day or night but are often preferred as night splints. This permits some corrective action while the patient sleeps and frees the hand for action during the day.

We wish to stress that in the use of static braces, *conformity supports; nonconformity corrects*. If we desire simple support, the orthosis is made to fit the segment exactly; if we desire to correct a deformity, the brace should be slightly nonconforming so that a corrective force is exerted. As the contracture responds to the force, the brace is readjusted to remain nonconforming and continually correcting.

To Provide Traction. When we use the word traction in this chapter, it has a different connotation from the use of external power to assist or substitute for a motion. The most common example of substitution or assistance is elastic traction for finger extension. Rubber bands or springs are suspended from an outrigger and attached to the fingers in such a manner that they pull the fingers into extension. Such a splint can be used to *substitute* for lost extensor function, to *assist* weak extensor function, or to provide *traction* or tension against the finger flexors. Traction can be recognized as a specific function of the rubber bands quite apart from the others mentioned. An understanding of this difference is essential to the proper prescription of upper limb orthoses.

To mobilize flexion contractures, the elastics are adjusted to pull each finger to the limit of its range and provide an additional increment of tension in that end position. The additional tension of this kind of adjustment differentiates it from elastic tension for substitution or assistance and determines the actual traction against the flexors or other soft tissues.

In traction braces, three fundamental principles must be followed to achieve the best results. First, *the amount of traction and the angle at which it is applied* are crucial. Traction, especially on fingers, must be applied gently. Light traction over prolonged periods is more effective and less damaging than strong traction over short periods. In general, traction should be just adequate to produce a detectable tension in the pulling device beyond that necessary to pull the segment to its limit of motion. The pull should be as nearly perpendicular to the end position of the segment as possible.

The second rule follows naturally from the first: *repeated adjustment of the tension* is essential to retain efficiency. As the segment increases its range of motion, the traction device (unless it is a weight over a pulley) will become slack, ineffective, and not remain perpendicular to the end position.

Third, *the patient must be permitted to develop tolerance to the splint.* A stretching device is not comfortable; the patient may not be able to wear it for more than a few minutes a day at first. Tolerance is developed by the gradual addition of a few minutes of wearing time each day. One self-adjusting way to develop such a tolerance is to have the patient apply the splint at bedtime; if discomfort awakens him during the night, he takes it off. If the patient cannot learn to sleep through the night with the splint, the pull is probably too great and should be reduced.

In every splint which permits motion there must be some attempt to *enforce specific, directional control.* Without it, the moving splint would require many different external and internal power sources to provide such control. Most orthoses have directional control to reduce the number of planes of motion or degrees of freedom requiring control by power sources. For example, movable wrist splints commonly permit motion in flexion and extension only; abduction-adduction and circumduction of the wrist are blocked. Power is required only for extension and flexion and not for other motions. In this sense, most moving splints exert some directional control.

In a more restrictive sense, certain splints are built solely to control the direction of motion, especially when adequate muscle power is available but directional control is abnormal. Such applications are quite rare in upper limb orthoses though common in lower. Examples include friction feeders for those with severe upper limb ataxia, or splints to prevent ulnar deviation of the rheumatoid hand. Little success has been met in attempting to transfer to the upper limbs the favorable results of bracing athetoid lower limbs. At the hip, passable function can be achieved only if flexion and extension control are possible with the rest of the limb immobilized. In the upper limb, analogous flexion-extension control of the shoulder would permit no functional use of a rigid limb.

Attachment of Devices. Many of the splints discussed in this chapter may be used with adaptive devices attached. Although these are discussed in Chapter 19, we shall mention splints which serve as foundations for adapted equipment or accessories.

Mechanical Principles

The mechanical principles of upper limb orthoses are not complicated but do require definition. Many authors have used different terms to describe the operation and components of these devices and a jargon has burgeoned in the literature. We do not claim to offer the last word in such definitions nor to fix them unalterably but rather to use the existing terms in a systematic fashion.

Static, dynamic, and *functional* are commonly used adjectives with upper limb orthoses. The term *static* implies that the splint does not permit motion of the segment but serves rather as a rigid support.

Dynamic and *functional* are used synonymously, each meaning that the segment is permitted a certain degree of motion and that the effectiveness of the splint depends upon that motion. An example of a static splint is a simple wrist support to maintain wrist position during the healing of an extensor tenosynovitis. An example of a dynamic or functional splint is the elastic extensor splint described above to assist weak extensor muscles (In Great Britain, the dynamic splint is usually called a lively splint.) A single splint may serve both static and dynamic purposes for two adjacent segments of the upper limb. For example, a basic wrist splint with extensor elastic attachments for the fingers may be a static splint at the wrist and a dynamic splint at the finger level. Although traction devices are basically static, they are not usually so considered and in this chapter they are classified as a kind of dynamic or traction splint. Similarly, adaptive devices, although technically static, are not generally classified as such.

EXTERNAL POWER

External power (1, 57) for substitution or assistance for absent muscle power may be elastic, pneumatic, electric, or transmitted. In elastic power we include rubber bands, springs, and elasticized plastics. Each of these may be graded according to length, breadth, and spring constant. The behavior of elastic varies according to this grading. In general, a long elastic permits constant force transmission over relatively large ranges of motion; a short elastic changes its tension markedly over short ranges. The importance of factors of elasticity will be discussed in greater detail in relation to splints where these factors are pertinent.

Elasticized plastic is increasingly supplanting the traditional rubber band as the elastic component in upper limb orthoses. Although many plastics can be elasticized, we shall use the term elasticized nylon or elastic nylon for this class of elastics.

Pneumatic power is one source of external power. There is a family of pneumatic power devices called pneumatic actuators. Each of these devices depends for its power on the transduction of expanding carbon dioxide either through a piston or into enclosed flexible tubing which shortens. The resultant mechanical energy is used directly as tension and motion to drive orthotic devices. In this chapter, the terms *McKibben muscle* and *artifical muscle* are used interchangeably. Special reference will be made to other pneumatic devices, such as the elevating feeder.

Electric power refers to electric motors which drive splints directly, or pull or push cables which in turn drive the orthoses. A high speed motor provides a source of instanteous external power which rivals pneumatic systems in versatility and application.

Transmitted power is any power which activates an orthotic segment by means of a cable. However, we restrict the use of the term cable power in this chapter to external power originating in voluntarily controlled muscles at a distance from the orthotic segment. An example is a shoulder harness which transmits the motion of a scapula (driven by muscles under good control) and transmitted by cable from the harness to a hand orthosis. The transmission of force from voluntarily controlled muscles by cables depends upon the application of the Bowden principle (52), the transmission of force across joints without affecting them (Fig. 8.1).

INTERNAL POWER

By internal power we mean power supplied by the patient's muscles within the segment whether under voluntary control or by electrical stimulation. It is customary to define a splint in terms of the direction of the splint control provided by internal and external power. For instance, a hand

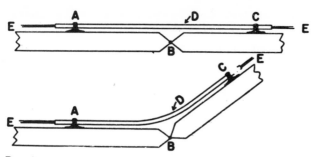

Fig. 8.1. Bowden cable, a device for transmitting tension forces applied at one end. although point *C* is brought closer to point *A* when rotation occurs about *B*, housing *D* prevents slack in cable *E* by preserving effective path length *A–C*. A counter force is required at opposite end to return flexible cable to original position. [Reproduced with permission of the American Academy of Orthopaedics (58).]

splint may be "voluntary closing, spring opening," implying internal power for flexion and external power for extension. Orthoses for other extremity segments may be defined similarly as at the elbow, "voluntary extension, rubber band flexion." Also, we may define doubly externally powered splints, as for example, "McKibben closing, spring opening."

This author and others have described special splints utilizing electrical stimulation for the control of muscles enclosed in braces (15, 41, 45). Two major types of these special splints are defined. Each depends on an exoskeletal structure which limits the movements of the braced segment to a controlled number of degrees of freedom. Within this framework, electrical stimulation of muscle provides motion in one direction while a spring manages return motion. The *electrophysiologic (EP) splint* consists of the splint itself, an electrical stimulator, and a graded control (discussed below) actuated by mechanical movement of some distant segment (for example, the shoulder) under voluntary control. The *myoelectric (ME) splint* consists of the same basic splint and a similar stimulator but is actuated by the electric potential output of a distant muscle which is innervated and voluntarily controlled. Some details of the control system will be discussed later. The EP and ME splints are experimental.

Another internally powered orthosis is the *tenodesis* splint. This term refers to the operation of a splint which resembles hand action following the surgical procedure of the same name. The principle involved refers primarily to finger flexion after tenodesis. In this surgical operation, the flexor tendons are attached to the radius so that dorsiflexion of the wrist produces finger flexion. The splint, which produces finger flexion on wrist extension, is called a tenodesis splint. It depends for its function upon the voluntary (internal) power of the wrist extensors.

ROLE OF GRAVITY IN CONTROL SYSTEMS

Gravity plays an important role in every upper limb orthosis but is most important in those joints where the heaviest masses must be moved—the shoulder and elbow. There has been great interest in multimotored, multi-segmental orthotic systems which embrace the entire upper limb which Engen (21) has shown to require a balance of three types of control: external power, internal power, and gravity. Gravity may influence the orthotic system in several ways: it may hinder motion, as in elbow flexion, where the weight of the forearm and hand resists moving the hand toward the mouth in the presence of weak elbow flexors. As we can see from the discussion above, there are several ways to overcome gravity. The weak elbow flexors may be overridden by an external power, such as elastics, or, the forearm may be counterbalanced to eliminate the effect of gravity and allow the weak elbow flexors to perform the desired motion.

In this reverse motion, gravity may assist rather than hinder. In elbow extension, the forearm falls with gravity and only the rate of fall need be controlled. Herein lies an advantage of elastic systems which both automatically assist the desired antigravity motion and control the rate of descent with gravity. Powerful pneumatic actuators are limited in their usefulness here by their "on-off" character. They cannot be used for smooth control or descent rate with gravity except with Engen's proportional flow valve. On the other hand, counterbalancing schemes, such as the ball bearing forearm orthosis, or feeder, are very adaptable for these purposes. Counterweighting can be exactly balanced against remaining muscle power so that motions in both directions are smoothly controllable.

If we consider the patient with completely paralyzed elbow flexors, the method of antigravity control is quite different. It is no longer possible for the patient to add his own weak voluntary control to elastic assistance, for he has no voluntary control. It thus becomes necessary to add some other form of external power such as the McKibben muscle or stronger elastic bands (if the elbow extensors are strong enough to overcome them).

A control system which may help to solve the problem of bidirectional control of heavy segments is an electric motor which reels wire like a fishing reel, allowing bidirectional motor control as long as there is an opposing force. In the orthosis, the opposing force is the weight of the segment or an opposing elastic (just as the fish is the opposing force to the reel). Alternately, directly geared motors can provide positive bidirectional drive (Fig. 8.39).

Even in the flail elbow or shoulder, counterbalancing schemes can be useful. In the absence of motor control of the upper limb, the patient may be able to shift his body weight to add or subtract weight to part of a counterbalanced system. This useful method of control is discussed under ball bearing forearm orthosis.

There are many different control systems available for upper extremity orthoses, the purpose of which is to allow the patient to communicate his desires to the orthosis. The control systems are varied as the appliances they control (see Chapter 20).

For external power, control systems must have a method for turning the power on or off and for grading the power application. For pneumatic and hydraulic systems the control is a valve which allows the input or exhaust of the controlling fluid, usually carbon dioxide. In elastic systems, control is achieved by the addition or subtraction of force from the system by voluntary contraction or relaxation of muscles through internal or transmitted power. Electric motors respond to various switches and rheostats.

Control systems for internal power require methods of grading the muscular contraction within the orthotic segment. If there is voluntary control, the system will, of course, respond to the central nervous system. If the patient is paralyzed and electrical stimulation is used, appropriate electrical controls are inserted. In the electrophysiologic splint, the control consists of a potentiometer which adjusts the stimulator output to the muscle. In the myoelectric splint, control is a function of the electrical output (integrated voltage) of a distant voluntarily controlled muscle which in turn modulates the stimulator output to the paralyzed muscle.

Electric switches and rheostats, control valves for pneumatic systems, and EP potentiometers can be mounted wherever convenient for the patient on the orthosis or the wheelchair; in general, the selection of the control site will depend upon the ingenuity of the designer and the requirements of the system.

Those accustomed to working with upper limb prostheses know the importance of routine cable checks. Similar checkouts should be applied to upper limb orthoses if externally powered through cables or pneumatic tubes. The route of power transmission must be free of unnecessary bends and kinks; cables must be of the exact length of the assigned purpose.

Patient Acceptance

The best possible orthosis is doomed to be ineffective if it is not accepted by the patient. The most important determining factor is *whether the orthosis permits the patient to perform activities which would not be possible without it and which the patient wishes to perform.* Unless these criteria are fulfilled by pre-prescription thought and discussion, the patient will waste much of his own and his therapist's valuable time in training to use a device which he will discard when he returns home, if not sooner.

Other factors which enter into patient acceptance include appearance and self-application. There are few orthoses so ugly that they will be rejected by a patient, who must have it to achieve a desired function; yet the patient is much more likely to accept a cosmetically attractive orthosis than an unattractive one. Sometimes the orthosis may be too difficult for the patient to apply himself, and there may be no one at home knowledgeable enough to apply it. For instance, one of the primary problems in the electrophysiologic splint is the difficulty encountered by families in applying the stimulating electrodes to good motor points. A splint cannot be useful if it cannot be put on.

Function of the opposite extremity is a major determinant in acceptance. Although good statistics are not available, many workers agree that most activities of daily living can be performed with on hand, especially if the remaining hand is the dominant hand. The presumption remains reasonably valid for the nondominant side after some practice. Hence acceptance of any orthosis for a single upper limb is greatly reduced by the existence of normal function on the opposite side. There is a delicate balance which determines acceptance in each case.

Patient acceptance is further influenced by the propriety of the original brace prescription. If the physician has ordered the wrong orthosis or prescribed one when none was needed, the patient notes at once the lack of improvement in function and rejects it. Functions which cannot be achieved by bracing should be avoided: for example, attempts to correct the position of a severely spastic upper limb segment, the control of dyskinesia or random motion of the upper limb, especially in the ambulatory patient, and real load-lifting ability at the shoulder or elbow.

The patient's feelings about his orthosis are greatly influenced by the physician's attitude toward it. Certain negative feelings about orthoses which deter the patient may be communicated by the physician. One of these feelings decried by Dr. Robert Bennett is that "a brace is an admission of defeat." Some physicians feel that the use of a brace signifies a failure of medicine, which is salvaged by orthotic supports or metal. The orthosis, if ever it signalized defeat, has become a symbol of progress which enables the patient to perform new activities and to take better care of himself. An orthosis is not a fixed solution to a problem; it may be applied during a period of recovery meaningfully for months or years yet one day be rightfully discarded by both patient and physician. Even if there is no recovery, a brace may become unnecessary for a patient who masters trick motions or when operative procedures achieve substitution.

The attitude of physicians toward bracing varies greatly. In the upper limb bracing of quadriplegics, opinions range from trying an orthosis on any patient who might benefit to the other extreme that such patients can function without orthoses. An intermediary school suggests that no patient should have an orthosis if surgery may permit the same functions. An orthosis should be tried on any patient whom it would theoretically assist toward better function; everyone in contact with the patient should encourage him to use it. The cost of such a device as a failure is a small price to pay for its possible success.

Prescription of the Upper Limb Orthosis

We present here those splints which offer the clinician a wide choice of orthoses of each upper limb segment in most clinical conditions.

Four basic orthotic families are represented: Rancho Los Amigos (Downey, California), the Bunnell series, the Bennett series (Georgia Warm

Springs Foundation) and the Engen series (Texas Institute for Rehabilitation and Research at Baylor University). It is extremely difficult to give credit where due since many braces were not reported in the literature by their originators; in some instances, the original idea can be traced to Dr. Sterling Bunnell (14).

How to Use This Chapter to Select an Orthosis

Since part of this chapter is meant to be a catalog, the reader should know how to use it to help him meet the needs of the patient. The requirements of the patient must be firmly extablished and the purpose of the device determined according to the criteria listed at the beginning of the chapter. The clinician should refer to Table 8.1 after he has determined whether the device is to be substitutive, assistive, supportive, for traction or control, or adaptive. The chart lists the upper limb segments in the following order: wrist, hand (thumb and fingers), shoulder, and elbow. Under each segment there is listed a group of orthoses classified by site of action (joint) and by desired function column until he reaches the level of the desired segment, joint and direction of action. At the junction of these coordinates he will list several suitable braces with the page on which they are listed in the left hand column. A study of each of the braces, their indications and contraindications, will allow the clinician to make his final choice. Using the orthotic prescription forms described in Chapter 1, Principles of Orthotics, may be helpful in using the catalog in this chapter.

Bennett (10) has given some guidelines to improve selectivity of orthotic devices. "1) The device must serve a real need. Applying unnecessary apparatus can be as dangerous as not applying necessary apparatus. 2) The device prescribed must be of a design that can be constructed, and, as necessary, repaired by a good orthotist. 3) The device must be as lightweight as possible, but capable of standing up under expected wear. 4) The device must be reasonable in cost. 5) The device must be sufficiently simple that it can be applied by the patient or his family. 6) The device must be acceptable in appearance, and 7) must in no way endanger the structural security of bodily segments through its use."

The orthoses described in this chapter have been screened to conform to these criteria. For example, most orthoses described in this chapter are made of aluminum or whatever material is lightest for the stresses to be encountered. Many may be equally useful when constructed of rigid plastics.

Fabrication and Fitting

After the clinician has selected an orthosis he must write the prescription and see that the orthosis is made and fitted correctly and that the patient receives proper training for its use.

Fabrication is generally entrusted to a certified orthotist. However, the occupational therapist may make certain orthosis with professional skill.

TABLE 8.1

Page	Splint	Substitution	Assist	Support	Traction	Control	Attach Devices
	WRIST						
	Static						
207	Bunnell spring			×			×
208	Bunnell basic dorsal			×			×
208	Long opponens (Rancho)			×			×
210	Bennett basic dorsal			×			×
211	Engen volar basic			×			×
	Dynamic						
213	Pope	×	×		×	×	
215	Other springs and stops	×	×		×	×	
204	Deviation	×	×		×	×	
	THUMB						
	Static						
222	Bennett basic hand	×		×			×
222	Short opponens (Rancho)	×		×			×
222	Engen basic hand	×		×			×
	Supports						
224	Opponens bar			×		×	×
224	C-bar					×	
224	Opponens dowel			×		×	
224	Thumb post			×			×
	Accessories						
225	Spring swivel thumb		×	×	×	×	
225	Thumb distal phalanx	×	×	×	×		
226	Thumb proximal phalanx	×	×	×	×		
	FINGERS						
	Static						
227	Troughs			×			
227	Platforms			×			
228	Hand sandwich			×	×		
228	Pancake			×	×		
228	Rheumatoid night			×			
	Dynamic						
	MP extension						
230	Extension outrigger	×	×		×		
230	Extension assist spring	×	×				
230	Extension assist pulley	×	×				
231	Thomas extension assist	×	×				
231	Reverse knuckle bender				×		
	MP flexion						
232	Knuckle bender			×	×		
232	Individual traction			×	×		
233	Control adjustable			×	×		
233	Spring flexion assist		×	×			
	Metacarpophalangeal						
	Abduction-Adduction						
234	Finger deviation (Rancho)			×	×		
234	Fifth finger adduction			×	×		
235	Smith ulnar deviation			×		×	
235	First dorsal assist	×	×	×	×	×	
	Interphalangeal joint						
	Extension						
236	MP extension stop					×	
237	IP extension assist	×	×				
237	Bunnell PIP traction				×		

TABLE 8.1—*Continued*

Page	Splint	Substitution	Assist	Support	Traction	Control	Attach Devices
	FLEXOR HINGE						
	MP-IP support						
241	Basic Rancho	×	×	×		×	
241	Short Rancho	×	×	×		×	
241	Artificial muscle	×		×		×	
243	Shoulder driven	×		×		×	
244	Electrophysiological	×		×		×	
245	Torque motor	×		×		×	
246	Myoelectric	×		×		×	
	FLEXOR HINGE						
	Tenodesis						
247	Rancho	×	×	×		×	
198	Warm Springs	×	×	×		×	
248	Engen reciprocal	×	×	×		×	
	SHOULDER						
	Static						
250	Airplane			×			
251	Biscapular support			×		×	
251	Single scapular support			×		×	
	Dynamic						
	Shoulder flexion-extension						
259	Workplane pitch adjustment	×	×	×		×	
263	Sling suspension, strap	×	×	×		×	
266	Ratchet lock	×		×		×	
261	Flexion rubber band		×	×		×	
261	Friction feeder			×		×	
	Shoulder abduction-adduction						
259	Workplane roll adjustment	×	×	×		×	
263	Sling suspension, overhead rod	×	×	×		×	
261	Friction feeder			×		×	
261	Elevating swivel arm		×	×		×	
262	Gas elevating feeder	×		×		×	
	Shoulder internal-external rotation						
255	X and Y adjustments	×	×	×		×	
263	Sling with rocker or trough	×	×	×		×	
267	Arm rotation spring	×	×	×		×	
	ELBOW						
	Dynamic						
	Flexion-extension						
259	Workplane pitch adjustment	×	×	×		×	
263	Double sling with strap	×	×	×		×	
261	Elbow flexion rubber band		×	×		×	
261	Elbow flexion artificial muscle	×		×		×	
261	Friction feeder			×		×	
262	Engen external power	×		×		×	
265	Double upright with elastic		×	×		×	
265	Double upright steel spring				×		
	Forearm rotation (attachments)						
271	Supinator assist	×		×		×	
272	Rotation assist	×	×	×		×	
273	Rotation springs	×	×	×		×	

Many orthoses mentioned in this chapter are commercially available in prefabricated form. Each orthotist has an excellent construction guide in Anderson's *Upper Extremities Orthotics* (3).

Fitting is the responsibility of the orthotist, but no person working with the patient and his orthosis can be relieved of the duty of continuously checking the fit, especially since fit may change with use.

Training

The following general steps should be taken in orthotic training. 1) If possible, the patient should see the proposed orthosis in action on other patients before his own prescription is complete. In rare cases, the patient may reject an orthosis as soon as he sees it, in which event training should be cancelled or at least not discussed for a while. More often, the early introduction to another patient with similar problems and orthotic solutions helps the patient to discuss his doubts and fears or at least those of his comrade. 2) Indoctrinate the patient before he receives his orthosis and include a discussion of its kinesiology, a valuable step which is often omitted because of the press of time.

We hear much about pre-prosthetic training but very little about pre-orthotic training. For externally powered devices, the patient should learn the use of the proposed control devices even before he receives his orthosis. The patient will save much time later if he learns early what is expected of him.

For internally powered devices, especially those run by voluntarily controlled muscles, *adequate strength must be present* in the segment to provide the required orthotic control. Muscle strength of good-minus to good is usually required to operate against elastic returns. Grades of poor-plus to fair can operate parts of assistive splints (as defined above) while muscles grading above fair-plus can be used in antigravity systems where gravity alone supplies the return force. For internally powered devices, the more strength available in the segment, the better. Hence, pre-orthotic isometric or isotonic exercises are an important part of orthotic training.

It may be necessary to stretch an involved segment before an orthosis can be applied effectively. For instance, the elbow may need to be stretched into enough flexion to allow the hand to reach the mouth in a balanced forearm orthosis; the web-space between the first two metacarpals may need stretching before a hand splint can be used efficiently. Stretching is prescribed in the usual manner, often preceded by some form of heat therapy. The intensity of stretching is prescribed as gentle, moderate, or forceful, along with the number of times per day and the amount per sitting. Forceful stretching is usually avoided in the upper limb, especially at the elbow and in the hand because of the danger of permanent damage and additional contracture. Sometimes, instead of stretching or in addition to it, traction splints may be prescribed preparatory to the application of other dynamic splinting.

In patients with severe trunk weakness, imbalance, or ataxia, additional pre-orthotic training may be necessary in "trunk balance." The patient is taught to maintain a stable base at the shoulders from which to operate his upper limbs most efficiently. The stable base can usually be achieved in physical or occupational therapy by supported (and later unsupported) balancing in a wheelchair or on a mat. It may be necessary to maintain external support (19) in the form of a corset or even a more firm support, such as molded trunk supports which may attach to the wheelchair, affording a very stable base of operation. Similar firm, lateral supports can be written into wheelchair prescriptions. Manufacturers' catalogues describe some of these.

The early phases of adjustment to wearing an upper limb orthosis are critical in determining ultimate acceptance. The personnel must have a positive attitude; good fit is crucial. The orthosis must be checked daily to make sure that pressure areas are not developing or that looseness is not reducing efficiency. If either of these deficiencies is noted, it must be corrected at once. Minor adjustments can often be made without tools or with a pair of moleskin-tipped pliers.

The orthosis cannot usually be worn full-time immediately; it is applied for short periods at the onset and these are increased as rapidly as tolerated. It does no good to have the orthosis in place 8 hours a day if the arm is idle for most of the time. Increased wearing time must be accompanied by increased use. Specific methods must be developed for each patient for carryover of trained performance to the hospital or home situation. The personnel who come into contact with the patient on the hospital floor, or in his home, must be trained in the application and removal of the orthosis if the patient cannot perform these tasks himself. They must be taught how the orthosis works and what the patient should be expected and urged to do with it. They and the patient must be taught the danger signs of pain, swelling, or redness which indicate that the orthosis should be removed and the physician or therapist responsible called.

Although increased use of the orthosis is a desirable, early goal, great care should be exerted to keep the operating muscles from becoming excessively fatigued. Pushing the patient too hard at the beginning may cause him to reject the splint because he becomes too tired to use it correctly. In externally powered devices, even the relatively normal muscles distant from the paralyzed segments may become fatigued from too early continuous operation of the control devices. Electrically stimulated, internally powered systems may fail due to fatigue of the stimulated muscles; internally powered assistive systems will fatigue rapidly because they often operate near their maximum capacity. The complexity of activity expected of the patient should be increased slowly. It is a mistake to expect the newly fitted patient to perform complex activities of daily living. The patient should be indoctrinated by the orthotist or occupational therapist in the basic motions and controls of the orthotic system and only after such an introduction should more complex acts be attempted.

The next step is post-orthotic supportive therapy. It is sometimes necessary to continue the pre-orthotic physical therapy into the post-orthotic training period. Stretching should be continued for tight segments until they reach normal range or until no further increase can be expected. Strengthening exercises of the muscles in the control system of externally powered devices or within the segment of internally powered devices should be continued until a plateau of strength is reached, after which the patient usually maintains a good level of strength by constant use. If, for some reason, the patient stops using the orthosis for a while, as for a major operation, it may be necessary to reinstitute exercises. The final step should include home evaluation (see Chapter 15). Many an orthosis has been discarded by its owner immediately after returning home from a structured, training environment. If the gains of the training period are to be maintained, the home environment must be adjusted to fit the needs of the patient.

The Wrist

The upper limb serves the functions of the hand. Its primary purpose is to locate the hand in space so that it can best carry out its owner's wishes. Within this basic framework, the wrist provides a fine adjustment of hand position by flexion, extension, radial or ulnar deviation, or any combination of these. As soon as a splint is placed on the wrist, this fine adjustment, this vernier action, is abolished. Although most functions of the limb can still be accomplished with little difficulty, the increased burden of substituted motion is thrown on the rest of the limb.

In the opening and closing motions of the hand, the wrist acts continually to adjust the opposing viscoelastic tension of the flexors and extensors. In the healthy hand, the wrist extends during finger flexion and flexes during finger extension through a range of 20° to 30°. This motion permits the hand to take advantage of the tenodesis effect of the long finger flexors and extensors thereby reducing the amount of voluntary contraction required to produce hand motion (23). This energy-saving reciprocation is lost when a static splint is worn.

SPLINTING THE WRIST

Effects of Wrist Position

Knowledge of the reciprocal action of wrist and fingers helps to determine the wrist position for weakness or disability of the fingers. If the finger flexors are weak, the wrist can be "set" in slight extension (10° or 20°) to stretch the flexors and thus assist hand closing. If the finger extensors are weak, the wrist should be splinted in the neutral position or in slight (10°)

flexion to assist the extensors. If the fingers are controlled by strong musculature so that they do not need the assistance of wrist splinting, the position of choice for the wrist is the *functional position,* a convenient designation for partial dorsiflexion assumed by the normal empty hand when the fingers are fully flexed. It is probably the most efficient position for tight grasp.

Although wrist position may be used to assist certain finger motions, *the distal effect of wrist positioning may also be detrimental to the fingers* and we must bear this in mind whenever a wrist splint is prescribed. Patients may present wrist and finger flexion contractures (or spasticity) simultaneously. There is a tendency to splint the wrist in neutral position or extension "so that it will be nearer the position of function." This ignores the fact that pushing the wrist from its flexed position into the neutral or extended position causes the fingers to flex further; nothing could be more detrimental to finger flexion contractures or finger flexor spasticity than the isolated splinting of the wrist in this manner. If the wrist is to be splinted, the fingers often must also be splinted. The decision to splint the fingers must always be considered along with the decision to splint the wrist. Since wrist bracing often commits the physician to finger bracing, he must determine whether this often bulky unit is really necessary. It is sometimes better to leave the wrist unbraced than encumber the patient with a combined wrist and finger splint.

Dorsal or Palmar

Wrist orthoses may be placed on either the anterior or posterior aspect of the forearm. For many years, there has been discussion of the merits of one or the other placement, and, as is so often the case in such prolonged controversy, there are advantages and disadvantages of each.

Anterior (or palmar) splinting of the wrist is probably used more often; it appears in simple cock-up splints and in trays made of plaster or plastic. It provides a very firm support for the hand, with even distribution of pressure in or across the palm, on areas accustomed to bearing some pressure. It has two disadvantages: a) it is difficult to apply most of the common devices for bracing of the thumb and fingers to an anterior splint, except for external power devices such as finger flexors, and b) it obstructs the palm. Some practitioners feel that blocking of palmar sensation and limitation of palmar gripping contraindicates all palmar wrist splints. This is probably an over-concern since such splinting can offer relatively rigid immobilization of the wrist under controlled conditions, when needed. For example, a temporary wrist splint for night immobilization of the rheumatoid wrist or the post-cast Colles fracture is logically placed anteriorly.

In an attempt to free the palm of encumbrance and to allow attachment of commonly used dorsal devices, the dorsal wrist splint has become the standard static base for many dynamic splints. As will be seen below, the whole family of Warm Springs and Rancho Los Amigos splints evolved from a base of static dorsal wrist splinting. The chief advantage of dorsal splinting is that it frees the palm for feeling and grasping, by the use of metal grips which curve around to the palmar surface of the second and fifth metacarpal heads (Warm Springs splint). The grips provide support to prevent wrist flexion but allow a clear palm and an open area in the central palmar arch. The Rancho splints have developed a compromise in palmar clearance. A pallar support passes under the entire breadth of the palmar arch thus slightly limiting palmar contact. What it loses in palmar clearance it gains in palmar arch support.

The metacarpal grips (or the C-bar which usually substitutes for the one under the second metacarpal head) of the Warm Springs dorsal splint do not supply good support for the entire hand and can be a source of pressure leading to skin inflammation. The palmar portion of the Rancho splint does not have this disadvantage since it permits pressure distribution across all the metacarpal heads. In common with the Warm Springs splint, it depends for rigidity on a "wrist extension bar" which passes over the dorsum of the wrist and virtually carries the whole weight of the hand. If not perfectly fitted, or, when old and bent, the wrist extension bar can press on the dorsal wrist and distal forearm, permitting the weight of the hand to be borne on this single area, and this often leads to skin inflammation or even skin breakdown. The pressure is most intense if spasticity or other forms of tightness forcefully flex the wrist and fingers and in such cases it is best to avoid dorsal splinting. Zislis (77) presents a convincing argument in favor of palmar splints in spastic hemiplegics. By means of electromyographic (also cf. 26) and clinical observations, he showed an immediate reduction in flexor muscle activity when a dorsal splint was replaced by a palmar splint, and considers skin receptors over the dorsum as the cause of spasticity. The general theory is reflected in clinical practice by McCoullough's use of plastic volar trays in hemiplegia (52).

Distal Limits of Wrist Orthoses

A major aim of effective wrist splinting is the control of wrist position or motion without encumbering the fingers. All wrist splints have one potential danger in common: their palmar supports may extend beyond the metacarpophalangeal joints, thereby restricting finger flexion at that joint. All properly designed wrist splints or casts avoid this restriction of motion; unfortunately, the design is often carried out imperfectly. Special care must be taken that splints do not impede metacarpophalangeal joint flexion, or that they do not slip distally, with the same effect. Plaster casts or plaster cock-up splints should be carefully inspected and revised if necessary.

Proximal Extent of Wrist Orthoses

The proximal extent of the wrist extension bar determines to a great degree the lateral stability of the brace. Radial and ulnar deviation of the wrist within an orthosis cause the orthosis to deviate with the hand and since this acts through a short lever arm proximal to the wrist it can cause the proximal end of the splint to slip off the forearm or slide about on the dorsum of the forearm. A long proximal extension of the wrist extension bar is necessary for good leverage and hence adequate control of radial and ulnar deviation tendencies at the wrist. In addition, it decreases the unit surface pressure. We recommend that the wrist extension bar extend proximally two-thirds of the forearm length.

Compromise of Rotation Centers and Axis in Dynamic Orthoses

The center of rotation of the dynamic splint should be placed to avoid interference with normal movement of the segment about its natural centers or rotation. It is usually necessary for the orthotic center to overlie the center of rotation of the segment.

In the wrist there are several centers of rotation corresponding to the different motions of the wrist. There is one axis for wrist extension (related to intracarpal movement), another axis for wrist flexion (radiocarpal movement) and still another for abduction movements (a combined proximal and distal row movement). It is difficult and unnecessary to have two separate centers of rotation for the two separate motions of flexion and extension. We usually use a compromise single center of rotation at about the midpoint of the side of the wrist corresponding to the approximate location of the proximal carpal row.

TYPES OF WRIST ORTHOSES (WHOs)

Static orthoses for the wrist are used a) to immobilize (support) the wrist and b) to serve as a base for the attachment of devices. All of these splints are stabilized by a forearm splint from which is extended a device to support and immobilize the hand in the chosen position. This family of orthoses is used so often that it is very large; representative types of each major group will be described.

Spring Cock-up Splint (Bunnell)

This supportive splint (Fig. 8.2) provides a broad trough in which the forearm rests and which is bound to the forearm by straps. The hand

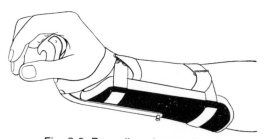

Fig. 8.2. Bunnell cock-up wrist splint.

support is made of spring metal and extends into the palm in the form of an oval support which occupies much of the palmar surface. The spring metal of the support extension is very stiff and does not permit significant motion. It can be bent a little and partially adjusted for proper wrist position although basically it is for use in the extended (cocked-up) position. This splint is strong enough to be used when there is marked spasticity of the wrist flexors. There is some danger of finger flexion contracture when this splint is used in spasticity but it can be used, for instance, to determine whether a patient will tolerate a proposed wrist fusion or when an adequate finger splinting is also used. It is made of padded steel and is commercially available as the Bunnell spring cock-up splint. Since it is relatively inexpensive and easily available it is one of the most frequently used splints for isolated wrist immobilization.

Dorsal Wrist Splint (Bunnell)

The Bunnell dorsal wrist splint (Fig. 8.3) consists of three flat steel plates joined by a wrist extension bar. The largest plate is over the posterior aspect of the forearm, with smaller plates over the dorsum of the hand and fingers. The wrist extension bar may be bent at any desired angle for positioning the wrist in flexion or extension. Significant abduction adjustment and control are not possible. Since it is designed to leave the palm free to manipulate objects, it is used only when there is enough strength in the finger flexors to permit dextrous activity. Otherwise, there are few limitations or unusual prerequisites for this very adaptable orthosis.

Basic Long Opponens Hand Splint (Rancho Los Amigos)

The purpose of this splint (Figs. 8.4 and 8.5) is to support the wrist and palmar arch while stabilizing the thumb in a functional position. However, the most common indications are not related to support of the wrist. It is an excellent basic positioning device for the thumb in substitutive or assistive splints; it is also a firm base for many substitutive, assistive, and tractive devices. This aluminum splint consists of a single wrist extension bar on the dorsal surface of the forearm, wrist and hand, to which is attached a curved bar which passes around the ulnar border of the hand, under the palmar arch, finally curving dorsally again to grip the head of the second metacarpal;

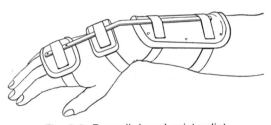

Fig. 8.3. Bunnell dorsal wrist splint.

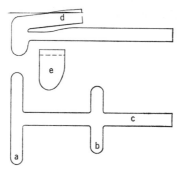

Fig. 8.4. Template for basic long opponens hand splint (Rancho Los Amigos). *a*, proximal tab; *b*, wrist extension bar; *c*, distol tab; *d*, opponens bar; *e*, C-bar.

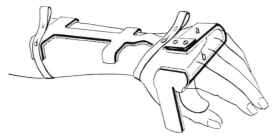

Fig. 8.5. Basic long opponens hand splint (Rancho Los Amigos). *a*, dorsal extension; *b*, volar support.

processes extend from the basic structure to support the web space of the thumb and to prevent excessive extension of the first metacarpal (Fig. 8.4). Indications for the use of this splint for wrist support (without required support of the thumb) are minimal when the total scale of indications for wrist splinting is considered. The splint is at its best as an isolated wrist support when supporting a relatively unloaded hand. It cannot be used to support a wrist with significant contractures or spasticity because of the light aluminum construction. Lightness is an advantage when devices are added to create a complex wrist, thumb, and finger support or for other purposes. This is probably the most commonly used basic splint for sophisticated, dynamic splinting. As mentioned above, it has the slight disadvantage of partial palmar obstruction. Although this support partially limits manipulation of objects against the palm, its great clinical success suggests that objections to it may be more theoretical than real. Unlike the Bunnell splints just described, this orthosis requires individual construction and fitting by a skilled person since an exact fit is critical; proper molding of the palmar support is especially important. The splint has a tendency to slide distally on the hand. This can be prevented, in part, by special attention to the location of the distal strap which should be anchored proximally enough (over the distal carpal row) so that when buckled it will seat firmly against the pisiform bone on the palmar aspect of the wrist, thus preventing distal excursion of the whole splint.

Basic Dorsal Wrist Splint (Bennett)

This light aluminum splint (Figs. 8.6 and 8.7) is similar to the one described above but differs through the absence of the palmar support bar. A single wrist extension bar traverses the entire length of the splint, from the proximal, dorsal forearm to the metacarpal heads. The distal dorsal bar crosses the entire dorsum, laps over the ends of the metacarpus to form on one side a hypothenar bar, and on the other side an opponens bar. The hypothenar bar supports the head of the fifth metacarpal; the opponens bar prevents excessive extension of the first metacarpal. To complete the support of the whole hand, the C-bar intrudes under the head of the second

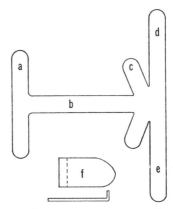

Fig. 8.6. Template of Bennett basic dorsal wrist splint. *a*, proximal tab; *b*, wrist extension bar; *c*, distal tab; *d*, opponens bar; *e*, hypothenor bar; *f*, C-bar.

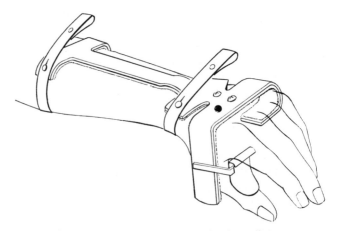

Fig. 8.7. Bennett basic dorsal wrist splint.

metacarpal; the opposite end of the C-bar extends along the webspace and proximal phalanx of the thumb.

This splint is almost identical with the Rancho Los Amigos basic long opponens splint in its uses. It is primarily a splint for the attachment of other devices and secondarily, it may be used as a simple wrist support. As a wrist splint it is limited to support of the unloaded hand; it is not indicated when there is significant contracture or spasticity. The advantage of the Bennett splint in this category is its lack of palmar encumbrance; the hand is gripped only by the hypothenar bar and the C-bar, leaving the palm free for manipulation of objects. In spite of this moderate advantage, it is usually advisable to use the basic Bunnell splints for simple, unloaded wrist support because of their cost and availability. If support of the unloaded wrist is desired for a long period, when comfort and freedom of the palm are important, the Bennett splint is useful.

The Bennett splint is difficult to fit but easily accepted when properly fit. Problems of fit include the danger of pressure under the second metacarpal head due to the C-bar, the proper fit of the hypothenar bar so that the hand will not slip out of its support, the need to squeeze the hand slightly between the opponens and hypothenar bars to create a palmar arch, and the tendency to develop pressure under the wrist extension bar as it crosses the distal forearm and dorsal wrist. As with the Rancho splint, the distal strap must be placed so that it will lock firmly under the pisiform bone on the palmar aspect of the wrist, preventing the splint from slipping distally. Distal slipping will cause the C-bar and the hypothenar bar to impinge under the respective proximal phalanges, limiting metacarpal flexion.

Engen Volar Basic Wrist Splint

This orthosis is one of a family of plastic hand and wrist orthoses which differ from those described above in that they combine plastic and metallic construction (20–23), thus combining strength and custom fit. Final adjustments are made with a heat gun which makes possible both weight-bearing support and individual control. From Figs. 8.8 and 8.9 it will be seen that the plastic portion is molded to support the palmar arch, provide a posted position for the thumb in opposition, and preserve the web space. Since there is minimal free palm space the splint does have some of the limitations inherent in other palmar splints.

The Engen splint is best for simple support of the unloaded wrist or as the base for adaptive or other attachments. For correction or holding of the spastic wrist, the strong and simple Bunnell spring splint or any of the many related cock-up splints seem superior. The Engen splint, when properly fitted, especially the palmar molding, is very comfortable and this means that the splint will be superior if made by a skilled orthotist or therapist. Velcro fasteners are convenient for application and removal with minimal muscle strength.

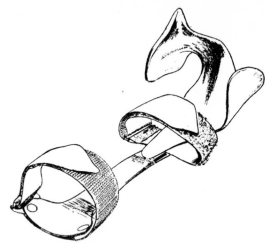

Fig. 8.8. Engen palmar basic wrist splint, dorsal view. (From a photograph supplied by Thorkild J. Engen, C.O.)

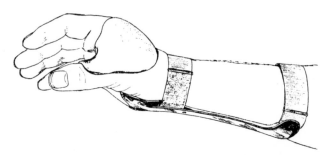

Fig. 8.9. Engen palmar basic wrist splint, lateral view.

Ulnar Deviation Stop

This device is used to prevent ulnar deviation of the wrist. In order to provide a corrective or preventive force, it has three points of contact with the forearm and hand; two of these are on the ulnar border of the segment, proximally and distally; the other is between the distal and proximal points. The distal point consists of a special metal trough adapted to the basic splint, extending along the ulnar border of the base of the fifth finger (Fig. 8.10). As an alternative the ulnar trough may extend proximally from the hypothenar bar along the ulnar border of the hand. The proximal point is represented by the medial proximal tab of the basic splint. The tab is lengthened beyond the normal to tolerate the greater pressures it must bear. The middle point is located at the wrist level, on the radial side of the splint and is a curved metal process of the wrist extension band. This structure is

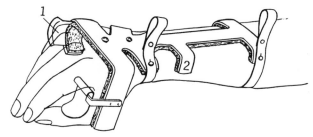

Fig. 8.10. Ulnar deviation stop. 1, ulnar trough; 2, radial stop.

a "radial stop" or "radial trough." This combination is useful in spasticity or muscle (weakness) imbalance.

DYNAMIC WRIST ORTHOSES

Dynamic orthoses for the wrist are more limited in use than static appliances; in many cases, dynamic splints are modifications of static splints. They are meant to allow or encourage motion and possess a joint corresponding, more or less, to the physiologic center of wrist motions. They may be used for substitution (absent muscle power), assistance (weak segments), traction, for directional control of the wrist and rarely, for simple support of the wrist or as the base for attachments.

Despite their theoretical usefulness we seldom use such splints because, in general, wrist splints are most often prescribed to subserve some requirement of the hand. When the hand cannot be helped by a splint, there is seldom much sense in applying a dynamic wrist splint; when the hand alone will profit from orthotic assistance, it is more desirable to use one of the compound splints described under the section on hand splints instead. Some examples of the dynamic wrist splint are discussed below.

The Pope Wrist Joint

The insertion of the Pope wrist joint in designs similar to those described above the static splints will produce an adjustable dynamic wrist splint for flexion and extension control, traction, or assistance. The joint is built on the same principle as the Pope ankle joint: a prefabricated joint which allows free motion in one direction but is restrained either by a solid stop or spring in the opposite direction. If a spring is present, it assists in the direction opposite to its stopping function. Pope joints are inserted in the lateral and medial side bars of a jointed wrist splint. The hand piece and forearm piece follow design principles mentioned above. Such a splint with a Pope joint in place is shown in Fig. 8.11.

If the Pope joint is used with a stop instead of a spring, the following considerations apply. A "stop" is a device to prevent motion beyond a certain point. A dorsal stop prevents extension; a palmar stop prevents flexion. If the Pope joint is mounted with its stop dorsally, it will stop

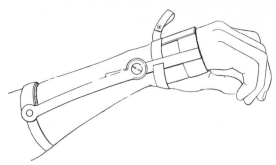

Fig. 8.11. Pope wrist joint.

extension; if it is turned upside-down and mounted with the stop on the palmar aspect it will stop flexion, providing substitution for absent wrist extensors. It also substitutes for the extensors in their essential function of antagonists to the finger flexors while they are in operation.

For example, if the wrist extensors are only of fair strength and can therefore just go through range of motion against gravity without further resistance, they will be able to lift the hand against gravity but would not be able to support the wrist while the finger flexors are making a tight fist. A dynamic splint might be indicated here to allow wrist extension by the wrist extensors but to take over the wrist extensors' function when the finger flexors come into forceful play. On the other hand, if the wrist flexors are weak, the weight of the hand is often enough to substitute for their usual function during action of the finger extensors, so that a dorsal stop is rarely used. Certain weaknesses about the hand and wrist may require dynamic splinting with free flexion range (with or without a dorsal stop). For instance, if the finger extensors are weak, at about the fair-minus level, the patient can often extend his fingers fully if he lengthens the finger extensors by permitting the wrist to fall into flexion. If such a patient is not permitted adequate range of wrist flexion, or even more maladroitly, held in the slightly extended "position of function," he will not be able to extend his fingers fully.

If the Pope joint is used with a spring, it usually serves for complete substitution of an absent muscle, assistance of a weak (and usually improving) muscle, or for mild traction. The spring's function may be directed either dorsally (extension) or toward the palm (flexion). A spring which is strong enough to be of assistance is usually strong enough to reposition the wrist and fingers. This new position must not be in the same direction as other factors tending toward finger contractures (such as flexor spasticity), or else exercises and stretching must be used when the splint is not worn to assure that contractures will not develop.

Other springs and stops for dynamic wrist flexion-extension splints have been described. Huddleston, Henderson and Campbell (32) connected dorsal metal plates on the hand and forearm with piano wire springs which supply the needed support or traction. The use of springs and stops in this and similar splints follows the principles described for the Pope wrist joint. The Rancho long opponens splint (Fig. 8.12) is an example, to which a hinged wrist joint and an extension assist spring (rubber band) have been added. An extension stop in the neutral position may be included, to prevent the elastic bands from keeping the wrist in an extended position. Such a splint may be used for a patient with weak wrist extensors but with good hand function and wrist flexors. With this arrangement the patient sacrifices strong grip (limited by the strength of the rubber bands) for range of flexion. If the patient needs stronger grip but can sacrifice the flexion range, a static wrist splint will fulfill his needs better.

Abduction-Adduction Wrist Splint

This compact splint (Fig. 8.13) for the control or correction of ulnar or radial deviation at the wrist (54) consists of a palmar bar beneath the forearm, with distal and proximal tabs, as on dorsal splints previously described. The palmar center of the brace has the form of an overlapping hinge. The hypothenar and radial bars grip the heads of the fifth and second metacarpals. This splint supports the wrist in the neutral or slightly extended position and was originally intended as a traction (rubber band) device to correct imbalance between radial and ulnar deviators. In addition to its use for the correction of imbalanced weakness (by assistance of weak muscles) it can be used as a basic traction device to overcome or prevent deformity.

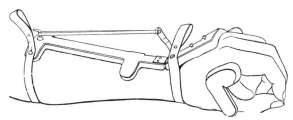

Fig. 8.12. Wrist extension hinge and elastic extension assist on long opponens hand splint.

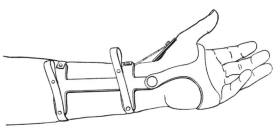

Fig. 8.13. Abduction-adduction splint for wrist.

dorsal interossei share bony and extensor mechanism insertion. The palmar interossei all insert into the extensor mechanism (24). There is no evidence to indicate that these differences in attachment result in functional differences.

The abduction-adduction control of the fingers by the interossei is most effective when the MP joint is in or near extension; in this position, the collateral ligaments are loose enough to permit satisfactory abduction-adduction range. When the MP joint is flexed, the collateral ligaments tighten and prevent that range, which suggests that any orthosis designed to correct or prevent finger deviation or to substitute for or assist weak fingers deviators operates most efficiently when the metacarpophalangeal (MP) joint is in extension. Orthoses have been constructed which permit some abduction-adduction assistance in most positions of the MP joint while it is in motion. Such a device is useful, but must assure that control is exerted at all points in the motion curve.

Power Grip, Precision Handling, and the Three-Jaw Chuck

The term "three-jaw chuck" (49) motion is used to describe a certain action of the fingers. Some observers feel that most daily activities involve the use of the thumb and first two fingers, with the thumb approximating a point midway between the fingers in closure. It is implied in the three-jaw chuck motion that the fingers move toward the thumb and the thumb toward the fingers. Along these lines, Landsmeer (37) divided hand motions into two theoretical classes: power grip and precision handling.

Precision handling and the three-jaw chuck concept are similar if not identical. Each implies thumb and two-finger motion with an interplay of intrinsic and extrinsic muscles. Landsmeer's concept suggests that the three-jaw chuck motion is confined to precision functions of the fingers, while power grip is another kinesiologic entity serving the further function of powerful grasp. In power grip, the major operators are the extrinsic flexors, with assistance from the interossei, as shown by our laboratory group (44, 45, 47, 50).

This discussion is pertinent to selecting a hand splint. The Bunnell concept of supporting each finger individually has been generally accepted with no attempt to differentiate between power and precision of the device or the patient's hand; it left the patient free to choose for himself the desired function. As an outgrowth of the three-jaw chuck pinch function in daily living activities, the flexor hinge splint and the flexor hinge hand (55), a surgical equivalent of the orthosis, were developed. The flexor hinge splint (Fig. 8.36) holds the first two fingers together as a unit articulating at the level of the MP joints; the thumb is held in opposition to contact these two fingers simultaneously. With this splint, the idea of using the splinted hand for power is virtually discarded. This is not a criticism of the concept, for there are relatively few instances in which power grip is essential or even the full hand but the lumbricales are active whenever the interphalangeal joints are extending. The interossei are active if the interphalangeal joints are extending or held extended at the same time as the metacarpophalangeal joints are flexing or held flexed. It is a major function of the lumbricales to draw the flexor profundus tendons distally, to relieve viscoelastic tension on the distal portion of the profundus. This tension would otherwise tend to flex the finger toward the clawed position. Since the interossei do not arise from the profundus tendons, they participate only when moving toward their shortest length—in the motions mentioned above for their participation. Further discussion of this theory can be found in the earlier works of Landsmeer and this author and his associates (37–41, 44–50).

The extrinsic extensor does include control of the interphalangeal joints as well as the metacarpophalangeal joints in spite of the lumbricales' major role in interphalangeal control. If a patient has no intrinsics but has a good extrinsic extensor, the interphalangeal joints can be extended if an artificial means can be found to prevent hyperextension at the metacarpophalangeal joints. Such control can be achieved by a bar or metacarpophalangeal (MP) stop applied dorsally over the proximal phalanges since that is the best position to prevent metacarpophalangeal hyperextension (Fig. 8.34).

Reciprocally, if the extrinsic extensor is absent, the intrinsic muscles can extend the interphalangeal joints if an artificial means can be found to extend or hold extended the metacarpophalangeal joints. The device, in this case, substitutes for the missing extensor digitorum. A good example is seen in the Thomas dorsal hand splint (Fig. 8.26).

The provision of extension assistance as dynamic splinting for the fingers requires that the assistance be properly placed. If the extrinsic extensor is weak, as above, but the intrinsics are strong, the support is placed under the proximal phalanges. If the extrinsics and intrinsics are weak or absent, the substitutive or assistive springs or elastics should act at the level of the distal interphalangeal (DIP) joint. The supporting rings, sleeves or cuffs should not impair touch on the finger pads; therefore, the level of the DIP joint itself is chosen. The cuff or ring prevents the joint from flexing as well as supporting the entire finger in extension. If the intrinsics are missing, but the extrinsics are present, the support again goes under the DIP joints. However, it is now necessary to add an MP stop bar (Fig. 8.34) to prevent MP hyperextension by the supporting brace (usually elastic "traction").

Abduction-Adduction

Abduction is movement away from the center line of the middle finger (dorsal interossei action); adduction is motion toward the center line (palmar interossei action). The attachments of individual interossei differ in the percentage of attachment of the muscle sub-bellies to bone (at the base of the proximal phalanx) or to the extensor mechanism (in the lateral bands). The first dorsal interosseus attaches entirely into bone while the other

The Hand

In the entire locomotor system, except for eye tracking movements, the hand demonstrates the most coordinated and sensitive control. A hand which is damaged severely enough to require orthotic assistance rarely regains full function with an orthosis. Our goal should be to return function to as near normal as possible with the knowledge that complete return cannot be expected. Even when the motion of the hand can be restored to nearly normal, the very application of a splint often reduces the sensitivity of the palmar surface and the tactile pads of the fingers by the interposition of a foreign material between the hand and the object of its touch or grasp. Thus, the hand orthosis is an easy mark for the reluctant patient or physician who looks for reasons not to use it. Hand orthoses are used less than they should be, partially because of the limitations we have mentioned and the resulting lack of enthusiasm with which they are prescribed. On the other hand, in some centers hand orthoses are not only well accepted but proliferating; an aura of enthusiasm and optimism surrounds the prescription of the orthosis. It is only necessary that this optimism be tempered with realism to achieve maximal usefulness for patient and physician.

Flexion-Extension

The kinesiology of the hand is based on a working relationship between the intrinsic (wholly contained within the hand) and extrinsic (muscle bodies outside, tendons extending into the hand) muscles. The two sets of muscles are linked by the "extensor assembly," a criss-cross linkage which transfers the intrinsic pull into the lateral bands of the expanded extrinsic extensor tendon. Landsmeer (40) has shown that the metacarpophalangeal and interphalangeal joints are so constructed that operation of the finger by extrinsic muscles alone would have to follow a pattern of metacarpophalangeal extension and interphalangeal flexion. This is the "intrinsic minus" hand, of Bunnell, seen in combined ulnar-median lesions at the wrist level, such as the claw hand. In order to prevent the collapse of the finger into the claw position under the influence of the extrinsics, the intrinsics must operate under certain conditions as borne out by electromyographic evidence (41). The interossei supply a metacarpophalangeal flexion and interphalangeal extension component to counteract the clawing effect of the extrinsic muscles. When the full hand opens, the extrinsic extensor and the lumbricales join to straighten the whole finger. When the whole hand is closed to a fist, the deep flexors flex the finger. The extensor participates as a brake during flexion; the flexor superficialis participates erratically in all flexing motions of the finger; it is most active if the wrist is in flexion and least in extension. The superficialis participates in major fashion only if flexion of the distal interphalangeal joint is prohibited voluntarily (not by a splint) during finger flexion.

The lumbricales and interossei are "silent" during unresisted closing of possible for the hand encased in an orthosis. When power grip is important or possible, for example, in radial nerve injury or disease in an otherwise strong individual, instead of the flexor hinge, a supporting system should be used for the individual fingers. This will give the patient a choice between power grip and precision.

Web Space and the "Posted" Thumb

Proper splinting demands proper positioning of the thumb, which is a compromise between the obvious desire to hold the thumb in a useful position and the severe encumbrance due to its immobility and the holding device. It is logical to place the thumb in a position to meet the first two fingers as demanded by the theories of precision handling and the three-jaw chuck. It is also logical to spread the web space as far as possible to permit large objects to be grasped or pinched. A thumb which is placed in response to these logical conclusions is called a "posted" thumb, for the thumb acts as a post against which the fingers operate. An immediate minor problem results: the thumb cannot move toward the center of the thumb-finger air space so the system does not act as a true three-jaw chuck. Some braces overcome this problem by allowing the thumb to move, but the complexity may not warrant the resulting benefit. Another problem is that the posted thumb gets in the way constantly. Although it is sometimes convenient for the patient to rest his hand and brace on the thumb or the opponens bar, it is more often inconvenient to have his thumb protruding constantly from his palm. This position makes it impossible for the braced hand to enter the pocket or go through the unaltered sleeve of a coat or shirt. No way has been found out of this dilemma for the thumb must be posted if the hand is to operate efficiently.

Another problem of the posted thumb is caused by the structures needed to hold the thumb in position; the supports are usually metal and extend around the thumb, especially in the flexor hinge splint. The metal extensions cause the same kind of difficulty as does a brace structure in the palm; it covers the palmar surface of the thumb making the thumb less sensitive and making it more difficult to pick up solid, smooth objects because of the lack of friction with the equally smooth metal of the post. This should be taken into consideration in choosing between, for instance, the Rancho long opponens splint and the flexor hinge splint. The former, and its relatives, leave the thumb partially free to move and uncovered by metal at the tip; the flexor hinge completely limits thumb motion and partially covers the tactile pad.

In order to post the thumb properly, the width of the web space must be maintained in one of the following ways: insertion of a C-bar or plastic or wooden dowel between the thumb and the second metacarpal; metallic fixation of the thumb in posted position, as in the flexor hinge splint; use of a "saddle" on the proximal phalanx of the thumb, connected by a strut to the basic brace at the level of the second metacarpal head (Fig. 8.14), or, application of a saddle with an expansion spring substituted for the strut. The differences in function and subsequent advantages and disadvantages of these types of structure follow from the reasoning above. The C-bar and its equivalent dowels maintain the web space but leave the thumb free to move (except in adduction) and to feel. They may be used for the completely paralyzed thumb but operate better when the thumb is powered, at least in part. The disadvantages of the metallic fixation of the fully posted thumb have been mentioned above; however, it is often advantageous to use this method of fixation for the paralyzed thumb to assure its continuous proper opposition to the fingers. The use of a saddle and strut construction implies that opposition of the thumb is powered; the saddle cannot be used on a completely paralyzed thumb. The saddle with the expansion spring implies not only that opposition is powered but also that there is voluntary adduction of the thumb strong enough to overcome the spring and bring the thumb toward the center of the thumb-finger air space.

MECHANICAL FEATURES OF HAND ORTHOSES

Bulkiness is the plague of the complex hand orthosis. There is little that can be done about the problem of the thumb which must be posted. The wearer must put the splint on after he is dressed and must remove the splint to put on his coat. This is not too difficult if the patient can apply and remove his own splint but the inconvenience may cause the patient and family to reject the splint. The second area of bulkiness problems concerns outriggers for substitution, assistance or traction for the fingers and thumb. Fortunately, many outriggers are removable so that the whole brace does not have to be removed to get the arm through the sleeve. Several splints have been designed to shorten outriggers and to use other methods of support (Fig. 8.25).

Cuffs and Rings

The methods of support for fingers and thumb range from metal platforms to carefully machined rings which slip on the fingers. The choice of sup-

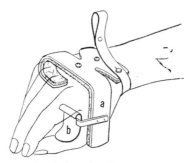

Fig. 8.14. Bennett basic hand splint. *a*, opponens bar; *b*, C-bar.

porting structure will depend upon two factors: the purpose and need for the splint and the limitations imposed on the patient's strength, range of motion and tactile ability in the splint. Platforms must be used only for static support; the splint is inherently nonfunctional. Leather or plastic cuffs are the most commonly used supporting structures in dynamic hand splints. Cuffs must be fairly wide to support the DIP joint or the proximal phalanx adequately; eventually, leather cuffs soften, stretch, and narrow, thus losing their wide area of support. When this happens they should be replaced; plastic cuffs stretch very little. Rings have the advantage that they can be machined to fit each finger and do not change their width. However, these great advantages are overshadowed by the tendency of the best rings to slip off the finger accidentally if they are loose enough to be removed easily by the patient and family. The choice of cuffs and rings often becomes a matter of local taste and practice.

Elastics and Springs

The most commonly used "traction" element in hand splints is the rubber band. Modifications, such as elasticized plastic, have been used but the rubber band remains the favorite because it is available, easily replaced, and adjusted. Springs, on the other hand, must be carefully selected for strength and length and a great number must be stocked by the orthotist or therapist for proper adjustment. *No elastic or spring should ever be stronger than that just necessary to perform the desired function in a hand splint.*

Metal and Plastic

The advantages which metal or plastic might have with respect to the other are still to be determined. Since plastics were introduced in the 1940's, there have been many attempts to use them for hand orthoses. The suggestion that plastic will replace metal in hand orthoses remains to be fulfilled for permanent orthoses although they are widely used for temporary orthoses and static splinting. With the notable exception of the excellent Engen splints, plastics are not commonly used for much dynamic splinting on a permanent basis. In general, most metal splints are durable, adaptable, and easy for the therapist, physician, or orthotist to handle and repair. Plastic splints do lend themselves well to static support, especially of the wrist, or of "platformed" fingers. Temporary dynamic splints of plastic have been widely used in nerve injuries and in burn orthoses. The new thermoplastics are much easier to mold and repair than the older thermo setting types of rigid plastic (see Chapter 3) and promise more extensive use in the future.

HAND ORTHOSES (HOs)

We have classified orthoses and attachments for the thumb and fingers as thumb, static and dynamic; fingers, static and dynamic. Finger splints are further subclassified by joint (see Table 8.1).

THUMB

Static thumb splints post the thumb in opposition to the index and middle fingers. They are used for substitution for absent or weakened thenar eminence muscles, for support for the thumb in the posted position. The differentiation between static and dynamic thumb splints is not very clear, but basically, static splints do not encourage or permit significant thumb motion. The problem of definition occurs because some static splints do permit significant opposition (Warm Springs basic hand splint with C-bar).

The basic hand splints are presented here to illustrate methods of thumb support. The basic hand splint is not encountered commonly in clinical practice because most hands which require splinting also require wrist splinting for stability. The structural support of the thumb in basic hand and wrist splints is identical within each family of splints.

Warm Springs Basic Hand Splint

This splint is easily constructed from aluminum stock by a skilled orthotist, therapist or physician (Fig. 8.14). It is a T-shaped piece of metal bent to form two supports (an ulnar bar and an opponens bar). The proximal tabs support the Velcro straps or other fasteners; the straps prevent the splint from sliding distally off the hand by fastening tightly just proximal to the protrusion of the pisiform bone. The thumb is supported by an opponens bar which prevents it from swinging radially (toward extension at the carpometacarpal joint) and by the C-bar which is the web space spreader. It is important that the C-bar nestle closely under the head of the second metacarpal to support the radial end of the palmar arch. The thumb end of the C-bar lies against the ulnar side of the proximal phalanx of the thumb and extends a little beyond the interphalangeal joint unless there is voluntary control of the interphalangeal joint.

The main purpose of the basic hand splint, including an opponens bar and a C-bar, is to maintain the web space and prevent the thumb from falling back into the "ape-hand" position. The splint without any attachments can be used for support of the thumb (as in the patient with a powered thumb with web space contracture) or as a substitution for absent thenar eminence muscles. It may also be used for the attachment of accessories for the fingers when wrist support is not needed.

Rancho Short Opponens Hand Splint

This can also be made from aluminum stock by skilled orthotists and therapists. It has the same functions as the Warm Springs splint but in addition it provides good support for the palmar arch because of the palmar bar (Fig. 8.15).

Engen Basic Hand Splint

This orthosis is a molded plastic impression of the palm and thenar eminence with the thumb in opposition (Figs. 8.16 and 8.17). This molded

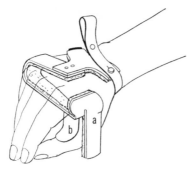

Fig. 8.15. Rancho short opponens hand splint. *a*, opponens bar; *b*, C-bar.

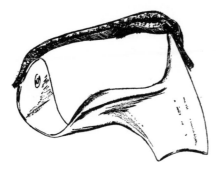

Fig. 8.16. Engen basic hand splint seen from distal end. (From a photograph supplied by Thorkild J. Engen, C.O.)

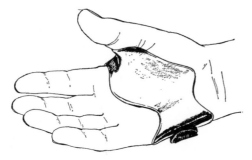

Fig. 8.17. Engen basic hand splint seen from palmar side. (From a photograph supplied by Thorkild J. Engen, C.O.)

palm plate is similar in appearance to the palm plate of the Engen basic wrist splint; it is strapped to the hand with an elastic strap. It supports the thumb in opposition, preserving the web space and preventing it from dropping back into the ape-hand position. The splint is best for support or to substitute for weak thenar muscles. It is seldom used for the attachment of accessories.

The splints presented thus far include the general families of hand splints which may be used with modifications or combinations. Further definitions and information are offered to assist the reader in prescription.

STATIC THUMB SUPPORT

The *opponens bar* is the portion of the splint which is the palmar extension of the radial bar (Fig. 8.14). It prevents the thumb from swinging into the ape-hand position; it holds the thumb in opposition. It prevents motion in one direction only but motion across the palm toward the little finger is still possible.

The *C-bar* is a C-shaped band of metal imposed between the thumb and the notch proximal to the second metacarpal head. It maintains the width of the web space and helps support the palmar surface of the proximal phalanx of the thumb. The C-bar is usually made of more malleable and thinner metal than the rest of the hand splint. It can be bent by hand to assume new and more appropriate dimensions as the web-space width slowly responds to splinting or other treatment. Two different types of C-bar which serve the same purposes are shown in Figures 8.14 and 8.15.

The *opponens dowel* is similar in its effect to the C-bar; it preserves web-space width (Fig. 8.18). It is less adjustable than the C-bar since it must be completely removed and replaced to conform to the patient's new requirements. In addition, the dowel does not fit the contours of the notch below the second metacarpal head as well as the C-bar, nor does it support the ulnar border of the first phalanx as well as the C-bar. The C-bar has the advantage that it can be built in the compound curved shape necessary to conform to both the second metacarpal and the proximal phalanx of the thumb.

Although each of the methods above more or less "posts" the thumb, there is one type which is specifically called a *thumb post*. It is exemplified in the flexor hinge splint to be described later (Fig. 8.36); a rigid band of metal which conforms to the dorsal surface of the thumb. It does not enclose the palmar surface of the thumb except over the palmar pad of the distal phalanx where an incomplete band of metal encircles the thumb to provide support. The thumb post, although shown in this chapter only in relation to the flexor hinge family, can be applied to either the Rancho or Warm

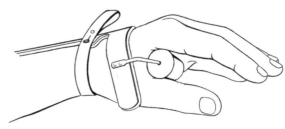

Fig. 8.18. Opponens dowel on Bennett basic hand splint.

Springs splints as full wrist and hand splints or as hand splints alone. It is generally most advisable to use opponens bar and C-bar combinations when possible instead of the thumb post because of the freedom permitted the thumb in the ulnar direction. However, in the completely paralyzed, unstable thumb, it may be necessary to use the thumb post. The post limits tactile sensation on the important thumb touch pad.

DYNAMIC THUMB SPLINTS

Spring Swivel Thumb

Swivels which have been described as attachments for splints follow a common principle. The swivel is an interlocking pair of loops, located at the base of the index finger (Fig. 8.19). The spring may be a curved or partially coiled piece of piano wire. It is always an expansion spring with its two points of attachment held away from each other. The point of attachment opposite the loop-swivel is usually a saddle which rests on the proximal phalanx of the thumb. In order to operate properly, this attachment requires a powered thenar eminence (or substitutive musculature such as long thumb flexor), plus reasonable range of motion of the carpometacarpal joint. A powered adductor permits full use of the three-jaw chuck, with fingers and thumb moving toward a central point. The reason this attachment is so little used is that most thumbs good enough to use the attachment are too good to need splinting at all. Also, the saddle tends to slip off the thumb during repeated movement.

A modification of the attachment was described by the Rancho Los Amigos group. In cases where there is an overactive deep flexor causing interphalangeal joint flexion during attempted pinch, a device called a stabilizer is used. This is a modified saddle which almost encircles the thumb and extends across the interphalangeal joint to stabilize it.

Thumb Distal Phalanx Extension Outrigger

This simple device has many modifications all of which serve the same

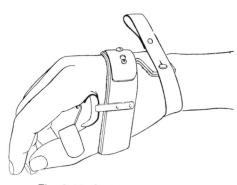

Fig. 8.19. Spring swivel thumb.

purpose, to assist extension of the distal phalanx of the thumb with springs or springs and elastics. It is used to substitute when there is no active extensor pollicis longus, or to assist when this muscle is weak. It may also be used if both thumb extensors are weak. A piano wire outrigger is fastened to the base of the hand or wrist splint, usually at the level of the opponens bar, and attached by a cuff to the distal phalanx. As an alternate, the piano wire may have a piece of elastic attached to it which is cuffed to the distal phalanx (Fig. 8.20).

Thumb Proximal Phalanx Extension Outrigger

This device is identical to that described above for the distal phalanx except for its attachment to the proximal phalanx; thus, its use is indicated in isolated weakness of the extensor pollicis brevis. It is very rarely used since patients substitute the long extensor if the short one is deficient.

FINGERS

Static splints for the fingers attempt to hold a single position, primarily for the prevention of contracture or for the production of a slow, steady, correcting force against an existing contracture. The correction of an existing contracture can be encouraged by the application of a slightly nonconforming splint. As the hand gradually changes to conform to the splint, the orthosis is adjusted to remain slightly nonconforming. If simple support is the purpose of the splint, no such continued readjustment is necessary.

In prescribing static splints for the fingers, we must bear in mind that all their joints depend upon each other and that the new position held by the splint is likely to cause new positioning problems elsewhere in the hand and wrist. This is true primarily for disorders of the extension or flexion mechanism as opposed to disorders of capsules and joints. If, for instance, a single proximal interphalangeal (PIP) joint is involved with mild rheumatoid arthritis and a supporting splint is desired for the night, it would be safe to apply such a splint without worrying about the effect on other joints. This

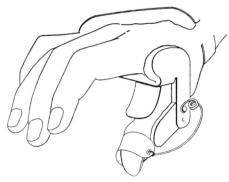

Fig. 8.20. Thumb distal phalanx extension outrigger.

safety is based on the lack of cross-coupling of the PIP joint contracture with the behavior of other joints as would be the case in tendon tightness.

What is done to one finger may affect other fingers. If, for example, a single finger is splinted straight, this limits strength and range of the flexor profundus to the other fingers. The profundus cannot shorten adequately, so the patient cannot make a tight fist. Most of the burden of hand closure is then thrown on the superficialis, which of course, cannot flex the distal joints at all.

Hand motion should be limited only to the extent necessary to serve the functions of the orthosis. Static splints for the fingers, especially of the platform variety, may immobilize all the fingers when this effect is only desired on one or two. In such an instance, the orthosis should be chosen to permit finger support or traction rather than the shotgun method of platform support. Some of the static attachments will be discussed along with the dynamic splints which they accompany. At this point we shall discuss only the most common static splints.

Finger troughs are simple gutters in which the fingers are placed and immobilized with fastening devices. They can be made of wood, plastic, aluminum, or plaster of paris. When they are to be used for immobilization only and are not to be connected to a basic hand or wrist splint they can be constructed with ease by the physician or therapist. Troughs may be attached to any splint when specific, positioning control of the IP joints is desired. If the problem is flexor tendon tightness, the MP joint must not be allowed to flex when the finger is splinted lest MP contracture result from IP immobilization.

An aluminum trough is attached to the finger by straps; a plaster trough is usually more temporary and may be attached with bandage. Troughs are generally used to maintain finger positioning during the healing period following a lesion of tendon or bone, or to prevent or slowly correct contracture of capsule or musculotendinous mechanisms.

Platform splints support all fingers simultaneously on a table-like flat surface (Fig. 8.21). The radial and ulnar edges are raised to prevent the fingers from sliding off the splint. Since the splint is so restrictive, it is often

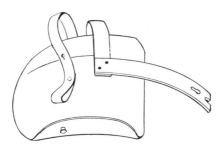

Fig. 8.21. Platform splint attachment.

used as a night splint for stretching or position maintenance. It is also used on hands which are completely paralyzed or not functional, in which case it can be worn in the daytime. The finger platform splint is often a good solution to the problems encountered when correction is required in a wrist flexion contracture due to tight wrist flexors or tight finger flexors. This situation, often seen in hemiplegics, requires splinting of the wrist and fingers simultaneously to prevent finger flexion contracture as would happen if the wrist alone were supported.

A strap is required across the backs of the fingers for control, but when spasticity is severe, a strap is inadequate and one of two picturesquely named orthoses may be used. The "pancake splint" and the "hand sandwich" are modifications of the platform splint which add a second, similar platform posteriorly so that the hand is squeezed between the two platforms. The double platform may be rigidly anchored to the wrist, as in the hand sandwich (Fig. 8.22) or attached to a basic Bunnell wrist splint by a steel spring which exerts additional extension force against the wrist flexors, as in the pancake splint (Fig. 8.23). These splints have been described as useful in cerebral palsy and hemiplegia (74). They fully position the fingers while correction is applied against wrist flexion contracture.

Rheumatoid Arthritis Night Splint (University of Michigan). Bender (9) described a static splint to be used at night for proper positioning of rheumatoid fingers. It is made of metal and consists of a palmar bar under the proximal phalanges of all the fingers, attached to a forearm anterior

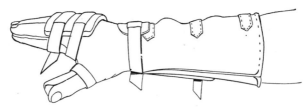

Fig. 8.22. Hand sandwich.

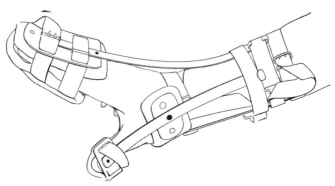

Fig. 8.23. Pancake splint.

trough by means of a palmar connection. Finger separator posts extend dorsally between the fingers to prevent ulnar deviation of the fingers during sleep, thus reducing the stress on the radial collateral supporting structures of the MP joint. Bender (8) credits the dynamic ulnar deviation splint of Smith as superior to his own in the prevention of ulnar deviation (see below).

Dynamic Finger Splints

Dynamic splinting of the fingers is one of the most challenging and complex aspects of upper limb bracing. Diverse problems may face the physician at different joints of different fingers on the two hands of the same patient. The physician must determine whether all the fingers have similar disabilities, by gross examination. If so, he may prescribe an orthosis which is relatively simple and operates on one basic principle. If he finds that the fingers or their separate joints present varied problems, he must prescribe an orthosis which reflects these differences and attempts to correct each disability as best possible. To assist in prescription, this section presumes basic knowledge of the subjects discussed earlier in this chapter—especially concerning basic wrist and hand splints. We shall discuss a series of brace attachments or accessories which serve specific functions at specific joints or in specific fingers (Table 1). In addition, we shall describe orthoses which act as total braces for wrist, finger, and thumb, including the flexor hinge splint and the tenodesis splint.

Dynamic splinting is usually used in the fingers for substitution for absent motor power, assistance for weak motor power or for traction against contractures or impending contractures.

DYNAMIC METACARPOPHALANGEAL JOINT ORTHOSES

Dynamic splinting is applied to the MP joint to affect one of the axes of movement. It must relate to extension-flexion or to abduction-adduction (deviation). Any splint listed as an extension splint is a splint which will also stretch the flexor system. Conversely, all flexion splints stretch extensors; all radial splints stretch the ulnar deviators and vice versa.

Splinting for Extension

The *MP extension assist* is one of the commonest attachments to hand orthoses. There are several varieties which attempt the same objective: to provide extension where the extrinsic extensors are weakened or absent, or to provide traction against a tight flexor system. If the point of support is beneath the proximal phalanx, the finger will tend to curl into flexion when extension traction is applied. The only counters to this tendency are the existence of good intrinsics to extend the IP joints, or the presence of ankylosed fingers. If either of these is present, traction or support can be placed under the proximal phalanx as a true MP extension assist, but if neither intrinsic control nor ankylosed IP joints are present, the support or traction must go under the DIP joint (as described below for IP extension assist). Traction (substitution or assistance, or true traction) is applied to the proximal phalanges through rubber bands, elasticized nylon or spring wires. Since this is a dynamic assist, permitting full range of motion of the MP joint, it is not possible to maintain the traction perpendicular to the proximal phalanx. A compromise is to allow the point of support to protrude a little distal to the MP line.

The *MP extension outrigger* is the most frequently used extension assist, probably because of its ease of construction (Fig. 8.24). The device consists of a removable arch of metal, extending from the distal portion of the wrist extension bar of the basic dorsal wrist splint or the dorsal bar of a basic hand splint over the fingers. From a cross-beam at the end of the arch are suspended the elastic (usually rubber band) devices which attach to the fingers by cuffs or rings.

The *MP extension assist by spring wire* is a modification of the MP extension assist and relies for its tractive assistance on spring wires instead of elasticized plastic or rubber bands. They are mounted on a T-shaped bar which attaches to the distal portion of the wrist extension bar of a basic hand splint, or to the dorsal bar of a basic hand splint. The spring wires are arranged so that their tension is exerted toward extension. This splint is less bulky than the extension outrigger and looks better but is more difficult to make.

The *MP extension assist with pulleys and elastic cord* has the dual advantage of long elastic support and reduced bulk (Fig. 8.25). It relies for its support on long strands of elasticized nylon which stretch almost the entire length of the basic wrist splint, from its proximal end to a bank of pulleys mounted on a short outrigger overlying the proximal phalanges. The amount of tension exerted by the very long elastics remains almost constant through the opening and closing range of motion of the hand. In shorter

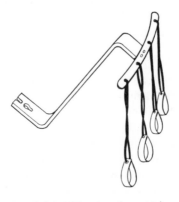

Fig. 8.24. MP extension outrigger.

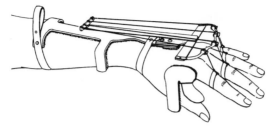

Fig. 8.25. MP extension assist with pulleys, elastic cord.

elastics, the amount of pull varies greatly from the fully extended to the fully flexed position of the MP joints. As can be seen in Fig. 8.25, the pulleys are covered by guides for the elasticized nylon to keep the elastic from jumping out of the sheave. This splint is cosmetically more acceptable and less bulky than the outrigger.

The *Thomas MP extension assist* in spite of its simplicity is very versatile and commonly used (Fig. 8.26). It consists of a fairly bulky outrigger from which is suspended a single strand of elastic supporting a cylindrical rod (about the diameter of a pencil) which passes under the palmar surface of the proximal phalanges of all the fingers, which it supports, mainly in the elastic between the outrigger and the palmar bar. The springiness of the outrigger also contributes to this support. The Thomas attachment, because of its assistance to all the fingers, may be used on a wrist splint to provide excellent substitution for absent muscles in radial nerve palsy. It then supports wrist and fingers on the extension side. The addition of a thumb distal phalanx extension outrigger to substitute for the missing thumb extensors completes the "radial nerve palsy splint."

The *reverse knuckle bender* (not illustrated) is a splint for extension traction to the MP joints which attempts to reverse the effect of the knuckle bender (Fig. 8.27). Its design is similar to that of the knuckle bender, but its rubber band traction is exerted against the *palmar* surface of the fingers to exert an extending force.

MP Flexion Splints

Dynamic splints for MP flexion usually provide traction against MP extension contractures. Since there is no single flexor of the MP joints, this type of splint is rarely used to provide substitution or assistance for the flexors of the MP joints. If for some reason the fingers are ankylosed, except at the MP joints, this splint may be a useful substitute for weak long flexors.

A common type of contracture in extension at the MP joints is caused by tightness of the MP capsule, especially the collateral ligaments, which are strong and resist passive stretching. Long periods of traction are required to produce any real effect; the general rules for tractive bracing (angle of pull, method of beginning, and so on) must be followed. To be effective, MP

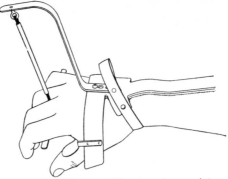

Fig. 8.26. Thomas MP extension assist.

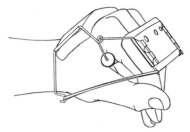

Fig. 8.27. Knuckle bender.

flexion traction requires some form of power to maintain the results of traction, either internal voluntary power (extrinsic flexors) or external power. It is often necessary to stretch the MP joints into flexion so they will have adequate range to be operated by a flexion splint, such as the artifical muscle. However, it is usually fruitless to stretch MP joints into flexion if they are not to be used functionally in flexion thereafter, for the contracture will recur unless repeated stretching is used.

The *knuckle bender* is the "old faithful" orthosis to stretch MP contractures. Described by Bunnell (14) it is a masterpiece of simplicity and effectiveness (Fig. 8.27). A metal plate on the back of the metacarpus and another over the proximal and middle phalanges dorsally are linked by rigid wires to a palmar bar passing under the heads of the second to fifth metacarpals. Elastic bands are rigged to the metal plates to apply flexion traction through the device. The traction is easily regulated by changing the size and strength of the rubber bands. The only significant disadvantage of this efficient splint is its equal treatment of all fingers. No provision can be made for individual fingers which lag behind the stretching process: all fingers must wait for the laggard. This disadvantage is partially balanced by the low cost of the splint, its commercial availability and minimal fitting requirements.

MP individual finger flexion traction is a commonly used attachment which relies on individual rubber band traction to assure that flexion traction can be given to different fingers in different amounts. Weight and length of elastic can be varied to provide this fine differentiation for individual fingers. The attachment can be applied easily to the Bunnell spring cock-up wrist splint (Fig. 8.28).

The *MP flexion control (adjustable)* is included here, although it permits no motion toward extension, because of the adjustable nature of this stop (Fig. 8.29). The device consists of a bar across the dorsum of the proximal phalanges set in a degree of flexion determined by the prescribing physician. Its purpose is to maintain any correction that may have been gained against an MP extension contracture through treatment or activities of daily living. The bar is used as an adjustable stop; it is moved into more and more flexion regularly as the contracture is stretched. It allows motion toward flexion, thus permitting use of the hand for daily living.

The *MP spring flexion assist* is the same as the MP flexion control except that it is fitted with a flexing spring (or elastic) instead of a stop. It maintains

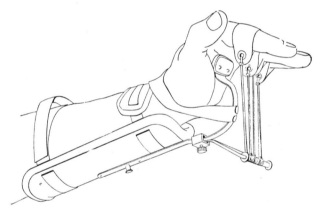

Fig. 8.28. MP individual finger flexion traction on Bunnell cock-up wrist splint.

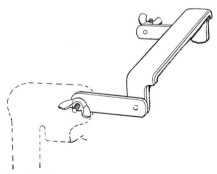

Fig. 8.29. MP flexion control, adjustable.

constant tension against extension contractures of the MP joint but also allows the hand to open by permitting MP extension. It is excellent for the long range, steady stretching of MP flexion contractures between treatment sessions.

Abduction-Adduction Splints

When introduced in the 1950's these splints were used for substitution or assistance for poliomyelitis-weakened muscles. They remain useful for this objective in peripheral nerve lesions and quadriplegia, but they have become increasingly useful in the treatment and prevention of rheumatoid arthritis deformities. They provide an abduction or adduction deviating force to prevent abnormal positioning of the finger and to control the finger through an undeviated track during flexion and extension. The use of these splints in rheumatoid arthritis is based on the hypothesis that continued improper use of the hand permits irreparable stretching of supporting structures; the prevention of this stretching is essential to the prevention of rheumatoid deformity.

The *finger deviation splint (Rancho Los Amigos)* is built on the principle of the basic hand splint previously illustrated. It does not have a C-bar but does have an opponens bar to help position the thumb (Fig. 8.30). The principle feature of the splint is a bar which passes dorsal to the proximal phalanges; the bar is hinged at the level of the MP joint centers of rotation. Suspended from the bar are separate supporting cuffs for each finger with a nonelastic, very short connection from the cuffs to the bar. Each cuff is slightly offset ulnarly from its point of suspension so that a continuous radial deviation pressure is exerted on each finger. Because of the hinge, the bar and deviating cuffs follow the fingers during opening and closing motions of the hand, thus supplying continuous corrective force against the ulnar-deviating tendency of the rheumatoid hand.

The *fifth finger adduction splint with spring wire* described by Bender (9), applies a radial-deviating force by means of a spring and saddle arrange-

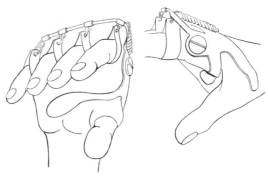

Fig. 8.30. Rancho finger deviation splint.

ment impinging on the ulnar side of the proximal phalanx of the small finger (Fig. 8.31). By supporting this finger, it supports, to some extent, the entire row of fingers against ulnar deviation. The splint permits normal opening and closing motions of the hand.

The *dynamic ulnar deviation splint* of Smith, Juvinall and Pearson (71) prevents ulnar deviation by stopping ulnar drift of the fifth finger in a manner similar to that of the Bender splint described above. This splint, however, has a rigid support hinged at the MP joint lying along the ulnar border of the fifth finger as far as the proximal interphalangeal joint. The splint may be made of either stainless steel or polyvinylchloride plastic (Fig. 8.32). Like the two preceding splints, it provides dynamic support during motion of the MP joints, preventing ulnar drift in the rheumatoid hand. A "fixed post" version of this splint is also described, in which the hinged fifth finger piece is replaced by a sheet of metal or plastic which serves as a stop against ulnar deviation throughout the range of the fifth MP joint.

The *first dorsal interosseus assist* is a simple, little outrigger which may

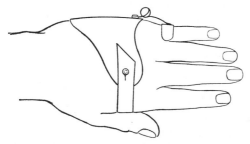

Fig. 8.31. Fifth finger adduction splint with spring wire.

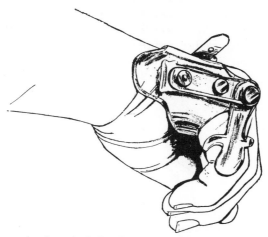

Fig. 8.32. Dynamic ulnar deviation (prevention) splint. [Reprinted with permission from: E. M. Smith, R. C. Juvinall, and J. R. Pearson (72).]

be attached to any basic splint to provide controllable radial deviation of the index finger (Fig. 8.33). It may substitute for or assist a weakened first dorsal interosseus. In isolated instances of beginning ulnar deviation of the ndex finger in rheumatoid arthritis it may be used as a preventive or corrective device, and this is important if, as some believe, the index is the first finger to deviate in this disease and then pushes the others into ulnar deviation.

INTERPHALANGEAL JOINTS

The major attention in splinting interphalangeal joints is usually directed to the proximal interphalangeal (PIP) joint. The distal interphalangeal (DIP) joint is not as important in hand function and so is rarely braced if it alone is affected. There are some times when it should be braced, for example, fracture of the tip of the middle phalanx (baseball finger). Because of the great interest in the PIP joint, this section will deal mainly with orthoses for that joint. Included in this section are braces for substitution, assistance and traction.

When the mechanical effect of a dynamic splint is directed at the PIP joints, the force must not be dissipated on the MP joints. If we desire extension of the PIP joints, we must block MP extension at some point to prevent action at the PIP level. If we wish flexion at the PIP joint we must stop it at the MP joint.

Splinting for Interphalangeal Extension

In order to assist IP joint extension we must combine extension "assist" and a stop to prevent MP extension.

An *MP extension stop* is a metal bar placed across the dorsum of the proximal phalanges, limiting MP extension. If the patient has an extrinsic extensor but no intrinsic musculature, he can still extend all of his finger joints with the extrinsic extensor when there is an MP extension stop. The extension stop is often used to assure that the more distally placed elastics will give distal action. The usual combination of MP extension stop and IP elastic traction is shown in Fig. 8.34. An example of the use of an MP

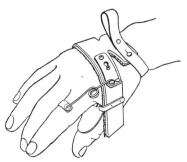

Fig. 8.33. First dorsal interosseus assist.

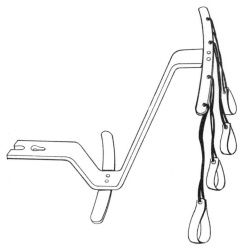

Fig. 8.34. IP elastic traction with MP stop.

extension stop as a "pure" extension stop is seen in the adjustable MP flexion control splint shown in Fig. 8.29.

The *IP extension assist* is very often used, especially in connection with the MP extension stop. It consists of an extension outrigger identical with that used for MP extension assistance, but a little longer. The cuffs or rings, attached by elastic to the outrigger, act at the level of the DIP joints (Fig. 8.34). This level of action assures some support for the DIP joint while allowing most of the effect of the brace to be felt at the PIP level. The MP effect is blocked by the MP extension stop. The splint is used for substitution or assistance, for combined weakness of extrinsic and intrinsic extensors, or for traction against the palmar side of the PIP joint or the flexor musculo-tendinous apparatus. Rarely, the cuffs may be allowed to support the fingers over the touch pads on the distal phalanges. This is indicated only if contractures on the flexor side of the DIP joint must be stretched. Since this splint is such an effective traction device, the rules for application of traction must be followed carefully. It is especially important to allow the patient to start wearing the splint gradually and to be sure that the traction is at an easily tolerated pain level.

The *Bunnell PIP extension traction splint* is a simple, ingenious device designed solely for traction at the PIP joint (Fig. 8.35). It may be applied to counteract flexion or extension contractures. It is similar in operation to the knuckle bender. For extension traction at the PIP joint, one saddle of thin steel sits under the palmar surface of the proximal phalanx; another rests under the distal phalanx. Counterpressure is exerted at the level of the PIP joint by a cloth strap with buckle. The required tractive tension is applied with two pieces of spring wire which join the saddles under the proximal and distal phalanges.

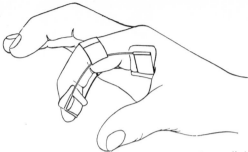

Fig. 8.35. Bunnell PIP extension traction splint.

Interphalangeal Flexion

Interphalangeal flexion is produced in a manner opposite to that used for extension; all of the palmar structures are made dorsal and *vice versa*. Dynamic splinting for IP flexion is usually for traction against tight extensors or the dorsal side of the PIP capsule.

The *Bunnell PIP flexion traction splint* can be visualized if that shown in Fig. 8.35 is turned upside-down. The metal plates go on the dorsum of the proximal and distal phalanges and the webbed strap goes around the palmar portion of the PIP joint.

An *IP flexion assist* usually uses elastic bands to flex the IP joints. If the elastics are to effect the PIP joints, the MP joint must be prevented from flexing with a metal bar crossing under the palmar surfaces of the proximal phalanges. Such a stop may be called a *metacarpal bar* or an *MP flexion stop*. This splint is difficult to construct and even more difficult to wear. The basic splint must be palmar, like the Bunnell spring cock-up wrist splint. To this must be attached the metacarpal bar after which the palmar traction outrigger is added as in the splint shown in Fig. 8.28. The presence of harp-like elastics strung across the palm makes the brace completely nonfunctional; its best use, if any, is as a night splint or a splint for a nonfunctioning hand.

THE FLEXOR HINGE HAND SPLINT

This splint is based on the principle of the flexor hinge hand as described by Nickel, Perry, and Garrett (55) in 1955 and developed by them and their co-workers in the years which followed. The principle is that of the modified three-jaw chuck, in which the index and middle fingers move, together, toward a posted thumb which falls between the touch pads of the two fingers. The flexor hinge is that part of the splint which hinges at the MP joint and envelops the index and middle fingers. It is free to move on its hinge from a position of at least full extension of the MP joint to the point where the fingers impinge upon the thumb. The splint is operated in one direction by internal or external power under voluntary control, and returned to the opposite position by external power, usually a spring.

It is important to determine, if a choice is possible, whether the orthosis is to operate as a voluntary opening or voluntary closing device. In almost all instances, the decision favors voluntary closing, automatic (spring) opening, since this assures that all available, controllable power will be used in three-jaw pinch or grasp. It also prevents continuous finger tip pressure inherent in most spring-closing splints. The more limited system (the spring) is then used to return the fingers to the open position.

The flexor hinge splint is more sophisticated than many of the splints discussed earlier. It requires expert training along with a basic knowledge of orthotics and metal-working to build one and should not be attempted by others. There are several critical points in the construction and fitting of the splint. First, the flexor hinge must be constructed meticulously with the axis of rotation correctly placed to avoid "bind" or excess motion between the splint and the fingers inside the splint. Binding limits the range of motion; excess motion within the splint may cause skin damage and lower grasping efficiency. The axis of rotation must lie exactly over the center of rotation of the MP joint which is approximately in the center of the MP head.

The thumb must meet the fingers between the index and middle fingers and this requires finger positioning which conforms with hand dynamics yet without undue strain on the hand. To achieve this the middle finger must articulate in a direct line with the third metacarpal. The index finger is then bound to it within the flexor hinge approximately parallel to the middle finger. In order to articulate properly with this index-medius combination, the thumb must be brought in under the fingers. If the thumb is held out in its normal relaxed position (to the palmar and radial side of the index), the fingers would have to be abnormally forced radially in order to make the tip of the thumb meet the touch pads of the index and medius and this is to be avoided.

Holding of the fingers and thumb must be done in relation to the function of the splint. Although it is basically a flexor hinge and three-jaw chuck, the splint must also allow for the best possible use of the touch pads. The basic structure precludes full use of the thumb touch pad but the finger pads should be left free. They may have to be covered to provide support for the DIP joint in the case of DIP joint contracture or severe long flexor spasticity.

Since the fingers are purposefully held rigid in this splint, the "joint stabilizers" of the index and middle fingers must fit fairly snugly, yet avoid circulatory embarrassment by encirclement or skin damage by compression.

In spite of the problems of construction and fit, the flexor hinge splint is widely used for it not only fulfills the purposes of the earlier Rancho and Warm Springs splints but is the base for a whole extended family of orthoses, a group characterized by the use of internal and external artificial power applications which include the electric motor, electrically induced muscle contraction, and the artificial muscle.

The flexor hinge splint is a way to control the direction of movement of a limited portion of the hand (three-jaw chuck) while permitting hinge operation with power from the muscles of the patient or from the outside. It can be used for substitution or assistance for weakened or paralyzed muscle and specific directional control of the index and middle fingers. It is not used for simple support of the wrist or fingers because of its dynamic nature, but it can be used as a traction splint under certain circumstances. Better splints at lower cost are available for that objective.

Although the flexor hinge is operated mainly through the index and middle fingers (Fig. 8.36), it is possible under certain circumstances to add the power of other fingers to drive the device. If the patient with extensor paralysis has good-minus long flexors all the way across the hand, the flexors of the ring and small fingers can be used to assist the index-middle combination for tight pinch, by extending a bar ulnarward beneath the DIP joints of the ring and small fingers. When the hand closes, the long flexors of all the fingers can assist in the process. The reverse motion is accomplished by a spring, as in any flexor hinge splint. Sometimes, especially if the long flexor is a little spastic or tight, it is necessary to substitute a small metal platform for the bar extension under the ring and small fingers which partially prevents curling of these fingers. It may be advisable to include the bar extension (flexor bar) under the ring and small fingers routinely even if these fingers are not powered. This is done to keep the fingers from dangling into the palmar area during attempted manipulation of objects. The bar can also be used on the extensor side. If the ring and small fingers are powered by extrinsic extensors, a bar across the dorsum of the proximal phalanges will transfer the power of the extrinsic extensors to the opening of the flexor hinge, with spring return closure.

The use of flexor or extensor bars on the flexor hinge makes it unnecessary for the index and middle fingers (two-thirds of the chuck) to be powered at all. It is possible to drive this splint very effectively through an extensor or

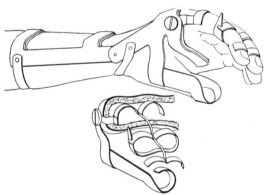

Fig. 8.36. Rancho basic flexor hinge splint.

flexor bar, driven by strong extensors or flexors of the ring or small fingers with no power in the three-jaw chuck itself.

The basic flexor hinge splints are included here along with their modifications.

Rancho Los Amigos Basic Flexor Hinge Splint

This orthosis is the lineal descendant of the original flexor hinge splint. Modifications of the basic wrist and forearm support have occurred during its use over the years (Fig. 8.36). The splint is available either as a basic flexor hinge (described here) or as a short flexor hinge—finger driven. The short flexor hinge splint is similar to the basic Rancho splint but is equipped with a flexor hinge mechanism identical with that of the basic flexor hinge splint. Since the hand splint has no support at the wrist, it requires a fully operational wrist but in other respects it follows the other rules for flexor hinges.

The Rancho basic flexor hinge splint consists of a forearm piece, bound to the forearm by straps, the distal one secured as usual beneath the pisiform bone. The thumb is posted in the appropriate position and held as described earlier. A palmar bar supports the palmar arch and a dorsal bar completes a narrow sandwich of the metacarpals just proximal to their heads. These bars must remain proximal to the metacarpal heads to permit full flexion and extension at the MP joints. The flexor hinge axis of rotation may be a screw (as shown) or simply a steel wire in a hole. The fingers of the flexor hinge are enclosed within stabilizers for both fingers, linked to a common bar which falls partially between the fingers. Dorsal metal arches control the position of the proximal and middle phalanges and prevent extension of the distal phalanx. The support of the fingers is completed by a single spring-steel band which passes to the palmar surface of the middle phalanx, to clip radially onto the middle phalanx dorsal bar. The clip is opened to permit the fingers to be inserted easily into the flexor hinge. The flexor hinge may be made without a clip so that the fingers must be slipped into the structure from the proximal end. In most cases, the clip is more convenient.

Short Flexor Hinge Splint

(See above.)

Basic Flexor Hinge Splint with Artificial Muscle

The artificial muscle and the flexor hinge splint owe their success, in part, to each other. For basic substitution of flexor power in the completely paralyzed hand with paralyzed wrist, the first form of reliable external power was the McKibben muscle, powered by carbon dioxide. The muscle (Fig. 8.37) is mounted along the forearm where it does not interfere with either the functional or cosmetic properties of the orthosis. The fairly inconspic-

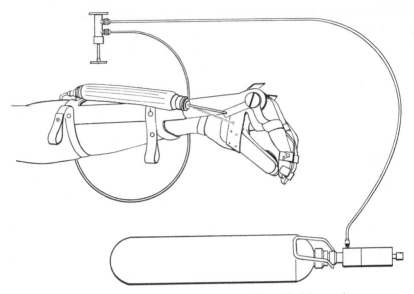

Fig. 8.37. Basic flexor hinge splint with artificial muscle.

uous McKibben muscle is used as a voluntary closing-spring opening device which virtually eliminated the need for a voluntary opening-spring closing device. Spring closing is dangerous due to the constant tension and constant pressure between the thumb and fingers in the closed position which can be harmful to skin and circulation. The logical use of voluntary closing-spring opening devices has obviated the previous need for "pressure relief devices."

With proper training the patient can exercise considerable control not only of the opening and closing of the hinge but also on the exact amount of pressure available between the jaws of the chuck. The patient learns to "feather" the valve control, fluttering the valve open and closed, allowing the passage of minute amounts of gas. The system is very efficient. Motion of the muscle follows entrance of gas with almost no measurable delay; however, the patient, in comparing this splint with others to be described, is able to detect delay times during entrance and exit of gas (valve passage time, not muscle response time). The delays do not occur in cable-operated splints driven by controlled, innervated muscles or in electric motor splints. Further engineering refinements of the McKibben valve system remove even this slight disadvantage (20). However, at the present time because of their accessibility and controllability, electric motors have replaced the artificial muscle in most applications. The valve control for the artificial muscle or an electrical switch for a motor may be mounted anywhere convenient for the patient; for example, under the rocker trough of a "feeder" on the opposite arm, under the toes of a partially controlled foot or above the shoulder in a quadriplegic patient.

Caution is necessary since artificial muscles may pull with a force as great as 60 pounds (27.2 kg), with a larger than normal pinch pressure. In the patient without sensation, such pressure may produce skin damage either from overpinch or compression against the thumb post or finger stabilizers.

The Shoulder-Driven Flexor Hinge Splint

The shoulder driven orthosis (Fig. 8.38) exemplifies many of the advantages and disadvantages of cable operation by innervated, voluntarily controlled muscles at a distance from the hand. The splint consists of a basic flexor hinge with a cable attachment for opening the fingers; a strong elastic closes the chuck.

Earlier cable devices required the distant muscle to remain contracted at all times when a load was held in the hand (as in writing) and this was very fatiguing. In order to avoid continuous contraction of the distant muscle, orthotists turned to voluntary opening, elastic closing devices. These required the addition of pressure-relief devices (Fig. 8.38) that permitted the hand to be held in a slightly opened position when not in use, to avoid constant pressure (by strong elastics against the fingers and posted thumb). This splint is included here in all its complexity because it may have an occasional application when nothing more sophisticated is available. The obvious advantages of later forms of external power preclude its use under most circumstances. Electric motors, for example, permit the hinge to remain tightly closed for indefinite periods without effort; complete pressure-relief occurs when the motor is reversed, opening the chuck. In the shoulder-driven splint, the cable supply may originate in one of several places, but most commonly in a shoulder harness (Fig. 8.38). This method permits transmission of voluntary power from a distant point to the splint.

Proximal control, by locks or power, is essential to hand operation by

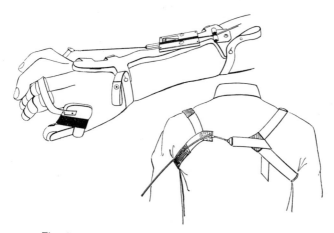

Fig. 8.38. Shoulder driven flexor hinge splint.

cable. If, for example, a naked cable passes in the common location anterior to the elbow joint and inferior to the shoulder joint, it will have a flexing effect on the elbow joint and an extending effect on the shoulder. Thus, the patient must have control of the opposing motions in order to limit motion of the elbow and shoulder while attempting to transmit power to the hand. In this case, he requires elbow extension control and shoulder flexion control. These controls must be strong enough to oppose the strong muscles which operate the cable from the shoulder level. If elbow and shoulder control muscles are not available, limits must be set on elbow and shoulder motion through stops or locks in exoskeletal supporting structures. Such stops at locks further complicate the proximal structure behind the hand splint and this is one reason why they are not popular. Further details about this splint and cable controls are found in Anderson (2, 3). Some of the complexities are avoided by using a sheathed (Bowden) cable (53) (Fig. 8.1).

Electrophysiologic Splint for the Hand (Flexor Hinge)

Following the suggestion of Liberson and Asa (42) that electrical stimulation could be harnessed to provide power in paralyzed muscles, Long and Masciarelli (49) reported on such a splint for the hand in 1963. The splint operated on the principle of electric stimulation of finger flexors, accompanied by spring opening (this was an internally powered "voluntary closing" spring-return splint). Stimulus spread in the flexors plus other technical details caused the discarding of this splint as a clinical entity.

Since the original development and discarding of the flexor hinge electrophysiologic splint, considerable work has continued at the Engineering Design Center at Case Western Reserve University and in the Rehabilitation Engineering Center at Case. Severe problems are inherent in electrical stimulation, including insufficient strength of partially denervated muscles, rapid fatigue, and unrepeatable responses. Several physiologic experiments with chronic electrical stimulation by Peckham and others (61–63) demonstrated a transition from Type II (fast) to Type I (slow) fibers. Systems have been developed to avoid fatigue of these fibers by rotating the stimulation among sets of fibers through multiple implanted electrodes.

Each site is stimulated at frequencies below those expected to produce tetanus; therefore, stimulation of multiple sites is staggered to produce fusion frequencies for the muscle as a whole.

Two types of splints are under clinical investigation by Peckham, one system stimulating the appropriate muscle for grasp and the other for lateral pinch. Stimulation strength is controlled either by myoelectric input or by proportional position control from shoulder or head. Energy for the stimulation crosses the skin via indwelling percutaneous electrodes. Investigation of totally implanted stimulators continues to be under animal evaluation (25).

Flexor Hinge Splint with Electric Motor

This splint (35) uses an electric motor as an on-off source of power. The speed of closing (motor speed) depends on the impressed voltage and the attached gearing. It is mounted in a convenient location, such as the wheelchair. Forward and reverse are possible. Although a cable reel may be used on the motor to drive the splint, the drive is more reliable with a rack and pinion gear (Fig. 8.39), avoiding delays in reeling cable. The splint can operate in nearly ideal fashion, since it can be voluntary (power) closing, spring opening and depends in no way on shoulder or elbow control for power transmission. Power is transmitted by a cable in a housing (Bowden, Fig. 8.1). The proximal end of the cable housing is firmly attached to the housing of the torque motor. The distal portion is attached to the hand splint. Shortening of the system can only occur between the distal end of the housing and the three-jaw chuck, so the effect of the shortening is not felt proximal to the hand splint.

The motor is most widely used and successfully tested external power source for the flexor hinge hand splint. Especially with rack and pinion

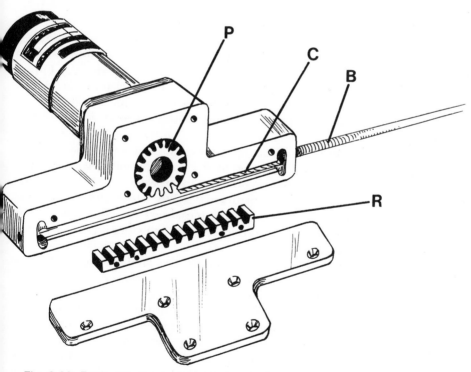

Fig. 8.39. Rack and pinion assembly for electric motor hand splint. *R*, rack; *P*, pinion; *C*, naked cable; *B*, Bowden cable housing.

linkage, it has the advantage that it starts and stops instantly; it reaches its full speed in so short a time that the patient regards it as instantaneous. Additionally, it permits almost infinite variations of pressure to be exerted at the fingertips. A 12-volt battery, a common source of power for this splint, is not only rechargeable, but may also provide simultaneous power for the wheelchair and for a wheelchair-based environmental control system.

Myoelectric Flexor Hinge Hand Splint

Although Battye, Nightingale, and Whillis's (7) brilliant idea of using myoelectric sources (voltages generated by muscles during contraction, *i.e.*, electromyographic) as control signals has been clinically applied to the below-elbow prosthesis, it has not found successful clinical application in arm or hand orthoses.

Myoelectric control has been tried in various ways to serve as the control unit for a flexor hinge hand splint. In general, three voltage levels (three-state system) are used from the myoelectric source; zero voltage stops the motor; intermediate voltage drives the motor in one direction; and higher voltage in the other. To date, the myoelectric control has proved unnecessary, since similar controls can be developed mechanically at less expense and with considerably less training.

In its "purest" form, the myoelectric system has been tried in tandem with an electrophysiologic splint. The myoelectric output from an innervated muscle (*e.g.*, trapezius in a quadriplegic) is used to modulate the output of a stimulator acting in turn on the paralyzed muscle. Future development of this system could lead to the use of myoelectric modulation of a stimulator system using the rotational stimulation system through implanted electrodes, in the electrophysiologic splint described by Peckham and others.

The whole area of myoelectric input remains a challenge. The reader is referred to the bibliography included in Scott and Paciga's report of three-state control (68). They also report that in experiments with five-state control (69), the probability of control error is from 3 to 20 times as great as in the three-state system. They identify muscles receptive of myoelectric training in the following order: biceps brachii, flexor carpi radialis, pectoralis major, and trapezius (see also 44).

Myoelectric control has a further major problem: electromyographic output of muscle has no conscious analog and so cannot be felt or detected by the person generating the signals. Electromyographic output relates most directly to muscle tension which in turn plays through the gamma system and extrapyramidal pathways without coming to consciousness. Therefore, the results of myoelectric outputs, especially when complex, must be fed back to the operator in an artificial way. Details of this dilemma are spelled out in a study by Radonjic and Long (64). Further comments are available in a book by Herberts and co-authors (27).

Rancho Los Amigos Flexor Hinge Tenodesis Orthosis

In 1954, Bisgrove (11) wrote of a new, dynamic, wrist extension-finger flexion hand splint, which, in its various modifications, has become the cornerstone of braces for certain disabilities of the upper limb. Its action relies on a simulated flexor tenodesis function. The surgical procedure of tenodesis anchors the tendons to a solid structure to allow opposing musculature to produce segmental motion through the passive action of the anchored tendons. In a flexor tenodesis, the flexor tendons are fastened proximal to the wrist so that wrist extension produces passive finger flexion. Fusions may be performed in finger IP and thumb carpometacarpal joints to assure proper use of a flexor hinge hand-driven by the tenodesis. The flexor tenodesis splints which developed from Bisgrove's splint, all utilize the principle of tenodesis action. When the wrist is extended actively, the fingers are flexed by the splint. C-6 quadriplegics present an ideal indication for the tenodesis splint. The extensor carpi radialis is often spared since it is innervated at the C-6 level; all the other wrist muscles are commonly innervated at C-7 or below; finger muscles are usually below C-6 (16). The spared radial wrist extensor can be harnessed by the prescription of a flexor hinge tenodesis splint. These splints work well if the radial wrist extensor rates good-minus or higher (lifts three pounds or more). Muscles in the fair-plus range fatigue much too rapidly to be useful. However, fair-plus muscles may gradually strengthen with appropriate therapeutic exercises to become useful and enduring muscles.

The Rancho Los Amigos flexor hinge tenodesis splint is reminiscent of the flexor hinge splint; its construction is virtually identical as far as finger and thumb support are concerned. The flexor hinge tenodesis splint (Fig. 8.40) operates on the three-jawed chuck principle. It opposes the thumb to the index and middle fingers. The flexor hinge consists of a pair of linked stabilizers identical with those in the flexor hinge splint; they articulate against a posted thumb. The major differences between the tenodesis and the straight flexor hinge splint are the hinged wrist and the connecting power bar.

In all types of tenodesis splints the hinges are in the side-bars at the wrist. They locate their axes of rotation between the proximal and distal carpal rows making the usual compromise to the compound physiologic center of

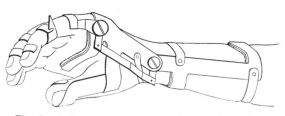

Fig. 8.40. Rancho flexor hinge tenodesis splint.

wrist rotation. The hinges are often simple, overlapping bars. The connecting power bar links the forearm portion of the splint with the flexor hinge portion holding the fingers. It causes finger flexion during wrist extension by holding the proximal end of the bar anchored while the distal drives the fingers into flexion. The bar may be located on the palmar or dorsal portion of the splint; the style has varied in each direction over the years.

The benefit of this splint in substituting for absent finger flexors in the presence of strong wrist extensors cannot be overemphasized.

Engen Reciprocal Finger Prehension Unit (with Adjustable Telescoping Unit)

Engen has also devised a flexor tenodesis splint (22). It is based on a shortened version of Engen's plastic flexor hinge splint. The molded plastic palm piece is typical of this family of splints. The flexor hinge consists of linked stabilizers with the addition of a telescoping unit which is an adjustment for the length of the connecting power bar (Fig. 8.41). By appropriate adjustments, it is possible to handle larger or smaller objects with maximum efficiency of wrist power and position for a particular sized object. The patient can make these helpful adjustments himself with his other hand or may push the adjustment button against a solid object for the same purpose. The range of activities possible with the tenodesis splint is increased by this modification.

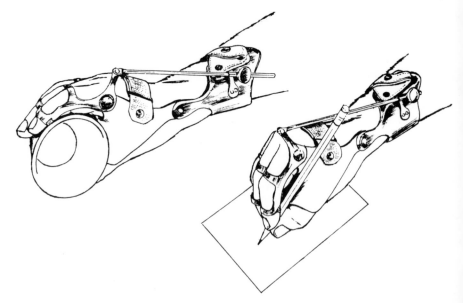

Fig. 8.41. Engen reciprocal finger prehension orthosis with adjustable telescoping unit. (From a photograph supplied by Thorkild J. Engen, C.O.)

The Shoulder

As the wrist serves to locate the hand in space, so the shoulder serves to locate the arm. Codman (17) likened the complexity of shoulder motion to that of backing a trailer into a driveway. He said that the shoulder must aim the multijointed segments of the upper limb toward their target as though controlling several trailers simultaneously. The complex, coordinating function is served by extrinsic and intrinsic muscle groups. The extrinsic muscles are the large prime movers extending from the thorax to the humerus with the exception of the deltoid which reaches from the scapula to the humerus. The intrinsics are the smaller muscles which arise on the scapula and clasp the humeral head and neck in their insertion on the musculotendinous "rotator cuff."

Inman and co-workers (33) describe the combined functions of these muscles as a continuously coordinated task in which the intrinsics serve to anchor the humeral head in the glenoid fossa and to provide a depressor force at the humeral head for completion of a necessary rotary force couple. The extrinsic prime movers provide the major force required to move the upper extremity against resistance. It is these large muscles for which external power is usually substituted in upper limb bracing. Function of the smaller, intrinsic muscles is taken over by the support property of the brace.

The shoulder is a compound joint; it is an anatomical area including several joints. The articulations which are involved in gross shoulder motions (flexion-extension, abduction-adduction) are the glenohumeral, the scapulothoracic, the acromioclavicular and the sternoclavicular. Inman and co-workers describe the interactions of these separate joints in abduction and flexion. Restriction of motion in any of the articulations will limit shoulder motion as a whole. Since shoulder braces do not usually permit rotations at each of these joints through their full range, these orthoses are necessarily restrictive. A compromise must be struck between the practical and the theoretically possible. Compromise at the shoulder often involves a single center of rotation for flexion-extension and a second center for abduction-adduction. The relation of these centers to the physiologic centers for these motions will be discussed under *dynamic support*. Provision for rotation at the sternoclavicular and acromioclavicular joints is not usual; however, adequate range of motion is available for the performance of daily activities.

STATIC BRACING OF THE SHOULDER

Static support for the shoulder is usually provided by simple means short of bracing. In most fractures, injuries of the rotator cuff or brachial plexus stretch injuries, it suffices to enclose the arm and shoulder in a Velpeau type of dressing or cast for immobilization. In special cases where immobilization in abduction is desired, an airplane splint may be made of plaster or may be purchased or fabricated as described below.

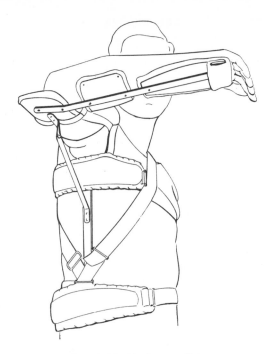

Fig. 8.42. Airplane splint.

The *airplane splint* derives its name from the resemblance of the patient's outstretched arm to the wing of an airplane (Fig. 8.42). It immobilizes the patient's arm at about 90° of abduction at the shoulder. The elbow is permitted a flexed position of about 90°. The weight of the outstretched arm is born primarily on the iliac crest in one of several forms of "pelvic rests." Care must be taken to avoid excessive pressure on the iliac crest in this family of braces. A strap holds the brace against the side of the trunk to assure proper seating on the ilium. A second strap crosses the chest to hold the brace firmly into the axilla. The arm is fastened loosely to the brace with straps. This brace is used mainly for support of the shoulder in abduction. It may be used for short periods to maintain correction after shoulder manipulation or surgery or after surgical repair of the brachial plexus.

Scapular fixation braces for serratus palsy are classified here as static since they contain no moving parts; however, they do permit virtually free movement of the upper extremity. They are used for support of the scapula in serratus anterior paralysis during the recovery of isolated neuropathy of the long thoracic nerve.

A major function of the normal serratus anterior is to provide a lateral rotation force at the inferior angle of the scapula during abduction and flexion movements. Together with the upper and lower trapezius the serratus forms a rotary force couple tending to rotate the scapula in the appropriate direction. In the absence of serratus function the scapula rotates in the opposite direction and is pushed posteriorly off the surface of the thorax (winging). Braces for scapular fixation prevent this counterrotation.

The *Biscapular support brace*, described by Russek and Marks (66) consists of two scapular supports fastened rigidly to a breast plate by metal bars passing over the shoulders. Straps under the axillae secure the brace to the thoracic wall. Even though there is biscapular support, this brace is intended for unilateral involvement. Modifications have been described by Truong and Rippel (75).

The *single scapular support brace*, described by Johnson and Kendall (34) has only one scapular support which applies pressure to the posterior and inferior portions of the scapula of the involved side (Fig. 8.43). Spring steel attaches the scapular plate to two supports over the anterior chest wall. Straps around the patient's waist further anchor the brace in place. This brace is lighter than the biscapular mentioned above.

DYNAMIC SUPPORT FOR THE SHOULDER

Dynamic shoulder support can be provided through "mobile arm supports" (54), including ball bearing, overhead sling, suspension and friction feeders, and "functional arm braces" (3) with specially molded plastic shoulder caps. As a general rule, the mobile arm supports, also called ball bearing forearm orthoses, are for the nonambulatory patient and are at-

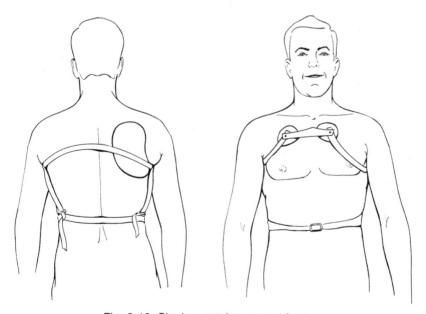

Fig. 8.43. Single scapular support brace.

tached to his wheelchair. Functional arm braces are useful for ambulatory patients.

The purpose of either form of dynamic shoulder support is to provide assistance for weak musculature or substitution for absent muscles. For assistance, the orthosis usually depends upon elastic band external power or on the ingenious use of gravity assistance or relief from gravity resistance. For complete substitution, external power is used to completely override the gravity or residual muscular components of the braced segment.

MOBILE ARM SUPPORTS

Mobile arm supports remove as much of the gravity effect from the weakened extremity as possibly and take advantage of gravity in assisting weak portions of the extremity, based on two principles. First, the mobile arm support is adjusted to take advantage of the principle of the inclined plane (see below). These devices are adjusted so that the arm will run "downhill" with gravity assistance and will be moved "uphill" by the patient's muscles or by muscles plus assistance or by external power substituting completely for these power sources. The second principle is that of the first class lever as seen in a child's teeter-totter. In such a system, the fulcrum is in the center, the force is at one end of the beam and the load at the other. This principle is seen at work in the forearm trough of the mobile arm support. The trough-lever is made either "hand-heavy" or "elbow-heavy" by adjusting the position of the fulcrum. The "heavy" end of the lever is carried downward by gravity; it must then be lifted by an internal or external power source.

The mobile arm support is much more than a shoulder supporting device; it virtually embraces the entire limb and is related to the function of both the shoulder and elbow (including forearm rotation).

Ball Bearing Forearm Orthosis

The ball bearing forearm orthosis (ball bearing feeder; balanced forearm orthosis, also called BFO) is the most commonly used orthosis for wheelchair patients with severe, proximal (shoulder and elbow) weakness or paralysis (Fig. 8.44). It can be constructed by any skilled orthotist but its effectiveness depends upon careful adjustment by the therapists and other persons in direct contact with the patient as he performs his daily activities. Since this is such a versatile device, the term "feeder" is perhaps belittling; the orthosis often enables the patient to do far more than feed himself. It may open a whole new world of typing, writing, grooming, recreation through board games and reading, kitchen activities, smoking, telephoning, and some vocational activities. The BFO is a therapeutic device which permits and encourages the patient to use his residual muscle power and enhance the development of increased strength and control by graded use. It also allows

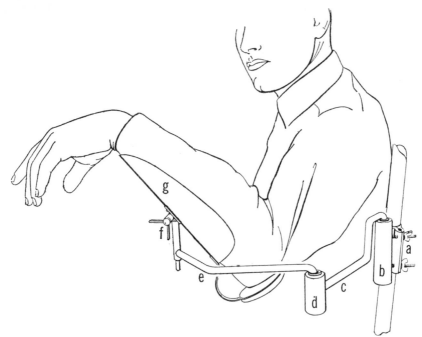

Fig. 8.44. Ball bearing orthosis on wheelchair. *a*, bracket assembly; *b*, proximal ball bearing; *c*, proximal swivel arm; *d*, distal ball bearing; *e* distal swivel arm; *f*, rocker arm assembly; *g*, trough.

the therapist to make continual adjustments in proportion with increase in patient strength, providing a form of graded, resistive exercise.

The BFO has advantages over its predecessor, the overhead sling suspension. While the sling suspension is unwieldy, extending far above the wheelchair, the BFO is more compact, will pass through doors more readily and is more appealing cosmetically. Once adjusted, the BFO will retain its adjustment until a change is desired; it is always ready for use. Sling suspensions, on the other hand, must be readjusted each time they are applied.

There are six prerequisites for the BFO.
1. Weakness must be severe enough to require assistance or substitution: either the elbow or shoulder function should be between zero and fair-plus, or have grades above fair-plus with limited endurance for sustained activity.
2. A power source must be available to drive the orthosis "uphill." Such sources are poor-plus to fair-plus shoulder and elbow muscles; or, neck or trunk muscles adequate to shift the trunk center of gravity; or, shoulder girdle muscles adequate to change scapular position (poor-minus to fair-

plus); or, an external source of power for complete substitution in shoulder or elbow motion or a better-than-good distant muscle for cable control.

3. Adequate range of passive motion: 90° of shoulder abduction and flexion for adequate elbow elevation; 60° of internal and external humeral rotation for rocker trough action; 130° of elbow flexion for the hand to reach the face; 80° of forearm pronation to allow grasp of object on surface; 85° of hip flexion to permit patient to sit fully upright.

4. Well-coordinated muscles in control segment since a BFO is free-moving with low friction.

5. Patient must be able to sit upright for several hours or lateral trunk supports provided.

6. Complex orthosis requires adjustment, training and high motivation. Trial with a temporary adjustable orthosis. Group training may be useful.

ADJUSTMENT, FITTING, MECHANICAL PRINCIPLES

Proper adjustment of the BFO determines whether the patient will use the device and whether it will be efficient. The mechanical principles on which adjustments are based are simple enough for engineers but when translated into terms understandable to physicians it is difficult to avoid oversimplification of these foreign, geometric concepts. Smith and Juvinall, a physiatrist-engineer team, wrote an interpretation of "feeder mechanics" geometry (71). Similarly, the Rancho Los Amigos group includes detailed "steps of adjustment" and geometric discussion in their Occupational Therapy Department training course (40, 60) as does Anderson (3). The following description applies the geometry of Smith and Juvinall to the Rancho and Anderson procedures. Although the procedure is arranged for minimal interference with preceding steps, areas of interference are reviewed at the end of the procedure.

PROCEDURE AND RATIONALE OF BFO ADJUSTMENT

1. Fitting

The details of fitting a patient with a BFO of appropriate size and relative dimensions (proximal and distal swivel arm length, trough size, depth and so on) may be found in the book of Anderson (3).

2. Positioning in Wheelchair

The patient should be positioned optimally in the wheelchair, upright, hips back in the seat and centered, with lapboard in place if the patient has one. All hand splint parts must be in place since these affect the balance of the feeder trough as well as the total weight of the upper limb. Lateral supports should be added to the wheelchair if the patient does not have trunk stability. A posture panel may be placed on the seat back to assist in upright maintenance if required.

Proper positioning and stability of the trunk provide optimum positioning of the shoulder, the central point for BFO operation. Smith and Juvinall point out that the feeder allows the shoulder and elbow to move in eight degrees of freedom (directions of primary and return motions); two at the elbow and six at the shoulder. Three of the degrees of freedom at the shoulder are "translational" movements. These are superior-inferior (up-down), antero-posterior (front-back) and medio-lateral (side-side) transla-tion. It should be determined for each patient whether these movements are essential to comfortable control, for if they are they must be permitted. Translation of the shoulder may be produced by scapular movement in relation to the thorax or by movement of the thorax and scapula as a unit, held together by the viscoelastic restraints between them. If the patient has scapular control musculature, it may be best to stabilize the trunk to permit the most efficient use of these muscles. If the arm is flail, the patient will depend upon trunk or neck movement for shoulder translation and must not have his trunk rigidly immobilized.

3. Height of Ball Bearing Assembly

The height of the ball bearing bracket assembly must be correct since it positions the whole BFO. According to Juvinall and Smith the purpose of this adjustment is to set the height of the work-plane (or "pivot height") by adjusting the vertical position of the pivot of the rocker arm assembly (Fig. 8.45). The work-plane should be set at the height which produces a forearm inclination of between 45 and 55° from the horizontal when the hand is at mouth level. This is optimal because it permits the hand to reach the mouth and to move up and down (shoulder axial rotation) with minimal impinge-ment on the viscoelastic restraint limits of the patient's shoulder. The elbow dial must not strike the lapboard and the shoulder must not be passively forced into superior translation. This and subsequent adjustments bring into play combinations of the remaining five (nontranslational) degrees of freedom of the system. They are all rotational: at the shoulder, axial rotation (internal and external), flexion-extension, and horizontal abduction-adduc-tion; at the elbow, flexion-extension and supination-pronation.

4. Forearm Trough Balance

The forearm trough is balanced for optimal range and force of vertical motion, depending on the nature of the rocker arm assembly. In the standard rocker arm there is only an adjustment which allows the pivot (fulcrum) to be moved toward the elbow or hand. The movement is called an adjustment of the X axis by Smith and Juvinall (Fig. 8.46). Moving the pivot toward the

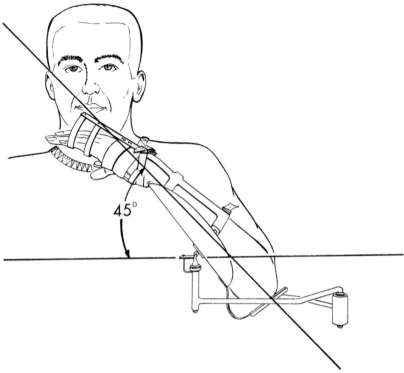

Fig. 8.45. Effects of vertical adjustment of bracket position. Height should be adjusted to approximately 45 to 55° angle of forearm to horizontal.

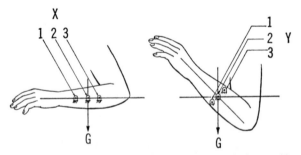

Fig. 8.46. Effects of X and Y adjustments on forearm balance. Hand heaviness is produced by moving X adjustment toward elbow with forearm horizontal. Moving the Y adjustment superiorly with forearm horizontal produces hand heaviness when the forearm is moved to vertical position. G, gravity.

elbow makes the forearm "hand heavy." In some feeder assemblies (Fig. 8.48) a second adjustment is possible, allowing the pivot to be placed above or below the forearm or a Y axis adjustment (Fig. 8.49). Moving the pivot superiorly makes the forearm "hand heavy."

It will be seen in Fig. 8.47 that the X and Y adjustments are sensitive to the position of the forearm. If the forearm is horizontal, the X adjustment is effective, the Y is not. If the forearm is vertical, the Y adjustment is effective, the X is not. The combined X and Y adjustments allow a hand-heavy or elbow-heavy condition to be effective throughout the range of motion of the rocker arm. If only one adjustment is available it must become decreasingly effective toward either the horizontal or vertical position.

The decision concerning hand or elbow heaviness might be made on theoretical grounds following muscle testing and range of motion examination. However, the best method of determination is with the patient in the

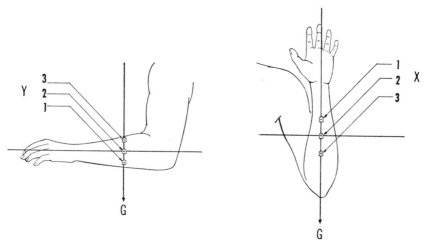

Fig. 8.47. Ineffective positions for X and Y adjustments of forearm balance. The X adjustment has no effect when the forearm is vertical. The Y adjustment has no effect when the forearm is horizontal. G, gravity.

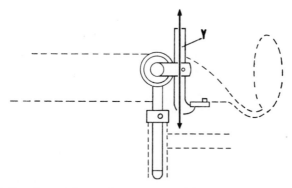

Fig. 8.48. Rancho outside rocker arm assembly permits Y adjustments in addition to X adjustment possible in standard rocker arm assembly. Y-Y adjustment.

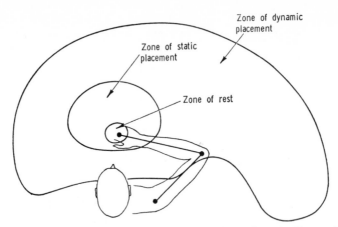

Fig. 8.49. Zones of hand positioning in feeder. [Reproduced with permission from Smith and Juvinall (71).]

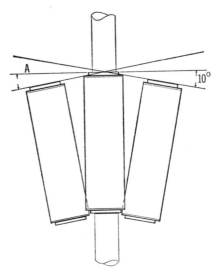

Fig. 8.50. Rotation of wheelchair bracket for workplane roll adjustment (front view). In starting position *A*, workplane is horizontal, bracket is straight and vertical, wheelchair post fixed about 10° posterior inclination (not shown here). As bracket is rotated to right or left, 10° discrepancy between bracket and post is translated into 10° slant of workplane. Intermediate positions produce intermediate degrees of slant.

BFO in a practical daily living environment. First, the patient should be able to actuate the BFO through full range without excessive trunk or shoulder motion. If the patient has enough musculature to lift the hand (for instance, shoulder external rotators) the forearm is made slightly hand heavy so that it will return to rest position with the hand down. Little power is required for down motions since little resistance is encountered in these motions in daily activities. However, up motions are often made against significant resistance, as in lifting food to the mouth or transferring objects in the horizontal plane. Therefore, if the up motion is poorly powered by musculature, there is a temptation to make the system quite elbow heavy. Smith and Juvinall advise that such adjustments are not useful for repetitive activities since they cause excessive braking motions by the down-moving muscles during unloaded motions. They suggest that an optimal energy expenditure of up- and down-moving muscles can be achieved by adjusting X or Y axes to a slightly elbow-heavy condition, just below that required for average loads. At average load levels, this requires the up-moving muscles to operate and takes the braking requirement off the down-moving muscles during up motions. With this adjustment, the hand still returns to an up rest position.

If adequate elevation cannot be achieved by these methods, a rubber band assist for hand elevation can be used on the "outside rocker arm" type of trough support (Fig. 8.48). This permits the axis to be moved closer to the elbow for a greater vertical range of hand movement. The rubber bands assist the up-moving musculature in lifting the excessive weight of the portion of the forearm distal to the X axis.

5. Pitch and Roll

Pitch and roll are nautical or aeronautical terms which have been applied to BFO adjustment. Pitch refers to work-plane deviation from the horizontal, front or back edges up or down. Roll produces deviation of the work-plane, lateral edges up or down. The work-plane is the plane in which the pivot-axis of the forearm trough may move. If the patient has poor horizontal control, the major purpose of adjustment of this plane is to control the "zone of rest" of the hand. In any condition of feeder adjustment the hand will return reproducibly to a relatively small zone of rest when all musculature is relaxed (Fig. 8.49). Adjusting the work-plane tilt in pitch and roll directions allows the hand to come to rest in a predetermined zone. This zone is logically the area where food or a typewriter might be placed.

The pitch and roll adjustments are made at the ball bearing bracket. Fig. 8.50 shows that although the bracket may be aligned vertically, the wheelchair post is not vertical (by about 10°). Thus, rotating the bracket laterally or medially slants the bracket any amount up to 10° off vertical and the work-plane any amount up to 10° off the horizontal. This rotational adjustment of the bracket affects the roll of the work-plane and positions the zone of rest of the hand to the right or left.

Pitch is adjusted by varying the vertical position of the bracket (Fig. 8.51). Anteroposterior changes in tilt of the bracket are reflected in horizontal changes of the work-plane. Tilting the top of the bracket backward moves the zone of rest backward; tilting the bracket forward moves the hand forward.

There is not a separate pitch adjustment at the bracket on each BFO. In these devices, rotation of the bracket to the right or left produces roll adjustment with a compound, secondary effect on the pitch adjustment of the work-plane. Experimentation with rotation of the bracket will demonstrate the pitch effect. When separate pitch adjustment at the bracket is not available, the work-plane can be tilted in a similar, although not identical, manner by tilting the distal ball bearing (at the end of the proximal swivel arm) either toward the hand or shoulder. Tilting toward the hand moves the hand away from the patient; tilting toward the shoulder moves the hand toward the patient.

These adjustments are critical to position the hand zone of rest for the patient who has poor horizontal control. The zone of rest may be with the hand down on the work surface, or the hand up near the mouth. In most cases the hand-up position is preferred since objects on the work surface are more easily moved than is the patient's head.

For the patient with good horizontal control, in whom hand rest control is less needed, the tilt adjustment (pitch or roll) may be used to assist weak muscle groups in producing motion of the limb in the BFO. For instance,

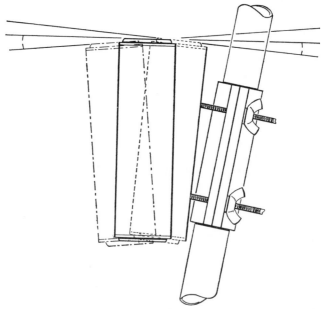

Fig. 8.51. Tilting of bracket for workplane pitch (side view). Changing angle between wheelchair post and bracket causes workplane to tilt so that front or back edges move up or down correspondingly (pitch adjustment).

forward pitch may be used to assist weak elbow extensors and lateral roll to assist weak horizontal abductors of the shoulder.

6. Order of Adjustments

We must check to see whether this order of adjustments has caused deviation in the preceding adjustments. Smith and Juvinall refer to the following interactions of adjustments: a) change in the hand rest position alters hand-heaviness because the elastic forces change with joint rotation. Such a change may throw off previously balanced X and Y adjustments; b) change in balance (pivot) point elevation alters the hand rest position; c) shift in the X adjustment affects balance (pivot) point elevation when the forearm is vertically inclined (Fig. 8.47); d) shift in the Y adjustment affects balance (pivot) point elevation as the hand moves over the workplane.

7. Need for Special Attachments

Special attachments may be necessary for individual patients. a) Outside rocker arm (Fig. 8.48) for use when elbow trough balance is critical with hand near mouth permits Y adjustment. Standard feeder trough with elbow dial (Fig. 8.44) has X adjustment only. b) Outside rocker arm with rubber band assist helps lift added apparent weight of hand if distal lever arm is made long to allow hand to reach face. c) Feeder trough with clip clamps the patient's hand splint to the feeder trough in cases where the arm tends to slide out of trough. It eliminates straps to hold arm in place. Because it prevents forearm rotation it should not be used if active supination-pronation control is available. d) Vertical stop (Fig. 8.52) added to feeder trough if patient has tendency to excessive range in hand-up position is especially useful with rubber band assist to prevent bands from raising hand too high. e) Horizontal stop (Fig. 8.52) is used for the patient with poor ability to stop horizontal motion. It limits the motion to ranges the patient can control but it is not always useful because of rebound (bouncing off the stop). Rubber bands may be used (rarely) with stop to assist weak horizontal motions. f) Lateral trunk support (Fig. 8.52) may be used unilaterally or bilaterally for the patient with poor trunk support. It is removable to allow patient to transfer in and out of chair. g) "Flying saucer" feeder trough (Fig. 8.52) has no pivot point and is supported by the distal bearings of the proximal feeder arm; no distal arm is needed. Patient's medial epicondylar and olecranon areas are supported by the saucer when only horizontal assistance is required. Patient must have good hand elevators (elbow flexors and humeral external rotators) to lift the hand out of the trough for activities in the head zone or between work surface and head zone. h) Elevating proximal swivel arm with rubber band assist (Fig. 8.52) for the patient with poor deltoid power uses rubber bands to assist the deltoid (and rotator cuff) in humeral abduction and flexion. It allows more hand elevation than the standard BFO. i) Carbon dioxide-powered elevating feeder assembly 21) consists of a

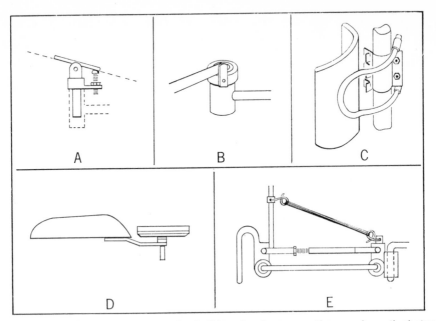

Fig. 8.52. Some attachments for ball-bearing forearm orthoses. *A*, vertical stop; *B*, horizontal stop; *C*, lateral trunk support; *D*, ''flying saucer'' feeder trough; *E*, elevating proximal swivel arm with rubber band assist.

parallelogram linkage which substitutes for the proximal feeder and may be used for the patient with no significant shoulder control (muscles less than poor). The example shown in Fig. 8.53 is powered by a carbon dioxide artificial muscle but other models are available with gas-powered piston elevators. Electric motors could also drive this device but specific applications have not been published.

The friction feeder (27) which resembles the ball bearing forearm orthosis (Fig. 8.44) possesses adjustable friction in the proximal and distal ball bearings and in the rocker arm assembly. The orthosis is used for patients who have adequate power to move the arm against gravity, but who have superimposed incoordination or spontaneous movements. The friction adjustments provide damping of the involuntary or incoordinated motions. Horizontal and vertical stops may be used to control the range of these movements.

Sling Suspensions

Sling suspension orthoses have been the workhorses of occupational therapy clinics since the 1940's. Their ease of management, low cost, and ability to support proximal weakness of the upper limb have contributed to their popularity. The overhead suspension by itself is a useful device, but it

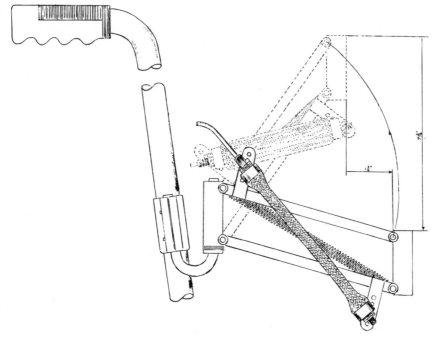

Fig. 8.53. Carbon dioxide-powered elevating feeder assembly.

is commonly used as a training apparatus prior to the application of ball bearing forearm orthoses.

The overhead sling suspension derives its name from support on a suspension rod above the patient's head. The upper limb swings, pendulum fashion, from straps attached to the suspension rod. The major purpose is to reduce the gravity load on the limb, permitting operation of the limb by muscles otherwise too weak to be functional.

Sling suspensions are used primarily for the assistance and support of subfunctional (poor-minus to fair-minus) muscles. They may also be used for gravity-eliminated exercise of muscles at the strength levels just mentioned or for the encouragement of increased range of motion through repetitive activities.

TYPES OF SLING SUSPENSION

In the double sling suspension (Fig. 8.54A) two supports which originate independently at the suspension rod hold the wrist and elbow (10). In the single suspension (6) the limb is supported by only one sling, usually at the elbow level (Fig. 8.54B). The single suspension with rocker bar (5a) has a single point of suspension from the overhead bar. A lever, with notches or holes for adjustment of the fulcrum, supports the suspension straps which in turn provide support for the wrist and elbow separately (Fig. 8.54C). In the single suspension with rocker trough (59) the limb is supported in a rocker trough similar to that used in the balanced forearm orthosis. It is suspended from a single point on the overhead bar (Fig. 8.54).

ADJUSTMENT OF SUSPENSION

Strap Adjustments. The strap which connects the overhead bar to the limb directly or via rocker bar or trough may be adjusted for length. This provides elevation control for the entire limb in the case of single suspension or for wrist and elbow separately when separate supports are provided. Adjustments for height in relation to work surface or head zone are similar to those discussed for ball bearing forearm orthoses described above.

Height. The higher the overhead bar, the longer the pendulum supporting the upper limb and the flatter the arc of motion traversed by the limb. Usually, the bar is kept as high as feasible for the patient's wheelchair to pass through the standard doorway. Lowering the bar shortens the pendulum arc and causes the upper limb to move "uphill" at each extreme of the arc. Lowering of the overhead bar can thus add resistance to muscles driving the upper limb during its activites.

Rotation. If the overhead bar is rotated outward, it causes the upper limb to move outward; if rotated inward, the extremity moves inward. This response can be used for either assistance or resistance to shoulder motions—horizontal adduction and abduction.

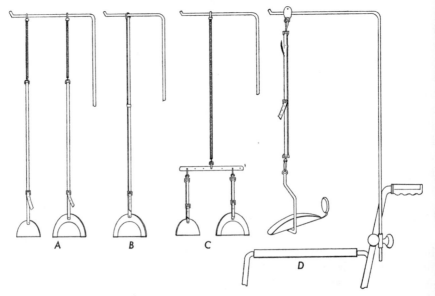

Fig. 8.54. Sling suspension. *A*, double sling; *B*, single sling; *C*, sling with rocker arm; *D*, sling with rocker trough.

Springs. Springs may be inserted in the straps supporting the upper limb to allow a certain amount of "give" as the patient reaches down toward the work surface and a limited amount of assistance as he moves toward the head zone. In early muscle re-education, springs allow the patient to produce movement by bouncing his limb up and down, a motion not as easily possibly with straps alone. The overhead suspension bar is usually made of moderately springy material so some bouncing is possible in all suspensions.

Counterbalanced suspensions are also frequently used. A weight over pulley serves to balance for weight of the arm. It provides the same "give" in downward motion of the arm that is characteristic of springs.

Reclining bracket. For all suspension devices, the overhead rod may be supported by a "reclining bracket" which permits the suspension to be adjusted to true verticality when the patient's wheelchair is partially reclining.

INDICATIONS FOR ADJUSTMENT

The double sling suspension is a versatile beginning suspension for the recovering patient or the patient destined to use ball bearing orthoses. Moving the distal (wrist) support distally or proximally along the suspension rod provides either resistance or assistance to the elbow flexors or extensors as desired. Also, rest position of the unloaded hand is determined partially by positioning this distal strap. The proximal strap is moved away from the patient to assist shoulder extension and horizontal abduction.

The single sling suspension is a relatively rarely used support. Since the suspension is at the elbow, it requires the patient to lift the forearm with his own muscles which means that the elbow flexors and external humeral rotators must be stronger than fair. Its analogy to the "flying saucer" mobile arm support is apparent.

The single suspension with rocker bar or rocker trough is recommended as an intermediate step for the patient who will later use a BFO. It permits the therapists to balance the forearm on an adjustable fulcrum, allowing control of elbow or hand heaviness. The training patient may start with double sling suspensions and move to the rocker systems or may start directly with rockers. These suspension systems are more adaptable to the reclining wheelchair than are ball bearing orthoses, which make them useful during the recovery of quadriplegics before trunk control and circulatory homeostasis have developed enough for the patient to sit upright.

Training

Since overhead slings are often used as training or interim devices before the prescription of ball bearing orthoses, training can be carried out in suspensions. These run the gamut of motions possible for the shoulder and elbow including scapular protraction and adduction, shoulder flexion and extension, elbow flexion and extension, and humeral internal and external rotation (especially in rocker devices). Functional activities (including those of daily living) can also be practiced in suspension slings.

Functional Arm Brace

The term *functional arm brace* generally refers to a complex upper limb orthosis for the ambulatory patient. It is a molded plastic support at the shoulder level on which are mounted combinations of exoskeletal supports and controls for the shoulder and the elbow. When the hand and wrist also require bracing, they are usually splinted separately from the functional arm brace according to the patterns described earlier. In this section, we shall treat the shoulder and elbow together since their actions are interlocked in the functional arm brace. Separate bracing for the elbow will be considered later. Barber (5) has reviewed some combinations of use of this device.

The locking joint functional arm brace (3) is founded on a plastic, molded shoulder cap which covers the scapular area and lateral, anterior chest as well as the superior portion of the shoulder (Fig. 8.55). This brace must be constructed by a skilled orthotist because the plastic shoulder cap must be expertly fitted for proper operation of the entire orthosis. The plastic shoulder cap and its locking joint orthosis has replaced suspension hoops because it is more comfortable and requires less care and adjustment.

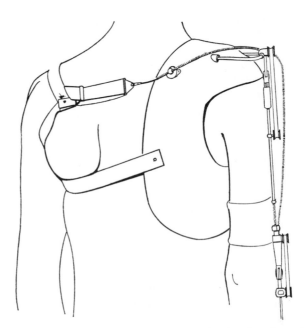

Fig. 8.55. Molded shoulder cap and harness for functional arm brace.

The locking joint functional arm brace (FAB) (with elastic elbow flexion assist or artificial muscle flexion substitution) is a versatile device which provides a strong, mobile base of support for elbow assistance or substitutive external power. Secondarily, it allows certain motions at the shoulder: abduction-adduction, which occurs at the FAB shoulder hoop (Fig. 8.56) and flexion-extension which occurs in the ratchet lock joint as the shoulder.

The shoulder ratchet lock joint is set so that its axis of rotation lies over the flexion-extension axis for the glenohumeral joint (approximately through the center of the humeral head). It allows unrestricted forward motion of the shoulder. In the unpowered or paralyzed shoulder this motion must be provided passively by the other arm or by bending forward or by propping the arm against a solid surface such as a table. If the patient has enough strength in the shoulder flexors to operate an assistive system (poor to fair-minus) elastic flexion assistance may be used. In the model shown by Anderson (Fig. 8.56) rubber bands for shoulder flexion assistance may be applied between the band posts above the ratchet lock joint and just above the elbow lock.

The ratchet lock joint has five separate stopping or locking points up to 110° of flexion. The device may be held at any of these positions without use of power by the patient. A cable control allows the ratchet to be unlocked. The cable does not require a separate control source but is linked by the brace construction with operation of the elbow, the shoulder ratchet lock automatically releasing when the elbow joint is extended.

The elbow joint in this orthosis is made to operate with external power (rubber bands or the artificial muscle). Rubber bands are used for assistance, the artificial muscle for substitution. The patient must have elbow extensors better than good-minus to stretch the elastic bands. If extensor strength is not great enough to meet this requirement, the artificial muscle must be used.

The elbow joint contains a ratchet lock similar to the shoulder mechanism; however, it is more sophisticated, permitting two modes of operation. It is controlled by a cable and harness (Fig. 8.55). In one mode of operation the cable locks or unlocks the elbow at given ratchet points of which there are six between full extension and full flexion. In the second mode, the patient need not maintain cable tension to keep the lock open but instead pulls and then releases to unlock, pulls and releases again to lock. The locked elbow permits the patient to carry heavier loads with a flexed elbow than he could otherwise handle. It also permits the carrying of loads for prolonged periods without the exertion of continuous muscle power, or above the carrying strength of elastic power.

When the artificial muscle is used as an external source of power at the elbow, there is some danger of rupture if its full strength is exerted against a locked elbow. To avoid this danger the elbow lock is always used in the simple pull-unlock, release-lock manner. The valve control for the artificial

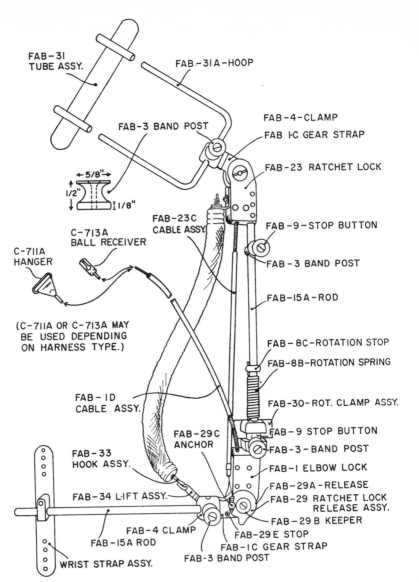

FAB-31
TUBE ASSY.

FAB-31A-HOOP

FAB-3 BAND POST

FAB-4-CLAMP

FAB I-C GEAR STRAP

FAB-23 RATCHET LOCK

←5/8"→

1/2"

1 1/8"

FAB-23C
CABLE ASSY.

C-713A
BALL RECEIVER

FAB-9-STOP BUTTON

C-711A
HANGER

FAB-3 BAND POST

FAB-15A-ROD

(C-711A OR C-713A MAY
BE USED DEPENDING
ON HARNESS TYPE.)

FAB-8C-ROTATION STOP

FAB-8B-ROTATION SPRING

FAB-1D
CABLE ASSY.

FAB-30-ROT. CLAMP ASSY.

FAB-29C
ANCHOR

FAB-9 STOP BUTTON

FAB-33
HOOK ASSY.

FAB-3-BAND POST

FAB-1 ELBOW LOCK

FAB-34 LIFT ASSY.

FAB-29A-RELEASE

FAB-29 RATCHET LOCK
RELEASE ASSY.

FAB-29 B KEEPER

FAB-4 CLAMP

FAB-15A ROD

FAB-29 E STOP

FAB-1C GEAR STRAP

WRIST STRAP ASSY.

FAB-3 BAND POST

Fig. 8.56. Locking joint functional arm brace. [Reprinted with permission from Anderson (3).]

muscles is attached in series with the cable, tension on which valves the gas into the muscle and unlocks the elbow. With this ingenious arrangement the muscle cannot operate against a locked elbow.

The *wrist strap assembly* (Fig. 8.56) attaches the distal portion of the forearm bar of the brace to the patient just proximal to the wrist joint leaving the wrist free for motion if desired. The wrist strap attaches to a *friction wrist control* which allows the forearm to rotate freely in the brace or be limited by varying degrees of friction up to complete locking. "Zero" friction is used if the patient's musculature can rotate the forearm. For the unpowered forearm, intermediate friction permits the patient or another person to set the forearm position as desired manually. For external power sources the friction is made maximal (locked).

External power for rotation of the two longitudinal axes of the device is available through coil springs mounted around the supporting rods parallel to the humerus or the forearm. The spring (Fig. 8.56) at the distal end of the arm rod may be wound either left- or right-hand for internal or external humeral rotation. A similar spring can be mounted at the distal end of the forearm rod to assist either supination or pronation.

These springs can be used only with better than good-minus strength in the opposing musculature. Their use presumes that the splint will assume a rest position in the direction of the spring action and can be controlled outside of that position only by the continuous use of opposing muscle power. Stops are used with the rotation springs to be sure that the "rest" position will not be abnormal or uncomfortable.

The Elbow

Much concerning elbow orthotics has been discussed in describing shoulder devices. This section will be limited to those orthoses specific to elbow bracing, but even these must in some way affect the shoulder because it is usually necessary to support the shoulder while supporting the elbow. To assure complete coverage and to make that coverage easily available, the Splint-Finding Chart (Table 8.1) has been included to help the reader select the appropriate apparatus when the desired result is known.

The elbow lengthens or shortens the arm and provides axial control of forearm position through supination and pronation. The elbow is flexed by the brachialis, assisted under certain conditions of supination or load resistance by the biceps brachii. The brachioradialis forms a reserve force (16) for elbow flexion under load (gravity, acceleration, or deceleration). The elbow is extended by the triceps brachii. Forearm pronation is performed by the pronator teres and pronator quadratus; supination by the biceps brachii and the supinator muscle.

The axis of rotation for flexion and extension at the elbow passes through the medial and lateral epicondyles, the articulation taking place at the ulnohumeral joint. The orthotic elbow articulation can accommodate well to this single axis joint when it is adjusted to overlie the epicondyles. Accommodation of an orthosis to the forearm axis of rotation (axial; pronation-supination) is not as simple, but is adequate for the purposes of most orthoses. However, the axial rotation line for supination-pronation does not lie down the center of the forearm, since the radius is anchored at its proximal end, orbiting at its distal end around the ulna. For this reason, when forearm rotation is desired as part of any linked, multiple arm control system, it is often best to leave the wrist free to rotate as it wishes (as when lying at the distal end of a feeder trough) or to disconnect the hand link of the system from the elbow control link allowing them to operate independently. In some systems it is necessary to discard the advantage of independent forearm rotation for other advantages such as the external power available in the Engen elbow flexion unit described below. In these cases, no forearm rotation is possible.

The elbow cannot provide extension forces without equal flexion force at the shoulder, nor can it apply flexion forces without balanced shoulder extension. These antagonistic forces, essential at the shoulder, can be applied by a shoulder locking device. The mechanism of action of such a device is exemplified in the description of the shoulder ratchet lock. Although the examples given above included only extension and flexion at the shoulder, any force tending to deviate the station of the elbow will require an opposing force at the glenohumeral and scapulothoracic joints.

STATIC BRACING

Static bracing of the elbow is seldom effected by orthotic devices. Stable positioning can be accomplished by using posterior shells of plastic or plaster, stretching from upper arm to wrist and adapted to the required elbow position. Within multi-linked upper limb orthotic systems, the elbow is sometimes temporarily held in a static position with locks, which can serve as both static and dynamic braces, as exemplified by the ratchet lock.

DYNAMIC BRACING

Elbow flexion can be assisted or substituted. This function is usually served within a multi-link system as in the mobile arm support or functional arm brace. However, a specific elbow flexion external power unit has been described by Engen (21) as shown in Fig. 8.57. The shortening of the artificial muscle transmits motion over a cable-wound reel to provide elbow flexion. The forearm is supported by a trough similar to that in a ball bearing orthosis. The hand is supported rigidly on a molded plastic palmrest. The unit is used for wheelchair patients and mounted in a manner similar to the ball bearing orthosis. It is useful for the patient with powered shoulder and paralyzed elbow. In patients with no significant shoulder or elbow control the elbow flexion unit is coupled with the shoulder abduction unit of Engen to produce a fully externally powered, two-link unit for shoulder and elbow control at the wheelchair level.

A *brace for elbow flexion alone* should be considered for patients with good upper limbs except for an isolated paralysis of elbow flexion, as in musculocutaneous nerve injury or neuropathy. In such a case it is possible to use a brace designed only for elbow flexion without need for a shoulder

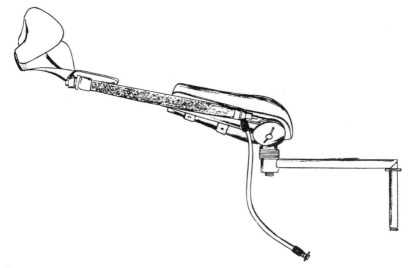

Fig. 8.57. Engen externally powered elbow flexion unit. [Reprinted with permission from Engen (21).]

support (Fig. 8.58). It consists of two uprights, one medial and one lateral, for the arm and two for the forearm, joined by a simple, 1° articulation at the elbow level. Elastic bands can be attached to this brace to provide elbow flexion, antagonized by the normal elbow extensors.

Elbow extension. Only rarely is an assistive or substitutive device needed for elbow extension. Usually, gravity assistance is adequate to control the extension side of the unpowered elbow. The most common need for elbow external extension power arises in balancing the power requirements of orthotic systems. The elbow flexion unit of Engen provides a flexion force primarily. For quick initiation of extension and to cushion the end of extension, a coil spring for extension is included in the elbow mechanisms. Sometimes, to speed the mechanism of extension in ball bearing feeders, it is necessary to use rubber bands or springs at the distal ball bearing.

Corrective brace for hemiplegic arm. In the presence of flexion contracture of the elbow a special brace has been described (65) to provide extension-traction in the hemiplegic. The brace has the same basic design as that described for elbow flexion alone (Fig. 8.58), but incorporates a long, steel spring running the length of the lateral uprights to produce a continuous extension force acting at the elbow. As described by the orignators, this brace is part of a multi-link unit which includes a "reverse" knuckle bender for correction of flexion contractures of the fingers.

Forearm rotation assistance, rarely substitution, can be provided in most of the families of orthoses which support the forearm and elbow. These include the three examples which follow.

Supinator assist for ball bearing forearm orthosis (Fig. 8.59). The forearm must be pronated to reach food on the plate but supinated slightly to place the food in the mouth. For the patient without powered supinators, this crucial lack may be just sufficient to prevent self-feeding in a ball bearing orthosis. The supinator assist takes advantage of the force derived from the elbow-down motion of the rocker trough to provide supination assistance through about 20 to 30°. As the feeder trough rocks into the elbow-down position, the entire trough is rotated into supination. As the hand returns to the down position, the trough and enclosed forearm move back into pronation. No elastic return devices are necessary since the device is powered by the movement of the rocker trough itself.

Rotation assistance for suspension feeders can be applied to a sling suspension feeder whenever the device includes a wrist supporting strap. Such assistance is therefore impossible in single suspension slings at the elbow. When wrist suspension is present, rotation assistance can be provided by clipping the supporting leather strap to either the radial or ulnar side of the wrist cuff. If support is given via the radial side, the forearm rests in a

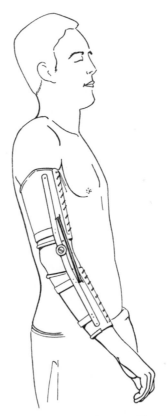

Fig. 8.58. Double upright elbow brace with elastic flexion assist.

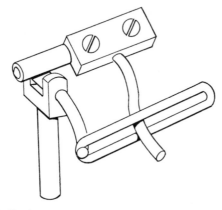

Fig. 8.59. Supinator assist for ball bearing forearm orthosis.

partially supinated posture requiring muscular effort to reach the prone posture. Suspension from the ulnar side produces a prone resting position of the forearm and voluntary supination is required to rotate out of that position.

Rotation assistance in the multi-link orthosis. Pronation and supination assistance is exemplified by the use of right- and left-hand springs on the forearm bar of the locking joint orthosis in the multi-link orthosis described elsewhere.

Upper Limb Orthotics Research

The impetus provided by the rapid growth of electronic knowledge in relation to space travel and other advances was transmitted to the medical profession as a refinement of electronic technique coupled with remarkable progress in the miniaturization of components.

Several research centers about the world were quick to apply new technologies to handicapped people. This was first apparent following Thalidomide congenital amputations. Several governments devised new technologies or refined old ones to meet the crisis, notably Germany (51), the Soviet Union (36), Canada (69), Italy (30, 31), and the United Kingdom (12). The solutions included the pneumatic Heidelberg arm (51) and the Bheograd arm (36), a myoelectric system (see below). At the same time, it was recognized that new technologies could be used to solve orthotic problems, but inevitably, the search for solutions led to more problems, as discussed below.

UPPER LIMB REQUIREMENTS

The upper limb has certain unique functions which challenge the investigator. It must function dextrously, with accurate placement and sensitive operation of the grasp and release mechanisms. It must be able to operate against heavy loads when desired and have adequate range of motion to perform the activities of daily living. The upper limb researcher is faced with the impossibility of control of the paralyzed upper limb to serve more than the most generic normal functions. Priorities must be established. For instance, the upper limb articulations can move normally in more than 20 describable directions simultaneously. The researcher must decide which of these motions will not be controlled in his system. Among each of the unique and generic attributes of the upper limb such a choice must be made since all the problems cannot be solved simultaneously.

Sequential and Simultaneous Control

In the standard orthotic systems of the 1950's and some of the more sophisticated systems of the 1960's (such as the ball-bearing forearm orthosis coupled with electric motor hand control) the patient was called upon to perform several functions *simultaneously*. These might include elbow extension, release of prehension and shoulder internal rotation. In these systems it was most likely that one or several of the anatomical segments included in the orthosis would be powered by the patient's muscles thus requiring no retraining for those motions. In considering the fully paralyzed extremity, the simultaneous control of these axes becomes complicated by the requirement that the patient learn new control methods for the transmission of external (or electrical stimulation) power to the segments in the orthosis. Even if the orthosis were to limit motion to five general directions (degrees of freedom) the retraining task would be complex if the patient were expected to operate the entire system simultaneously. In such systems the theoretical advantage of sequential control becomes important. If the patient can operate one orthotic degree of freedom at a time, he can perform any complex motion, broken down into its component parts. However, the concomitant disadvantage is the severe limitation of total orthotic response time to the patient's over-all demands. It is therefore generally preferable, in the design of sophisticated systems to concentrate on simultaneous control systems permitting control of many degrees of freedom in a single, coordinated system.

Control Sites. Sophisticated control systems for orthotic devices are born of need, usually severe paralysis. In the severely paralyzed patient, the researcher is limited by the small number of control sites available for the input of a signal to the orthotic device. The quadriplegic, for instance, may have only neck muscles and a small number of shoulder muscles to provide a message source. These muscles and their anatomic segments are further limited because any contraction of muscle or consequent movement of segment may cause a motion which is not part of the desired orthotic pattern of feeding or performance of other function. It is therefore of primary importance to the orthotic researcher to solve this problem of limited availability of control sites.

One avenue of approach is the use of a computer to simulate central nervous system control of the upper limb. Such a computer could permit the patient with limited control sites to use them as signal areas for the control of more degrees of freedom than would be possible through the simultaneous use of all controls. Several methods have been developed for the transmission of signals from the control sites into the computer: myoelectric, mechanical, and photoelectric.

Myoelectric systems utilize the electrical output of contracting muscle as a control signal. This electrical signal can be used to modulate or activate the power source of an orthotic system. The Russian myoelectric prosthesis (70) uses such a control to turn off and on the electric motor which drives the hand. A similar system quantitatively regulates the output of the electrical stimulator in the myoelectric splint described above (45, 76), and the below-elbow prosthesis designed by Bottomley (13). Myoelectric control sites can be used similarly as the input to computer control systems at the man-machine interface.

It is important to the flexibility of the computer system that it be able to receive information from the patient concerning his desires. The computer must know what the patient wants to do. It must know this in some detail; for instance, it might be told that the patient wants the hand to move from one position in a coordinate system to another position in the system. A relatively large number of bits of information must be communicated, compared with the number of control sites available. The researcher has a choice of using sequential information input, which is slow, or shifting to a more efficient utilization of existing sites for simultaneous input. The answer to efficient use may lie in the input of *patterns* of signals from the control sites. For instance, if there are five control sites, the patient might fire 1, 4 and 5 simultaneously with one meaning, 1 and 2 for another and so forth. The number of combinations possible in such a system is 2^n, or in the case of five sites 2^5, that is, 32.

Mechanical systems may be used to supply computer input. A good example is the "joy stick" method. This system is mounted like the control stick in an airplane to make contact or combinations of contacts in an electrical system if the stick is moved to and fro, sideways or diagonally. The system can also provide up and down motion. A relatively simple computer circuit can be built to make the hand move in directions analogous to that of the joy stick. The disadvantages include the coupling of the joy-stick movement with the arm movement. This is particularly opprobrious when the joy stick must be moved by the head; it then becomes impossible to move the arm while the head is still.

In *photoelectric systems*, photic energy is converted to electrical energy for signalling. One of the research devices was the Case Research Arm Aid (4, 18) which used an infrared source on the patient's eyeglasses to signal a computer program for a desired activity. The patient aimed the infrared beam (with a visible monitor) at the photo cell programed for the desired motion. Photoelectric systems have limited use because of the small amount of information rapidly transmissible in a necessarily sequential system.

The Computer. The orthotic computer may vary from the relatively simple device required for *coordinate conversion* in the joy-stick system to the immensely complex instrument required for tape storage and retrieval or for a *decision-making system.* The Case Institute Cybernetic Systems Group experimented early with a tape recorder device in which was stored a family of digital programs. These digital programs represented different coordinated motions of the arm and could be "played back" through the orthotic device. The computer received its orders from a combination of on-off input signals combining photoelectric and mechanical switching devices. The tape recorder system proved extremely slow (up to 5 seconds delay) while operating in the "search mode" seeking the program desired by the patient. Patient and engineer rejection was high.

A second computer type can be programed with environmental information concerning the location of the arm segments. It can then be signaled, concerning the desired goal of the hand. It is up to the computer to determine what combination of power sources must be activated in the orthosis to bring the hand to the desired position. Such a computer unit may be called a multi-level, multi-goal (MLMG) computer. The delay can be within the patient's tolerance (under 0.1 second).

SOURCE OF INPUT TO COMPLEX SYSTEMS

Position input is becoming increasingly accepted in relation to the patient's ability to generate meaningful input for an upper extremity computer. The ultimate goal of the multi-axis orthosis is to provide a positional change in the hand. Although numerous coded methods, including myoelectric switching, can be used to signal the computer of the patient's intentions, it is most simple to enter a direct position signal. Ideally the patient should enter "up" to move the orthosis up, "right" to move it right, and so forth. This can be accomplished by using a segment of the body attached to relatively normal nervous system, to provide a direct, positional input to a logic device. For instance, a set of receptors (potentiometers or similar) attached to the patient's chin can signal the desired direction (and even speed) of motion to an arm orthosis via a logic device. This method of chin control, and where appropriate, shoulder control, is now in clinical use for some purposes, such as driving complex wheelchair mobility systems. The extension of its application to complex orthoses is only a matter of time. The same principle of position input can be applied to non-arm-based manipulators (see below). Extensions of these and similar principles of complex upper extremity control systems can be found in other publications by this author (45, 64).

POWER SOURCES

Research orthotic systems use power sources significantly different from those used in conventional orthoses. In general, research power sources are more difficult to control than the clinical sources, requiring more sophisticated engineering to assure repeatable performance.

Pneumatic and Hydraulic Systems

A carbon dioxide (pneumatic) system operating at 600 psi formed the power source for the actuators of arm motion in the Case Research Arm Aid. The actuators contained small control valves with a total travel of about 0.003 inch between full-open and full-close. The valves were driven open and closed by torque motors. The extreme accuracy necessary in constructing and operating such a system is apparent. It is possible that some day a hydraulic system will operate at even higher levels of pressure (up to 20,000 psi) and even smaller valve clearances. Such systems will require major engineering revisions in existing control systems as well as in the power source. Precautionary protective systems for the patient in the presence of these high fluid pressures will assure safety.

Electric motors behave with reasonable accuracy in driving a single axis orthosis, but such motors will not be suited for multi-axis operation where repeated performance to small positional tolerance is required. Further development of electric motor drive systems will have to await the perfection of a better transducer.

Electrical stimulation presents an intriguing and perhaps fruitful source of orthotic power for the future. In contrast to the pneumatic and electric motor systems, the electrical stimulation system can operate without a supporting exoskeletal structure. It is theoretically possible to stimulate the muscles of the paralyzed limb to produce coordinated, useful motion for the patient. A computer can provide the necessary coordination of multiple axes of motion. Pilot systems of this type have been used on dogs by Kantrowitz for lower limb control and in upper limbs of men by the Case Institute-Highland View Group (76, 61). It is also possible to implant stimulating electrodes, with or without external connections, in the prime-moving muscles of the upper limb to permit the use of lower stimulation energy levels than necessary with transdermal stimulation. A further possibility is the radio-powering of implanted stimulators so that the patient would not even have to be in contact with the original signal generator (computer-controlled). This dream-like description of an electrical stimulation system is not without excellent opportunities for failure. For instance, the nature of the denervation process may render skeletal muscle uncontrollable by electrical stimulation after the passage of months or years of denervation.

Sensory feedback from the de-afferented limb within an upper limb orthosis would be theoretically beneficial. It might be especially desirable to have feedback to the patient concerning the pressure he is exerting between his anesthetic or astereognostic figners. It has not been necessary to include feedback devices in many research orthoses because of the relative efficiency of visual feedback as a proprioceptive substitute. Suggestions have been made through various laboratories of ways for the possible transduction of pressure and position sensation into meaningful signals. Pressure between the fingers could be transduced and then simulated elsewhere, for instance, as an analogous amount of pressure exerted in a non-anesthetic area elsewhere in the body. This system is only hypothetical but could be produced easily. When a computer is used in closed-loop fashion, as in the Case Research Arm Aid, position encoders may be used to inform the computer of the direction and magnitude of movement effected by the orthosis. This produces an error signal between the computer's desires and its actual effect, allowing the computer to correct this error continuously.

IDEAL MULTI-AXIS ORTHOSIS

The ideal multi-axis orthosis for the upper limb must have, first of all, Bennett's primary requirements of low cost, portability, utility, and cosmetic acceptability. In addition, it will include a computer for the conversion of a relatively small number of simultaneous input signals into a large variety of coordinated motions. Communication with the computer must be relatively simple and absolutely reliable. This communication should not cross-couple with other motions of the patient. Response time of the entire unit, from command to action should be less than 0.1 second. It should use an electrical supply source for the computer which is either self-contained and rechargeable or else available or installable in all homes. It should operate with minimal, if any, exoskeletal structure surrounding the upper limb. Its power source should be inexpensive, easy to repair or replace, and have little possibility of causing damage to the patient by accidental excesses above normal operation. Although these total requirements are rigorous, there is reasonable hope that the talents and resources of those engaged in research will fulfill them.

MULTI-AXIS ORTHOSIS vs. ENVIRONMENTAL CONTROL SYSTEMS (ECS)

Since the early days of research in man-machine interface communications, we have been seeking to improve the patient's control of his environment. This chapter has dealt heavily on the manipulation of objects in the environment. It is equally, if not more, important to be concerned with the patient's actual mobility in his wheelchair and his ability to control environmental items which pertain to activities of daily living and comfort. In recent years, these latter factors are transcending the simple, manipulatory functions of the patient.

Initially small devices were used to allow severely paralyzed patients to control the nurses' call button, the television or radio switch, and room lights. Today there are commercially available, reasonably priced, sophisticated systems which attach to the patient's electric wheelchair. For example these allow a C-4 quadriplegic patient to drive into a dark room, preceded by his headlight, switch on the room lights, activate his "no hands" telephone, dial a number, speak and listen to the telephone, turn on a radio, set the station and the volume, and then to tape-record and play back any part of the input received. This input may be from radio or television in the room, from the telephone, or from a speech or lecture. Thus, in the electronically oriented world of today, the patient is far less dependent on actual physical manipulation of objects, and this makes him less dependent also on such devices as the multi-axis orthosis. For this reason, it is very difficult to convince high level paralytic patients that the immense amount of training time in the use of multi-axis orthoses, plus the mechanical inconveniences, are indeed worth the effort. The situation is even more compelling when we realize that the training time for a multi-axis orthosis may exceed 100 hours while the time for a very complex environmental control system may be 1½ hours. For further discussion of some of these environmental control devices see Chapter 20.

MULTI-AXIS ORTHOSIS vs. THE MANIPULATOR

Although manipulators have been applied primarily to the handling of radioactive or other dangerous materials, the possibility is growing of applying "non-arm-based" manipulators to the care of severely paralyzed patients. Arm-based manipulators have numerous design problems, as discussed in this chapter; simply being "arm-based" is the major deterrent to an efficiently operating system. The system must make manipulations in three degrees of vertical and three degrees of rotational freedom, corresponding to up-and-down, front-and-back, and side-to-side movement, plus rotations around these axes. In addition to manipulating the desired object, the arm-based system must fit each center of rotation of the arm, must avoid undue forces on the arm itself, and must carry the arm wherever it goes.

Because of these considerations, future research may lead in the direction of table-based or wheelchair-based manipulators that do not conform to the arm. Once the psychological barrier is broken by moving away from anthropomorphism, and away from the necessity to move the patient as well as the object, a great step will be taken toward the efficient manipulation of objects by severely paralyzed patients.

REFERENCES

1. ALLEN, J. R., KARCHAK, A., JR., SNELSON, R., AND NICKEL, V. L. Design and application of external power and control of orthotic devices. Am. Soc. Mech. Eng. J., 84: 52, 1962.
2. ANDERSON, M. H. Functional Bracing of the Upper Extremities. Charles C Thomas, Springfield, Ill., 1958.
3. ANDERSON, M. H. Upper Extremities Orthotics. Charles C Thomas, Springfield, Ill., 1965.

4. BAHNIUK, E., RESWICK, J., *et al.* A progress report on a programmed orthotic arm. *Med. Electron. Biol. Eng., 1:* 509, 1963.

5. BARBER, L. M. Combined motor and peripheral sensory insufficiency. II Use of orthoses in treating adult brachial plexus injuries. *Phys. Ther., 58:* 287, 1978.

6. BASMAJIAN, J. V., AND LATIF, A. Integrated actions and functions of chief flexors of elbow. *J. Bone Jt. Surg. (Am.), 39:* 1106, 1957.

7. BATTYE, C. K., NIGHTINGALE, A., AND WHILLIS, J., JR. The use of myo-electric currents in the operation of prostheses. *J. Bone Joint. Surg., 37B:* 506, 1955.

8. BENDER, L. F. Personal communication, 1965.

9. BENDER, L. F. Prevention of deformities through orthotics. *J.A.M.A., 183:* 946, 1963.

10. BENNETT, R. L. Orthetics for function. *Phys. Ther. Rev., 36:* 721, 1956.

11. BISGROVE, J. G. A new functional dynamic wrist extension-finger flexion hand splint. A preliminary report. *J.A.P.M.R.,* September, 1964.

12. BOTTOMLEY, A. H., AND COWELL, T. K. An artificial hand controlled by the nerves. *New Sci., 21:* 668, 1964.

13. BOTTOMLEY, A. H., KINNIER-WILSON, A. B., AND NIGHTINGALE, A. Muscle substitutes and myo-electric control. *J. Br. Inst. Radio Eng., 26:* 6, 1963.

14. BUNNELL, S. *Surgery of the Hand,* 4th ed. Lippincott, Philadelphia, 1964.

15. BURKE, J. F., POCOCK, G. S., AND WALLIS, W. D. Electrophysiological bracing in peripheral nerve lesions. *J. Am. Phys. Ther. Assoc., 43:* 501, 1963.

16. CHUSID, J. G., AND McDONALD, J. J. *Correlative Neuroanatomy and Functional Neurology.* 11th ed. Lange Medical Publications, Los Altos, 1962.

17. CODMAN, E. A. *The Shoulder.* Thomas Todd, Boston, 1934.

18. CORRELL, R. W., AND WIJNSCHENK, M. J. Design and development of the Case research arm aid. Engineering Design Center Report No. 4, Case Institute of Technology, April, 1964.

19. DORANDO, C., AND NEWMAN, M. K. Bracing for severe scoliosis of muscular dystrophy patients. *Phys. Ther. Rev., 37:* 230, 1961.

20. ENGEN, T. J. Description of upper extremity orthotics including externally powered systems. Unpublished report, 1965.

21. ENGEN, T. J. Development toward a controllable orthotic system for restoring useful arm and hand actions. *Orthop. Prosthet. Appl. J., 17:* 184, 1963.

22. ENGEN, T. J. A modification of reciprocal wrist extension, finger flexion orthosis. *Orthop. Prosthet. Appl. J., 14:* 39, 1960.

23. ENGEN, T. J. A plastic hand orthosis. *Orthop. Appl. J., 13:* 38, 1959.

24. EYLER, D. L., AND MARKEE, J. E. Anatomy and function of intrinsic musculature of fingers. *J. Bone Jt. Surg. (Am.), 36:* 1, 1954.

25. HAMBRECHT, F. T., AND RESWICK, J. B. *Functional Electrical Stimulation, Applications in Neural Protheses.* Marcel Dekker, New York, 1977.

26. HASTINGS, A., GERSTEN, J. W., SCHOMBURG, A. AND KIME, L. The effect of hand bracing on function and electromyographic patterns in the hemiparetic. *Arch. Phys. Med. Rehabil., 45:* 262, 1964.

27. HERBERTS, P., KADEFORS, R., MAGNUSSON, R., AND PETERSEN, I. *The Control of Upper-Extremity Prostheses and Orthoses.* Charles C Thomas, Springfield, Ill., 1974.

28. HICKS, D. J., SCALISI, S., WOODY, F., AND SKINNER, B. Increasing upper extremity function. *Am. J. Nurs., 64:* 59, 1964.

29. HOLSER, P. An upper extremity control brace. *Am. J. Occup. Ther., 13:* 165, 1959.

30. HORN, G. W. *Elettronica e Automazione negli Apparecchi di Protesi Orthopedica.* A. Naz. Prod. Protesi Otoped, Treviso, 1963.

31. HORN, G. W. Electromyographic signal produced by muscle movement controls grasp of prosthetic fingers. *Electronics, 36:* 35, 1963.

32. HUDDLESTON, Q. L., HENDERSON, W., AND CAMPBELL, W. The spring wrist cock-up splint. *Am. J. Occup. Ther., 12:* 58, 1958.

33. INMAN, V. T., SAUNDERS, J. B. DEC. M., AND ABBOTT, L. C. Observations on function of shoulder joint. *J. Bone Jt. Surg. (Am.)*, *26:*, 1944.

34. JOHNSON, J. T. H., AND KENDALL, H. O. Isolated paralysis of the serratus anterior muscle. *Orthop. Prosthet. Appl. J.*, *18:* 201, 1964.

35. KARCHAK, A., JR., ALLEN, J. R., NICKEL, V. L., AND SNELSON, R. The electric hand splint. *Orthop. Prosthet. Appl. J.*, *19:* 135, 1965.

36. KOBRINSKI, A. Y. Bioelectric control of prosthetic devices. *Herald, Acad. Sci. U.S.S.R.*, *30:* 7, 1960.

37. LANDSMEER, J. M. F. The anatomy of the dorsal aponeurosis of the human finger and its functional significance. *Anat. Rec.*, *104:* 31, 1949.

38. LANDSMEER, J. M. F. Anatomical and functional investigations on the articulation of the human fingers. *Acta Anat.*, *25:* suppl. 24, 1955.

39. LANDSMEER, J. M. F. The coordination of finger joint motions. *J. Bone Jt. Surg. (Am.)*, *45:* 1654, 1963.

40. LANDSMEER, J. M. F. Power grip and precision handling. *Ann. Rheum. Dis.*, *21:* 164, 1962.

41. LANDSMEER, J. M. F., AND LONG, C. The mechanism of finger control, based on electromyograms and location analysis. *Acta Anat.*, *60:* 330, 1965.

42. LIBERSON, W. T. AND ASA, M. M. Further studies of brief isometric exercises. *Arch. Phys. Med. Rehabil.*, *40:* 330, 1959.

43. LIBERSON, W. T., HOLMQUEST, H. J., SCOT, D., AND DOW, M. Functional electrotherapy: stimulation of the peroneal nerve synchronized with the swing phase of the gait in hemiplegic patients. In *Proceedings of the Third International Congress on Physical Medicine,* Washington, D. C., 1960. Chicago, American Congress of Physical Medicine and Rehabilitation, 1962.

44. LONG, C., II. Intrinsic-extrinsic muscle control of the fingers. *J. Bone Jt. Surg. (Am.)*, *50:* 973, 1968.

45. LONG, C., II. Normal and abnormal motor control in the upper extremities. Final Report, Social and Rehabilitation Services, Grant No. RD-2377-M, December 1, 1966 to April 30, 1970. Cleveland, Ohio, June, 1970.

46. LONG, C., II. Physical medicine and rehabilitation. In Ray, C. D.: *Medical Engineering,* chap. 43, edited by C. D. Ray, pp. 516–541. Year Book Medical Publishers, Inc., Chicago, Ill., 1974.

47. LONG, C., II, CONRAD, P. W., HALL, E. A., AND FURLER, S. L. Intrinsic-extrinsic muscle control of the hand in power grip and precision handling. An electromyographic study. *J. Bone Jt. Surg. (Am.)*, *52:* 853, 1970.

48. LONG, C. II, AND EBSKOV, B. Research application of myoelectric control. *Arch. Phys. Med.*, *47:* 190, 1966.

49. LONG, C. II, AND MASCIARELLI, V. An electrophysiologic splint for the hand. *Arch. Phys. Med. Rehabil.*, *44:* 449, 1963.

50. LONG, C. II, AND BROWN, M. E. Electromyographic kinesiology of the hand; muscles moving the long finger. *J. Bone Jt. Surg. (Am.)*, *46:* 1683, 1964.

51. MARQUARDT, E. *Pneumatic Arm Prosthesis for Children.* Heidelberg, 1963.

52. McCOLLOUGH, N. C., III. Orthotic management in adult hemiplegia. *Clin. Orthop.*, *131:* 38, 1978.

53. MICHAEL, R. R., AND CRAWFORD, F. R. Myo-electric surface potentials for machine control. *Elec. Eng.*, *82:* 11, 1963.

54. NATIONAL FOUNDATION. Brochure accompanying exhibit on orthetic devices for upper extremity bracing. August, 1958.

55. NICKEL, V. L., PERRY, J., AND GARRETT, A. L. Development of useful function in the severely paralyzed hand. *J. Bone Jt. Surg. (Am.)*, *45:* 933, 1963.

56. NICKEL, V. L., PERRY, J., AND SNELSON, R. *Handbook of Hand Splints.* Downey, Calif., 1960.

57. NICKEL, V. L. Investigation of externally powered orthotic devices. Progress Report, V.R.A. Project No. RD-518, Washington, 1964.
58. *Orthopedic Appliances Atlas,* vol. 2. J. W. Edwards, Ann Arbor, Mich., 1960.
59. OCCUPATIONAL THERAPY DEPARTMENT, Rancho Los Amigos Hospital. Mobile arm supports; ball bearing, suspension and friction feeders; parts and their function. Rancho Los Amigos Hospital Document OT/OL-711, Part I, 1964.
60. OCCUPATIONAL THERAPY DEPARTMENT, Rancho Los Amigos Hospital. How to fit and adjust a ball bearing feeder. Rancho Los Amigos Hospital Document OT/OL-711, Part IV, 1964.
61. PECKHAM, P. H., AND MORTIMER, J. T. Restoration of hand function in the quadriplegic through electrical stimulation. In *Functional Electrical Stimulation, Applications in Neural Prostheses.* Mercel Dekker, New York, 1977.
62. PECKHAM, P. H., MORTIMER, J. T., AND VAN DER MEULLEN, J. P. Physiologic and metabolic changes in white muscle of cat following induced exercise. *Brain Res., 50:* 424, 1973.
63. PECKHAM, P. H., MORTIMER, J. T., AND MARSOLAIS, E. B. Alteration in the force and fatigability of skeletal muscle in quadriplegic humans following exercise induced by chronic electrical stimulation. *Clin. Orthop., 114:* 326, 1975.
64. RADONJIC, D., AND LONG, C. Why myo-electric control is so difficult. In *Advances in External Control of Human Extremities,* edited by M. M. Gavrilovic and A. B. Wilson, Jr. pp. 59–67. Yugoslav Committee for Electronics and Automation, Belgrade, 1970.
65. RUDIN, L. N., CRONIN, D. J., AND CROUCHER, J. S. Corrective brace for upper extremity in hemiplegia. *J.A.M.A., 153:* 479, 1953.
66. RUSSEK, A. S., AND MARKS, M. Scapular fixation by bracing in serratus anterior palsy. *Arch. Phys. Med. Rehabil., 34:* 633, 1953.
67. SCHOTTSTAEDT, E. R., AND ROBINSON, G. B. Functional bracing of the arm. *J. Bone Joint. Surg.,* June, *38A:* 477, 1956.
68. SCOTT, R. N., AND PACIGA, J. E. Clinical evaluation of UNB 3-state myoelectric control. Progress Report No. 16, University of New Brunswick, Canada, 1978.
69. SCOTT, R. N., PACIGA, J. E., AND PARKER, P. A. Operator error in multistate myoelectric control systems. *Med. Biol. Eng. Comput., 16:* 296, 1978.
70. SHERMAN, E. D. A Russian bioelectric-controlled prosthesis. Report of a research team from the Rehabilitation Institute of Montreal. *Can. Med. Assoc. J., 91:* 1268, 1964.
71. SMITH, E. M., AND JUVINALL, R. C. Theory of feeder mechanics. *Am. J. Phys. Med., 42:* 3, 1963.
72. SMITH, E. M., JUVINALL, R. C., AND PEARSON, J. R. Dynamic ulnar deviation splint. Unpublished report, 1965.
73. SNELSON, R. AND CONRY, J. Recent advancements in functional arm bracing, correlated with orthopedic surgery for the severely paralyzed upper extremity. *Orthop. Prosthet. Appl. J., 12:* 41, 1958.
74. STAMP, W. G. Bracing in cerebral palsy. *Orthop. Prosthet. Appl. J., 17:* 354, 1963.
75. TRUONG, X. I., AND RIPPEL, D. V. Orthotic devices for serratus anterior palsy; some biomechanical considerations. *Arch. Phys. Med. Rehabil., 60:* 66, 1979.
76. VODOVNIK, L., LIPPAY, A., STARBUCK, D., AND TROMBLY, C. A. A single channel myoelectric stimulator. Case Institute Report EDC 4-64-9, November, 1964.
77. ZISLIS, J. M. Splinting of hand in spastic hemiplegic patient. *Arch. Phys. Med. Rehabil., 45:* 41, 1964.

9

Lower Limb Orthotics

JUSTUS F. LEHMANN, M.D.

The most commonly used category of orthotic device is the lower extremity orthosis. While design features changed slowly over many decades, in recent years, engineering skills were applied to their design, and new plastic materials became available, leading to a bewildering and rapidly changing variety of orthotic designs. The purpose of this chapter is to furnish guidelines for the evaluation of a patient and the selections of an orthotic design through an understanding of the functional biomechanical principles used in orthotics. Such an understanding simplifies the approach to the patient (38). A detailed description of the biomechanics of normal human locomotion is beyond the scope of this chapter.

Orthoses for Neuromuscular Conditions

Orthoses for neuromuscular disorders are designed to permit safe and effective ambulation by patients with weakness resulting from upper and lower motor neuron disease or muscle pathology (26, 79, 80, 85). They may also prevent the development of deformity and require modifications in design to accommodate spasticity and/or muscle imbalance.

Ankle-Foot Orthoses (AFO)

Most patients with weakness around the ankle and foot are able to ambulate without an orthosis; however, they may fall or turn an ankle and injure themselves. Therefore, the most common purpose of bracing is to ensure safe ambulation. The orthosis should provide mediolateral stability at the ankle during the stance phase to prevent an inadvertent turn of the ankle and toe pickup during the swing phase to prevent a stumble caused by toe drag during the swing. In addition, the orthosis can be equipped with features which simulate pushoff to further approximate a normal gait pattern—the closer to normal that the gait is, the less excessive the energy expenditure. The orthosis also has a significant effect on knee stability (38).

The biomechanical function of AFOs is best discussed in terms of the standard double-upright metal orthosis. The principles thus illustrated can be used to evaluate any other orthosis, regardless of design or material used.

Components

The orthosis should be attached to a firm Blucher type shoe for ease of donning and doffing. Various stirrups are commonly used and incorporated into the shoe. The *conventional stirrup* (Fig. 9.1) is a steel plate bent in a U-shape. It is fastened to the shoe between sole and heel, and the upper end forms part of the ankle joint. The *split stirrup* allows the detachment of the stirrups and the uprights from the shoe, thus making possible the exchange of shoes so equipped (Fig. 9.2). A *long flange stirrup* or a *sole plate* riveted to the stirrup extending to the metatarsal head area may be used, and the stirrup thus equipped may have an additional strut. An alternative to the stirrup with ankle joints is the use of a *round calipers*, a device which connects the brace uprights to a metal plate that is attached to the shoe and to which a bushing is added to receive the calipers (Fig. 9.3). This device also allows detachment of the uprights from the shoe; however, a disadvantage is that the axis of the brace movement is significantly distal to the axis of the anatomical ankle, a problem of less significance in small children.

The conventional ankle joints allow motion only into plantar or dorsiflexion. The so-called *free ankle* does not significantly limit motion in either direction. A *posterior or plantar flexion stop* may be added by inserting a

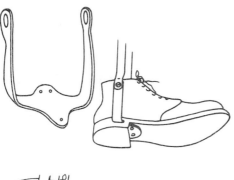

Fig. 9.1. Conventional stirrup.

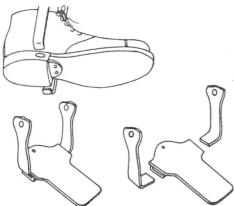

Fig. 9.2. Split stirrup.

steel pin into the channel so that the pin stops plantar flexion by resting against a flange of the stirrup. A set screw allows setting of the angle at which plantar flexion is stopped. If a spring is used instead of the steel pin, it is also called a *"lift assist."* A *double-stopped ankle joint* (or dual channeled double-upright adjustable ankle-locking device, "Bicaal") adds a similarly constructed *dorsiflexion or anterior stop.* It usually is used together with a sole plate or long- flange stirrup. Most of these joints are manufactured by the Pope Foundation (Klenzak joint), the Becker Co., or the U. S. Manufacturing Co. (Fig. 9.4). The *uprights* are usually made of stainless steel bar stock, but aluminum is used where light weight is important. The two uprights are held rigidly together at the top by a padded and leather-covered posterior steel *calf band* and an anterior soft closure.

Biomechanical Function

The standard double-upright orthosis attached to a firm shoe often provides sufficient mediolateral stability, except in those patients with significant spasticity, such as stroke patients who tend to invert one foot. In such cases, a T-strap attached to the outside of the shoe covering the lateral

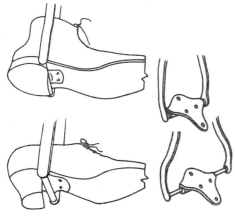

Fig. 9.3. Round caliper.

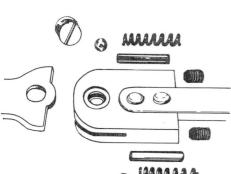

Fig. 9.4. Double-stopped ankle joint.

malleolus and cinched around the medial upright can be added (Fig. 9.5). When cinched, the lateral malleolus is pushed medially, thus correcting the varus position. If there is a tendency toward eversion, the valgus position can be corrected by attaching the T-strap to cover the medial malleolus and cinching it around the lateral upright.

The plantar flexion stop at the ankle joint is a substitute for weak foot dorsiflexors; it prevents toe drag and stumbling during the swing phase. In moderate-to-severe spasticity, a firm pin stop may be required to prevent a lapse into the equinus position. In flaccid paralysis or mild spasticity, a spring assist may be adequate. The type of stop also has a significant influence on knee stability. Instead of letting the foot down slowly from heelstrike to foot flat by a contraction of the foot dorsiflexors, the patient rocks over the posterior portion of his heel. In this position, the ground-reactive force is extended behind the knee joint (Fig. 9.6) with the moment

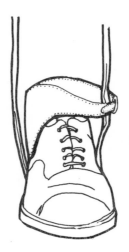

Fig. 9.5. Outside T-strap correcting varus position.

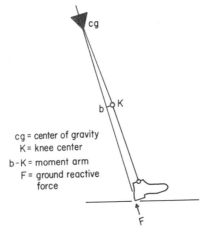

cg = center of gravity
K = knee center
b - K = moment arm
F = ground reactive force

Fig. 9.6. Knee bending movement at heelstrike.

arm (perpendicular distance from knee axis to force line) posterior to the knee, creating a bending moment at the knee greater than that produced by the normal lengthening contraction of the foot dorsiflexors. This bending moment must be overcome by knee extensor musculature. In many cases of significant weakness around the ankle, the muscles which extend the knee are also affected, making it essential for the orthotic design to minimize this bending moment.

This can be accomplished in the following ways: (a.) The minimal force necessary to pick up the toe (*i.e.*, prevent plantar flexion) during the swing phase should be used. If a spring assist is adequate, it should be used rather than the pin stop. (b.) The angle of the ankle at which plantar flexion is set has an influence on the magnitude and duration of the bending moment at the knee (44). Fig. 9.7 shows that the bending moment is less if more plantar flexion is allowed than if the ankle is set in slight dorsiflexion. There is direct tradeoff—the more dorsiflexion provided at the ankle, the better toe clearance during the swing phase but the greater the bending moment at the knee which the patient must overcome through voluntary muscle effort. The more plantar flexion provided, the more toe drag during swing phase but the less bending moment at the knee. This implies that no more toe pickup than necessary should be provided by the stop.

The anterior dorsiflexion stop may be combined with a sole plate extending to the metatarsal head area. Then, as the center of gravity of the body moves forward, the heel rises, the shoe pivots over the end of the sole plate, and pushoff is simulated. The result is an elevation of the lowest point of

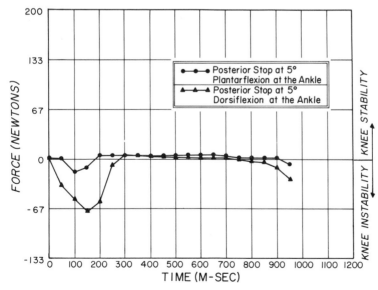

Fig. 9.7. Force between leg and ankle-foot orthoses at the calf band during stance (average of five consecutive steps).

the center of gravity pathway during the phase of double support, *i.e.*, a reduction in the total amplitude of the center of gravity pathway. If the ankle joint has free dorsiflexion, the center of gravity moves forward, and the entire shoe stays flat on the ground.

Thus, the dorsiflexion stop is a substitute for the plantar flexion musculature, the gastrocnemius, and soleus. It also has an effect on knee stability (Fig. 9.8) (38). As the foot pivots over the metatarsal head area during the latter part of the stance phase, the force on the ball of the foot creates a moment arm extending in front of the knee. This is in the opposite direction of the moment arm during heelstrike and produces knee extension. Since the posterior capsule and check ligaments prevent hyperextension, the knee is locked in extension. Too much extension moment may result in genu recurvatum because the posterior capsule and check ligaments are not particularly strong structures. This possibility should be kept in mind when the patient is fitted with such an orthosis, and the stop adjusted. A spring plantar flexion assist is rarely used, since the forces needed to simulate pushoff easily compress a spring causing the foot to stay flat on the ground.

The extension moment at the knee depends on the angle at which the dorsiflexion stop becomes effective (Fig. 9.9) (38). If the angle at the ankle is fixed at 5° plantar flexion, the dorsiflexion stop increases knee stability over most of the latter part of the stance. The extension moment is of large magnitude while the effect of the plantar flexion stop is of short duration and small magnitude. Thus, in this position, the stability is gained during the rest of the stance. On the other hand, if the ankle is fixed at 5° dorsiflexion by plantar and dorsiflexion stops, the bending moment at the knee during heelstrike is of long duration and large amplitude. Consequently,

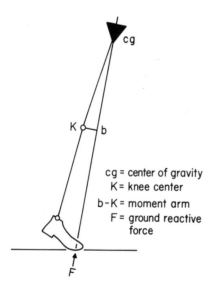

Fig. 9.8. Knee extension moment during pushoff.

cg = center of gravity
K = knee center
b-K = moment arm
F = ground reactive force

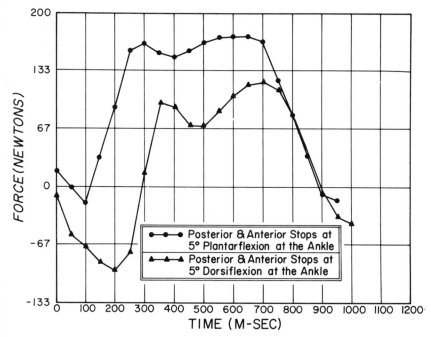

Fig. 9.9. Force between leg and ankle-foot orthosis at the calf band during stance (average of five consecutive steps).

the stabilizing extension moment is of subsequently shorter duration and less magnitude. The tradeoff between toe pickup and knee stability is as follows: the more toe pickup, *i.e.*, dorsiflexion of the ankle needed to adequately clear the ground during the swing phase, the more knee instability is produced by the plantar flexion stop during the heelstrike phase, and the less knee stability and pushoff simulation can be gained from the dorsiflexion stop, and *vice versa*. If, during the swing phase, significant spasticity forces the foot into the equinus position, a solid posterior plantar flexion pinstop is needed to prevent the toe from dragging. If, at the same time, the adjustment of the stop, *i.e.*, the angle at which it becomes effective, is such that the knee buckles during the heelstrike phase, the bending moment can be changed. This is accomplished by moving the location of the ground-reactive force forward (Fig. 9.10) (38), either by cutting off part of the heel at a 45° angle or by inserting a cushion wedge into the heel (58).

EVALUATION OF ORTHOSES BY BIOMECHANICAL PRINCIPLES

In prescribing a lower extremity orthosis, it is most important that the patient's need for mediolateral stability at the ankle, toe pickup, knee stability, and simulated pushoff be determined. A gross assessment of the forces required, especially for toe pickup, is desirable. The orthotic design which best corresponds to the patient's need should be selected. The many recent orthotic designs and modifications using new materials such as plastics can be readily evaluated using the biomechanical principles discussed. Several examples of these designs and principles of application are described in the following section.

An orthosis with a single metal upright and a posterior plantar flexion stop is shown in Fig. 9.11. The plastic laminated shoe insert allows shoes to

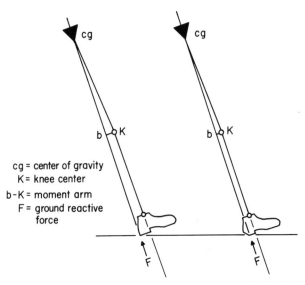

cg = center of gravity
K = knee center
b - K = moment arm
F = ground reactive force

Fig. 9.10. Reduction of knee bending moment during heelstrike by heel cutoff.

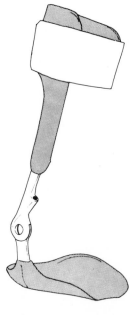

Fig. 9.11. Single-upright plastic ankle-foot orthosis with metal plantar flexion stop.

be changed. If an anterior dorsiflexion stop were added, the insert would also serve as a sole plate equivalent for pushoff. The absence of a medial upright makes knocking of the medial malleolus by the opposite leg less likely, but the orthosis obviously does not provide as much mediolateral stability as a double-upright design. Although this design could be used as a toe pickup orthosis, the patient using it should not have much spasticity driving the foot into an equinovarus position.

The so-called *Seattle Orthosis* (Fig. 9.12) was the first plastic orthosis described in the literature (30, 83). Lamination over a positive mold taken from a cast was used in its manufacture. The orthosis is rigid, encasing the

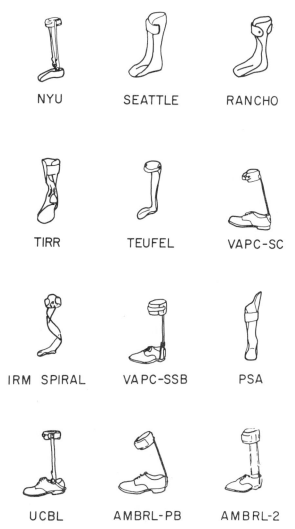

Fig. 9.12. Small selection of recent orthotic designs. [Modified from Rubin (71).]

ankle, and therefore is a biomechanical equivalent to an anterior and posterior pinstop with a sole plate extending to the metatarsal head area. It provides maximal mediolateral stability. Since knee stability is dependent on the degree of plantar or dorsiflexion at which the foot is fixed, casting at the correct angle of the ankle is important and must take into account heel and sole height of the shoe. Change of shoes is possible only so long as heel and sole height remain the same. To reduce the bending moment at the knee during heelstrike, a cushion wedge (58) or cutoff heel can be used. If it is desirable to reduce the extension moment at the knee, the anterior portion of the brace can be trimmed back slightly.

This design has been modified by Lehneis and by Rancho Los Amigos (71), using plastics such as polypropylene (Fig. 9.12), therefore reducing the cost of manufacture since vacuum-forming techniques can be used with these plastics. Depending on the thickness of the plastic used and the trim lines, the rigidity of these orthoses is somewhat less than the Seattle orthosis, but the biomechanical function is basically the same.

Another orthosis which is available in different sizes as a stock item is the *Teufel orthosis* (Fig. 9.12) (11, 38, 74). Its appearance suggests that it provides limited mediolateral stability. If the orthosis is manually stressed, it is fairly rigid in resisting plantar flexion, but if the same force is applied to push the orthosis into dorsiflexion, it yields easily. Therefore, it is effective in patients needing a moderate amount of force for toe pickup but needing little additional knee stability during the latter part of the stance. Because of available dorsiflexion and the fact that the orthosis acts as a posterior leaf spring, the center of rotation in the orthosis is different from the location of the anatomical axis of the ankle. The discrepancy produces some relative motion between the orthosis and the limb, which may be a problem in some patients.

Another plastic orthosis made of polypropylene and designed by Engen (also called the *TIRR orthosis*) is shown (Fig. 9.12) (71, 74). This orthosis is corrugated posteriorally to gain greater strength. Depending on thickness of plastic and trim line, it resists moderate-to-mild forces pushing it into plantarflexion but barely resists being pushed into dorsiflexion. Depending on trim line, it provides limited mediolateral stability. Therefore, this orthosis is commonly used for patients with flaccid paralysis or mild spasticity, primarily to give toe pickup through the swing phase. It adds little increase to knee stability during pushoff or the latter part of the stance phase.

The *VAPC shoe clasp orthosis* (Fig. 9.12) (38, 71, 80) is a plastic leaf spring orthosis attached to the heel counter of a shoe via a clasp and loosely to a calf band to absorb the relative motion of brace against the limb. The centers of rotation of the ankle and the orthosis are in different locations, but pistoning of the plastic bar within the calf band is allowed. The main advantage of the orthosis is that it is "ready made" and that no more than a firm shoe is required to apply it. The orthosis provides only moderate force for toe pickup and provides no significant mediolateral stability, and even without stress it collapses readily into maximal dorsiflexion, thus contributing no additional knee stability (Fig. 9.13).

These examples show the value of understanding the basic biomechanical function so that it becomes easier to match patient need to appropriate orthotic design. Fig. 9.12 shows only a small selection of the many orthoses available. By using biomechanical principles, prescription of orthoses is made far easier than by relying on rote memorization of indications and contraindications. Biomechanical considerations also allow more individualization.

An excellent example of applying biomechanics can be demonstrated by considering the *plastic spiral orthosis* designed by Lehneis (Fig. 9.12) (38, 48, 49, 71). By manual stressing and application of biomechanical principles, its function can be readily assessed. Without this knowledge, the following indications developed by Sarno (76) would have to be memorized: (1) severe weakness or absence of ankle dorsiflexors and plantarflexors; (2) mild-to-moderate defect in mediolateral stability during stance or swing; (3) tendency toward varus or valgus during stance; and (4) flaccidity or mild-to-moderate spasticity.

Another consideration in prescription should be whether the orthotic design increases functional ambulation capability and decreases energy expenditure. A comparison was made between normal subjects and hemi-

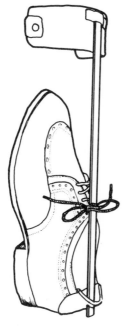

Fig. 9.13. VAPC shoe clasp orthosis, no resistance to dorsiflexion. [Redrawn from *Atlas of Orthotics* (1).]

plegic patients walking without an orthosis, with the Seattle orthosis, and with a double-upright ankle foot orthosis with anterior and posterior pin-stops and sole plate. The oxygen consumption was least in normal subjects for a given walking speed, and it was highest when the hemiplegics were walking without an orthosis. When walking with the orthosis, the oxygen consumption was reduced but was considerably higher than in normals. There was no difference in the oxygen consumption for various speeds between a patient using the Seattle or the double-upright AFO. The use of either one of the orthoses increased the comfortable walking speed, *i.e.*, the walking speed at which the minimum amount of energy is required to cover a given distance and also the maximum walking speed, as compared with the same patient walking without the orthosis. In this respect, there was no difference between the two types of orthoses used (Fig. 9.14) (15, 16). Most important, perhaps, the patients walking without the orthoses had to be guarded against falls but walked safely with either one of the orthoses.

To summarize, proper bracing improves the patient's safety, increases

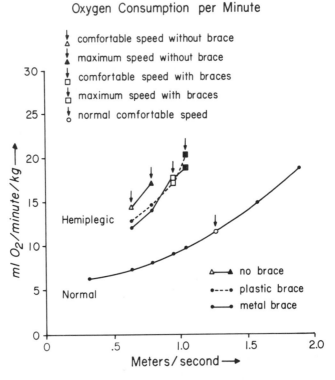

Fig. 9.14. Oxygen consumption at different ambulation rates of a patient walking without orthoses and using a plastic laminated ankle-foot orthosis and ankle-foot orthosis with double metal uprights, anterior and posterior stops, and sole plate extending to the metatarsal head area. [From Corcoran *et al.* (9, 10).]

functional ambulation, and decreases energy consumption. If the same biomechanical design is used in orthoses, the results are quantifiably similar, even though materials used and appearances may be very different. Even minor differences in the weight of the orthosis are not as important in influencing energy consumption as biomechanical function and its influence on the center of gravity pathway.

CHECKING ORTHOSES USING BIOMECHANICAL PRINCIPLES

Once the patient is fitted with an orthosis, it should be checked. It is of greatest importance, irrespective of the material used, that the orthosis not create any intolerable pressure areas. The calf band should not impinge on the peroneal nerve below the fibular head, and the orthosis should follow the contour of the leg with adequate clearance from the skin, especially around the ankle. In plastic orthoses, especially the Seattle or Rancho types, and in patients with spasticity or impaired sensation, it is important to check the skin frequently for pressure areas. The proper fitting of these orthoses is as important as the fitting of a prosthetic socket to an amputee, and initially the orthosis should be worn only for short periods of time.

If the orthosis allows any ankle movement, it is important to align the axis of the ankle joint for plantar and dorsiflexion approximately to coincide with the location of the anatomical joint axis. Inman and associates (28) determined this axis, which can be approximated by connecting the tips of the medial and lateral malleoli. This alignment prevents forces from developing between the orthosis and the limb. It is a special problem in plastic or posterior spring orthoses, in which the center of rotation in the orthosis differs from that of the ankle joint.

Dynamic loading of the orthosis is essential for checking its function. When the patient is standing, the sole and heel of the shoe should be flat on the floor. When walking, this should be observed at midstance. The entire gait cycle should be observed to see whether or not there is inadequate knee stabilization from heelstrike to foot flat and hyperextension of back knee from heel rise to the toe off and whether the toe drags during the swing phase. These undesirable features can be related to the biomechanical function of the orthosis and its adjustments, such as the ankle. Buckling of the knee during the heelstrike phase can be related to the plantar flexion stop, i.e., if it engages at more dorsiflexion than is necessary for toe clearance or if a rigid stop is used where a spring assist may be adequate to pull up the weight of the foot during swing. Back knee during push off will be observed if the anterior stop is set at too much plantar flexion or the sole plate or long flange of the stirrup extends too far forward.

Only a few orthoses specially designed for unusual conditions can be discussed here. One example is the University of California at Berkeley dual axis ankle brace (33). Inman and associates (28, 29) determined that the axis of inversion and eversion of the subtalar joint is 42° from the horizontal plane and 23° from the midline of the foot. These measurements served as the basis for the development of an orthotic design (Fig. 9.15) which allows combining of an axis for plantar and dorsiflexion with an axis located posteriorly at the heel of the shoe to allow inversion and eversion. The ankle joint is a standard joint which can be stopped or modified as in other orthoses. This orthosis is applicable to only a small number of patients, as it can rarely be used in patients with weakness of the anterior leg musculature. If a stopped ankle joint for toe pickup is necessary, this implies that the foot dorsiflexors are nonfunctioning or weak. Since these muscles are also part of the inversion and eversion group, most patients need mediolateral stability of the ankle and cannot use the additional freedom to invert and evert that is provided by this orthosis.

Another special orthotic design is the spring-loaded telescoping section of a single-bar ankle joint which allows some rotation of the foot and absorbs any pistoning action of the orthosis against the leg in case the ankle joint is not perfectly aligned (Fig. 9.16) (54).

Finally, a more commonly used orthosis is the spring wire orthosis (1, 23) for toe pickup, which is now frequently replaced by plastic orthoses.

KNEE-ANKLE-FOOT ORTHOSES (KAFO)

KAFOs are prescribed for patients with lower limb weakness from upper and lower motor neuron lesions. Most commonly, they are used in spinal cord injuries including conus and cauda equina injuries. However, these orthoses may also be prescribed for patients with other neuromuscular diseases. They may be used for either functional ambulation or exercise. In

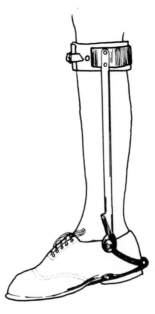

Fig. 9.15. University of California Biomechanics Laboratory dual-axis ankle-foot orthosis.

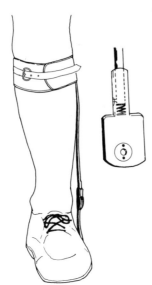

Fig. 9.16. Spring-loaded telescoping ankle joint for single-upright orthosis. [Redrawn from *Atlas of Orthotics* (1).]

spinal cord injuries, it has been suggested that only those patients with lesion levels below T_{10} become functional ambulators (53, 78). Aside from lesion level, the ability to functionally ambulate depends on age, strength, and coordination.

Patients with upper and lower motor neuron lesions require knee-ankle-foot orthoses for mediolateral stability at the ankle during the stance phase, and they must further provide knee stability during this phase. An anterior dorsiflexion stop in combination with a rigid sole plate extending to the metatarsal head area can simulate pushoff. During the swing phase, the orthosis should ensure toe pickup. In the standard double-upright orthosis, a posterior plantar flexion stop at the ankle will be sufficient to guarantee this clearance. Patients with bilateral involvement usually use a swing-to gait, or the more effective swing-through gait. Those patients who are able to walk functionally can move at normal walking speeds using a swing-through gait with crutches. At higher lesion levels, patients may not walk functionally, but limited ambulation using crutches or parallel bars may be beneficial for maintenance of upper limb strength, joint mobility, and prevention of orthostatic hypotension.

The problems encountered with knee ankle foot orthoses are of several types. Improper knee alignment may occur within the orthosis due to improper fitting design, or application of the orthosis. In the standard double-upright design, the ischium may rest on the upper thigh band, especially when the orthosis is too long. Also, excessive forces on bands or straps may be applied, and such forces can affect skin integrity. The design of the orthosis may also produce excessive anatomical knee shear, loosening the ligaments and occasionally creating a "back knee" if the patient wears the orthosis regularly. Some orthoses may have unnecessary structural components which increase weight and may be cumbersome during transfers or when the orthosis is donned or removed.

Other issues in lower limb orthotics include the use of the pelvic band and the introduction of such novel structural elements as plastic and pneumatic tubes. Further considerations in application are energy consumption and the practicality of each type of KAFO.

The principles used in proper design of the knee-ankle-foot orthoses will be discussed using the standard double-upright orthosis and its variations. In general, these principles are applicable irrespective of materials. As a basis for further discussion, it is necessary to review common components of standard double-upright orthoses.

Components

Shoes, stirrups, ankle joints, uprights, and calf bands are the same as those used in AFOs. The commonly used knee joints are: a *free knee*, a knee joint with a *drop lock (ring lock)* or *bail lock (Swiss lock)* (Fig. 9.17). For stability, it is advisable that both uprights be locked at the knee. The two uprights are connected on top by a rigid, padded *upper thigh band* with an anterior soft closure. This band should clear the ischium by approximately 1 to 1½ inches. Usually, a second lower thigh band is used with a soft front closure.

Knee stabilization is provided by a number of different devices (Fig. 9.18). Three common designs feature two straps to stabilize the knee, one combining a *suprapatellar* and a *patellar tendon strap* applying the forces to the musculature above the patella and to the patellar tendon below the knee

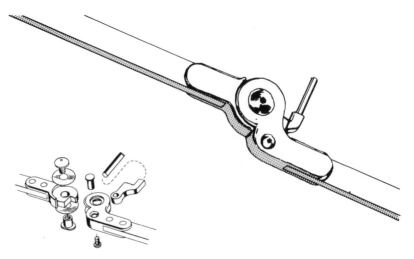

Fig. 9.17. Bail or Swiss lock for knee joint.

and a second combining lower thigh band closure with a calf band closure. The third design combines the lower thigh band closure with a patellar tendon strap. Three other common designs apply the entire stabilizing force with just one strap—a suprapatellar strap, a patellar tendon strap, or a so-called *knee cap strap* or "spider" which applies the forces to the patella itself (43).

Most hip joints limit motion to flexion and extension; a few allow adduction and abduction. The joint may be locked, for instance, with a drop lock (Fig. 9.19). These joints are attached to a pelvic band (1), and the posterior and lateral portion of this band is made of steel and padded. In front, a soft belt closure is used. The band should be located between iliac crest and greater trochanter.

KAFOs should provide the following: (a) mediolateral stability at the ankle during the stance phase, as in the AFOs (an anterior dorsiflexion stop may be used at the ankle, as in the AFOs); (b) knee stability in cases in which AFOs are not adequate for that purpose; and (c) a posterior plantar flexion stop at the ankle for toe pickup during the swing phase, as in the AFO.

Thus, the only additional functional features from AFOs is the stabilization of the knee joint during weight bearing. This requires a three-force application to keep the knee from buckling (Fig. 9.20) (43). While the

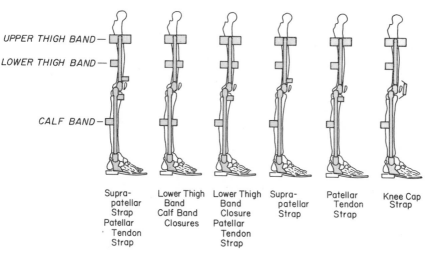

UPPER THIGH BAND—

LOWER THIGH BAND—

CALF BAND—

| Supra-patellar Strap Patellar Tendon Strap | Lower Thigh Band Calf Band Closures | Lower Thigh Band Closure Patellar Tendon Strap | Supra-patellar Strap | Patellar Tendon Strap | Knee Cap Strap |

Fig. 9.18. Six common variants of knee-ankle orthoses.

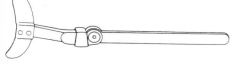

Fig. 9.19. Drop lock hip joint.

counterforces are applied at the level of the foot and the upper thigh band, the knee-stabilizing force in front may be applied by a variety of designs. It is desirable to keep this force and, consequently, the counterforces to a minimum in order not to exceed tolerance limits.

When the forces against the upper thigh band were measured in paraplegics using a swing-through gait, no differences were found, irrespective of which of the six previously described variants of knee-stabilizing force application were used. However, if the amount of total stabilizing force was determined, whether one or two straps were used, the highest force was required when a lower thigh band and calf band combination was used. Thus, in order to minimize the required stabilizing force, it is best to apply the force close to the knee center since this provides a better leverage to counteract the bending moment at the knee; in other words, the greater the distance the strap is from the knee center, the greater the force required for knee stabilization. For this reason, the force applied by a lower thigh band and calf band combination was 30 to 50% greater than that applied by a kneecap strap.

In addition, not only must the orthosis be designed to keep the knee straight, but also it must be applied correctly if it is to function as intended. If the straps are not evenly cinched, which often occurs if the patient's orthosis is applied while he is sitting, or if no special attention is given to the force applied to the straps, the orthosis will allow the knee to bend. If such flexion is allowed, the force required to stabilize the knee will be double that required with a correct application of the orthosis.

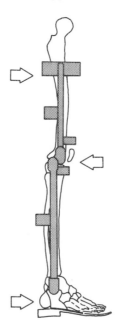

Fig. 9.20. Principle of three-point force application to stabilize the paralyzed lower extremity.

Furthermore, it is important to know how much pressure or force per unit of surface area is applied by each strap. Since the straps are of approximately the same size and configuration, one can equate pressure with the force measured at each strap. In testing, there was more than a 100% difference between the forces measured at some straps and those measured at others (Fig. 9.21). The highest forces were measured if single straps were used, such as a suprapatellar strap or a patellar tendon strap used alone, followed by the kneecap strap or "spider." Lesser forces are measured in strap combinations where two straps provide the stabilization of the knee. The least forces were measured with the combination of a suprapatellar and patellar tendon strap.

It is, therefore, advisable to use two straps to keep the knee straight, thus distributing the force over a wider area or to enlarge the single strap so that forces are applied over an area equivalent to two straps. The combination

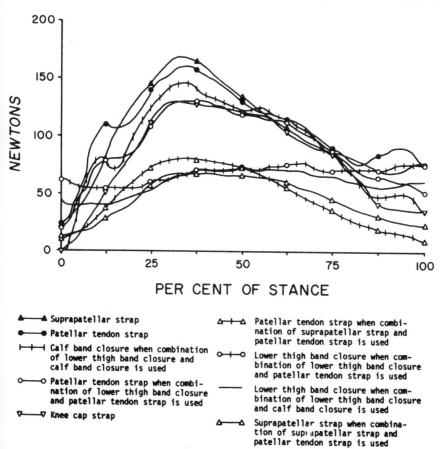

Fig. 9.21. Forces on each of the individual strap closures stabilizing the knee in the same patient, using the six orthoses.

of suprapatellar and patellar tendon straps is advantageous because these two straps apply the forces to very tolerant tissues—the patellar tendon and the musculature above the patella.

To estimate whether the forces measured were of biological significance, the range of bending moments created by the forces applied to the upper edge of the upper thigh band were measured. During paraplegic ambulation, the moments ranged from 5 to 3 newton-meters. To estimate the actual forces applied to the tissues, one would need to know the precise area of interaction at the upper edge of the posterior thigh band. Since this information is difficult to obtain experimentally, the forces were calculated assuming force interaction in any location from 0 to the total length of the band. This calculation showed forces of a very large order of magnitude: 1000 mm of mercury pressure. These forces are large enough not only to occlude blood flow but also to significantly shear the tissue.

This calculation is consistent with the clinical experience that patients ambulating often get abrasions or sores at this upper edge of the thigh band if the orthosis is poorly fitted. When the patient's ischium sits on this upper edge, these forces are particularly high. If one properly applies the orthosis, the tissue will interact with the flat surface of the band.

The extremes encountered in paraplegic ambulation at this flat surface interaction were also measured, and the forces developed at this or other bands were between 170 and 100 newtons. By calculating the forces at various band widths, these forces were found to still be quite significant, 1 to 10 newtons per square centimeter, or 100 mm mercury pressure, still large enough to occlude blood flow. They are tolerated without much apparent difficulty because the blood flow to these tissues is shut off only intermittently. If very narrow straps are used, these forces are increased, and they may produce tissue damage, especially if the strap is applied to a bony area covered by little soft tissue. This conclusion is also confirmed by clinical experience.

Anatomical knee shear was also measured, and the shear curves of the six orthotic modifications were found to vary significantly (Fig. 9.22). During early stance phase, the shear is in a positive direction, i.e., after heelstrike, the femur shears forward on the tibia. Later, this direction changes to a negative shear, i.e., the femur shears posteriorly on the tibia. As in Fig. 9.18, the suprapatellar strap used alone or the kneecap strap produced very uneven distributions of shear (the two lowest curves in Fig. 9.22). In these two strap designs, the positive shear is relatively small and of short duration; however, the amplitude of the negative shear is great and lasts over most of the stance phase. The total amplitude from the maximum positive to the maximum negative is also larger than the amplitude in the other orthotic configurations, which have a more even distribution between positive and negative shear in both amplitude and duration.

A relatively even type of shear curve is produced by the combination of the suprapatellar and patellar tendon straps (Figs. 9.18 and 9.22). Other straps which produce this type of curve include the patellar tendon strap in combination with the lower thigh band closures and the calf band in combination with lower thigh band closures. One concludes that a better shear distribution can be obtained if all or a major portion of the knee stabilizing force is applied below the knee center.

To understand this principle, examine Fig. 9.23 (*A* and *B*) showing forces during the pushoff phase of gait. In pushoff, the shear against the floor is in a posterior direction, and that measured in the orthosis is anterior. The shear transmitted through the skeletal system is equal to floor shear minus the shear measured in the orthosis. Since these shear forces are vectors, the shear in the orthosis is added to the floor shear in the opposite direction. Therefore, the shear in the skeletal system is large and posterior. This large amount of shear is transmitted up the skeletal leg column until another force is met. If this force is applied by a patellar tendon strap, as shown in Fig. 9.23*A*, shear is markedly reduced. Therefore, reduced shear is trans-

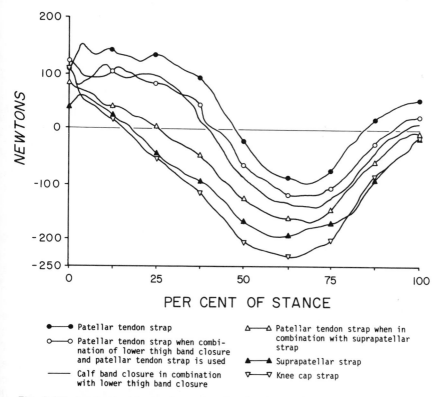

PER CENT OF STANCE

●——● Patellar tendon strap

○——○ Patellar tendon strap when combination of lower thigh band closure and patellar tendon strap is used

——— Calf band closure in combination with lower thigh band closure

△——△ Patellar tendon strap when in combination with suprapatellar strap

▲——▲ Suprapatellar strap

▽——▽ Knee cap strap

Fig. 9.22. Anatomical knee shear showing force interaction between femur and tibia. *Positive* values indicate the femur shearing forward on the tibia; *negative* values indicate the femur shearing backward on the tibia.

mitted to the knee ligaments, as compared with Fig. 9.23B, where the force is applied above the knee. Since the amount of shear is small and evenly distributed between positive and negative directions, the chance of loosening these ligaments is less with the patellar tendon strap. Similar observations have been made during the heelstrike phase.

From these observations, biomechanical principles used in the optimal design for the application of the knee-stabilizing force may be summarized as follows. Forces should hold the patient's knee straight, should be applied close to the knee, and should be distributed over two straps or one large strap. They should be applied to tolerant areas such as the patellar tendon and suprapatellar areas and applied at least in part below the knee to reduce shear.

Unnecessary Structural Components

The question has been raised as to whether the standard orthotic designs contain unnecessary components, increasing weight and making the orthoses difficult to don and doff. The Craig-Scott brace (Fig. 9.24) (21, 46, 77) was designed with this problem in mind. This orthosis eliminates the lower thigh and calf bands and retains the bail at the knee. It uses an anterior pretibial rigid piece, which may be hinged and locked into position or may be permanently attached to the uprights. This orthosis has four rigid connections between the two uprights: the posterior rigid thigh band, the bail at the knee, the anterior shin piece stabilizing the knee, and the stirrup at the

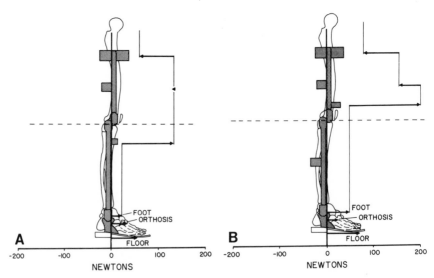

Fig. 9.23. A, schematic representation of shear distribution in limb and orthosis during pushoff, with stabilizing force below the knee; B, schematic representation of shear distribution in limb and orthosis during pushoff, with stabilizing force above the knee.

lower end. Like the other orthoses, it uses an anterior and posterior stop at the ankle and a rigid sole plate extending to the metatarsal head area.

A comparison of forces applied by the straps was first made (Fig. 9.25). Total knee-stabilizing force applied by the Craig-Scott was low, comparing favorably with the other orthoses. If, however, forces from the shin piece were compared to forces from single straps, they were relatively high and were applied to a bony area covered by little soft tissue (Fig. 9.26). Func-

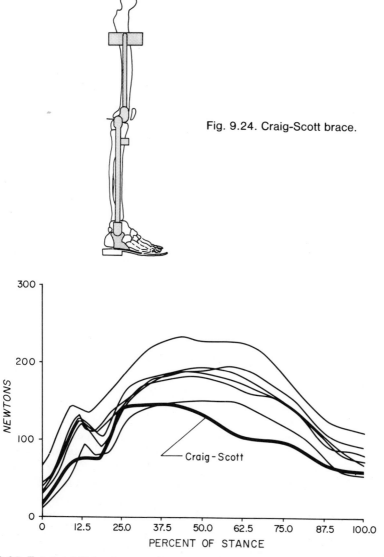

Fig. 9.24. Craig-Scott brace.

Fig. 9.25. Total stabilizing force on knee as compared with six other configurations.

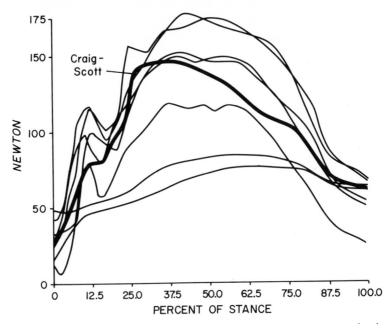

Fig. 9.26. Force on pretibial shell, as compared with forces per strap in six other orthotic configurations.

tionally walking paraplegics who walked for more than half an hour in this orthosis had reddened skin which lasted over an extended period of time. Some of them even had abrasions, although the pretibial piece was well padded and constructed according to the original design. When the piece was widened and molded so that a major portion of the force was applied to the patellar tendon, this eliminated the problem.

The amount of shear in the Craig-Scott orthosis was of favorably low total amplitude, and there was an even distribution between anterior and posterior shear. This observation is consistent with designs which apply stabilizing forces below the knee center.

The rigidity of the orthosis was tested by removing the lower thigh and calf bands. It was placed in a jig which stressed the brace structures to the same magnitude as those forces generated by normal ambulation, close to the knee center. Mediolateral displacement at the upper thigh band level, anterior-posterior displacement at the knee level, and rotation at the upper thigh band were measured. The results are shown in Fig. 9.27A when calf band and lower thigh band, but not the bail, are removed from the standard double-upright configuration. The minimal deformation shown in Fig. 9.27A is essentially the same as obtained in orthoses with all cross-connections intact (Fig. 9.27B). However, when all bands and bail are removed, a major deformation of the orthoses does occur as shown in Fig. 9.27c. Thus, the

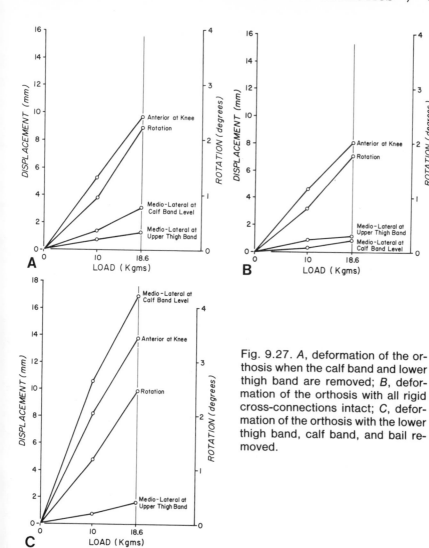

Fig. 9.27. *A,* deformation of the orthosis when the calf band and lower thigh band are removed; *B,* deformation of the orthosis with all rigid cross-connections intact; *C,* deformation of the orthosis with the lower thigh band, calf band, and bail removed.

Craig-Scott orthosis with a bail and anterior rigid pretibial shell should have adequate structural rigidity.

In conclusion, maintaining the structural rigidity of a KAFO requires at least one rigid cross connection between the two uprights in addition to the upper thigh band and the stirrup.

Energy Consumption

The energy consumption required by the various orthotic designs was also assessed. One indication of consumption is the amount of change in the center of gravity pathway since these changes necessitate corresponding energy expenditure. Design features which influence the center of gravity pathway are the construction of the ankle, the stirrup and the sole plate as in the AFO.

The orthotic designs surveyed used an anterior (40) and posterior rigid pinstop at the ankle in combination with a rigid steel sole plate extending to the metatarsal head area, i.e., the same basic design used in the Craig-Scott orthosis. Another common design uses an ankle joint with a posterior pinstop alone to provide toe pickup but allows free dorsiflexion at the ankle and, therefore, does not simulate pushoff. Pushoff resulting from the dorsiflexion stop occurs when the patient leans forward on crutches in preparation for swing-through; the anterior stop prevents dorsiflexion at the ankle, the orthosis pivots over the metatarsal head area, and the heel rises off of the ground. As its lowest point, the center of gravity pathway stays at a higher elevation from the floor with the two-stop design than with the design using the posterior stop only. The difference between the two designs in amount of center of gravity pathway lift necessary to clear the ground during the swing phase is shown in Table 9.1. The double-stopped ankle joint requires less lift.

The amount of mechanical work required can also be measured by having the patient walk with crutches over force plates. The force that the patient exerts against the ground through the crutches is multiplied by the displacement of the center of gravity. When one thus estimates the mechanical work necessary during the lift phase and compares it in different designs (Table 9.2), it can be seen that the double stop requires less work.

The amount of oxygen consumed measures energy consumption required, both for the amount of mechanical work during lift and also for the muscular control required to lower the center of gravity and absorb the shock of

TABLE 9.1. *Comparison of vertical lift (in centimeters) of center of gravity area.*

Patient No.	Sex	Level of Lesion	(n=10) Post. Stop	(n=10) Post. and Ant. Stop	t value (p*)
1	F	T12	13.2	9.0	5.998 (0.0001)
2	F	T7-8	12.0	6.85	6.414 (0.0006)
3	M	L2-3	21.6	13.3	5.534 (0.00002)

*p = probability

heelstrike. Table 9.3 shows a comparison of energy consumption for orthoses with and without anterior stops and sole plates. The total oxygen consumption dropped rapidly during the rest period and was almost normal after 4 minutes of rest. If the same patient walked with an orthosis with a posterior stop only, maximum oxygen consumption occurred late in the rest period, indicating that the person incurred a significant oxygen debt which he must then repay.

A marginal ambulator may be able to ambulate only with an orthosis with both stops and sole plate; if the orthosis has only a posterior stop, oxygen consumption may be prohibitively high to sustain ambulation over more than a short period of time. Even though the orthosis with two stops and sole plate is heavier by an average of 0.6 kg, the difference in center of gravity pathway amplitude is more important than the weight of the orthosis.

TABLE 9.2. *Comparison of work done during lift phase of swing-through (in centimeters).*

Patient No.	Sex	Level of Lesion	(n=10) Post. Stop	(n=10) Post. and Ant. Stop	t value (p*)
1	F	T12	548.1	399.3	2.083 (0.0449)
2	F	T7-8	631.5	340.0	2.634 (0.0144)
3	M	L2-3	1526.4	1081.9	4.409 (0.00086)

*p = probability

TABLE 9.3. *Comparison of energy consumption of patient ambulating with each brace.*

	Post. ankle stop		Post. and ant. ankle stop	
Intervals of O_2 Consumption	Run 1	Run 3	Run 2	Run 4
Rest 1 min.	0.42 liters	0.44 liters	0.67 liters	0.66 liters
Ambulation 200 feet..............	2.48 liters	2.49 liters	2.56 liters	2.04 liters
Min. 1 and 2 rest	1.56 liters	1.58 liters	1.82 liters	2.22 liters
Min. 3 and 4 rest	3.35 liters	3.38 liters	1.01 liters	0.95 liters
Total O_2 consumed*	7.39 liters	7.45 liters	5.39 liters	5.21 liters
Total caloric* equivalent	36.95 Cal.	37.25 Cal.	26.95 Cal.	26.05 Cal.
Ambulation time	1 min., 11 sec.	1 min., 19 sec.	1 min., 13 sec.	1 min., 17 sec.

*Prerun rest not included in totals.

In summary, the dorsiflexion stop in combination with sole plate or long flange stirrup reduces center of gravity vertical excursion with a resulting reduction in energy consumption, thus making an oxygen debt less likely.

Practicality

Ease of donning and doffing was compared for all the orthoses investigated, including the Craig-Scott. Time required to put on and take off an orthosis was used as a measure of the difficulty encountered. As an example, the Craig-Scott was compared with a standard KAFO with patellar tendon and suprapatellar straps; the average donning time was 111 seconds for the Craig-Scott and 153 seconds for the standard orthosis, and doffing time was an average of 28 seconds vs. 33 seconds. However, the Craig-Scott orthosis slid several inches forward on the thigh whenever the patient sat down. Therefore, it was necessary to add a posterior soft closure in lieu of a calf band, which added an average of 4 seconds to the donning and doffing times (37). The conclusion can thus be drawn that one posterior connection between the uprights below the knee is essential to keep the orthosis from slipping off of the thigh.

Transfer activities were accomplished with equal ease with a standard double-upright orthotic design using a patellar tendon-suprapatellar strap combination or the Craig-Scott design with the anterior tibial band hinged. Standing balance was also identical as long as the comparison was between orthotic designs with both stops and the long sole plate. A brace with free dorsiflexion (no anterior stop) produced much poorer standing balance (38). Thus, the anterior stop and sole plate provide a firmer standing platform over which the patient can better balance his center of gravity.

HIP-KAFOs IN NEUROMUSCULAR CONDITIONS

The indications for bracing the hip and trunk have been controversial. A pelvic band design with a lockable hip joint is the most frequent means of stabilizing the hips. However, patients can use a swing-through and swing-to gait without this band and be quite stable. When crutches are in front, stability is achieved by the forces of gravity pulling the hips into extension. Hypertension is checked by extremely strong ligaments. After swinging through, the patient is stable with his crutches behind him. If he has learned to arch his trunk, the center of gravity force line falls behind his hip joints into an area of support between his legs and crutches. His hips are again locked by the extension moment created by the force line falling behind the hip joint. Thus, patients can ambulate effectively without the encumbrance of a pelvic band.

The literature suggests that the pelvic band reduces excessive lumbar excursion and also controls the forward swing of the legs, especially in cases of uneven spasticity (13). These claims were tested experimentally by applying an electrogoniometer to the backs of paraplegic patients to estimate the maximal excursion of the lumbar spine throughout the gait cycle. The hips were somewhat limited by the pelvic band. Since the lumbar spine compensated for lack of mobility at the hip, lumbar excursion was significantly increased, contradicting earlier claims. When the patient walked with the pelvic band mean stride and the center of gravity pathway, amplitude was increased. Removing the pelvic band reduced the amplitude of center of gravity pathway, and mobility increased at the hip, allowing the patient to clear the ground more easily during the swing phase (Table 9.4).

From these measurements, it may be assumed that energy consumption will be greater when the patient uses a pelvic band. The donning and doffing times were greater if the orthosis included this band. The pelvic band had one advantage—standing balance was slightly improved, particularly if the patient had some spasticity. Even though a patient's forward leg swing may be better controlled with a pelvic band, all of those tested learned to overcome their initial difficulties without one, and all decided against the pelvic band when they chose permanent orthoses. Thus, for most paraplegic patients, pelvic bands are probably not necessary; however, in some exceptional cases of spasticity, they may still be useful.

In summary, the pelvic band should not be used on a routine basis. It is of limited help in controlling uneven leg swing and scissoring in patients with spasticity and may control excessive rotation of the legs. It is more effective in children because of their shorter legs. In order to control rotation of the legs, the pelvic band may also be used, together with a twister cable (Fig. 9.28) attached to a modified stirrup for a unilateral upright orthosis.

NEW DESIGNS AND MATERIALS

Once one understands the basic principles in an orthotic design, one can look at new designs using new materials and easily recognize their functions. For instance, consider a design developed by Lehneis (Fig. 9.29) (12). In this

TABLE 9.4. *Comparison of lumbar excursion, stride length, and center of gravity amplitude with and without pelvic band.*

	With pelvic band	Without pelvic band	Wilcoxon Test*
Mean Maximum Range of Lumbar Excursion (degrees)	29.0	26.8	$p < 0.05$
Mean Stride Length	0.96 m	1.03 m	$p < 0.05$
Mean Center of Gravity Amplitude	10.8 cm	8.7 cm	$p < 0.05$

*Matched-pairs signed-ranks test

plastic knee-ankle-foot orthosis, the knee-stabilizing force is applied in the suprapatellar and patellar tendon areas. The ankle is rigid and is functionally equivalent to an anterior and posterior stop, with sole plate extending to the metatarsal head area. The malleoli are encased to provide maximal mediolateral stability. The posterior soft closure prevents the orthosis from sliding off of the thigh when sitting. The upper closure is equivalent to the posterior thigh band. Thus, the orthosis can be related to known functions.

Pneumatic orthoses were recently introduced into the U. S. by Silber and

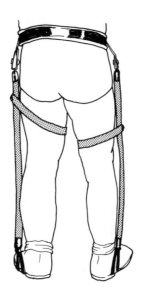

Fig. 9.28. Twister cables attached to pelvic band and modified stirrups.

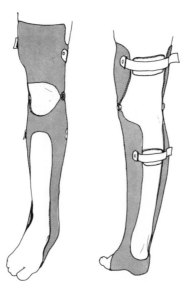

Fig. 9.29. Molded plastic knee-ankle orthosis. [Redrawn from *Atlas of Orthotics* (1).]

his associates (81) for use by paraplegic patients, and they were more recently tested by Ragnarsson (69). The orthoses are manufactured in both long and short versions and consist of a garment with inflatable tubes both anteriorly and posteriorly (Fig. 9.30). When these tubes are inflated, they provide rigidity; when deflated, the patient can easily bend his hips and knees.

The long orthosis covers the hips and a portion of the trunk, increasing hip and trunk stability. Toe pickup during the swing phase is provided by boots covering the ankle which must be worn with this orthosis. The shorter version of this orthosis extends only as far as the standard metal double upright orthosis, 1 to 1½ inches below the ischium. Mediolateral stability, as well as toe pickup, can be improved by using a plastic AFO of the Seattle or Rancho types as an insert. This will also increase the efficiency of ambulation because of simulated pushoff.

These orthoses were tested by patients who were either functional or marginal ambulators, walking primarily for exercise purposes. The shorter pneumatic orthosis could only be used if more stability at the ankle was added and, even with a plastic polypropylene AFO, relatively few patients could really use the orthosis.

These several versions of the pneumatic orthoses were compared with standard metal double upright orthoses in patients with T_{12} paraplegia for the following functions (42):

1. Amplitude of change of center of gravity during the gait cycle.
2. Angulation changes at the knee and ankle.
3. Oxygen consumption while ambulating 300 meters.
4. Distance walked at a prescribed rate until speed slows down.

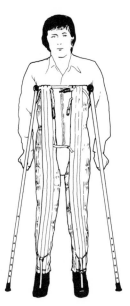

Fig. 9.30. Long pneumatic orthosis.

A detailed description of the results of these studies can be reviewed in Ref. 42. The results of these studies are summarized as follows: The long pneumatic orthosis provides hip and trunk stability with reduced oxygen consumption when used in conjunction with a plastic AFO (Seattle or Rancho type). This results in increased effectiveness of ambulation documented by increased distances walked at lower speeds. At higher rates of ambulation, buckling at the knee becomes so pronounced that it reduces the effectiveness of walking. For a functional ambulator, the standard double-upright orthosis was preferred. Difficulties in inflation and donning/doffing of the pneumatic orthosis added to this preference. The long pneumatic orthosis can be effectively used during early mobilization of the spinal cord injured since, as an adjustable stock item, it can be applied immediately. It also reduces tendency towards orthostatic hypotension and adds to the ease of ambulation. However, the pressures are significant enough to create pressure sores in anesthetic area; therefore, the garment should be not only carefully applied but also checked at short intervals. The proper size should be selected and appropriately adjusted for each individual. The cost of the orthosis is also reduced by its repeated use for different patients.

Several new design features have been experimentally used to allow a free knee movement during the swing phase to foreshorten the swinging leg, thereby more nearly approximating a normal gait pattern. The orthosis, however, firmly stabilizes the knee during heelstrike and stance.

The *UCLA functional long leg brace* was developed for the flaccid paralysis resulting from poliomyelitis (4). The orthosis used an offset knee joint and a hydraulic cylinder(s) at the ankle (Fig. 9.31). Some weight bearing through the upper plastic cuff made the offset knee joint more

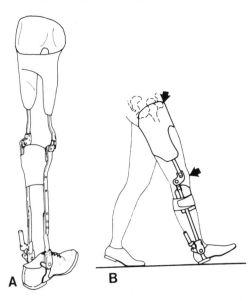

Fig. 9.31. UCLA functional long leg brace.

A   B

effective in providing stability at the knee during stance. In addition, the hydraulic cylinder(s) resisted dorsiflexion at the ankle to create a knee extension moment. Strohm and associates (87) evaluated this orthosis in 55 poliomyelitis cases. They found that knee flexion contractures of 10° made it impossible to use this orthosis. Valgus deformity of the knee and the absence of all hip extension musculature also represented contraindications.

This design works only when the knee is straight during weight bearing. Since many patients with upper motor neuron lesions with some spasticity have difficulty keeping the knee straight during the stance, orthotic designs with a lock that engages even when the knee is slightly bent during the stance but allows free motion during the swing have been suggested (55, 57, 63). An evaluation of such an experimental design (41) showed that energy savings were significant only at ambulation rates at or above 73 meters/minute, (Figs. 9.32–9.34), a speed which could only be attained by normal subjects.

In order to achieve such high rates of ambulation, a patient's hip flexors must be quite strong, yet a KAFO is required only when the patient's knee extensors are weak. In patients with spinal cord injuries, this pattern of muscle strength is rarely encountered. The innervation of hip flexors and knee extensors overlap, so voluntary control of these muscles will either be present or absent for both muscle groups. Therefore, most spinal cord injured persons who need a KAFO would not greatly benefit from this locking mechanism, although there may be other conditions in which this device will prove valuable.

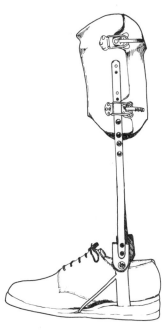

Fig. 9.32. Patellar tendon-bearing brace for limiting weight bearing, incorporating bivalved patellar tendon-bearing cuff closed by ski boot buckles, standard uprights, double-stopped ankle joint, and sole plate extending to the metatarsal head area.

Orthoses for Bone and Joint Pathology

Orthoses for disorders of the bones and joints are designed mainly for two purposes: to limit weight bearing of the lower extremity through the skeletal system and to maintain or correct joint and bone alignment.

PATELLAR TENDON BEARING ORTHOSIS

The patellar tendon bearing orthosis uses a cuff which incorporates the design principles of the patellar tendon bearing socket for amputees (Fig. 9.32). It is intended that skeletal weight bearing below the knee be relieved by transmitting the majority of the force from the patellar tendon area into the cuff. This force is then transmitted through the uprights and the shoe to the ground. Clearance between the patient's heel and the shoe is provided to minimize unloading of the orthosis through contact of the limb against the ground.

Orthotic Components

Stirrup, ankle, stops, and sole plate or long flange stirrup may be used, as in the AFO. The patellar tendon bearing cuff is attached to the two uprights. It is bivalved for easy donning and doffing and closed by rigid ski boot-type buckles (Fig. 9.32). A soft closure such as leather or Velcro yields enough to decrease the weight bearing function of the orthosis. In order to allow

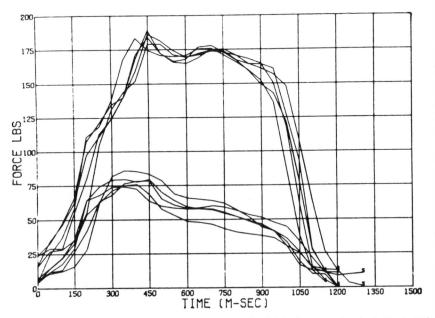

Fig. 9.33. Patellar tendon bearing brace with rigid closure, short shell at 10°, fixed ankle at 7°, heel clearance ⅜ inch. *Upper curves*, force plate force; *lower curves*, brace forces.

proper weight bearing, the patellar tendon bearing shell should be flexed to approximately 10° in relation to the uprights. If a fixed ankle joint is used, the stop should be adjusted to 7° dorsiflexion from the 90° neutral position.

Biomechanical Function

The weight bearing function of the orthosis depends on variation in its design, on the amount of heel clearance, and on training patients in its use. When the orthosis is fitted with a 3/8-inch heel clearance, it is found that up to 43% of the total force to the ground is transmitted through the orthosis (Fig. 9.33). Maximal load bearing of the orthosis occurs during the heelstrike phase and drops off during pushoff. The heel clearance provided in fitting the orthosis reduces the possible force transmission from heel to ground during heelstrike; however, a patient with normal musculature can still actively push against the ground using gastrocnemius, soleus, and other plantar flexors during the pushoff.

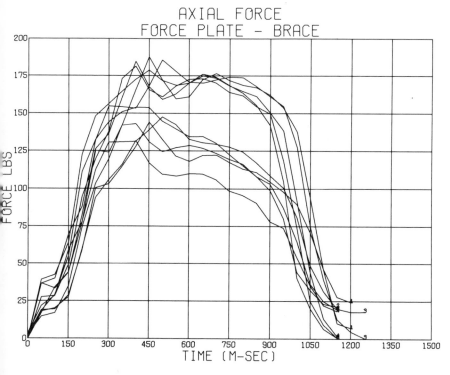

PTB BRACE   MAXIMAL LOADING

SHELL – SHORT 10°   ANKLE – FIXED, 7°   HEEL CLEARANCE –

Fig. 9.34. Patellar tendon-bearing brace used with training, short shell at 10°, fixed ankle at 7°, dorsiflexion, heel clearance 1 inch. *Upper curves,* force plate force; *lower curves,* brace forces.

If the patient is also trained not to push off actively in the orthosis and to kneel against the patellar tendon shelf of the cuff, and if the heel clearance is increased, weight bearing can be still further improved (Fig. 9.34) (47, 89) until at least 50% of the patient's weight is borne through the orthosis during the entire stance. Patients who are unable to avoid active pushoff may be fitted with a rocker bottom under the shoe, which makes active pushoff even more difficult, therefore preventing the drop-off in weight-bearing function of the orthosis during pushoff.

The design features of the ankle joint are another determinant of the weight bearing function. A free ankle joint reduces weight bearing through the orthosis primarily during the latter part of the stance phase (Fig. 9.35).

A *cable ankle joint* (Fig. 9.36) has the same effect. This joint has been used by Sarmiento and Sinclair (75) and others in fracture cast bracing because it accommodates its center of rotation to the location of the

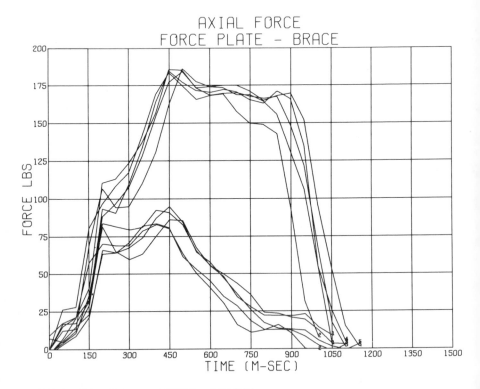

PTB BRACE   FREE ANKLE

SHELL - SHORT, 10°   HEEL CLEARANCE - 3/8"

Fig. 9.35. Patellar tendon-bearing brace with free ankle joint, short shell at 10°, heel flexion clearance ⅜ inch. *Upper curves*, force plate force; *lower curve*, brace forces.

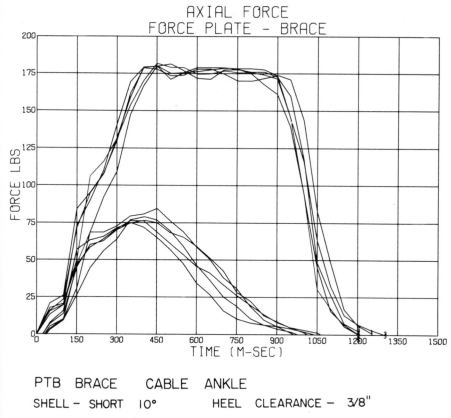

AXIAL FORCE
FORCE PLATE - BRACE

PTB BRACE   CABLE   ANKLE

SHELL - SHORT 10°   HEEL CLEARANCE - 3/8"

Fig. 9.36. Patellar tendon-bearing, cable ankle joint, short shell at 10° flexion, heel clearance ⅜ inch. *Upper curves*, force plate force; *lower curves*, brace forces.

anatomical ankle axis, yet provides mediolateral stability. This is important when plaster is used because a poorly aligned conventional ankle joint generates enough force between limb and orthosis to cause a plaster shell to be rapidly destroyed.

In summary, the weight-bearing function of the patellar tendon-bearing orthosis depends on training, heel clearance, ankle design, and the use of a rocker bottom.

Indications and Contraindications

The indications for the use of the patellar tendon bearing orthosis, according to Davis and associates (12) on a short-term basis (up to 6 months) are as follows:

1. Healing of os calcis fractures
2. Postoperative fusions about the ankle

3. Painful conditions of the heel which have been refractory to conservative management and for which surgery is contraindicated.

The orthosis is recommended for long-term use in:

1. Delayed unions or nonunions of fractures and fusions
2. Avascular necrosis of the talar body
3. Degenerative arthritis of the subtalar or ankle joint
4. Osteomyelitis of the os calcis
5. Sciatic nerve injury with secondary anesthesia involving the sole of the foot
6. Chronic dermatological problems, such as diabetic ulceration
7. Other chronic and painful conditions of the foot not amenable to surgery.

Contraindications include conditions of the skin and peripheral circulation in which pressure about the patellar tendon and popliteal regions cannot be tolerated.

ISCHIAL WEIGHT BEARING ORTHOSIS

The ischial weight bearing orthosis is intended to transmit force from the ischium into the orthosis and down through the uprights to the ground. The amount of weight borne through the orthosis will depend on variations of the design with regard to the weight bearing cuff, the function of the knee and ankle, and the clearance between the heel and ground. Like the patellar tendon bearing orthosis, its effectiveness also depends on training the wearer.

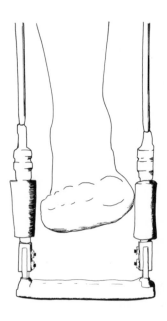

Fig. 9.37. Patten bottom for weight-bearing orthoses.

Components

Either an *ischial (Thomas) ring* (2) or a rigid plastic *quadrilateral cuff* following the design of the quadrilateral socket for the above-knee amputee is used (50, 62, 64, 72). Standard stainless steel bar stock is usually used for the uprights. Free or bail lock knee joints are used as well as a calf band below the knee. Stirrup and ankle joints are the same as those used in the patellar tendon bearing orthosis. A rocker or a patten bottom may be used as well (Fig. 9.37).

Biomechanical Function

The Thomas ring offers a relatively small contact area between the ischium and the orthosis. Patients often loosen the thigh lacer to get relief from this discomfort and, as a result, the ischium drops into the ring and the weight bearing function of the orthosis is lost (Fig. 9.38) (45). A better design than the Thomas ring is the quadrilateral rigid cuff (Fig. 9.39). The use of this design markedly improves the weight bearing function of the orthosis. Maximal weight bearing occurs during the heel strike phase when over 50% of the forces are transmitted through the orthosis. A marked drop in the weight bearing function of the orthosis is observed during pushoff

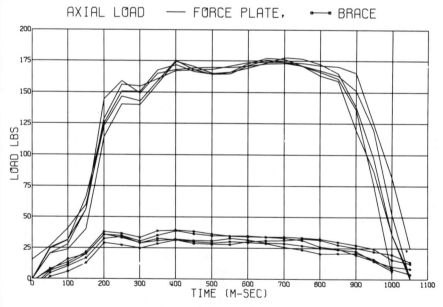

FREE ANKLE. FIXED KNEE. THOMAS RING - LOOSENED

Fig. 9.38. Axial loads developed on force plate and in uprights of a brace with free ankle, fixed knee, and Thomas ring with thigh lacer loosened during five stance phases.

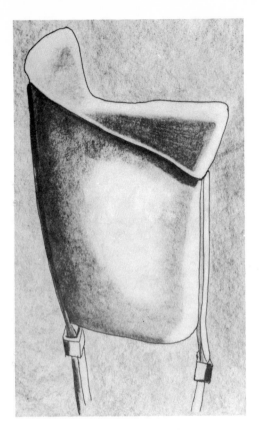

Fig. 9.39. Rigid quadrilateral cuff for ischial weight-bearing orthoses.

because the patient actively plantar flexes, pushing against the ground. If the patient is trained to avoid active pushoff and to use the ischial seat of the quadrilateral cuff, weight bearing through the orthosis occurs throughout the stance phase at a level of more than 50% of body weight (45, 89).

It should be noted that these figures were all obtained in orthoses with a locked knee, a free ankle joint, and ⅜-inch heel clearance, as measured in midstance. When a fixed ankle is used with an anterior and a posterior pinstop and a sole plate extending to the metatarsal head area, the weight bearing function of the orthosis becomes more reliable (Fig. 9.40) and occurs at approximately 56% of body weight throughout the stance phase. If the patient is trained to avoid pushoff with a fixed ankle, weight bearing can be achieved through the orthosis at a level of approximately 86% (Fig. 9.41). If a rocker bottom is added, making active pushoff virtually impossible, more than 90% of the body weight is borne through the orthosis (Fig. 9.42). If a patten bottom is used, 100% of the weight is borne through the orthosis, as can be anticipated since there is no limb contact with the ground.

If a free ankle joint in combination with a free knee joint is used, about 55% of the weight may be borne through the orthosis. However, there is

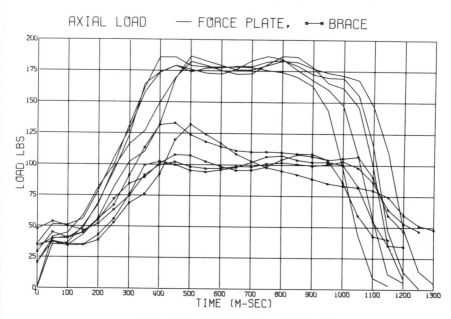

FIXED ANKLE, FIXED KNEE, QUADRILATERAL SHELL

Fig. 9.40. Axial loads developed on force plate and in uprights of a brace with fixed ankle, fixed knee, and quadrilateral shell during five stance phases.

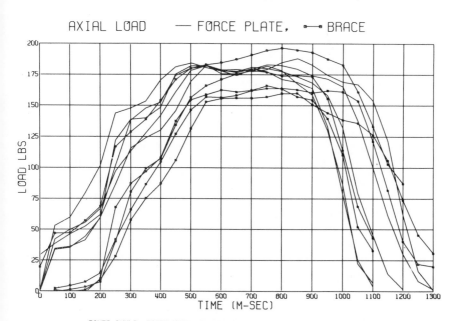

FIXED ANKLE, FIXED KNEE, QUADRILATERAL SHELL - ACTIVE DORSIFLEXION

Fig. 9.41. Axial loads developed on force plate and in uprights of a fixed ankle brace with a volunteer attempting active dorsiflexion to avoid pushoff during five stance phases.

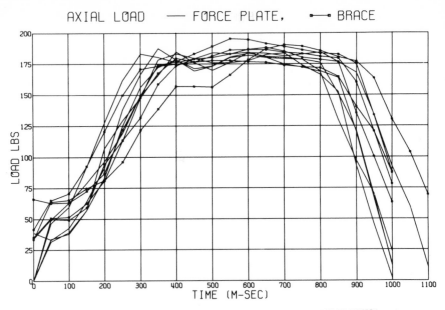

Fig. 9.42. Axial loads developed on force plate and in uprights of a brace with fixed ankle, fixed knee, quadrilateral shell, and rocker bottom during five stance phases.

extensive variability (Fig. 9.43), and in an active and vigorous walker the stress on the orthotic brace components is so great that the orthosis quickly breaks or deforms. Although the same biomechanical principles apply to fracture cast bracing, the pain associated with the treated condition usually prevents early destruction of the orthosis.

Theoretically, if all weight is transmitted from the ischium into the ischial seat of the quadrilateral cuff, the orthosis should provide 100% protection for the hip joint since no force should be transmitted through the hip joint. Actual measurements with an instrumented ischial seat show that only approximately 40% of the force is transmitted through the ischial seat. The rest apparently passes from the quadrilateral cuff through the soft tissue mass of the thigh into the skeletal structure. Therefore, an ischial weight bearing orthosis is not an appropriate means of protecting the hip and crutches, or canes should be used instead. A three-point gait with crutches can eliminate 100% of weight bearing by a hip joint.

In conclusion, the older design of the Thomas ring has become obsolete through the use of the quadrilateral cuff. The weight bearing function of the orthosis depends on design and training as follows:

(1) The orthosis with a fixed knee, free ankle joint, without training,

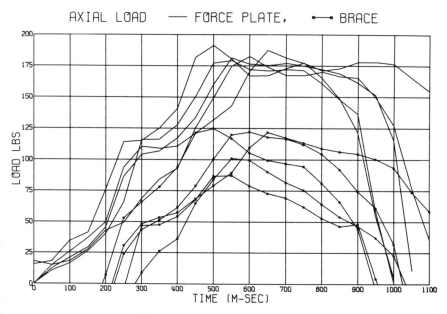

Fig. 9.43. Axial loads developed on force plate and in uprights of a brace with free ankle, free knee, and quadrilateral shell during five stance phases.

produces 50% plus weight bearing through the orthosis only during heel strike.

(2) The orthosis with a fixed knee, free ankle joint, with training, produces 50% plus variable weight bearing through the orthosis throughout the stance phase.

(3) The orthosis with locked knee and fixed ankle, without training, produces weight bearing through the orthosis at 50% of body weight with little variation.

(4) The orthosis with locked knee and fixed ankle, with training, produces weight bearing through the orthosis at approximately 86% of body weight.

(5) The orthosis with locked knee, fixed ankle, rocker bottom, and training produces weight bearing through the orthosis at 90% plus of body weight.

(6) The orthosis with fixed knee and patten bottom produces 100% weight bearing through the orthosis.

FRACTURE CAST ORTHOTIC DESIGNS

In the past 10 years, the principle of minimizing weight bearing in lower extremity fractures by specially designed casts with patellar tendon or ischial weight bearing has been successfully utilized in many programs. The biomechanical function of the critical design features is the same in fracture cast bracing as it is in weight-bearing orthoses. The indications also overlap. The basic differences are that in fracture cast bracing the material originally used was plaster of Paris and that the entire segment of the lower extremity, which had to be kept in alignment, was tightly encased. Sarmiento (74) suggests that the fluid column of the soft tissue thus encased adds to the weight-bearing function (74). However, this requires further investigation since no significant difference in weight bearing function was found between the patellar tendon-bearing orthosis which tightly encases the entire leg to the ankle and a short patellar tendon-bearing cuff. The distinction between fracture cast bracing and weight-bearing orthoses is even further blurred since Sarmiento replaced plaster of Paris with heat-forming plastic.

The success of using a weight-bearing orthosis *vs.* traditional methods in the treatment of fractures is indicated by the shortening of the immobilization period and satisfactory healing time using fracture bracing. Nickel and associates (62) describe healing of 102 femoral fractures after traction in an average of 12 weeks (62). Sarmiento (73) used 382 patellar tendon-bearing orthoses in patients with an average healing time of 14.5 weeks. These and other authors did not observe any significant shortening of the limb associated with this treatment method. They found that both delayed and nonunion fractures also responded well.

In conclusion, it is likely that this type of treatment of fractures is effective because it maintains bony alignment and limits weight bearing through the fracture site to a tolerable level which promotes bone healing and allows the patient to be active and ambulatory early. The quantity of weight bearing through the fracture cast orthosis depends on the same biomechanical principles and design features of the above-described weight-bearing orthoses.

MODIFICATION OF WEIGHT-BEARING ORTHOSES TO MAINTAIN OR CORRECT JOINT ALIGNMENT

In cases of joint pathology such as rheumatoid arthritis or degenerative joint disease, orthoses are designed to limit weight bearing and/or maintain joint alignment. The basic design used is that described under patellar tendon- or ischial weight-bearing orthoses. In order to provide mediolateral stability at the ankle, plastic laminates can be extended across the ankle for maximal stability, as described under AFOs for paresis or paralysis.

One of the major problems in maintaining proper alignment is most commonly at the knee, especially in rheumatoid arthritis, where destruction and loosening of the medial collateral ligament leads to valgus deformity. The deforming force increases as the deformity progresses. The more valgus deformity exists, the more the center of rotation for medial deviation of the knee is forced medial to the extension of the ground reactive force line, *i.e.*, the more the knee is deformed, the greater the moment arm bending the knee further into valgus position. To counteract this bending moment, a corrective force must be applied medially to the knee which is countered by two forces, one applied to the limb above and one below (Fig. 9.44) (84). This force is usually supplied by a *corrective pressure pad* applied to the medial side of the double-upright orthosis. This can be designed to rotate in order not to rub against the skin when the patient sits down.

The alternative construction is to use a plastic-contoured insert which is extended slightly above the knee level (supracondylar extension) to better distribute the correcting force (1, 49). A plastic rigid shell may be used instead of thigh bands to control femoral position (22). The plastic shell, both above and below the knee, must be manufactured from an accurate plaster cast made when the limb is in its optimally corrected position. Lamination or vacuum-forming techniques are used.

In cases when the knee joint of the orthosis is free, it is equally critical to maintain optimal alignment and locate the center of rotation of the orthosis coincident with the knee joint. Special care must be taken since the instantaneous center of rotation of the knee changes its location (16). Only an approximation can be achieved with a single axis brace joint. A commonly used method to align the orthotic knee joint with the anatomical joint axis

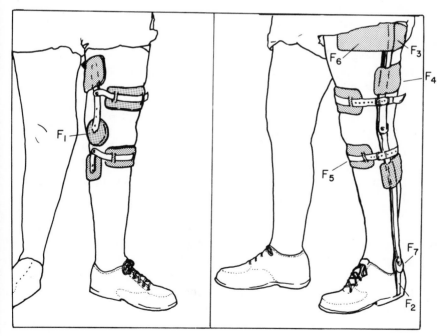

Fig. 9.44. Free knee brace utilizing seven forces for control of valgus and anterior tibial displacement. [Redrawn from Smith *et al.* (74).]

is as follows. The axis of the orthotic joint is located over the maximum bony prominence of the medial femoral condyle, or a line encircling the knee joint horizontally at the midpatellar level is subdivided into halves. If the midpatellar point is extended posteriorly backwards, two-thirds of the medial half is the location of the joint axis. The accuracy can be checked with the finished orthosis. When the patient sits down, there should be no relative motion between the orthosis and limb. If the brace axis is too high, the lower thigh band will dig into the thigh. If it is too low, the calf band will bite into the calf (5). If the orthotic joint is not properly aligned, the forces created between limb and orthosis may substantially aggravate pain in an arthritic joint, and the orthosis consequently will not be worn.

Smith *et al.* (84) evaluated single- and double-upright orthoses in patients with rheumatoid arthritis and valgus deformity at the knee and found that the use of a single upright is limited to a correcting force of 18 to 20 pounds. Both the single- and double-upright orthoses could only be worn if flexion contracture was less than 15 to 20°. They found that of 50 patients thus fitted, 38 patients wore their orthoses successfully for 7 to 48 months.

If there is no knee flexion contracture, a newly introduced orthosis to correct either valgus or varus deformity called a "C.A.R.S."-U.B.C. (Canadian Arthritis & Rheumatism Society-University of British Columbia) knee varus-valgus orthosis has proven very successful in early reports (11). It requires a minimum of measurement and adjustment for fitting and thus is relatively inexpensive. It also has a definite cosmetic advantage over more elaborate designs and so is better accepted by patients.

Another common alignment problem at the knee is "back knee," or genu recurvatum. This is frequently encountered in neurological lesions which have led to a muscle imbalance or where the patient has stabilized his knee during the stance by constantly manipulating extension, the ground-reactive force vector in front of the knee to create an extension moment. This is checked by the posterior joint capsule and the extension-limiting ligaments. These may gradually yield, and a back knee may produce the same result. If there is a mild tendency to genu recurvatum and the patient can safely ambulate with an AFO. as is commonly observed in hemiplegics soon after a stroke, an AFO with plantar and dorsiflexion stops and sole plate can be used as a training device to prevent hyperextension of the knee. For this purpose, the ankle is usually set in some dorsiflexion in order to create a strong bending moment at the knee during the first part of the stance and to minimize any extension moment produced by the orthosis. In some cases, even the dorsiflexion stop may be removed. It is obvious that the patient must have enough voluntary control of the knee musculature to keep the knee from buckling.

The most common way of managing a more severe genu recurvatum is with a KAFO which is designed to position the knee in slight flexion to control the back knee. Hopefully, the posterior capsule and check ligaments can be tightened so that the patient may not have to wear the orthosis permanently. Bennett (5) has pointed out that the knee position in the orthosis depends on the relative depth of upper and lower thigh bands; with the upper thigh band relatively deep and the lower thigh band relatively shallow, the knee is put in a flexed position. The thigh bands may be replaced by a contoured rigid plastic cuff. In addition, orthotists feel that even better alignment and force distribution can be achieved if a similar plastic posterior shell is used below the knee, instead of the calf band (82).

Several older and newer orthoses of various designs have also been advocated to control recurvatum. These include the "Swedish" knee cage (2), which has a rigid connection between the orthotic upright posteriorly and two counter forces applied by elastic straps just above and below the knee. Many modifications of this design have been attempted (49), but none of them are as effective as the KAFO. Knee orthoses (such as the Swedish knee cage) have a tendency to slide along the leg, and the force application is not as favorable as in the KAFO. Such designs include the hinged knee cage and the double-anterior loop knee orthosis (2). More recently, plastic models of these designs have been advocated (49, 82).

Special orthoses for the hip joint include the Toronto abduction orthosis for Legg-Perthes disease (Fig. 9.45) (15). This orthosis maintains the hip in 45° abduction and 18° internal rotation, yet allows ambulation and knee and hip flexion. An angle of 90° is maintained at all times between the two legs. The treatment rationale is that the femoral head will reform if weight bearing is allowed only in the abducted position.

Orthoses Using Electrical Stimulation

Functional electrical stimulation has been introduced by Liberson and his associates (51). Since in upper motor neuron lesions, the lower motor

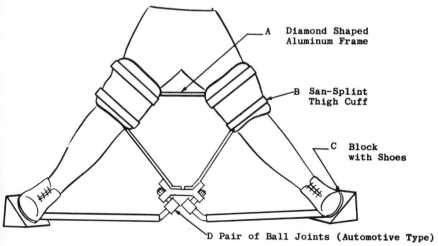

A   Diamond Shaped Aluminum Frame

B   San-Splint Thigh Cuff

C   Block with Shoes

D Pair of Ball Joints (Automotive Type)

Fig. 9.45. Toronto Legg-Perthes orthosis. [From Fifth Workshop Panel (15).]

neuron including the axon survives, the peripheral nerve can be stimulated electrically, producing a contraction of the muscles innervated by this nerve. Stimulation must be phased properly to produce a functional result. Practical application of this concept has been primarily in hemiplegic patients to control foot drop during the swing phase.

Two types of stimulators are available—one uses external stimulation of the peroneal nerve through the skin, the other uses an implanted electrode surgically applied to the nerve. A miniaturized electrical stimulator produces currents with pulses between 20 and 300 microseconds in duration. The frequency of repetition is 30 to 100 cycles/second, and the peak current is below 90 milliamperes. The voltage requirements vary between 0 and 50 volts (18, 51, 91).

With the first type of stimulator, a power pack is worn on a waist belt. The skin electrode is applied to the peroneal nerve below the fibular head and the inactive electrode to the leg below. A foot switch is incorporated into the shoe which turns the stimulator on when the heel comes off of the ground and turns it off on heelstrike (61).

The surgically implanted electrode is placed directly on the nerve, and a flexible wire lead is connected to a subcutaneously implanted receiver located over the anteromedial aspect of the thigh. According to Waters et al., (92) nerve conduction velocity in the nerve is not significantly affected by the stimulation. Fuhrer (88) found that repetitive stimulation slightly decreased skin impedance and slightly increased current levels. The stimulator and transmitter are worn with power pack at the waist. The transmitter is connected to an antenna which is placed on the surface of the skin over the receiver implant. A heel switch with transmitter is incorporated into the shoe to control phasing of the stimulation. Its signal is received by the receiver part of the stimulator-transmitter assembly attached to the waist belt (Fig. 9.46) (84).

These types of functional orthoses have been applied to hemiplegic patients who were also able to ambulate without any orthosis. As a matter of fact, Waters et al. (91) felt that the patient should be able to walk without an orthosis faster than 25 meters per minute and should have good balance and that the major gait problem should be foot drop which could also be corrected by an AFO. In addition, proprioception should be intact, and the patient's ankle should not be plantar flexed more than 10° during the stance. Takebe and his coworkers (88) have found that if the stimulation is externally applied, the patient should have no manual difficulty in applying electrodes and should be able to tolerate discomfort from stimulation (88).

Liberson et al. (51) suggested that this therapy would increase strength of foot dorsiflexors and could be used as a means of reeducating the patient's muscles on a long-term basis, even without continued use of the electrophysiologic orthosis. Lee and Johnston (37), rather than stimulating the peroneal nerve, applied a train of electrical pulses to a single skin area to

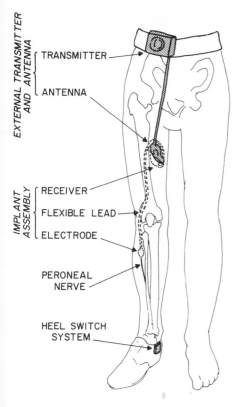

Fig. 9.46. Relative location of neuromuscular assist equipment on patient with right-sided hemiplegia. [Redrawn from Waters *et al.* (91).]

induce a flexion reflex in order to improve gait pattern during swing phase. Finally, Dmitrijevic *et al.* (14) have claimed that stimulation of the foot dorsiflexors produces a reciprocal inhibition of the triceps surae. Therefore, the electrophysiologic orthosis prevents undesirable ankle clonus.

The same principle used in these electrophysiologic orthoses has been applied experimentally to major hip and thigh muscle groups in spinal cord injured patients (94) and has also been tried in the upper extremity to reduce wrist drop and improve functional grasp (7, 61).

Conclusions

Understanding the biomechanical function of orthoses has improved the proper selection of a specific orthosis for an individual patient's need. Better designs and new materials have also resulted from understanding these biomechanics. The new orthoses may have much higher cosmetic value and thus may enhance patient acceptance. However, an orthosis should always be used as an integral part of a comprehensive management strategy. To solve problems arising from spasticity solely by orthoses when there are also drugs and motor point blocks available or to gain patient acceptance by improving cosmesis at the expense of psychologic treatment of the patient's problem are not sufficient to obtain the best results from orthotic management of the lower extremity.

REFERENCES

1. AMERICAN ACADEMY OF ORTHOPEDIC SURGEONS. *Atlas of Orthotics,* pp. 209, 216, 226, and 232. St. Louis, C. V. Mosby Co., 1975.
2. AMERICAN ACADEMY OF ORTHOPEDIC SURGEONS. *Orthopedic Appliances Atlas.* vol. 1, pp. 398–399. J. Edwards, Ann Arbor, 1952.
3. ANDERSON, M. H., BECHTOL, C. L., AND SULLAR, R. E. *Clinical Prosthetics for Physicians and Therapists.* Charles C Thomas, Springfield, Ill., 1959.
4. ANDERSON, M. H., AND BRAY, J. J. The UCLA functional long leg brace. *Clin. Orthop., 37:* 98–109, 1964.
5. BENNETT, R. L. Orthotics for function. Part I. Prescription. *Phys. Ther. Rev., 36*(11): 1–25, 1956.
6. BOWERS, J. A., AND LASSEN, E. G. Use of short leg braces with patellar tendon bearing cuffs. *Arch. Phys. Med. Rehabil., 45:* 436–437, 1964.
7. BURKE, J. F., POCOCK, G. S., AND WALLIS, W. D. Electrophysiological bracing in peripheral nerve lesions. *J. Am. Phys. Ther. Assoc., 43*(7): 501–504, 1963.
8. CASSON, J. Advanced designs of plastic lower limb orthoses. *Orthotics Prosthet., 26:* 23–30, 1972.
9. CORCORAN, P. J. Evaluation of a plastic short leg brace. *M. S. Thesis,* University of Washington, Seattle, 1968.
10. CORCORAN, P. J., JEBSEN, R. H., BRENGELMANN, G. L., AND SIMONS, B. C. Effects of plastic and metal leg braces on speed and energy cost of hemiparetic ambulation. *Arch. Phys. Med. Rehabil., 51:* 69, 1969.
11. COUSINS, S., AND FOORT, J. An orthosis for medial or lateral stabilization of arthritic knees. *Orthotics Prosthet., 29:* 21–26, 1975.
12. DAVIS, F. J., FRY, L. R., LIPPERT, F. G., SIMONS B. C., AND REMINGTON, J. The patellar tendon bearing brace: report of 16 patients. *J. Trauma, 14:* 216–221, 1974.
13. DEAVER, G. G. Lower limb bracing. In *Orthotics Etcetera,* edited by S. Licht. Elizabeth Licht, New Haven, 1966.
14. DMITRIJEVIC, M. R., GRACANIN, F., PREVEC, T., AND TRONT, J. Electronic control of paralyzed extremities. *Biomed. Eng. 3*(8): 14, 1968.
15. FIFTH WORKSHOP PANEL ON LOWER EXTREMITY ORTHOTICS. Subcommittee on Design and Development Committee on Prosthetics Research and Development. Division of Engineering, National Research Council, National Academy of Sciences, National Academy of Engineering, Atlanta, Georgia, April 3–4, 1968, p. 17.
16. FRANKL, V. H., AND BURSTEIN, A. H. *Orthopedic Biomechanics.* Lea & Febiger, Philadelphia, 1970.
17. FUHRER, M. J., AND YEGGE, B. Effects of skin impedance changes accompanying functional electrical stimulation of the peroneal nerve. *Arch. Phys. Med. Rehabil., 53:* 276–281, 1972.
18. GRACANIN, F., AND TRNKOCZY, A. Optimal stimulus parameters for minimum pain in the chronic stimulation of innervated muscle. *Arch. Phys. Med. Rehabil., 56:* 243, 1975.
19. GLANCY, J., AND LINDSETH, R. E. The polypropylene solid ankle foot orthosis. *Orthotics Prosthet., 26*(1): 14, 1972.
20. GRYNBAUM, B. B., SOKOLOW, J., AND FLEISCHMAN, E. P. An adjustable ischial weight bearing brace for early ambulation in lower extremity fractures. *Arch. Phys. Med. Rehabil., 54:* 566–568, 1973.
21. HAHN, H. Lower extremity bracing in paraplegics with usage followup. *Paraplegia, 8*(3): 147–153, 1969.
22. HEIZE, D. Bracing design for knee joint instability. In *Principles of Lower Extremity*

Bracing, edited by J. Perry and H. Hislop, pp. 92–96. American Physical Therapy Association, 1967.

23. HEIZER, D. Short-Leg brace design for hemiplegia. In *Principles of Lower Extremity Bracing*, edited by J. Perry and H. Hislop. American Physical Therapy Association, 1967.

24. HILL, J. P., BENSMAR, A. S., DOZIER, A., AND STUBE, R. W. Epoxy-fibreglass short leg brace. *Arch. Phys. Med. Rehabil.*, *52*: 82–135, 1971.

25. HILLT, J. T., AND FENWICK, A. L. A fiberglass-epoxy drop-foot brace. *Orthotics Prosthet.*, *22*: 1–8, 1968.

26. HINES, T. F. Indications and principles of bracing. In *Orthotics Etcetera*, edited by S. Licht. Elizabeth Licht, New Haven, 1966.

27. INABA, M. Bracing the unstable knee and ankle in hemiplegia. In *Principles of Lower Extremity Bracing*, edited by J. Perry and H. Hislop, pp. 70–75. American Physical Therapy Association, 1967.

28. INMAN, V. T. *The Joints of the Ankle*. Williams & Wilkins Co., Baltimore, 1976.

29. INMAN, V. T. UC-BL dual axis ankle control system and UC-BL shoe insert. *Bull. Prosthet. Res., Spring:* 130–145, 1969.

30. JEBSEN, R. H., SIMONS, B. C., AND CORCORAN, P. J. Experimental short leg brace fabrication. *Arch. Phys. Med. Rehabil.*, *49:* 108–109, 1968.

31. KIRKPATRICK, G. S., DAY, E. E., AND LEHMANN, J. F. Investigation of the performance of an ischial load bearing leg brace. *Exp. Mechanics*, 1–5 1969.

32. KLOPSTEG, P. E., AND WILSON, P. D. *Human Limbs and Their Substitutes. Hagner Publishing Co.*, New York, 1968.

33. LEBLANC, M. A clinical evaluation of four lower limb orthoses. *Orthotics Prosthet.*, *26:* 27–43, 1972.

34a. LEE, K. H., AND JOHNSTON, R. Bracing below the knee for hemiplegia: biomechanical analysis., *54:* 466–510, 1973.

34. LEE, K. H., AND JOHNSTON R. Biomechanical comparison of 90 degrees plantarflexion stop and dorsiflexion assist ankle braces. *Arch. Phys. Med. Rehabil.*, *54:* 302–306, 1973.

35. ROBIN, G. C., MAGORA, A., ADLER, AND SALTIEL, J. Dynamic stress analysis of plastic below-knee drop foot braces. *Med. Biol. Eng.*, *9*(6): 631–636, 1971.

36. LEE, K. H., AND JOHNSTON, R. Effect of below knee bracing on knee movement: biomechanical analysis. *Arch. Phys. Med. Rehabil.*, *55:* 179–182, 1974.

37. LEE, K. H., AND JOHNSTON, R. Electrically induced flexion reflex in gait training of hemiplegic patients: induction of the reflex. *Arch. Phys. Med. Rehabil.*, *57:* 311–314, 1976.

38. LEHMANN, J. F. The biomechanics of ankle foot orthoses: prescription and design. *Arch. Phys. Med. Rehabil.*, *60:* 200–207, 1979.

39. LEHMANN, J. F., DELATEUR, B. J., WARREN, C. G., AND SIMONS, B. C. Trends in lower extremity bracing. *Arch. Phys. Med. Rehabil.*, *51:* 338–353, 1970.

40. LEHMANN, J. F., DELATEUR, B. J., WARREN, C. G., SIMONS, B. C., AND GUY, A. W. Biomechanical evaluation of braces for paraplegics. *Arch. Phys. Med. Rehabil.*, *50:* 179–188, 1969.

41. LEHMANN, J. F., AND STONEBRIDGE, J. B. Knee lock device for knee ankle orthoses for spinal cord injured patients: an evaluation. *Arch. Phys. Med. Rehabil.*, *59:* 207–211, 1978.

42. LEHMANN, J. F., STONEBRIDGE, J. B., AND DELATEUR, B. J. Pneumatic and standard double upright orthoses: comparison of their biomechanical function in three patients with spinal cord injuries. *Arch. Phys. Med. Rehabil.*, *58:* 72–80, 1977.

43. LEHMANN, J. F., AND WARREN C. G. Restraining forces in various designs of knee ankle orthoses: their placement and effect on anatomical knee joint. *Arch. Phys. Med. Rehabil.*, *57:* 430–437, 1976.

44. LEHMANN, J. F., WARREN, C. G., AND DELATEUR, B. J. A biomechanical evaluation of knee stability in below knee braces. *Arch. Phys. Med. Rehabil.*, *51:* 687–695, 1970.

45. LEHMANN, J. F., WARREN, C. G., DELATEUR, B. J., SIMONS, B. C., AND KIRKPATRICK, G.

Biomechanical evaluation of axial loading in ischial weight bearing braces of various designs. *Arch. Phys. Med. Rehabil.*, *51:* 331–337, 1970.

46. LEHMANN, J. F., WARREN, C. G., HERTLING, D., McGEE, M., AND SIMONS, B. C. Craig Scott orthosis: a biomechanical and functional evaluation. *Arch. Phys. Med. Rehabil.*, *57:* 438–442, 1976.

47. LEHMANN, J. F., WARREN, C. G., PEMBERTON, D. R., SIMONS, B. C., AND DeLATEUR, B. J. Load bearing function of patellar tendon bearing braces of various designs. *Arch. Phys. Med. Rehabil.*, *52:* 367–370, 1971.

48. LEHNEIS, H. R. New concepts in lower extremity orthotics. *Med. Clin. North Am.*, *53:* 3, 1969.

49. LEHNEIS, H. R. New developments in lower-limb orthotics through bioengineering. *Arch. Phys. Med. Rehabil.*, *53:* 303–310, 1972.

50. LESIN, B. E., MOONEY, V., AND ASHBY, M. E. Cast bracing for fractures of the femus. *J. Bone Joint Surg.*, *59A*(7): 917–923, 1977.

51. LIBERSON, W. T., HOMQUEST, H. J., SCOT, D., AND DEW, M. Functional electrotherapy: stimulation of the peroneal nerve synchronized with the swing phase of the gait of hemiplegic patients. *Arch. Phys. Med. Rehabil.*, *41:* 101–105, 1960.

52. LINDSETH, R. E., AND GLANCY, J. Polypropylene lower-extremity braces for paraplegia due to myelomeningocele. *J. Bone Joint Surg.*, *56A*(3): 556–563, 1974.

53. LONG, G., AND LAWTON, E. B. Functional significance of spinal cord lesion level. *Arch. Phys. Med. Rehabil.*, *36:* 249–255, 1955.

54. LOWER EXTREMITY ORTHOTICS, VAPC RESEARCH. *Bull. Prosthet. Res.*, *Spring:* 220–222, 1967.

55. McGEE, R. B. Electrically controlled knee joint for long leg braces. Eighth Workshop Panel on Lower-Limb Orthotics of the Subcommittee on Design & Development, Los Angeles, October 2–4, 1972.

56. McGEE, R. B., TOMOVIC, R., YANG, P. Y., AND MacLEAN, I. C. An experimental study of a sensor controlled external knee locking system. *IEEE Trans. Biomed. Eng.*, *25*(2): 195–199, 1978.

57. McGEE, R. B., TOMOVIC, R., YANG, R. Y., AND MacLEAN, I. C. An experimental study of a sensor-controlled external knee locking system. *IEEE Trans. Biomed. Eng.*, *25*(2): 195–199, 1978.

58. McILMURRAY, W., AND GREENBAUM, W. The application of SACH foot principles to orthotics. *Orthop. Prosthet. Appl. J.*, *13:* 37–40, 1959.

59. McILMURRAY, W. J., AND GREENBAUM, W. A below knee weight bearing brace. *Orthop. Prosthet. Appl. J.*, *12*(2): 81–82, 1958.

60. MARX, H. W. Lower-limb orthotic designs for the spastic hemiplegic patient. *Orthotics Prosthet.*, *28*(2): 14–20, 1974.

61. MERLETTI, R., ACIMOVIC, R., GROBELNIK, S., AND CVILAK, G. Electrophysiological orthosis for the upper extremity in hemiplegia: feasibility study. *Arch. Phys. Med. Rehabil.*, *56:* 507–513, 1975.

62. MOONEY, V., NICKEL, V. L., HARVEY, J. P., AND SNELSON, P. Cast brace treatment for fractures of the distal part of the femur. A prospective controlled study of one hundred and fifty three patients. *J. Bone Joint Surg.*, *52A:* 1563–1578, 1970.

63. NATIONAL ACADEMY OF SCIENCES. Committee on Prosthetics Research and Development. Rehabilitation Engineering: Plan for Continued Progress.

64. NICKEL, V. L., AND MOONEY, V. The application of lower extremity orthotics to weight bearing relief. Final narrative report. Rancho Los Amigos Hospital, Downey, Calif.

65. NITSCHKE, R. O. A single bar above-knee orthosis. *Orthotics Prosthet.*, *23*(2): 20–25, 1969.

66. NITSCHKE, R. O., AND MARSCHALL, K. The PTS knee brace. *Orthotics Prosthet.*, *22:* 46–51, 1968.

67. PERRY, J. Lower extremity bracing in hemiplegia. *Clin. Orthop.*, *63:* 32–38, 1969.

68. POST, B. S., FOSTER, S., ROSNER, H., AND BENTON, J. G. Use of functional electrotherapy in neuromuscular diseases. *N. Y. State J. Med*, *63:* 1808, 1963.

69. RAGNARSSON, K. T., SELL, G. H., MCGARRITY, M., AND OFFIR, R. Pneumatic orthosis for paraplegic patients: functional evaluation and prescription consideration. *Arch. Phys. Med. Rehabil.*, 56: 479–483, 1975.

70. ROBIN, G. C., MAGORA, A., ADLER, E., AND SALTIEL, J. Dynamic stress analysis of below-knee drop foot braces. *Med. Biol. Eng.*, 6(5): 533–546, 1968.

71. Rubin, G., and Dixon, M. The modern ankle foot orthoses (AFO's). *Bull. Prosthet. Res.*, Spring: 20–40, 1973.

72. RUSSEK, A., AND ESCHEN, F. Ischial weight bearing brace with quadrilateral wood top—preliminary report. *Orthop. Prosthet. Appl. J. 12*(12): 31, 1958.

SATTIEL, J. A one-piece laminated knee locking short brace. Orthotics Prosthet., *23*(2): 68–75, 1969.

73. SARMIENTO, A. A functional below the knee brace for tibial fractures. A report on its use in 135 cases. *J. Bone Joint Surg.*, 52A: 295–311, 1970.

74. SARMIENTO, A. A functional below-the-knee cast for tibial fractures. *J. Bone Joint Surg.*, 49: 855–975, 1967.

75. SARMIENTO, A., AND SINCLAIR, W. F. Application of prosthetics-orthotics principles to treatment of fractures. *Artif. Limbs, 11:* 28–32, 1967.

76. SARNO, J. E. Below knee orthoses: a system for prescription. *Arch. Phys. Med. Rehabil.,* 54: 548–552, 1973.

77. SCOTT, B. A. Engineering principles and fabrication techniques for Scott-Craig: long leg brace for paraplegics. *Orthotics, Prosthet.*, 28: 14–19, 1974.

78. STAUFFER, E. S. Symposium on spinal cord injuries. *Clin. Orthop.,, 112:* 1–165, 1975.

79. SIEGEL, I. M. Orthopedic correction of musculoskeletal deformity in muscular dystrophy. *Ad. Neurol.*, 17:343–364, 1977.

80. SEIGEL, I. M. Plastic-molded knee-ankle foot orthoses in the treatment of Duchenne muscular dystrophy. *Arch. Phys. Med. Rehabil.*, 56: 322, 1975.

81. SILBER, M., CHUNG, T. S., VARGHESE, G., HINTERBUCHNER, C., BAILEY, M., AND HIVRY, N. Pneumatic orthosis: pilot study. *Arch. Phys. Med. Rehabil.*, 56: 27–32, 1975.

82. SIMONS, B. C. Personal communication.

83. SIMONS, B. C., JEBSEN, R. H., AND WILDMAN, L. E. Plastic short leg brace fabrication. *Orthotics Prosthet. Appl. J.*, 21: 215–218, 1967.

84. SMITH, E. M., JUVINALL, R. C., CORELLL, E. B., AND NYBOER, V. J. Bracing the unstable arthritis knee. *Arch. Phys. Med. Rehabil.*, 51: 22–36, 1970.

85. SPENCER, G. A., AND VIGNOS, P. J. Bracing for ambulation in childhood progressive muscular dystrophy. *J. Bone Joint Surg.*, 44A(2): 234–242, 1962.

86. STILLS, M. Thermoformed ankle foot orthoses. *Orthotics Prosthet.*, 29(4): 41–51, 1975.

87. STROHM, B. R., BRAY, J. J., AND COLACHIS, S. C. Checkout evaluation and clinical experience of the UCLA functional long leg brace. *J. Am. Phys. Ther. Assoc.*, 46: 829–834, 1966.

88. TAKEBE, K., KUKULKA, C., NARAYAN, M. G., MILNER, M., AND BASMAJIAN, J. V. Peroneal nerve stimulator in rehabilitation of hemiplegic patients. *Arch. Phys. Med. Rehabil., 56:* 237–40, 1975.

89. WARREN, C. G., AND LEHMANN, J. F. Effect of training on the use of weight bearing orthoses. *Phys. Ther.*, 55(5): 487–492, 1975.

90. WARREN, C. G., LEHMANN, J. F., AND DELATEUR, B. J. Pelvic band use in orthotics for adult paraplegic patients. *Arch. Phys. Med. Rehabil.*, 56: 221–223, 1975.

91. WATERS, R. L., MCNEAL, D., AND PERRY, J. Experimental correction of foot drop by electrical stimulation of the peroneal nerve. *J. Bone Joint Surg.*, 57A(8): 1047–1054, 1975.

92. WATERS R. L., MCNEAL, D. R., AND TASTO, J. Peroneal nerve conduction velocity after chronic electrical stimulation. *Arch. Phys. Med. Rehabil.*, 56: 240–243, 1975.

93. WATERS, R. AND MONTGOMERY, J. Lower extremity management of hemiparesis. *Clin. Orthop.*, 102: 133–143, 1974.

94. VARKEN, E., AND JEGLIC, A. Application of an implantable stimulator in the rehabilitation of the paraplegic patient. *Int. Surg.*, 61: 335–339, 1976.

10

Orthotic Management of Children

GABRIELLA E. MOLNAR, M.D.

The principles of orthotics for children are the same as those for adults in terms of design and biomechanical characteristics. There are only a few devices that were designed specifically for children. As in adults, improvement of function and prevention of deformities constitute the two major reasons for the use of orthoses. From a clinical viewpoint, this conceptual distinction is often artificial since both functional and preventive purposes may be achieved simultaneously. Prescription of an appropriate orthosis for children is based on the universally applicable principles of biomechanics and is determined by the extent of functional loss, kinesiologic abnormalities, and anticipated musculoskeletal complications.

In the clinical application of orthotics there are differences between children and adults. They stem from the fact that throughout childhood growth and development act as dynamic forces although their influence is modified or curtailed by a handicap of early onset. The element of change created by the pervasive effect of these processes is a distinctive feature in the rehabilitation of children. The intention of this chapter is to discuss orthotic management in the perspective of growth and development.

Rehabilitation goals and, within this framework, orthotic intervention are contingent on developmental expectations. They must be consistent with the child's current level of function and adjusted as maturation proceeds. The well known standards of normal child development that relate accomplishment of certain milestones to chronological age are helpful only as a limited guide for handicapped children and need to be individually adapted in each case.

To define appropriate expectations a number of factors are considered: 1) anticipated deviations in motor development commensurate with the nature and extent of physical dysfunction; 2) personality development, in view of restricted mobility which tends to perpetuate dependence and emotional immaturity; 3) mental age, in case of intellectual deficit, which affects learning ability, adaptive and cognitive function; 4) possible medical complications associated with the motor disability that may influence the child's health and development. It should be apparent that the physical deficit is significant in the sense that it determines the pace and the highest attainable level of motor development. To what extent this potential is fulfilled will depend, however, on the interaction of some or all of the aforementioned factors. One should also be cognizant of the role of parents and family. Their contribution is crucial in fostering the child's development and independence toward realistic goals and without their consistent participation professional efforts are doomed to fail.

An important aim in the rehabilitation of children is to provide experiences that simulate or approximate the usual developmental sequence. In this context, an orthosis is a functional device for sitting or standing in infancy and early childhood as much as it is for walking at a later age. Bracing may be used to assist in less advanced gross motor skills when the likelihood of achieving more complex function is slight or perhaps nonexistent. An example is standing braces for a child who is not expected to ambulate. Although it would be difficult to measure the effect of this intervention, the assumption seems reasonable that handicapped children in the sensorimotor stage of development (45) also need to be exposed to a variety of new experiences, such as the sensation of being in the upright position and viewing the surrounding environment from different perspectives. It seems hardly necessary to mention that prevention of contractures and the physiologic effect of weight bearing on bone metabolism and on the formation of hip joints are additional benefits of this activity. A standing device may be, particularly, desirable and satisfying for a young child with normal intellectual endowment and severe physical impairment. Clinical experience indicates that eventually both parents and children are inclined to give up the use of an orthosis for such limited functional gain, usually by the end of early school years.

For a bright, well motivated young child, training in ambulation may be initiated in spite of the possible need for extensive orthosis and the fact that functional walking is not within the scope of long range projection. A primary motivation for young children is to achieve physical mobility. The importance of this desire is well illustrated by youngsters with spinal cord injury who often surpass adults with similar neurologic lesion in actual achievement and functional level of ambulation. Small stature, low center of gravity, and shorter leverage are mechanical factors in favor of greater mobility. One should be aware, however, that when walking is marginal and requires extensive bracing and other assistive devices a regression tends to occur around adolescence. At this age, intellectual, vocational, and other pursuits take priority, emotional turmoil may set in and the earlier interest in walking is lost. Also, the changing relationship between strength and forces of gravity as a result of sudden growth spurt seems to make the effort of ambulation increasingly more strenuous. Progression of deformities which cannot be controlled successfully in all cases can be an additional adverse influence.

That longstanding or permanent neuromuscular deficit, if untreated, leads to soft tissue contractures is a well known fact. These complications are more prone to appear in a growing child and tend to progress rapidly when the rate of growth is physiologically accelerated. A combination of sudden increase in stature with functional decline enhances the threat of progressive deformities in adolescents. The skeletal frame is molded by muscular and gravitational forces. In childhood, when bone tissue is more malleable and the epiphyseal plates are not ossified, bone and joint deformities can develop if these forces are unbalanced or abnormal. Protective orthotic stabilization of the lower limb may be needed to decrease skeletal changes resulting from neuromuscular dysfunction, defects or diseases of the joints, or their connective tissue support. For these reasons, there is a greater emphasis on the preventive use of orthoses in children than in adults. The same considerations account for the tendency to apply more extensive bracing which is decreased gradually as neuromuscular coordination and strength develop or at the cessation of growth. Night splints and braces represent a form of preventive orthotic intervention used more often in children than in adults. The term "night brace" is actually a misnomer since few children tolerate these devices through the night. Rather than to deprive the whole family of peaceful sleep, it is more practical to incorporate the use of resting braces in afternoon nap or evening play activities.

A comment on the role of orthotics in correcting deformities seems appropriate since it is sometimes mentioned as a feasible goal. While braces are very useful for prolonged stretching of tight soft tissues it is rarely, if ever, possible to expect correction of significant fixed contractures. Instead, the aim is to restrain their further deterioration. The orthosis should accommodate deformities that cannot be corrected by passive manipulation; otherwise, children do not tolerate the device and their tender skin can easily develop pressure ulcers.

A question, frequently raised, is the appropriate age when an orthosis should be provided for a child with delayed development as a result of motor disability of early onset. Understandably, there are no hard rules that can be applied to every case since there is a great variety in motor and associated deficits. When bracing is contemplated for functional purposes, one useful consideration is the level of gross motor accomplishments rather than chronological age. If the child has attained, at least, fair or preferably good head control, an orthotic device may be indicated for sitting or standing. Active trunk control or an ability to maintain passive alignment of the torso above the weight bearing surface in the erect position is needed to plan functional ambulation with braces and crutches. Aside from the physical attributes, a mental age of 2 to 3 years is usually required to learn the skill of crutch walking although a few exceptional children in our population were able to master it by 18 months of age. In children who have a relatively slighter delay of motor development and the outlook for unassisted walking is good, one can usually wait until they pull to stand and begin to cruise to decide whether an orthotic device is necessary. Normal children sit, pull to stand, and walk approximately at 6, 10, and 12 months of age, respectively. Keeping the previously mentioned developmental and physical requirements in mind, the chronological age when orthotic assistance would be considered is around the third or fourth quarter of the first year for passive sitting and 12 to 18 months for passive standing. Walking requires active participation under any circumstances and defies similar suggestions in terms of chronological age. The timing of orthotic intervention solely for preventive purposes depends primarily on the changing status of the musculoskeletal system. Evidently, the more severe the motor deficit the earlier and the faster will deformities occur. Splints made from plastic or other easily workable materials can be used in infancy or in older children as a substitute for costly and cumbersome orthoses when functional gains are not feasible. It is beyond the scope of this chapter to dwell on the difficulties of early prognostication of function in physical disabilities of prenatal, perinatal, or early postnatal onset or to discuss uncertainties of predicting exact life expectancy in some progressive neurologic diseases of variable course. Suffice it to say that these considerations stress the importance of instituting proper and timely measures for averting or delaying deformities regardless of the ultimate outcome.

The choice of various materials for orthotic devices is discussed in Chapter 3. Only a few points pertinent to pediatric patients will be mentioned here. In small children, light weight is a desirable feature. From this viewpoint plastic and some other synthetic materials have an advantage over metal. The cosmetically more acceptable appearance of a plastic orthosis is preferred by older girls. However, the need for durability is an important consideration for active ambulatory youngsters. Conventional metal orthoses usually wear better under excessive stress. They also allow greater possibility of adjustment for growth. Prescription of extensible upright bars is a standard procedure in pediatric orthotics. These advantages may outweigh the benefits offered by synthetic materials. In some cases, a combination of plastic and metal components can decrease weight, enhance durability, and provide greater accommodation for growth.

All children who wear braces should be periodically reevaluated. Progress in motor function may permit decrease or discontinuation of braces. In other cases changing musculoskeletal findings warrant modification of the orthosis. Proper fitting of braces and shoes should also be regularly examined since adjustment for growth is necessary. Generally, evaluation every 6 months is advisable but the exact frequency depends on the rate of growth, which is fastest in the earliest years of childhood and from about 10 years on through adolescence (6). However, some primary or secondary diseases of the skeletal system, neurologic deficits of cerebral origin and, especially, lower motor neuron lesions are associated with growth disturbances. In the rapid phases of growth conventional metal orthoses can usually accommodate length and girth increase for 2 to 3 years and those made out of synthetic materials for much shorter period of time. Similarly, in the fitting of shoes, growth should be taken into account. Correct shoe size should leave ¼ to ½ inch distance between the tips of the toes and the toe box. When the toes touch the end of the toe box new shoes are needed. Width should be appropriate for both the hindfoot and the forefoot. Shoes should be fitted in the standing position since foot configuration changes on weight bearing. The examiner should palpate the tip of first and second toes for proper length; feel the tension at the first and fifth metatarsal heads, over the instep and heel to determine correct width. During the fast growing phase of early childhood new shoes may be needed every 3 months. Some active youngsters with pathologic gait wear out their shoes in a matter of weeks and should be provided with two pairs. In young children high top shoes are used with orthoses. For older ones or when braces are less extensive Oxford shoes can be adequate. Split-size shoes are required if the difference between the two feet is in excess of one shoe size. For further details of shoe types and modifications the reader is referred to the following chapter.

Parents must be carefully instructed when the orthosis is first worn and these recommendations are reinforced in physical therapy. It is suggested that the brace should be applied for gradually increasing periods, that the skin be inspected for evidence of pressure marks, and that these measures be taken with special care when there is a sensory deficit. Although it may seem superfluous to mention this point, repeated counseling is needed about the implications of absent sensation. Benefits expected from the use of orthosis should be clearly explained. In the case of limited goals, the parents must be advised in specific practical terms about how and when the brace can be best used. It usually requires several weeks before braces can be tolerated by a child for the desired length of time. Parents should also be reminded that adjustments and changes due to growth have to be initiated on time to avoid problems caused by ill-fitting orthosis and shoes during the waiting period.

Cerebral Palsy

Cerebral palsy is defined as a nonprogressive damage to the immature brain which can occur in the prenatal, perinatal, or early postnatal period (37). The leading clinical sign is a neuromuscular dysfunction. There may be associated deficits when cerebral structures other than those contributing to motor function are impaired. Among these, mental retardation and seizure disorder are the most frequent. In some instances, impairment of vision and hearing may be present; the latter is most likely in the athetoid type. Cortical sensory deficit of the affected extremities, found in about half of the cases with hemiplegia, represents a limiting factor in functional use. It is often accompanied by a growth disturbance of central origin. Clinical classification is based on neurologic signs and their topographic distribution. Spastic clinical types have the highest incidence and include hemiplegia, diplegia, and quadriparesis. Dyskinetic clinical types are less frequent and encompass a range of athetoid-dystonic movement disorders. There may be a mixture of spasticity and athetosis. Ataxic and atonic clinical types are rare. In spite of the static brain lesion, the natural history of cerebral palsy is characterized by changing clinical findings. In addition to delayed motor development, hypotonicity is a frequent early sign. Spastic hypertonicity usually makes its appearance between 6 to 12 months of age whereas definite dyskinetic movements may not become evident until 18 months or later. These changes are related to maturation of the defective central nervous system. Natural development leads to functional progress over the years; its pace and final outcome reflect the extent of cerebral damage. Musculoskeletal sequelae of the neurologic dysfunction represent a simultaneous potentially opposing influence. Cerebral palsy is not a homogeneous disease entity in respect to etiology, pathology, clinical manifestations, and course. From the viewpoint of ultimate prognosis, severity of motor deficit, intellectual function, and emotional adjustment were found to have the most significant influence. As in all childhood disabilities where the presence of multiple handicaps is a possibility, planning of overall management is based on all aspects of function.

The motor deficit in cerebral palsy is a disturbance of central movement control. Defective coordination of selective muscle action is compounded by tone abnormalities, pathologic reflex activity, and persistent primitive infantile reflexes (7). Undifferentiated synergistic movement patterns are more prevalent in the spastic clinical types. From an orthotic standpoint, the goal is to control abnormal and excessive muscle activity that can lead to deformities and causes biomechanical abnormalities of stance and gait. Surgical lengthening of spastic muscles and correction of deformities is an effective method to improve postural deviations. Although this aspect of treatment is not discussed here, it should be understood that coordinated use of bracing and surgery is an essential part of management plans.

The greatest changes in orthotic management of children have probably occurred in cerebral palsy. The past trend of using long leg braces with pelvic band, often with spinal attachment (15), has been replaced by less extensive and more selective action orthoses (21, 22).

CONGENITAL AND ACQUIRED HEMIPLEGIA

Children with congenital hemiplegia are generally 4 to 6 months behind in early motor achievements. Attainment of walking may be delayed somewhat longer but the majority walk by 2 years and virtually all by the age of 3 (38). Rare exceptions are youngsters with profound mental retardation who achieve this milestone much later or in some cases do not walk at all. A cortical sensory deficit in the leg tends to prolong the delay of walking and is often accompanied by underdevelopment of the extremity. Size and length discrepancy usually become evident between 12 to 18 months and continue to increase until 6 to 8 years of age. Length difference rarely exceeds 1 inch. A shoe lift is not necessary for this amount of discrepancy since the resulting functional lateral curvature of the spine is mild and nonprogressive. Moreover, in the presence of plantar-flexor hyperactivity length difference makes toe clearance easier during swing phase. However, leg length has to be measured regularly and spinal alignment should be observed. Underdevelopment of the affected foot necessitates split-size shoes in some cases.

In general, an orthosis is not required until the child pulls to stand and begins to cruise around while holding on since range of motion can be maintained by other means prior to the stage of upright mobility. From this time on, a brace may be needed to correct ankle and foot abnormalities.

Gait deviations in children with hemiplegic cerebral palsy resemble the familiar kinesiologic features of extensor synergy. Plantar-flexor overactivity results in spastic equinus attitude of the ankle which makes toe clearance difficult; weight is borne mostly or completely on the forefoot. Inadequate knee flexion and, consequently, circumduction are particularly marked when walking is first started but decrease as coordination improves. Contrary to the usual synergistic pattern of hip adduction and internal rotation, a more common postural attitude in the early stages of walking is abduction and external rotation at the hip. One might assume that this is an adaptation of the normal toddler's walk superimposed on a pathologic gait. External rotation-abduction posturing needs no corrective bracing, such as a twister or other cumbersome device. It merely requires patience on the part of the examiner and reassurance of the parents that this is a temporary phenomenon.

Orthotic Management of Hemiplegic Cerebral Palsy

The most universal problem of orthotic concern is plantar-flexor spasticity and, consequently, assistance for toe pick-up. Hemiplegic children are very active walkers and generally require a conventional double-bar short-leg brace (AFO). When there is considerable heelcord tightness a posterior 90° ankle stop is preferable (16). Otherwise, a spring ankle joint to aid dorsiflexion is sufficient and biomechanically more satisfactory (31–33). Plantar-flexion motion can be limited to 10° (1). Inversion or varus attitude of the foot is a component of the extensor synergy and often accompanies the plantar-flexion contracture. However, some hemiplegic children have a combination of foot pronation and plantar-flexion. One might speculate that the duration of early walking pattern has some influence on subsequent foot deformity. When the limb is in abduction and external rotation, most of the weight is transmitted to the medial border of the foot causing pronation.

Usually, a mild degree of mediolateral ankle and foot malalignment can be controlled by adding appropriately placed Y straps and shoe modification to the conventional double-bar orthosis. Our experience has not been very satisfactory with the plastic molded shoe insert attached to the standard short-leg brace which has been recommended for foot and subtalar joint stabilization (17). Since corrective pressure is distributed over a relatively small area, the children complain of considerable discomfort.

A plastic solid ankle posterior orthosis (28, 49) which encases the foot and ankle is more effective in controlling foot pronation or supination, particularly when there is a visible tilt of the os calcis and some talar displacement. Children seem to find the polypropylene ankle-foot orthosis (AFO) (46) more comfortable than other rigid synthetic materials probably because it allows some flexibility at the ankle and foot joints. This material is durable enough for the younger child but not for older active youngsters. An additional advantage of polypropylene over plastic laminates is that it allows easy reshaping for some degree of growth. A fitted lining which is eventually removed extends the length of time before children will outgrow this type of orthosis.

In hemiplegic children knee instability rarely indicates orthotic correction. When there is spasticity of the triceps surae a few children compensate with knee hyperextension to achieve total foot contact in stance rather than by resorting to the characteristic toe walking. For the most part, genu recurvatum is correctable by plantar-flexion control with an AFO, although it may take several weeks or perhaps months until gait readjustment occurs. Understandably, correction cannot be expected if there is fixed equinus deformity. In more than 150 cases we have found a need for orthotic stabilization of severe persistently hyperextended knee posture in less than a half dozen instances. A conventional long-leg brace was used with shallow wide thigh and knee bands placed close to the free knee joint. The ankle joint had a dorsiflexion spring which allowed limited or no plantar-flexion. Among the more recent designs a plastic supracondylar knee-ankle-foot orthosis (KAFO) (11, 34) or combination of metal long-leg brace with plastic pretibial sheel (23) may be appropriate for this problem. Three additional children with hemiplegia acquired in infancy were braced above the knee for a different reason. They had extensive parietal lobe damage with apraxia and profound cortical sensory deficit, including absence of position sense. There was complete disregard for the lower limb which collapsed on weight bearing. A locked knee joint was needed in these cases and ambulation was achieved only after long training. In all cases it was possible to discard the long-leg brace within a few years except for one child who had sensory deficit.

SPASTIC DIPLEGIA AND QUADRIPARESIS

These clinical types show a wide range of neuromuscular dysfunction. The clinical course and orthotic management are less uniform than in hemiplegia. Approximately 85% of diplegic children walk independently or with assistive devices, the majority by 4 years of age. Two-thirds of those with quadriparesis become ambulatory with or without appliances, the majority after age 4 years (38, 39). Sitting at 2 years or earlier is a good indicator that the child will walk, while youngsters who do not sit by 4 years are not expected to ambulate.

Postural deviations of diplegic stance and gait have been observed by Little a long time ago and studied by others since then (43, 48). As a result of increased adductor tone the legs are approximated. The supporting base is narrowed and there is a scissoring gait. When this is severe the feet cross and it becomes difficult or impossible to take a forward step. Often there is increased internal rotation at the hips because of spasticity and possibly femoral anteversion (51). This will cause the knees and feet to turn inward and adds to the difficulties of advancing the leg in swing phase. The relative weakness of hip abductors produces a gluteus medius lurch. There is usually inadequate knee flexion in the swing phase creating the impression of a stiff gait. Yet, the child stands and walks with flexed hips and knees (19). The feet are in equinus attitude and toe clearance is impeded; weight is supported mostly or entirely on the forefoot. Additional foot deformities, either varus or valgus attitude, can be observed. Over the years abnormal muscular and gravitational forces lead to progressive deformities with predominance of different components of this basic pattern. It is not possible within the confines of this chapter to elaborate on the many complex postural deviations that can evolve (5, 19, 43, 48, 51). Only a brief description will be given of those that are most commonly of orthotic concern.

The so-called vase stance is initiated by excessive adductor spasticity pulling the thighs so close that they are virtually propped against each other. The associated rather marked genu valgum (19) allows the feet to be farther apart than the knees, hence the descriptive term. There may be internal hip rotation and equinovarus attitude of the feet. A perhaps more common accompanying foot abnormality is equinovalgus as a result of medial displacement of the weight bearing line associated with genu valgum. In the supple foot of a child, valgus deformity of the hindfoot can hide plantar-flexion contracture (5). In stance the foot appears plantigrade and the heel may be in contact with the supporting surface. However, on observation it becomes evident that there is a lateral angulation between the vertical axis of the calf and heel and that the plantigrade position is possible only because the contracted heelcord is displaced laterally.

Another frequent pattern, the crouch gait, is an exaggeration of the abnormal hip and knee flexion. In part, this may be a maturational phenomenon related to the cerebral dysfunction. Early predominance of extensor posturing and subsequent evolution of flexor pattern have been described as the natural course of spastic diplegia and quadriparesis (27). Once this reversal occurs, biomechanical forces come into play and the combined effects of relative weakness and contractures enhance the postural malalignment. Crouched posture and gait can either develop or become more severe after surgical overcorrection of heelcord contractures with resultant excessive ankle dorsiflexion (19, 43). Lastly, it should be noted that a compensatory mechanism more frequent in this group than in hemiplegia is genu recurvatum in the presence of plantar-flexion deformity. The severity and extent of postural abnormalities depend on the degree of neuromuscular deficit. In mild cases when spasticity around proximal joints is minimal pathologic features are confined to the ankles.

Children with milder degrees of spasticity rarely require braces until they stand with support. Since they have active motor function and move about in a variety of ways, contractures are unlikely to develop in early years. Orthoses may be needed for correcting abnormalities of stance and gait and to prevent deformities which appear, sometimes insidiously, once the upright position is attained. Many less affected children gradually acquire better volitional control, and braces worn in early years can be discarded later as postural deviations ameliorate. In other cases this becomes possible after corrective surgical procedures.

Orthotic Management of Spastic Diplegic Gait

Considerations for orthotic management of spastic equinus are identical with those in the hemiplegic type. The rather frequently seen equinovalgus deformity is an indication for polypropylene or plastic AFO extended over the medial malleolus (46, 49). An elevation for the medial border of the hindfoot and longitudinal arch support are incorporated in the foot extension making shoe corrections largely unnecessary. Varus deformity affecting the hindfoot is also more controllable by plastic AFO. Otherwise, for active children conventional short-leg braces are used with the usual components to control mediolateral malalignment primarily involving the forefoot.

In children who are or are expected to become functional ambulators, either independently or with crutches, the use of long-leg braces with pelvic band (hip-knee-ankle foot orthoses, HKAFO) is hardly ever warranted even if there is evidence of some adductor spasticity. These cumbersome and heavy braces do not promote earlier achievement of walking and for children who already do so they are a hindrance rather than a help in mobility. Severe overactivity of the adductors causing actual crossing of the legs does not occur in this group. Milder degrees of adducted gait will either be overcome by maturation or eventually require other means of correction. It is more unlikely that one can avoid some type of orthosis to control excessive hip adduction in youngsters with limited ambulatory potential. A pelvic band attached to conventional long-leg braces is a traditional method (15) but reservations regarding weight, restriction of mobility and increased energy cost still apply.

Another solution is offered by the hip action brace (21, 22). It consists of a pelvic band and wide thigh cuffs attached to it by lateral bars. The hip joint has a selective action permitting free flexion, extension, and abduction.

Its mediolateral alignment is adjustable so that the brace can be set at a desired degree of abduction, and adduction is not possible beyond that position. The hip action brace provides mediolateral hip stabilization and effectively widens the supporting base. In spite of some claims, it is not suitable to control rotational deformities at the hip. Reduction in the weight of the device and unimpeded active knee function which allows crawling are definite advantages. If necessary, the child can also wear a separate unattached AFO.

Excessive internal rotation of the hip causes a very unsightly gait because of the resultant intoeing. Although it rarely occurs as a single deformity, the problem often draws special attention on account of cosmesis. To control abnormal rotational attitude of the leg arising from the hip joint derotational moment is applied around the longitudinal axis of the limb. To be effective it has to act at least along the length of the femur and be transmitted to the foot. Moreover, the derotational moment has to be counteracted by balanced forces on the opposite side of the body. Otherwise, compensatory realignment of the pelvis and contralateral limb or rotation of the device occurs and makes corrective attempts ineffectual. Conventional long-leg braces with a pelvic band can achieve these requirements (15), but, again, they would be too extensive and unjustified for children who are active functional walkers (Fig. 10.1A). For these situations twister orthoses are available.

The initial version of these devices was the wraparound twister which consisted of a webbing strap (16) (Fig. 10.1B). To effect external rotation the strap is attached to the lateral border of a pelvic band and winds anteromedially around the thigh. For the second loop of the twist it courses

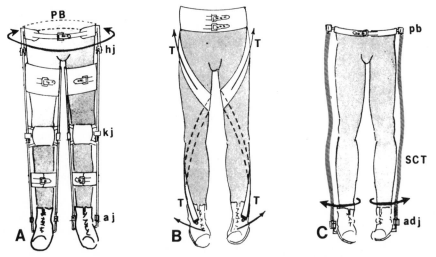

Fig. 10.1. A, Long-leg brace with pelvic band (HKAO). PB, pelvic band; hj, hip joint; kj, knee joint; aj, ankle joint; B, wrap around twister of webbing strap; C, cable twister. SCT, steel cable twister; adj, adjustable unit.

in a posterolateral direction and its distal end is attached anterolaterally to the dorsum of the shoe or calf cuff of short-leg brace.

A more sophisticated construction is the cable twister (Fig. 10.1C). Steel cables tightly coiled in a helical pattern are enclosed in a rubber housing (1, 21, 22). As they uncoil an external rotation moment is generated. The twister extends over the lateral side between the pelvic band and shoe caliper or the upright bar of a short-leg brace. Webbing straps hold them against the limb to keep them from flopping about in the swing phase. The rotational force can be adjusted with a key that winds or unwinds the cables at their proximal end. Easy breakage may be a problem when the twister spans the entire limb length but is uncommon if it is attached to a short-leg brace. In the rare event that a twister is used only for one leg, the pelvic band should be firmly anchored by a thigh corset on the contralateral limb in order to prevent derotation. The cable twister is helpful in producing cosmetic gait improvement in younger children, but its effectiveness decreases as they grow. Generally, after 10 years of age no significant change can be achieved by it. When twisters are used, possible sites of rotation other than the hips should be observed regularly, specifically, the knee joints and tibial alignment. More often than not internal hip rotation is caused by femoral anteversion rather than by muscle imbalance alone although the latter has been contributing as an initiating factor. Rotational laxity of the knee joints and external tibial torsion can develop, particularly when there is an underlying bony hip deformity. These considerations have significantly decreased the initial enthusiasm for using twisters in children.

For genu valgum, a prominent feature of vase stance, orthoses of the knee cage type (KOs) are not capable of providing the necessary stability due to the accompanying adducted hip position. Hip action braces (21, 22) with extension below the knee or different types of metal (42) or plastic (11, 22) KAFOs recommended for mediolateral knee stabilization are more suitable. Development of genu valgum should be preventable to a great extent if proper measures are taken on time to decrease adductor spasticity.

The flexor pattern of crouch gait is the most difficult problem to manage and results are the least satisfactory with an orthosis or by any other means of treatment (19, 43). This posture is sometimes caused, or possibly is aggravated, by surgical overcorrection of tendo Achilles contracture. The simplest and preferred method for effective walkers is to increase plantar-flexion in order to promote knee extension. Short-leg braces (AFOs) with a 90° anterior stop or with plantar-flexion spring assistance are appropriate. At the present time there is no effective orthosis acting on the knee itself that would selectively control unwanted bent knee attitude in stance and yet allow free flexion in swing phase. The eccentric free knee joint long-leg brace (24, 35), different types of plastic KAFOs (11, 23, 34), or the knee extension plastic floor reaction short-leg brace (50) require full joint extension before their mechanical assistance can come into effect and are not useful in spastic diplegia. To place these children in long-leg braces (KAFOs) with the notion of improving their gait is a desperate measure which serves no useful purpose since only with locked joints can knee flexion be eliminated. The same considerations apply to the use of HKAFOs. When faced with the dilemma of an orthotic device for crouch gait in a functional ambulator less is usually better than more, a decision that probably requires greater experience than prescribing extensive braces.

As stated previously genu recurvatum is more frequent in bilateral spastic cerebral palsy than in hemiplegia and can be a result of a spastic quadriceps muscle as well as of a spastic foot equinus posture. Principles of correction are identical and bracing above the knee is a rare exception.

Orthoses for Postural Training

When spasticity is more severe and ambulation is not a realistic expectation, braces can serve limited functional purposes and assist in less advanced gross motor activities. For lack of head control in supported sitting the possibility of a cervical brace with or without a halo type of overhead device is sometimes entertained. These appliances may be useful for training purposes when the child is able to hold his head momentarily. However, when total passive support is needed for hours on end, the risk of skin breakdown from excessive pressure is too great. In addition, parents usually find an overhead apparatus unacceptable in everyday situations. We generally resort to positioning and other wheelchair adjustments although no completely satisfactory solution is available for this most difficult problem. In this group of children extensor thrust, a total body extension pattern including strong hip extensor spasticity, may be a serious hindrance to assisted sitting. Aside from proper wheelchair modifications, a sitting brace may help to overcome hip extensor overactivity. It consists of a spinal brace, pelvic band and wide thigh cuffs extending just above the knees, and hip joints with flexion locks. When head control is somewhat precarious, it is better to adjust the hip lock at 100° rather than at 90° of flexion. Otherwise, the head tends to slump forward when the trunk is in vertical position.

In the past, conventional bilateral long-leg braces with pelvic band and spinal attachment (HKAFO) were the usual devices for passive standing of severely affected children. The parapodium (41) which was designed as a standing brace for high myelomeningocele lesions is suitable for this purpose in spastic cerebral palsy as well (Fig. 10.2). The principles and use of this orthosis are described later in this chapter. Suffice it to say that faster and more efficient donning and doffing offered by the parapodium is a definite advantage when a device is used only for a few hours daily. Moreover, simplicity of design makes fitting easier, particularly when there are asymmetrical thoracopelvic rotational deformities or leg length discrepancy, complications not uncommon in these youngsters.

Training braces are used sometimes as an adjunct in physical therapy or home program to alleviate a specific abnormal postural attitude. They are

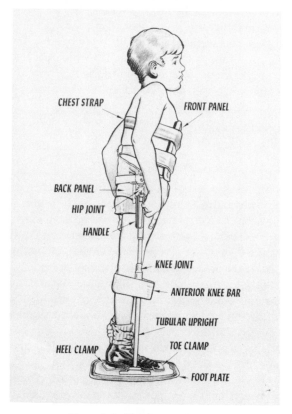

CHEST STRAP

FRONT PANEL

BACK PANEL

HIP JOINT

HANDLE

KNEE JOINT

ANTERIOR KNEE BAR

TUBULAR UPRIGHT

HEEL CLAMP

TOE CLAMP

FOOT PLATE

Fig. 10.2. The parapodium.

temporary devices intended to aid in learning to overcome or, at least, partially control these deviations. In the crouch posture a long knee cage (22) with anterior support worn alternatingly on one leg can be tried during gait training sessions with the hope that extensor pattern will be facilitated eventually. A hip abduction splint (22, 26) may be of help to practice crawling when spastic adductors interfere with this activity. The device consists of two thigh cuffs and an adjustable spreader bar. It allows free flexion and extension while adduction and abduction are controlled.

The role of resting splints or braces in delaying contractures or in preventing their recurrence after surgical procedures is more important when spasticity is moderate to severe. A hip abduction brace maintains prolonged stretching of tight adductors and may contribute to a more satisfactory development of the hip joints. Subluxation or dislocation of the hip is a serious threat in cerebral palsy, most frequently in severely affected nonambulatory children (51). It is caused by hip flexor and adductor overactivity that leads to coxa valga and femoral anteversion with shallow sloping acetabulum (20). There are several types of abduction braces, the previously mentioned crawling brace being one of them (26). Another simple method is a spreader bar attached to the soles of the shoes (1). In this device hip rotation and mediolateral ankle-foot alignment can be also varied by setting the wing nut and serrated bolt at different angles. A somewhat more elaborate abduction brace is the A frame (12) which consists of three bars arranged in a triangle shape. It is fastened to the legs by thigh and calf cuffs and holds the knees in extension. Night splints or braces may be recommended for stretching of tight heelcords. Padded metal foot plates with rigid ankle and laced sandal top can be attached to the A frame when the aim is to control the position of both hips and ankles.

DYSKINETIC TYPES

The role of orthoses is relatively insignificant in this clinical category. Involuntary movements, most often athetosis or dystonia, accompanied by fluctuating tone seem to avert the appearance of fixed contractures. Tightness of soft tissues occurs sometimes by adolescence when the predominant feature is dystonia. Control of involuntary movements is the usually stated reason for braces. More precisely defined, orthoses provide joint stabilization rather than actual movement control. As in the bilateral spastic types, the severity of neuromuscular impairment varies a great deal. Approximately three-fourths of these children achieve independent ambulation, the majority by 3 years of age (38, 39).

Unlike spasticity, dyskinesias do not present typical gait patterns with predominant specific postural abnormalities. Each child develops his own way of walking that may look awkward and is not economical, but it is effective from a functional standpoint. Some severely affected youngsters use alternative means of locomotion in their home or in other familiar situations, such as positions resembling crawling or knee walking.

Prevention of deformities is not an important consideration. On occasion, braces may be helpful from the time when erect position and incipient stages of assisted walking have been achieved. The usual problem that needs to be and can be successfully controlled is mediolateral ankle instability often combined with plantar-flexion attitude of the foot. A conventional double-bar short-leg brace is generally the most suitable because of sturdiness. Little, if anything, is gained from more extensive bracing. It may appear that involuntary movements are restrained, but there is no functional benefit and, in fact, the child usually finds it more difficult to move about. Braces cannot make the more severely affected children ambulate, particularly since upper extremity impairment usually precludes crutch walking.

OTHER CLINICAL TYPES

A combination of spasticity and dyskinesia increases the chances of contractures although they tend to appear later than in the spastic types. In these cases orthotic management is similar to that discussed in conjunction with diplegia and quadriparesis.

In the rare true atonic type prognosis is generally very poor. However, these children can develop contractures much like those in extensive flaccid paralysis. Most frequent are foot deformities and contractures around the hips and knees consistent with the so-called frog position in which they usually lie. Anterior hip dislocation can be an eventual consequence of this posture. Preventive positioning combined with splinting is needed before deformities occur. If the child has at least some head control, a parapodium (41) can be used as a standing brace.

Spina Bifida with Myelodysplasia

Spina bifida represents a congenital dysraphism of the vertebral canal with or without an underlying malformation of the spinal cord (9). The most common site of defect is the lumbosacral area. Thoracic and cervical segments are less frequently affected. The spectrum of clinical manifestations includes spina bifida occulta and cystica. The occult type is generally symptomless. Only in rare instances is it accompanied by partial defects of the spinal cord. These are usually located in the lumbosacral segments and cause mild gait abnormalities. Spina bifida cystica is associated with malformation of the spinal cord. An exception is the very rare simple meningocele. As a result of the myelodysplasia and determined by its location and extent, there is motor paralysis, partial or complete absence of sensation which predisposes to decubitus ulcers, and neurogenic impairment of bowel and bladder control, the latter resulting in recurrent or chronic urinary tract infection. Characteristically, muscle weakness is of the lower motor neuron type. Less frequently, one may find a combination of upper and lower motor neuron signs (57) as a consequence of other neurologic complications or malformations, particularly in myelomeningocele at higher thoracic levels. Additional neurectodermal defects (9) that may accompany the spinal cord abnormality include Arnold-Chiari malformation and aqueductal stenosis leading to hydrocephalus, dilatation of the lateral and third ventricles, and abnormal cerebral gyri and sulci. Among the associated mesodermal malformations, skeletal and urinary tract malformations are the most common (9). Particularly significant are vertebral anomalies, congenital kyphosis and hemivertebrae with relentless progression of scoliosis. Hypoplasia, agenesis, horse-shoe configuration of the kidney, and ureteral abnormalities may contribute to deterioration of neurogenic bladder dysfunction and renal status. There may be an intellectual deficit especially in the presence of hydrocephalus. The extent of paralysis is an important prognostic factor in that it curtails the upper limit of physical accomplishments but by no means does it ensure their achievement (3). Recurrent problems related to hydrocephalus, the urinary system, and decubiti can interrupt the child's development and functional training. Intellectual endowment, emotional adjustment, and home environment were also found to be of significance with respect to ultimate prognosis. Obesity is frequent among older inactive children and compounds other complications (3, 10). The management of children with myelomeningocele is a complex undertaking. Bracing is an important aspect of this process and has to be integrated with other therapeutic considerations.

The aim of orthoses is to provide mechanical substitution for weak or paralyzed muscles and to restrain the forces of those with unbalanced action. Orthotic prescription is based on accurate assessment of neurologic deficit which enables the examiner to project expected function and to anticipate musculoskeletal complications. Different mechanisms contribute to the development of deformities (62) in this condition: 1) selective paralysis and significant muscle imbalance at certain joints as a result of specific segmental neurologic lesions; 2) combined effect of gravity and poor positioning in the presence of complete or severe flaccid paralysis; 3) associated malformations of the skeleton; and 4) intrauterine position and lack of movement which may be responsible for some deformities present at birth seemingly inconsistent with the neurologic deficit. Preventive orthotic treatment when conscientiously applied is most successful in deterring contractures related to faulty positioning. Braces alone are less effective in complete prevention of deformities caused by significant muscle imbalance although they may delay the appearance and progression of these complications. Fixed deformities present at birth or caused by underlying skeletal malformation do not respond to orthotic correction.

In this particular handicap, the importance of standing with braces, regardless of the outlook for higher function, has to be stressed. Extensive flaccid paralysis is accompanied by significant osteoporosis. The increased frequency of long bone fractures in conjunction with minor unnoticed trauma among those children who were never subjected to weight bearing and, especially, after immobilization following corrective surgical procedures is clinical evidence of the benefit of standing. The spinal cord malformation is not always a well defined transverse lesion which leads to some variations in both motor and sensory findings. Such cases may permit the use of different orthoses than those which would be required in complete lesion of a specific spinal segment. This possibility should be kept in mind when, subsequently, the role of orthotics will be discussed in relation to segmental levels of deficit.

THORACIC LESIONS

Myelodysplasia in the thoracic segments spares the arms; there is a variable degree of trunk weakness and complete paralysis of the legs. Faulty positioning in supine and prone lying can lead to hip abduction, external rotation and flexion contractures with iliotibial band tightness and equinus deformity of the feet. During infancy these are preventable by exercises and do not require bracing. Unless there is significant hydrocephalus or other complications, head control and upper extremity use develop as expected.

These children can neither assume nor maintain active independent sitting. Eventually, they learn to sit up pulling with their arms and lean on them for support while sitting in a kyphotic or lordotic position. Many children can do this by 1 to 1½ years of age. A trunk corset or well padded plastic shell can help to free up the arms for play in a proper seating arrangement. This device merely serves as support but does not prevent scoliosis. Bracing of spinal deformities is discussed in another chapter.

Once sitting is begun, spinal deformities and hip flexion contractures must be watched. Children with this level of paralysis require braces for activities in the erect position. In most cases, standing with an orthosis is started between 12 and 18 months of age in conjunction with daily activities, such as feeding or play. The conventional long-leg braces with pelvic band and spinal attachment used in the past for this purpose (2) have been replaced by the parapodium (41) (Fig. 10.2). Simplicity and versatility of design, application, and functional use make this orthosis a generally preferred choice. The parapodium consists of a footplate, sidebars, back panel extending from the sacrum to the crease of buttocks, and padded anterior cross bar at the level of the patellar tendons. These components act as a continuous frame which ensures mediolateral and anteroposterior stability. An anterior pad placed over the xyphoid process provides counterpressure on the thorax. A unique constructional feature different from usual mechanical joints is the mechanism for locking and unlocking the hips and knees. A pair of folding handles rotate the upright bars and with them the orthotic joints. When the joint axes are aligned anteroposteriorly hips and knees are held extended. Ninety degree rotation places them in mediolateral alignment and allows flexion. The shoes are not attached permanently to the parapodium but are held in place by tight fitting clamps. For this reason and because there are no straps and buckles, donning and removing takes about 1 to 2 minutes instead of the 10 to 15 minutes required for the conventional orthosis.

A number of adaptations can be added to the basic design for increased knee and hip stability or when there are contractures, leg length discrepancy, or postural deviations. The standard back panel can be adjusted when the spinal lesion extends distally. It can also be replaced by a custom-molded plastic body jacket if there are severe asymmetrical deformities of the trunk and pelvis. Fitting in these problem cases is easier than it is with conventional braces. The parapodium is available in the form of modular kits. It comes in various sizes adjustable for growth.

There are other standing orthoses that utilize biomechanical principles similar to the parapodium (59, 60). Unlike the parapodium, they cannot be used for sitting since they have no provision for hip and knee flexion. The parapodium is the most innovative and successful advancement in the management of children with extensive paralysis. It is simpler to fit and is more comfortable than the conventional orthosis which would be required under these circumstances. Although it is recommended for adolescents and adults, in our experience and that of others (4), its usefulness and safety are limited by increase in body size. A principal factor for maintaining stability in the upright position is the surface area of the supporting footplate in relation to height and weight. In spite of larger footplate dimensions stability tends to decrease when adult stature is approached and in obese older children. Moreover, the bulky footplate required for taller patients is awkward for sitting in a wheelchair. These problems arise around adolescence at which time the orthosis is usually abandoned if it was used only for standing.

In thoracic lesions, a wheelchair is needed for unlimited functional mobility. The skate board, low cart, and other devices used by young children for getting around are discussed in Chapter 13. Ambulation as an exercise may be attained by a few youngsters with upper thoracic deficit and its likelihood increases in lesions below T-6 (2, 10). Some children in the latter group are household ambulators while young, most likely those with T-10, 11 segmental lesion. Functional community ambulation is not expected (25). Young children are able to use the parapodium not only for standing but also for ambulation with the aid of a walkerette or crutches. Forward progression is achieved by pivoting, drag or swing type gait.

Extrapolating the results of a study (61) on 53 normal children aged 11 to 36 months who were trained to walk with walkerette and Verlo orthosis, a device similar to the parapodium, it was suggested that ambulation with these appliances can be learned most expeditiously at approximately 24-month developmental level. The chronological age when some children with thoracic myelodysplasia can learn to ambulate in this manner varies greatly depending on their physical and mental attributes. The range extends from 3 to 10 years, with peak incidence of accomplishment around 5 to 7 years. As the child grows, increasing size of the footplate makes floor clearance more difficult or impossible. Therefore, it is well to bear in mind that the parapodium which may be a suitable walking device for younger children can hardly serve this purpose later on. In those few children with lesion in the lowest thoracic segments who show continuing promise of maintaining some degree of useful ambulation braces of conventional design are more applicable. This level of function can be expected only if the child has well developed upper extremity strength, lean body build, stable spine, and no significant lower extremity contractures. The decision of choosing or changing to standard walking orthosis should be made as early as possible since readjustment to the difference in construction and use becomes more difficult with increasing age. There is some controversy as to the optimal type of conventional orthosis for these youngsters (2, 10). One approach (2) advocates more extensive bracing with HKAFO, sometimes with spinal attachment, to minimize hip flexion contractures and to provide stability. The opposing view holds (10) that the pelvic band cannot control anterior pelvic tilt, and it presents a hindrance on account of added weight and is unnecessary when trunk control is sufficient to permit walking. Therefore, it is added only on occasion to ensure mediolateral hip stability. Our experience suggests that the need to apply pelvic band commonly arises for the latter reason.

Progressive hip flexion contractures represent one of the principal causes responsible for gradual regression of ambulation. The consequence on the growing spine is demonstrated by the wedge-shaped vertebral bodies usually seen in children with significant lordotic deformity which can occur in spite of the pelvic band. Studies on adult spastic paraplegics (64) showed that excursions in lumbar flexion and extension are enhanced rather than decreased by the pelvic band and refute the contention of anteroposterior alignment control. The long term merits and disadvantages of the two orthotic approaches in children require further examination. Regardless of whether HKAFO or KAFO is selected, it is generally of conventional design made out of metal. Ten degree limited motion or double action spring loaded ankle joints substitute for push off and facilitate toe clearance. For knee stabilization single lateral drop ring locks are adequate in children. Bail locks are not used as their safe handling cannot be learned at this age. Pressure exerted on the patella by the anterior knee pad is intolerable in some cases and has to be modified to double straps located over the patellar tendon and suprapatellar area. Wider thigh cuffs may also be helpful to distribute pressure to a larger area. Mediolateral knee instability necessitates varus or valgus pads or pullers. The pelvic band may need recontouring around a protuberant back lesion or ileoureteral diversion stoma. Butterfly attachments (16) or posteriorly placed webbing straps intended to assist hip extension can decrease lumbar lordosis only if there are no flexion contractures.

UPPER LUMBAR LESIONS

A lesion between the first and third lumbar segments leaves the hip flexors and adductors partially or completely innervated. There may be partial knee extensor activity and weak knee flexion performed by the gracilis muscle. Hip abductors and extensors are not functioning and the paralytic muscle imbalance leads to contractures and hip dislocation (9, 62). Surgical intervention is needed to prevent this problem. The hip abduction brace is used at night as a temporizing measure until surgery can be performed. The ankles are flail and equinus foot deformities develop as a result of faulty positioning or may be present at birth. Active trunk control and hip flexion enable these children to sit, usually between 12 to 18 months, provided that the medical course is uncomplicated. The characteristic sitting position is that of increased lordosis.

In L-1 lesions developmental and functional achievements requiring upright posture are similar to those in deficits of the lowest thoracic segments.

However, in this group unopposed hip flexion makes standing even more important. A parapodium (41) (Fig. 10.2) may be the preferred choice unless the child proves to be a limited functional ambulator in which case a standard orthosis is more applicable. Considerations in prescribing a conventional orthosis are as described under thoracic lesions.

Children with L-2 and particularly with L-3 intervention have the advantage of active knee extension. This makes pulling up to the standing position possible and most youngsters do so between 18 to 24 months. Unassisted standing and walking is not possible in the absence of active hip extension and abduction. Crutches or canes will be needed. Differences in orthotic management are probably the greatest in this group both with respect to the extent of bracing and the age when it should be initiated. One approach (2) is to use HKAFO from about 1 year on when possible. This is used as a standing device to prevent contractures. Ambulation training with walkerette or crutches begins later, its onset depending on developmental and medical status. Bracing is decreased to KAFO, preferably after cessation of growth when deformities are less likely to develop, and they are retained as definitive orthoses in most cases.

Another viewpoint (10) is that children with L-2 and L-3 lesions use crawling or scooting as the primary mode of mobility in early years and extensive braces interfere with these activities. Therefore, bracing may be deferred until after 2 years when walking with assistive devices becomes a more realistic functional goal. Exceptions are made if warranted by threatening contractures or when braces are used to help standing. The tendency is to emphasize the functional rather than the preventive role of orthoses from early age on. A pelvic band is not recommended and knee stabilization is attempted by devices acting distal to this joint. No rigid rules can be set about the approach one should follow since there is considerable diversity in clinical findings and course. The fact remains, however, that in some cases with hip instability pelvic bands cannot be avoided but most children who need this extent of bracing will be limited ambulators regardless of the type of orthosis used. More often than not KAFO with locked knee joints are needed because of quadriceps weakness.

When L-3 segmental innervation is present one would expect fair knee extension strength. Under these circumstances the question of eliminating the rigidly locked knee joints is an intriguing but, unfortunately, not always feasible option. One would particularly strive for less extensive bracing when the gracilis muscle is capable of initiating some knee flexion. There are several biomechanical solutions to enhance knee stability in case of partial knee extensor weakness. The problem can be approached by direct action on this joint and indirectly through ankle alignment. The eccentric free knee joint used with a standard metal orthosis (24, 35) does not eliminate bracing above the knee but allows a more economical and cosmetic gait. Other possibilities are the plastic supracondylar KAFO (11, 34) or one with a pretibial shell (23) using free knee joints. The laminated knee extension floor reaction short-leg brace (50) utilizes a somewhat similar principle of aiding extension by anterior support. Plastic braces require very careful fitting to avoid breakdown at the site where supportive pressure is exerted since these children have absent sensation. These devices are suitable only if passive range of lower extremity joints is normal, and the child is capable of maintaining a near vertical hip-trunk alignment with crutches so that in stance the line of gravity passes in front of the knee and behind the hip joint. Only in selected cases of L-3 lesion are these criteria adequately met to allow successful use of these orthoses either from the onset of walking or later on. Anteroposterior knee stabilization is enhanced by ankle plantar-flexion which decreases flexion torque on that joint from heelstrike to midstance. The free knee joint metal orthosis has a limited motion ankle joint with stop at 90° allowing 10° plantar-flexion. Plastic orthoses can have a similar ankle joint or a solid foot extension set in plantar-flexion. Before changing from locked knee orthoses, observing the gait with open joints during evaluation in the clinic is hardly sufficient to decide whether the child is a candidate for different devices. Walking in this manner should be practiced for several weeks in different situations before final decision is made.

Genu recurvatum is encountered sometimes when hamstring weakness deprives the knee of its posterior support while quadriceps function is preserved. In extreme cases of this imbalance knee extension contracture can develop. Mediolateral knee instability is not as frequent as in thoracic lesions. Knee support should be provided by KAFO with biomechanical features appropriate for the presenting problem.

Equinus deformity is not unusual among these children either from birth or acquired thereafter (10, 62). Shoe and brace fitting needs special care in these cases. Shoe inserts, heel lifts, and ankle joint adjustment are necessary to avoid breakdown over the heel. Increasing with the degree of plantar-flexion contractures there is greater pressure exerted on the tips of the toes, particularly on the hallux. Also, it becomes difficult to lace the shoe over the instep. To avoid pressure sores in these areas, it is possible to make adjustment on the regular high top shoes rather than to order costly custom-made shoes that the child will soon outgrow. The hard toe box is cut off and a soft higher and somewhat looser padded toe box is sewed on. A lace stay extension is added so that the shoe can be properly closed without constricting the instep. Shoe fitting requires as much attention and time as a complex brace. However, the benefits in return make this effort worthwhile since braces and other treatment plans will do no good if the child cannot be mobilized because of pressure sores on his feet.

Absence of hip extension and abduction necessitates other assistive devices for standing and walking in addition to orthoses. Children with L-2 or L-3 lesion may cruise holding on to furniture by 2 to 3 years. A weighted push cart gives greater freedom of mobility until they can learn to use a walkerette, crutches, or canes. Efficient crutch walking with KAFO can be learned by about 5 years if the lesion is at L-1 and around 3 to 4 years if the deficit is one or two segments lower. In the long range perspective about half of the patients will be functional household or community ambulators (25). Medical and musculoskeletal problems are responsible for failure to walk. Among the latter, hip dislocation is the most serious hindrance that in itself virtually eliminates the possibility of useful ambulation, a fact to be considered in orthotic plans. Unilateral (2, 62) hip dislocation is not unusual and leads to particularly severe asymmetrical pelvifemoral and spinal deformities which make orthotic fitting a most difficult task. In view of prognosis and fitting problems, a parapodium for standing may be the most appropriate orthosis in this situation regardless of the level of lesion.

LOW LUMBAR LESIONS

In L-4 lesion knee extensors are strong, there is a slight hip abductor and knee flexor function, and ankle dorsiflexion and inversion are largely unopposed. If the deficit spares the fifth lumbar segment hip extensors, abductors and knee flexors are gaining strength, foot everters are working, but plantar flexion remains weak. Hip flexion contractures and dislocation are still threatening possibilities and will require surgical intervention. Calcaneovarus foot deformity and knee extension contracture occur in L-4 lesion while a calcaneus foot is more characteristic of L-5 deficit.

Children in this group have the physical capability of pulling to stand and to cruise at an age close to the expected. Independent standing and walking tends to be delayed but is generally accomplished by 2 years. Due to the triceps surae weakness standing either on one or two legs is more difficult than walking.

An orthosis is prescribed when the child pulls to stand. Although the use of HKAFO is mentioned in the literature (2), primarily for younger children, such extensive bracing does not seem necessary. Crutches and canes assist in hip stability. Main concern is ankle stabilization which can be achieved by AFO. Conventional metal braces (2, 10) are used with anterior stop at 80° or 90°. Double bars are needed for durability. To decrease excessive inversion lateral Y straps are attached to the shoes. In some cases when L-4 function is incomplete less than normal knee extensor strength and plantar-flexion weakness tends to promote a knee flexion attitude. In such cases the laminated knee extension short-leg brace (50) may be useful provided that there is no fixed calcaneous deformity. A calcaneus attitude of the foot is a notoriously difficult problem to control by an orthosis and surgical correction is usually needed. Decubiti over the plantar surface of the heel are not uncommon in active children and are often accompanied by chronic osteomyelitis of the os calcis.

The majority of these children maintain functional ambulation (2, 10, 25).

Medical complications and hip dislocation which is less likely in this group than in upper lumbar lesions account for unfavorable outcome.

Sacral lesions are most frequently associated with pes cavus. Shoe modifications may be necessary.

Other Neuromuscular Diseases

DUCHENNE MUSCULAR DYSTROPHY

Duchenne muscular dystrophy affects boys and is the most frequent and severe type among the myopathies. It leads to wheelchair existence usually by adolescence and demise in the third decade of life. Symptoms appear in early childhood with predominant proximal weakness, most marked in the musculature of shoulder and pelvic girdle. Characteristics of stance and gait (29, 30, 52) are increased lumbar lordosis and trunk extension, hip and knee flexion, broad supporting base, gluteus medius and maximus gait, and toe walking. These changes occur both as a result of and as compensation for muscle weakness and eventually lead to contractures. In the past, orthoses have not been used in Duchenne muscular dystrophy. Recently it was suggested that as weakness progresses and deformities occur the above described compensatory biomechanical changes will reach a point when maintenance of upright posture is no longer possible. Percutaneous tenomies (52, 54) are recommended to release hip flexor, tensor fasciae latae and triceps surae contractures if weakness is not severe enough to prevent ambulation. Surgery is followed by early mobilization and bracing. Since surgical releases eliminate the previously utilized biomechanical compensation long-leg braces are needed to provide a stabilizing system for the lower limbs. Upright position is maintained by sitting on this passive support. In a conventional brace the knee joints are aligned in 5° knee flexion, ankles are held in neutral position and an additional upper gluteal contoured thigh cuff is included. Careful fitting is needed for proper length of the braces. Slumping and falling forward occurs if they are too long and backward tilt with severe compensatory kyphosis develops if they are too short. More recently, a high strength polypropylene ischial weight bearing long-leg brace with metal knee joints (KAFO) was suggested (53). This material gives weight reduction from one-half to one-third in comparison to conventional metal braces which is an important consideration in the presence of severe weakness.

It should be noted that there are as many enthusiastic advocates as opponents of the combined surgical-orthotic intervention in Duchenne muscular dystrophy. It has been stated that this approach can prolong ambulatory status by several years (63). However, to date there are no controlled clinical studies to compare the results of this method as opposed to conservative management.

Regardless of which approach is followed while the child is ambulatory, attempts should be made to slow down progression of deformities which often develop rapidly once the patient has become wheelchair bound. It is important, therefore, at this stage to try and prevent them by a system of resting orthotic devices with careful attention to recheck the fit of these as the child grows or joint configurations change. Development of severe equinocavovarus foot deformities in a wheelchair-bound child would eventually preclude wearing shoes. While proper positioning of the feet on the foot pedals can delay plantar-flexion contractures, it does not prevent varus deformity. Therefore, the use of AFO with lateral Y strap is advisable during the day. If fixed deformity is already present or occurs in spite of preventive attempts the orthoses should be aligned in a tolerable position of correction. Heel lift and long lateral bias-cut Y straps may be added. When regular shoes do not fit, sneakers, soft slippers with a strap over the instep, or thick woolen socks with soft leather sewn on the sole can serve as foot protection.

Hip and knee flexion contractures inevitably develop if the child is allowed to sit for prolonged periods with his legs dependent in the wheelchair. Resting splints made of plastic material such as Plastazote, Orthoplast, or polypropylene keep the knees in extension and the feet in neutral position and are helpful in preventing contractures of the knees and ankles. Unfortunately, it is not possible to apply splints to the hips. In advanced stages of the disease, flexion and abduction deformities of these joints make lying in bed very uncomfortable. A soft contoured mattress insert or pad is useful in relieving discomfort. Hip abduction deformities also present difficulties while sitting in a wheelchair. Lateral pads or cushions can relieve pressure on the thighs. A thermoplastic molded jacket which retains lumbar lordosis can help prevent the scoliotic deformities of the spine. A solid seat insert which provides a more stable sitting base than the usual soft sling type wheelchair seat also seems to delay this complication. Molded seat and back insert offers passive support, stability, and comfort on sitting in case of advanced trunk weakness and spinal deformities. As there is also weakness of neck musculature the insert should extend slightly above the occiput to provide head support.

OTHER MYOPATHIES

The application of braces has not been recommended in limb-girdle or fascio-scapulohumeral types of muscular dystrophy. For the predominantly proximal distribution of muscle weakness there are no satisfactory orthoses available and shoulder girdle weakness excludes the possibility of crutch walking. In rarer, less severe and more slowly progressive forms of myopathies braces can be of benefit for specific biomechanical problems such as foot drop or knee instability. In these cases light weight should be a primary concern. In some instances when generalized muscle weakness was evident in infancy but subsequent course proved to be rather stable we have used the parapodium (41) as a standing device and later for limited ambulation with walkerette.

MUSCULAR ATROPHIES

Infantile progressive muscular atrophy, Werdnig-Hoffmann disease, is the most severe form of these degenerative disorders. Prognosis is usually poor, and death is anticipated between 2 to 7 years depending on the onset of symptoms. However, there are more benign variants of this disease and the course may be less predictable in some cases, especially, when weakness becomes first evident after 2 to 3 years of age. We have been following a few children who now reached young adulthood, although muscle weakness was generalized and rather severe already in early childhood. As there may be a chance of longer survival, proper measures including bracing should be instituted to prevent contractures and to assist in mobility, limited though it may be. This is particularly indicated because these children are bright and alert. The parapodium (41) is very appropriate in this situation. An occasional youngster may be able to move around with this device and walkerette for very short distances perhaps for a few years. Orthotic devices such as those described to prevent contractures in Duchenne muscular dystrophy should also be provided for these children.

A more benign course is seen in Kugelberg-Welander disease. Muscle weakness, at least initially, is predominantly proximal in distribution which creates biomechanical abnormalities similar to Duchenne or limb girdle dystrophy. In a few cases, primarily on the insistence of the family, we have provided HKAFO when advancing muscle weakness made continuing ambulation impossible. No functional benefit was derived from bracing.

In the various forms of neuropathies that affect children splints or braces are used to prevent contractures. Orthoses to improve function are selected on the basis of developmental considerations and biomechanical abnormalities.

Arthritis and Collagen Diseases

In the acute and subacute stages of juvenile rheumatoid arthritis and other collagen diseases associated with pain and weakness splinting is the generally applied method for protective support and for maintaining or increasing range of motion. In the chronic stage of juvenile rheumatoid arthritis, an orthosis is sometimes used as a last resort when progression of a deformity cannot be controlled by other means. Contracture of the knee joint is the most likely problem requiring such treatment. In these cases the knee joint of a long-leg orthosis must be adjustable to permit controlled flexion-extension range. There are several types available. The polycentric knee joint (1) with spring to assist extension exerts continuous stretching. Placement of the mechanical joint must be most carefully determined so that its position corresponds to the axis of rotation of the anatomical joint. The dial lock (1, 23) restricts motion in one direction. To accommodate fixed knee flexion contracture the lock can be set at a desired degree of extension. It allows free movement through the rest of the range. The fan lock (23) does not permit motion, but it can be also adjusted to different joint positions. The choice of knee lock depends on whether the primary aim is stabilization or prevention of progressive deformity. Attempts to decrease knee flexion contractures are contraindicated if posterior subluxation of the tibia develops.

In the past this type of brace was used for hemarthrosis of the knee joint with progressive loss of range of motion in hemophilia (1). It was often combined with wide molded leather thigh and calf cuffs to decrease weight bearing and further trauma to the joint. The current preventive hematologic treatment has, to a large measure, eliminated the occurrence of this problem.

Disorders of the Skeletal System

Congenital hip dislocation under 3 months of age is treated with abduction splints (26, 36) or pillow.

Legg-Calvé-Perthes disease or juvenile coxa plana is an avascular necrosis of the femoral capital epiphysis which often occurs bilaterally. The treatment of this disease has undergone several changes over the years. Originally, it consisted of non-weight bearing until the stage of regeneration was completed. In bilateral affection this meant bed rest, at times as long as 1 to 2 years. In unilateral cases non-weight bearing was achieved by crutch walking and using a waist belt with sling loop that held the affected extremity suspended in flexion (56). Subsequently, ischial weight bearing long-leg braces (KAFOs) were developed. In the first model an ischial ring seat was incorporated (16). By virtue of a shoe extension platform the leg was freely suspended within the brace. The child could walk with crutches wearing this orthosis on one or both legs. In the unilateral case a shoe lift was added on the unaffected side to compensate for leg length difference created by the platform. The ischial ring was eventually replaced by a quadrilateral socket with ischial seat (47). Current treatment is ambulation in the abduction brace after the synovitis and pain have subsided (44). The walking brace maintains the hips in 45° abduction and 20° internal rotation. This position provides concentric coverage of the femoral head and promotes spherical reossification as regeneration occurs. The simplest device consists of long-leg plaster cylinders abducted by a broomstick (44). The casts are not removable but can be adjusted.

There are a number of removable abduction braces for bilateral hip pathology utilizing similar principles of design (8, 13, 14) (Fig. 10.3). All have two medially situated upright bars which are held in the desired position of abduction and internal rotation by two cross bars. One cross bar is located at the ankle and the other at the knee or at the proximal end of upright bars. Shoe platforms or shoe wedges provide flat weight bearing surface. An important consideration when using these braces is to avoid stress on the medial collateral knee ligament and development of genu valgum. The trilateral socket hip abduction orthosis (58) has a quadrilateral plastic

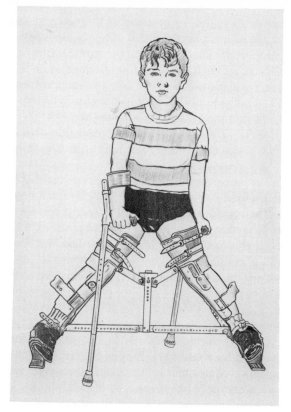

Fig. 10.3. Abduction brace for bilateral hip pathology.

laminated ischial weight bearing brim and a metal upright with a walking heel. Weight bearing is transmitted through the medial upright. In children over 7 years of age or when there is more severe involvement the orthopaedic surgeon may elect operative rather than conservative treatment.

Osteogenesis imperfecta is a rather rare disease but should be mentioned because of orthotic interest. The pneumatic orthosis described in Chapter 8 was originally designed for children with this disease (40, 55).

Genu varum and, particularly, genu valgum in mild form are a developmental phenomenon in normal children. Spontaneous correction occurs by 5 to 7 years of age. In the absence of neuromuscular impairment severe knee deformities can be caused by generalized primary or secondary metabolic diseases of the skeletal system, localized pathologic processes or injuries, and syndromes associated with ligamentous laxity. Progressive deformities occur because epiphyseal growth is uneven as a result of asymmetrical compression forces. Progression becomes especially fast when the weight bearing line passes either medial or lateral to the knee joint. Support for mediolateral knee instability can be incorporated in conventional metal braces with free knee joints using varus or valgus condyle pad and puller (16). Combination of a standard metal brace with plastic pretibial shell disperses the supportive force over a larger surface area and may be more comfortable (23). A metal KAFO with single medial or lateral bar (42) is lighter in weight but it may not provide adequate support for obese children. A plastic KAFO similar in design to the supracondylar type with free knee joints (11, 34) is more cosmetic in appearance but accommodation for growth is limited. In selecting the most appropriate orthosis it should be remembered that these children are not neurologically impaired, that they are very active and grow at a normal pace.

Foot deformities occur sometimes in otherwise healthy infants and may necessitate the use of a corrective brace either by itself or as an adjunct to other treatment modalities. The bilateral shoe clamp foot orthosis (1) is a spreader bar with footplate attached to the sole of shoes. Axial limb rotation can be varied by the position of footplate on the bar. Length of the bar determines limb abduction. If the bar is curved with its apex proximally or distally the foot will be in varus or valgus position, respectively.

Upper Extremity Orthoses

The need for upper extremity orthoses seems to arise less frequently in children than in adults. Clinical experience also suggests that these devices are not well accepted by youngsters. It appears that they prefer substitutive patterns of their own choice and reject interference with sensory feedback. Hand braces have certainly not gained significant application in the treatment of upper extremity impairment in neuromuscular deficits of early onset. Construction and proper fitting of orthoses or splints is often difficult for the small hand size, particularly, the more complex types used for functional assistance. It may well be that if these practical problems were eliminated, application at an early age would give better results similar to the experience with prostheses in congenital upper limb deficiency. When the purpose is to prevent contractures, hand splints or braces worn at night are better tolerated. Indications and biomechanical principles of upper extremity orthotics are the same in children as in adults (see Chapter 8).

REFERENCES

1. AMERICAN ACADEMY OF ORTHOPAEDIC SURGEONS. *Atlas of Orthotics*, pp. 197, 205, 206, 232, C. V. Mosby, St. Louis, 1975.
2. BADELL-RIBERA, A., AND SWINYARD, C. A. Rehabilitation of children with spina bifida cystica. In *Proceedings of Fourth International Congress of Physical Medicine*, International Congress Series No. 107, p. 625. Excerpta Medica Foundation, Amsterdam 1966.
3. BADELL-RIBERA, A., SWINYARD, C. A., GREENSPAN, L., AND DEAVER, G. G. Spina bifida with myelomeningocele: evaluation of rehabilitation potential. In *Comprehensive Care of the Child with Spina Bifida Manifesta*, ed. by C. A. Swinyard, Rehabilitation Monograph XXXI. New York University, New York, 1966.
4. BADELL-RIBERA, A. Personal communication.
5. BANKS, H. H. The foot and ankle in cerebral palsy. In *Orthopaedic Aspects of Cerebral*

Palsy, ed. by R. L. Samilson, Clinics in Developmental Medicine No. 52/53. J. B. Lippincott, Philadelphia, 1975.

6. BAYER, L. M., AND BAYLEY, N. *Growth Diagnosis: Selected Methods for Predicting and Interpreting Physical Development from One Year to Maturity.* University of Chicago Press, Chicago, 1959.

7. BOBATH, K. *The Motor Deficit in Patients with Cerebral Palsy,* Clinics in Developmental Medicine No. 23. Spastics Society/W. Heinemann, London, 1966.

8. BOBECHKO, W. P., McLAURIN, C. A., AND MOTLOCH, W. M. The Toronto orthosis for Legg-Perthes' disease. *Artif. Limbs, 12:* 36, Autumn 1968.

9. BROCKLEHURST, G., ed. *Spina Bifida for the Clinician,* Clinics in Developmental Medicine No. 57. J. B. Lippincott, Philadelphia, 1976.

10. BUNCH, W. H., CASS, A. S., BENSMAN, A. S., AND LONG, D. M. *Modern Management of Myelomeningocele.* W. H. Green, St. Louis, 1972.

11. CASSVAN, A., WUNDER, K. E., AND FULTONBERG, D. M. Orthotic management of unstable knee. *Arch. Phys. Med. Rehabil., 58:* 487, 1977.

12. CHALLENOR, Y. B. Orthoses for children. In *The Child with Disabling Illness,* ed. by J. A. Downey and N. L. Low. W. B. Saunders, Philadelphia, 1974.

13. COCCHIARELLA, A., CHALLENOR, Y., AND KATZ, J. F. Orthosis for use in Legg-Calve-Perthes' disease. *Arch. Phys. Med. Rehabil., 53:* 286, 1972.

14. CURTIS, B. H., GUNTHER, S. F., GOSSLING, H. R., AND PAUL, S. W. Treatment of Legg-Perthes' disease with the Newington ambulatory abduction brace. *J. Bone Joint Surg. (Am.), 56:* 1135, 1974.

15. DEAVER, G. G. Cerebral palsy, methods of treating the neuromuscular disability. *Arch. Phys. Med. Rehabil., 37:* 363, 1956.

16. DEAVER, G. G., AND BRITTIS, A. L. *Braces, Crutches, Wheelchairs,* Rehabilitation Monograph No. V. New York University, New York, 1953.

17. DOLAN, C. M. E., MEREDAY, C., AND HARTMAN, G. *Evaluation of NYU Insert Brace.* New York University, New York, 1969.

18. DUBOWITZ, V. Progressive muscular dystrophy: prevention of deformities. *Clin. Pediat., 3:* 323, 1964.

19. EVANS, E. B. The knee in cerebral palsy. In *Orthopaedic Aspects of Cerebral Palsy,* ed. by R. L. Samilson, Clinics in Developmental Medicine No. 52/53. J. B. Lippincott, 1975.

20. FUJIWARA, M., BASMAJIAN, J. V., AND IWAMOTO, M. Hip abnormalities in cerebral palsy. *Arch. Phys. Med. Rehabil., 57:* 278, 1976.

21. GARRETT, A., LISTER, M., AND BRESNAN, G. New concepts in cerebral palsy bracing. *J. Am. Phys. Ther. Assoc., 46:* 728, 1966.

22. GUESS, V. S. Control of lower extremity movement in cerebral palsy. In *Principles of Lower Extremity Bracing,* ed. by J. Perry and H. J. Hislop. American Physical Therapy Association, New York, 1967.

23. HEIZER, D. Bracing design for knee joint instability. In *Principles of Lower Extremity Bracing,* ed. by J. Perry and H. J. Hislop. American Physical Therapy Association, New York, 1967.

24. HEIZER, D. Brace design for flaccid paralysis. In *Principles of Lower Extremity Bracing,* ed. by J. Perry and H. J. Hislop. American Physical Therapy Association, New York, 1967.

25. HOFFER, M. M., FEIWELL, E., PERRY, R., PERRY, J., AND BONNETT, C. Functional ambulation in patients with myelomeningocele. *J. Bone Joint Surg. (Am.), 55:* 137, 1973.

26. ILFELD, L. W. The management of congenital dislocation and dysplasia of the hips by means of a special splint. *J. Bone Joint Surg. (Am.), 39:* 99, 1957.

27. INGRAM, T. T. S. *Paediatric Aspects of Cerebral Palsy.* E. S. Livingstone, Edinburgh, 1964.

28. JEBSEN, R. H., CORCORAN, P. J., AND SIMONS, B. C. Clinical experience with plastic short leg brace. *Arch. Phys. Med. Rehabil., 51:* 114, 1970.

29. JOHNSON, E. W. Pathokinesiology of Duchenne muscular dystrophy: implications for management. *Arch. Phys. Med. Rehabil., 58:* 4, 1977.

30. Johnson, E. W., and Kennedy, J. H. Comprehensive management of Duchenne muscular dystrophy. *Arch. Phys. Med. Rehabil., 52:* 110, 1971.

31. Lee, K. H., and Johnston, R. Bracing below the knee for hemiplegia: biomechanical analysis. *Arch. Phys. Med. Rehabil., 54:* 466, 1973.

32. Lee, K. H., and Johnston, R. Effect of below knee bracing on knee movement: biomechanical analysis. *Arch. Phys. Med. Rehabil., 55:* 179, 1974.

33. Lehman, J. F., Warren, C., and De Lateur, B. A biomechanical evaluation of knee instability in below knee braces. *Arch. Phys. Med. Rehabil., 51:* 688, 1970.

34. Lehneis, H. R. New developments in lower limb orthotics through bioengineering. *Arch. Phys. Med. Rehabil., 53:* 303, 1972.

35. Lister, M. J. Bracing the unstable knee in flaccid paralysis. In *Principles of Lower Extremity Bracing,* ed. by J. Perry and H. J. Hislop. American Physical Therapy Association, New York, 1967.

36. Mendes, D. G. A night splint for congenital dislocation of the hip. *J. Bone Joint Surg. (Am.), 52:* 588, 1970.

37. Minear, W. L. A classification of cerebral palsy. *Pediatrics, 18:* 841, 1956.

38. Molnar, G. E., and Gordon, S. U. Cerebral palsy: predictive value of selected clinical signs for early prognostication of motor function. *Arch. Phys. Med. Rehabil., 57:* 153, 1976.

39. Molnar, G. E., and Taft, L. T. Pediatric rehabilitation. Part I. *Curr. Probl. Pediatr., 7:* 3, 1977.

40. Morel, G. Un nouveau type d'appareillage orthopedique: l'appariellage a attelles pneumatique. *Rev. Clin. Orthop., 57:* 409, 1971.

41. Motloch, W. The parapodium: an orthotic device for neuromuscular disorders. *Artif. Limbs, 15:* 36, Autumn 1971.

42. Nietschke, R. O. A single bar above knee orthosis. *Orthot. Prosthet., 25:* 20, Dec. 1971.

43. Perry, J. The cerebral palsy gait. In *Orthopaedic Aspects of Cerebral Palsy,* ed. by R. L. Samilson, Clinics in Developmental Medicine No. 52/53. J. B. Lippincott, Philadelphia, 1975.

44. Petrie, J. G., and Bitenc, J. The abduction weight-bearing treatment in Legg-Perthes disease. *J. Bone Joint Surg. (Br.), 53:* 54, 1971.

45. Piaget, J. *The Origins of Intelligence in Children.* W. W. Norton and Co., New York, 1963.

46. Rubin, G., and Dixon, M. The modern ankle foot orthoses (AFOs). *Bull. Prosthet. Res., 10:* 20, Spring 1973.

47. Russek, A., and Eschen, F. Ischial weight bearing brace with quadrilateral wood top. *Orthop. Prosthet. Appl. J., 12(3):* 31, 1958.

48. Samilson, R. L., and Perry, J. The orthopaedic assessment of cerebral palsy. In *Orthopaedic Aspects of Cerebral Palsy,* ed. by R. L. Samilson, Clinics in Developmental Medicine No. 52/53. J. B. Lippincott, Philadelphia, 1975.

49. Sarno, J. E., and Lehneis, H. R. Prescription considerations for plastic below knee orthoses. *Arch. Phys. Med. Rehabil., 52:* 503, 1971.

50. Satiel, J. A. One piece laminated knee locking short leg brace. *Orthot. Prosthet., 23:* 68, June 1969.

51. Sharrard, W. J. W. The hip in cerebral palsy. In *Orthopaedic Aspects of Cerebral Palsy,* ed. by R. L. Samilson, Clinics in Developmental Medicine No. 52/53. J. B. Lippincott, Philadelphia, 1975.

52. Siegel, J. M. Pathomechanics of stance in Duchenne muscular dystrophy. *Arch. Phys. Med. Rehabil., 53:* 403, 1972.

53. Siegel, J. M. Plastic molded knee-ankle-foot orthosis in the treatment of Duchenne muscular dystrophy. *Arch. Phys. Med. Rehabil., 56:* 322, 1975.

54. Siegel, J. M., Miller, J. E., and Ray, R. D. Subcutaneous lower limb tenotomy in treatment of pseudohypertrophic muscular dystrophy. *J. Bone Joint Surg. (Am.), 150:* 1437, 1968.

55. SILBER, M., CHUNG, T. S., VARGHESE, G., HINTERBUCHNER, C., BAILEY, M., AND HIRVY, N. Pneumatic orthosis: a pilot study. *Arch. Phys. Med. Rehabil.*, *56:* 27, 1975.
56. SNYDER, C. H. Sling for use in Legg-Perthes disease. *J. Bone Joint Surg.*, *29:* 524, 1947.
57. STARK, G. D., AND BAKER, G. C. W. The neurologic involvement of the lower limb in myelomeningocele. *Devel. Med. Child Neurol.*, *9:* 732, 1967.
58. TACHDJIAN, M. O., AND JOVETT, L. O. Trilateral socket hip abduction orthosis for the treatment of Legg-Perthes disease. *Orthot. Prosthet.*, *22(2):* 49, 1968.
59. TAYLOR, N., AND PEMBERTON, D. R. The Verlo: an orthosis for children with severe motor handicaps. *Arch. Phys. Med. Rehabil.*, *53:* 534, 1972.
60. TAYLOR, N., AND SAND, P. Verlo brace use in children with myelomeningocele and spinal cord injury. *Arch. Phys. Med. Rehabil.*, *55:* 231, 1974.
61. TAYLOR, N., AND SAND, P. Verlo orthosis: experience with different developmental levels in normal children. *Arch. Phys. Med. Rehabil.*, *56:* 120, 1975.
62. TZIMAS, N. A. Orthopedic care of the child with spina bifida. In *Comprehensive Care of the Child with Spina Bifida Manifesta*, ed. by C. A. Swinyard, Rehabilitation Monograph No. XXXI. New York University, New York, 1966.
63. VIGNOS, P. J., AND ARCHIBALD, K. C. Maintenance of ambulation in childhood muscular dystrophy. *J. Chronic Dis.*, *12:* 273, 1960.
64. WARREN, C. G., LEHMANN, J. F., AND DE LATEUR, B. J. Pelvic band use in orthotics for adult paraplegic patients. *Arch. Phys. Med. Rehabil.*, *56:* 221, 1975.

11

Shoes and Their Modifications

ISIDORE ZAMOSKY, C.P.O.
S. LICHT, M.D.
J. B. REDFORD, M.D.

There was a time when no one wore shoes, but that was before recorded history. There are many people in the world who do not wear shoes; for some it may be a matter of choice, but for most the lack of shoes is economic. Those who live in a climate where the temperature does not make the feet uncomfortably cold, where the terrain is sandy, or where the walking surface is not painful to the naked foot may do without shoes, but for all others, well-fitting shoes offer many advantages.

In addition to the primary functions of shoes (to protect the sole from rough terrain and the sole and upper part of the foot from heat, cold, dampness, and dirt and to aid in walking and standing), Thornton (23) lists these advantages: (a) to assist the foot in abnormal functions, such as kicking a football; (b) to overcome abnormalities of the foot; and (c) to complete a costume.

Thornton (23) names two basic foot coverings, the sandal and the moccasin, and says that all other footgear are combinations of these. A sandal is a flat piece of material cut to the approximate shape of the foot and held onto the foot by straps, thongs, or pegs. Primarily, a sandal is for hot climates and a moccasin is for cold, but in the temperate climate each is needed and so the shoe, a combination of the two, resulted.

Shoemaking as a craft was advanced in ancient Egypt (25) and Greece. Until the 19th century, the method of making shoes remained virtually unchanged. Parts were cut from animal hides and sewn with waxed thread, by hand, over a model which corresponded roughly to a foot, either foot. Although there have been instances, over the ages, of shoes made in "pairs," that is, right and left, it was not until the 19th century that "rights" and "lefts" were generally available (3). In ancient times, shoes were not worn by all people. By law, slaves were not permitted to wear shoes in Egypt, and the penalty for attempting to achieve such comfort was severe (25).

The most ancient footgear of which there is record was the Egyptian Tabteb, a sandal of plaited papyrus strips or hide secured by thongs. In the time of Cleopatra there were curriers and tanners; skins and leather were used by early Babylonians to make foot coverings. Much later, a favorite leather was made from the Corsican goat, which was tanned in Cordova, Spain, and gave the name of cordovanner or cordwainer to shoemakers.

Shoemaking came to the U.S.A. through religious persecution. Phillip Kirtland of Sherrington, England, emigrated to Lynn, Massachusetts, where he founded a shoe trade which for many years made that city the most important in the industry.

Early in the 19th century, the apprentice worked in a small training shop until he learned the trade and then traveled the countryside, "living in" with a family until he made a year's supply for every member in the family. In 1810, the itinerant shoemakers of America produced a million pairs of shoes; in 1965, American shoe manufacturers produced more than 600,000,000 pairs of shoes and 300,000,000 pairs of other footgear.

In this chapter we shall discuss shoes for the disabled and nondisabled foot. From the standpoint of aids to living and making a living, the shoe is possibly the most important article of clothing. A shoe may be essential to the livelihood of certain workers: miners and all who work outdoors in cold weather.

Why should a shoe be considered a functional aid to the disabled? First, because a large number of people have serious foot problems and suffer their discomfort in silence until they learn that shoe alterations may reduce their daily discomforts to subthreshold level. Second, more attention to better fitting of shoes may not only relieve pain but also may prevent the progress of deformities and other problems. A shoe of improper design or fit may disfigure a foot and exaggerate a tendency to the formation of the bunion, flat foot, hammer toe, ingrown toenail, and other foot problems. Variations in shoe construction, adaptations through inserts, or sole and heel modifications may not only stop the progression of a pathology but also may improve the function and relieve pain. The distinction between a shoe and an orthopedic shoe may be one of degree. For most foot sufferers, a shoe is an orthotic device, that is, it supports, controls or aids a part of the body. However, it is important to distinguish between a shoe that is simply accommodating in character, that is, that causes no pain or deformity, and a corrective shoe, which is actually actively designed to try and prevent or correct a deformity through changing the forces around the foot.

It is safe to say that during a lifetime, 20% of all people have a foot problem of sufficient importance so as to cause discomfort ranging between unbearable symptoms and moderate pain. Most shoe problems are discussed with and settled by the shoe salesman. The more serious problems are frequently discussed with the family physician, orthopedist, or physiatrist. Since we believe that a physician should be willing and able to assist foot sufferers, he should be well informed about all aspects of shoes. He should also distinguish between someone who simply sells shoes and a trained shoe fitter or pedorthost who knows the details of how to fit feet with shoes. In this chapter, we shall discuss the manufacture, fitting, and modification of shoes in sufficient detail so that physicians and others may understand most problems of foot discomfort in relation to shoe applications.

The first requisite of a shoe is that it fits, that is, that it is comfortable and will not lead to pain or deformity.

Empirical standards have not been set for shoe fitting and little scientific research has been devoted to this subject. The foot has a "funny" shape. It is not symmetrical, has no geometric pattern, alters with growth and, after growth, alters with age and weight. Its dimensions change with the season, daily temperature, and time of day. More important is that the size changes with lying, sitting, and standing. The foot is narrow in the heel, wide near the front, and irregular in the toes. The feet of a person may be of different size. Variations in length, width, and shape are so great that a compromise must be made.

Fortunately, a shoe does not have to fit like a glove; it should fit like a shoe, that is, not too snugly, since the size of the foot changes while walking and running. A shoe must be snug enough not to fall off and loose enough to permit the parts of the foot to move in walking. If a shoe is too tight, it will cramp parts into misshape; if it is too loose, friction of the shoe against the skin will cause hypertrophy (corns and calluses), irritation, and even fissures in the skin. Almost no one buys a shoe that is a "perfect" fit. More often, the foot fills out the shoe that is worn; it expands or is compressed. That is why new shoes are sometimes uncomfortable and have to be "broken in" and why an old shoe is so often comfortable. But the shoemaker must start somewhere, and he starts as did his counterpart more than 2,000 years ago, with a form on which to build—on a last.

Lasts

Last is an Anglo-Saxon word meaning a footprint or boot. It is supposed to be a replica of a human foot, a three-dimensional outline of a foot. Before the nineteenth century, a last was usually carved of solid rock maple in the general shape of a foot, either foot. It was not until the 19th century that the "straight" last gave way to a "right" and a "left" last. Since the 1950's, lasts have been made increasingly of polyethylene in the U. S. The general shape of the last is based upon a standard which was adopted in the fourth quarter of the last century (26) (Fig. 11.1). The last is of great importance in the shoe industry because (a) a shoe cannot be made without one, and (b) the final dimensions of the shoe will be intimately associated with the exact shape of the last. Since style is of paramount importance to women and of more-than-passing importance to men, there is much competition

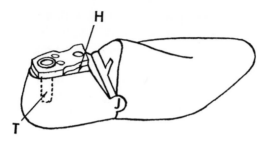

Fig. 11.1. Shoe last. *H*, heel cone; *T*, thimble; *J*, hinge joint. (Reproduced with permission from brochure of United Shoe Machinery Corporation of Boston.)

among last makers to achieve a "new" style each year and as much secrecy as with the new styles of automobiles (16). The back portion of the shoe is not "seen", so it remains almost the same from year to year, but the front part of a shoe is the shoe, and each year many changes, so minor as to be unrecognized by the average layman, are offered to the shoe manufacturer.

A style model is carved for a man's shoe in sizes 7 C and 10 C and for a woman in size 4 B. By means of an adjustable pantograph lathe from these models of lasts, as many as 70 different sizes of lasts of each model may be produced. Polyethylene is granulated, melted, poured into a mold of the approximate shape of a last, and cooled. The solid block of plastic is turned on a lathe—one, two, or four at a time. The rough last is sanded and polished since, unless it is very smooth, the shoe will not slide off at the end of manufacture. The last is also split and rejoined with a hinge for final removal. On the top of the heel, holes are drilled for the "thimble," a threaded cylinder for mounting on different machines. The sole tip and heel bottom are plated with a thin layer of metal to prevent tacks from penetrating the wood or plastic during assembly; instead, the nail turns under (is clinched). Lasts may vary no more than $\frac{1}{32}$ inch in length from the shoe manufacturer's specifications.

During World War II, the U. S. Army ordered millions of pairs of shoes. Only about 60% of people are truly happy with the fit of their shoes. Forty percent of millions was quite a number, and following the war, the government decided to learn more about "fit." Twenty-four measurements were made on each foot of many thousands of soldiers to determine which, if any, of the measurements most closely reflected the "size" of a man's (women were not measured) footshoe. It was found that the traditional measurement of heel to toe was not as important as that of heel to ball (widest part of the foot). In addition it was agreed that the dimensions of a foot did not increase arithmetically as feet became larger but more nearly geometrically. Increase in three-dimensional measurements is called "grading" in the shoe trade. A last is graded by combining measurements of the width, girth, and length of a shoe in "points." In the U. S. there are three sizes to the inch; in Europe there are four sizes to the inch. Width is measured in letters of the alphabet. Each higher letter indicates an increase in width of one-quarter inch. If a man's foot measures 11 inches long and 3 inches wide at the "joint," it is called size 8 B in the U. S. and size 40 in France. In France in 1965, more than 90% of the shoes manufactured were sold by length only; there is only one width per size, and the size is measured from heel to toe.

The grading of a last, which is based on a uniform increase (3% in all dimensions) is called *geometric*. The United Shoe Machinery Company has long sought for a method of shoe fabrication which has fewer hand operations and more automated steps (26). Because of the great expense entailed in tooling for shoe machines and the investment in machines by manufacturers of the U. S. (who in 1960 turned out more than 600,000,000 pairs of shoes), automation was delayed until the report of the army was released. Automated shoe manufacture in the U. S. is geared to the geometric last.

There is one other last which should be mentioned because of the amount of study entailed in its development. The Genesco Corporation continued along the lines of the army research and announced that it is possible to obtain a more accurate fit with a smaller stock of shoes by using a three-dimensional measurement correlating the distance from the heel to the ball joint, with the circumferential measurement at the ball. They call the measurement the DFC (dynamic fit concept) and began to manufacture shoes on lasts graded according to such measurements in 1964 (17).

In addition to regular lasts there are stock lasts with orthopedic features such as (a) a straight inner border which accommodates for several lesions such as hallux valgus, hallux rigidus, splay foot, metatarsalgia, and pes planus; (b) an inflare which accommodates an adducted forefoot or a foot in slightly fixed varus; (c) an outflare (pronator last) which accommodates an abducted forefoot or painful bunion, before or after surgery; (d) a bunion last, with slight outflaring which accommodates the exostosis and renders close conformity at the medial waist level to assist in hallux realignment, and (e) a stub last which accommodates an arthritic or otherwise contracted foot requiring depth in the toe and instep areas.

The moderately misshapen adult foot can usually be fitted with shoes made from a stock last, but the severely deformed adult foot cannot be contained in a stock shoe without expensive modifications. Often, it is economically more reasonable to custom-make a last which will be a faithful replication of the deformed foot, including the intended pressure reliefs and supportive features which are accomplished by adding or removing plaster. The shoe can be made directly over the cast, depending on the type of shoe that is to be made, or a duplicate wood or plastic last is made on a duplicating lathe. If the disability does not require gross reshaping, the stock last can be used as a base. It can be shaved or added to as required. Pressure reliefs can be installed by adding cutout pieces of leather or cork to alleviate pressure on such deformities as protruding interphalangeal joints, flexed toes, hallux valgus, etc.

For infants, stock lasts are used for correction and its maintenance. Correction can be achieved either by the use of selective lasts or by surgery. In either case, an adequate shoe will be required to maintain the improvement. Where surgery is not done, each new pair of shoes should approach a lesser degree of correction until a regular shoe can be worn. For the infant, there are two stock lasts with orthopedic features, one for talipes equinovarus and the other for talipes planovalgus.

Another method for measuring the foot for orthopedic shoes or modifications is recommended by the British Standards Institution. It consists of a pencil outline of the foot with some circumferential measurement from which a last can be modified (6). However, to obtain a correct picture of the topography of the sole, a plaster impression should be taken.

One unique type of custom-made shoe has been developed by Mr. A. E. Murray; it is called the "Space Shoe." These shoes can be ordered through orthotic facilities, and although they are more expensive than stock shoes, they have unique qualities. The appearance is somewhat unorthodox because people are not used to seeing shoes that are the shape and size of their foot. However, many people find a degree of comfort in this shoe that they never knew in the past (19).

As the dynamic forces of the sole are the most important factors in correction of faulty areas of pressure, various methods of recording these forces have been developed. Doctor Paul Brand has worked for years with leprosy and is intimately acquainted with the problems of faulty unbalanced pressure forces on feet. He and his associates have reported extensively on this problem. They recommend the Harris mat and the Microcapsule Sock as inexpensive methods of recording degrees of pressure on the foot when the patient stands and walks. Observations on footprints made in these shoe inserts can then be incorporated into the shoe (5). Another method of recording abnormal pressures in feet has been infrared themography. Brand and Bergtholdt have reported on the value of such recordings in fitting shoes to patients with poor sensation and potential skin damage (4).

Manufacture of Shoes

In many parts of the world there are craftsmen who make shoes or other foot coverings by hand, either because the people do not have the machines to make shoes or because the price of imported shoes is greater than that of locally handcrafted shoes. Regardless of how a shoe is made, a last must be used to build a shoe which will retain its shape. Most articles of apparel are made from patterns or pieces of material which are joined by sewing or cementing, and the shoe is no exception. It is made by a combination of hand and machine operations. Even the most highly automated shoe factory requires hand operations. In general, the finer the shoe, the more manual operations there are. Some shoes require up to 200 different steps (1).

The last determines the size and style. A last is usually made of two sections joined by a device which will permit the two parts to be separated at the end of the manufacturing process so that the last may be removed from the finished shoe (Fig. 11.1). Although shoes for men, women, and children are made in basically the same manner, there are differences. We shall describe first the manufacture of men's shoes and then mention those variations in the process which characterize the fabrication of other shoes.

A man's shoe may be high (covering the foot above the ankle) or low (lower than the ankle on the inner border). Although boots and high shoes were popular before the 20th century, the low-cut shoe, or oxford, has been preferred by most American and European men for a long time. There are two principal types of oxford, the blucher and the balmoral (bal). In a blucher shoe, the lace laps and tongue are formed from one piece; in the bal, the tongue is a separate piece of leather, and the lace laps are part of the body (upper) of the shoe (Fig. 11.2).

The usual last is made from maple wood in some countries but largely of plastic in the U. S. A wooden last may be built up by cementing or nailing on appropriate-sized pieces of wood or plastic, leather, or cork, or the last may be shaved to reduce its size. On the heel bottom there is a thin plate of steel which deflects the tips of nails as they arrive through the leather sole, so that they will not later pierce the shoe and penetrate the skin.

A shoe is made from the inside out. The insole, the part that will be closest to the foot, is nailed to the last. Pieces are added until the shoe is virtually complete. Then, the last is removed, and an inner lining is cemented

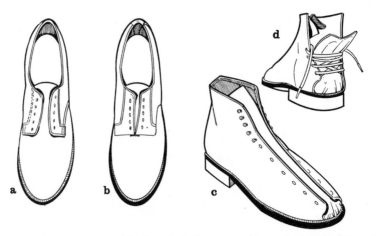

Fig. 11.2. Shoe styles. a, blucher; b, bal; c, convalescent; d, convalescent with posterior closure.

in place. In order for all pieces to come together and look "right" on such an irregular form, much planning is required. Each shoe factory has at least one patternmaker. He applies heavy brown paper (or some other material) to the contours of the last and by marks and cuts, makes outlines of the many parts of a shoe. The parts, mostly of leather, are "clicked" or stamped out of a large sheet of hide (22).

PARTS OF THE SHOE

There are three principal and very different parts of a shoe (Fig. 11.3). The part that bears most of the weight is called the sole. The part of the sole that touches the ground is called the outer sole; the part that comes closest to the foot is called the inner sole. In some shoes there is a layer of leather or other material between the forepart of the two soles.

The part of the sole between the widest point (ball or waist) and the heel is called the shank. Since much of the weight of the body is carried by the shank, it is usually reinforced with a strip of metal or with leather fiberboard. Sole leather is made of steerhide or other very strong leather. Its thickness will vary.

The part of the shoe that does not touch the ground is called the upper. It may be made of any leather or firm fabric. The upper consists of several pieces which are sewn together before being joined to the sole.

The front portion of the upper which covers the instep and toe is called the vamp. The rear portion of the upper is made of one, two, or more pieces or "quarters" which are not symmetrical since the inner border is lower than the outer border. These are sewn together to form the back seam. Usually, the outer quarter has a flap which caps the inner quarter. The inner surface of all parts of the upper is fitted with a lining of woven fabric in the vamp and leather in the quarters, or the entire inner surface may be made of leather.

The third element of a shoe is the heel. This may be made of leather, wood, plastic, rubber, metal, or a combination of these.

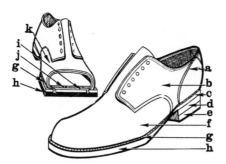

Fig. 11.3. Parts of a shoe. *a*, foxing; *b*, quarter; *c*, heel seat; *d*, heel base; *e*, heel; *f*, vamp; *g*, welt; *h*, outsole; *i*, filler; *j*, insole; *k*, waist.

MAKING A SHOE WITH A GOODYEAR WELT

The shoe last is fitted with a slotted or threaded thimble in the upper back. This opening fits over a spindle and permits the shoemaker to use both hands while working on a clamped inverted last (Fig. 11.4). The innersole is nailed to the last with a single nail in front and two or more in the heel. The lining of the shoe is tacked to the innersole rim. The lining may be thin soft leather, such as horsehide, or it may be canvas. Canvas is advisable for people whose feet perspire excessively. At this point, sturdy shoes receive vertical support—counters which will be concealed in the finished shoe. To the front of the shoe, over the vamp lining, is attached a toe box, a firm piece of leather or plastic which will be covered by a "doubler" cemented to the flesh side before it is covered by the outer part of the upper. To the back of the shoe, over the quarter lining, is attached a U-shaped piece of leather, the counter.

The upper and lining are mulled (softened for shaping in a high-humidity room) and fitted snugly to the last by pulling with a hand instrument called a lasting pincer. The upper is first secured around the heel piece of the last. Then the leather of the toe end is pulled over the toe of the last. Since it requires great strength to pull this taut and well-shaped, the pull, started by hand, is quite taxing for the custom shoemaker, who completes the operation by hand, but in the factory this step is completed by a machine which not only pulls the leather but also simultaneously tucks it under the innersole and nails it to the innersole with tacks. The next step will depend on the manner in which the shoe will be made. The sewing machine, invented by Elias Howe in 1846, was adapted for sewing soles to uppers by Lyman Blake in 1858. In 1875, Goodyear invented a welt method of attaching uppers to soles, and most quality shoes for men are made in this manner.

If the shoe is to be welted, a welt or strip of leather about one-eighth to three-sixteenths inch thick is nailed around the border of the front half of

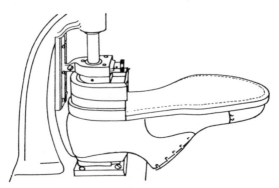

Fig. 11.4. Many steps in shoe manufacture are performed with last inverted. This step is heel alignment. (Reproduced with permission of United Shoe Machinery Corporation of Boston.)

the sole. Its primary benefit is to afford a smooth top innersole surface for comfort and strength. The welt, uppers, and innersole are pierced by an awl or sewing needle threaded with a freshly waxed multi-stranded linen thread. In hand-sewn shoes, the sewing needle is made from the split hair of a hog. Once the upper welt and innersole have been sewn to each other, the tacks are removed.

A rectangular piece of steel, about ⅟₁₆ inch thick by about 4 inches long and 1 inch wide, with a gentle curve resembling that of the natural arch, is placed on the innersole over the arch of the last. This is nailed into place through predrilled holes into the steel piece, which is called the shank (27) (Fig. 11.5). The shank is then covered with a piece of leather called the shank piece. A layer of leather, plastic, or composition is often applied from heel to toe, between the innersole and outersole, as a bottom-filler surface leveler and to reduce squeak in walking. Then, the outersole, which is cut slightly larger than the innersole and welt, is stitched to the welt or cemented to it, after being rough trimmed. Rubber or plastic cement is used. The heel base is nailed to the outersole heel seat area. If the shoe has been mulled, it is air dried. The outersole edge is trimmed, and the heel and sole bottom are buffed, inked, waxed, burnished, and stained. The front portion of the last is unlocked and the last is removed, and a heel pad is glued in place to cover heel nails and cushion the foot.

WOMEN'S SHOES

The manufacture of women's shoes is not very different from that of men's shoes. The primary difference in the U. S. is that whereas most men's shoes are welted, very few shoes for women are. Women's shoes contain a considerable amount of sewing thread, but almost all is used to join parts of the uppers or in decoration. The use of synthetic materials for heels has increased greatly from none in 1945 to about 75% in 1965. The sole of the women's shoe is usually applied with a synthetic cement such as Neoprene or Hycar. Cement is used on the heel, but nails are also used. When the sole and upper are finished, a hole is driven into the heel area from above through the heel portion of the sole into the heel. The two are held together with a screw bolt which is removed later when the cement is dry. Four or

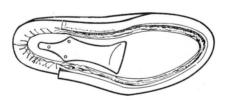

Fig. 11.5. Steel shank placement. (This illustration and most of those which follow in this chapter are reproduced with the permission of the U. S. Veterans Administration, Bulletin of Prosthetics Research, Fall, 1964, from an article by I. Zamosky.)

more nails are driven into the heel from the innersole side. The innersole of the shoe is covered with a sock liner which is made of very thin leather, kid for the finest shoes and sheepskin for less expensive shoes.

There are three principal types of shoes for women: the sandal, the oxford, and the pump (12). The sandal is primarily a sole which is held onto the foot with thongs, straps, or similar devices. It would fall off of the foot if the ties were completely undone. A pump has no ties, a very short vamp or no vamp, and it is low in the instep. It remains on the foot by virtue of the fact that the foot fills it as though the foot were poured into a funnel; in other words, by snugness of fit alone. The oxford appears to be a cross between a pump and a man's oxford. It has at least one pair of ties, and unless these are tied, the shoe will fall off during walking.

CHILDREN'S SHOES

Shoes for older children are made in a fashion quite similar to that of adults. Shoes for infants and younger children differ in three major respects; the heel is very low, the leather is soft, and the shape is that of the child's foot—straight inner border and broad toe (1). Soles and heels are made increasingly of a polyvinylchloride plastic. Uppers of expensive shoes are made of kid imported from India. Leather for uppers is classified by weight; leather which is $\frac{1}{64}$ inch thick is called 1-ounce leather. Some soles are made from leather-chromed bull hide. Shoes are lined with square weave duck to absorb perspiration. Instead of a heel in the shoe of the young child, an insert of leather is placed between the outer sole and the inner sole. Such a heel is called a *spring* heel. The heel of an older child's shoe is breasted, that is, cut to a desired or special shape for left or right or for support as in a Thomas heel. The height of a heel for a young child is usually $\frac{3}{32}$ inch. The height of the heel for growing girls should be about 1½ inches. The height of the heel for a boy will vary from ⅝ to 1 inch.

The shank of the shoe should be fairly broad at the waist of the foot, and firmness is supplied with a reinforced steel shank extending from the heel to the ball of the foot. The heel and counter should fit snugly around the heel to hold it in correct alignment.

Fitting of Shoes

A properly fitting shoe should fit the foot trimly. There should be no deep wrinkles. The joint of the large toe should be directly over the inner curve of the sole, where it starts to curve under the arch. When the toes are dorsiflexed, the break of the shoe should be indicated by lines running straight across. The upper should fit snugly around the ankle. There should be proper support for the arch, and the weight of the foot should be evenly distributed over the bottom of the foot. Depending upon the shape of the toe, there should be free space between the end of the great toe and the front of the shoe. A shoe that is comfortable will hold the back part of the foot firmly in place and will provide ample room for the toes and the ball of the foot (9).

The best test of proper fit is comfort during the period when the shoe is worn. The best immediate test is to run a dozen steps and stop short in the new shoe.

Shoe pressure may result in proliferation of the skin, commonly called corns; these may be hard or soft. Calluses or corns of upper portions of the foot may be treated by removing the source of the friction with a soft leather shoe until such time as they have disappeared and a proper fitting shoe has been supplied. Short and narrow fitted shoes distort the toes, causing them to curl with painful irritated surfaces where the skin rubs against the shoe. If the error is detected early enough in life, progress may be halted, and some correction can be gained with properly fitting shoes. Otherwise, the distortion is likely to become permanent.

It is not known whether bunions result from ill-fitting shoes alone. If shoes are too short or too narrow, the great toe, in its search for room, bends outward and may eventually overlap the adjacent toe or toes. Surgery often gives permanent relief. For those who will not accept surgery, a soft "bunion last" with a straight inner border and rounded toe of adequate size may give comfort for a long time.

If shoes are worn too short, the second toe may develop a corn on top, caused by friction. Another corn is often found on the tip where it rubs against the innersole.

The leather of a shoe is pliable largely because of the animal oils in it. When the feet perspire a great deal, the constant wetting of the lining dissolves oils from the leather, which becomes hard and cracks and which, by its increased rigidity, prevents previous comfort and adds more friction. The counters may bulge and wear away, the insole may become brittle, and the leather fibers may rot in any part of the shoe. When a shoe is short to begin with, the effects of perspiration are seen even earlier.

The fit of a shoe is of greatest importance during weight bearing, especially in walking. When fitting a shoe, the subject should be asked to walk in the shoes and to stand in them. The length of the ligaments will determine whether an A width expands to a B or C on standing. Changes in foot dimensions are greatest in feet with lax ligaments. An inspection of the old shoe will give much information about areas of pressure and need for larger sizes. Many adults demand the same size as before, and this often means a smaller size than adequate. The old shoe should be examined before a new shoe is fitted to see where it has lost its shape, for that is where the fit is wrong.

Another problem in fitting is related to the fixed idea of some people that the foot size remains constant in adult life. Many women who are style conscious remember their foot when it was a 4 B and go through life demanding that size (12). Some shoe departments will not stock shoes of C width because so many women will not wear a shoe with such a size stamped in. Pumps are fitted narrow to stay on. Nylon stockings are slippery. Therefore, when women try on a shoe, they sometimes complain that the shoe slips in the heel area, that they have a narrow heel. A chief complaint of women is that the heel of the shoe is not narrow enough.

In relation to the foot, the shoe can be considered under a number of criteria. In length, the shoe should be of sufficient length so that the end of the great toe is not against the end of the shoe. If the shoe is too long and too deep, the foot slides forwards and backwards with each walking cycle, resulting in abnormal pressures on the toes. Provision must be made for variation and length of the foot as it changes in function and length during the day. As styling is primarily done over the front part of the shoe, it is obvious that the great toe should be quite near to the tip in a square-toed shoe but about two-thirds inch away in a pointed shoe.

Just as in length, the width of the shoe should be such that the forefoot will not slide about. Basically, there should be no compression of the toes at the sides or the top. The width of the shoe should be such that the head of the first metatarsal should be free on the medial border and the head of the fifth metatarsal should be free on the lateral border.

A point on the vamp where the opening is located at the front of the shoe has a critical role in the "foot opening," the portion of the shoe that opens to accomodate the foot. The vamp point should correspond with the midpoint of a line drawn from the apex of the first metatarsphalangeal joint to the apex of the fifth toe joint. This location will ensure that the great toe joint will be positioned in a manner to secure for the foot the maximum possible support from the shank and medial aspect of the shoe upper.

Another critical factor in fit is the height over the instep. This should be of sufficient height to prevent impingement or irritation at or near the apex of the first metatarscuneiform joint. Inadequate height in this area, combined with snug lacing, will tend to push the arch downward, mechanically elongating the foot, perhaps eventually leading to symptoms of foot strain.

The height of the shoe is very critical, as painful symptoms will develop almost immediately if the height of the outside quarter exceeds that of the crease of flesh immediately under the lateral malleolus. If the height of the back part of this shoe is inadequate, the shoe will not be held securely on the foot. On the other hand, excessive height at this point will cause biting, blisters, and irritation. Elevation of the fore end of the shoe above the ground, or the toe spring, is obviously a critical factor in the locomotor function of the foot. The site of this point is often determined by the position of the toes: Do they curl up or down or are they flat? If the toe of the shoe slants down too much in the front and has little toe spring, the shoe will be uncomfortable for a person whose toes curl up.

The out-toeing of normal feet is about 7°. When the foot deviates further, the weight and pushing power are not distributed evenly, and the inner longitudinal arch receives the flattening forces of the body weight on forward motion. This tends to break down the arch. The progress of this out-toeing may be lessened by wearing a shoe with a straight inside border and an arch support to prevent swinging out and to permit the pushoff to be made with the first and second toes instead of the inner border of the foot. Pointed shoes push the large toe to the outside and encourage walking on the inner border, with callus formation on the side of the great toe. Soon the shoe follows the shape dictated by the pressures.

For the foot with a high arch, blucher shoes usually prove a more comfortable and better fit than bals. Proper fitting of the transverse arch of the foot is also important. Weakness in the metatarsal arch is seen more often in women than in men. If there is weakness, on weight bearing the metatarsal hits closer to the ground, the result being pain and soreness behind the ball of the foot. If the shoe is too short, as the foot lengthens with each step the toes strike the end of the shoe and are forced to pull or bend backward. The contracted toes press the heads of the metatarsals downward and increase the problem.

Narrow shoes also prevent the wide expansion of the foot and force the metatarsal heads downward. Increased height of the heel will also force this situation. The resulting pain and calluses under the metatarsal heads force a change in gait and may result in further foot problems.

THE HEEL

Elevated shoes and heels were worn by women in ancient times but disappeared until the Middle Ages. It was probably Louis XV, however, who was chiefly responsible for renewing the popularity of the high heel. He was a short man who did not enjoy being looked down upon by others. He demanded high heels. A form of high heel is still called the Louis heel, presumably after the monarch. The high heel has been the subject of much controversy. Dickson and Dively (8) and other physicians have condemned high heels for many reasons and point to the tottering gait of many ladies with very high heels. In view of the relatively few foot problems which can be blamed on the high heels worn by millions of women, it would seem that the high heel is not a high cause of foot problems. When women remove their shoes at the theatre or under the dining table, it is to obtain relief from tightness.

It has been said that high heels may shorten the gastrocnemius, with resultant pains and aches in the calf muscles. If such is really the case, the remedy is to lower the heel gradually and to give stretching exercises to the gastrocnemii. The heel should be lowered no more than two-eights inch at a time. It is claimed that high heels may lead to stretching and weakening of the ankle ligaments. If so, weakness leads to sprain, turned ankle, and other symptoms, and the wearer should be urged to lower the heel. A motion picture of walking feet in high heels taken from the rear should convince some wearers of the potential harm and immediate poor appearance a turned ankle makes at every step. It is said that a high heel interferes with mobility of the upper ankle because it creates an artificial equinus. Also, by increasing the slope of the sole, the foot slides forward into the waist of the shoe with poor pressure distribution.

According to Chernina and Davidowa (7), the pressure on the forefoot is approximately the same whether the subjects tested wear heels 2, 4, or 6.5 centimeters high. It would seem that it requires more than a high heel to cause a disability—perhaps frequency of use, the manner of walking, posture, and accommodation have much to do with the results of wearing high heels.

That elevated heels are not essential is proven by the fact that throughout the world, aborigines get about without them. This observation has led to the current fad of a negative heel "Earth shoe." Runners wear heel-less shoes, as man runs faster without them. However, anyone who has tried to walk without heels will recognize that they do offer several advantages. Since walking is heel-to-toe, the heel wears out before the toe, and adding a piece of leather in that position was probably first used to prolong the life of the shoe. Whether we accept the theory that heels were first introduced by Julius Caesar so that his legionnaires could walk farther and faster without fatigue or whether we believe that heels are devised for use with stirrups, it seems obvious that the heel is with us to stay, certainly in women's fashions. The high heel accentuates the curvature of the instep and arch and makes the foot seem smaller. It also shortens the step, draws attention to the foot and leg, and makes the calf appear slimmer. The most important characteristics of heels from the mechanical standpoint are the taper and the striking point. The narrower the point, the less secure the balance. Of equal importance is whether the ground contact of the heel is forward or in line with the postural plumb line. In general, the heel is used as a stilt and placed in line with the leg. Usually, heels have a wedge shape, with about ⅛ inch more in front, and are about ⅛ inch higher on the inner than on the outer side. In relation to the heel, the shank of the shoe should be molded to form a definite arch, with the highest point under the anterior half of the os calcis so that the foot may be adequately supported on its medial side to prevent pronation.

Size

Measurement of shoe size was established in 1324 by King Edward II. He decreed that three barleycorns taken from the center of the ear, placed end to end, equalled 1 inch. It was found that 39 barleycorns so placed, equalled the length of the longest "normal" foot. Because 39 was divisible only by 3, the longest normal foot was called size 13, and all other sizes were graded down by one barleycorn or ⅓ inch (22). This was later modified so that a foot of 8⅛ inches equals size one, and below this figure, the size range again starts at 13 and becomes 0 for 4 inches. Zero is the size of the shoe for an infant who is not yet walking; 3½ is for the first walking shoe. From birth to the time of walking, the shoe should be flexible to avoid restriction of movement; it should have a soft sole and no support. When weight bearing begins, little or no covering is needed, but climate and custom demand a covering. The young child needs protection from traumatizing surfaces and to have the feet held in balance (8).

In the U. S., the size of shoes varies from infant's sizes 000 to man's size 16. There are 12 widths ranging from AAAAA to EEEE, but the sizes most frequently required are A to D. The size stick listing the different sizes for men's and women's shoes is shown in Fig. 11.6. The Brannock Device (Fig. 11.7) for measuring foot size is used in most shoe stores to determine sizes by a sliding notch to fit on the ball of the great toe and a scale to read the distance. This third dimension should improve foot comfort. Unfortunately, shoes are not labeled for this particular length. For the patient who has problems being fitted, it is possible to achieve the best fit in a store that has a person knowledgeable about the anatomy of the lower extremity, the various lasts, and types of shoes and their construction. Most metropolitan areas have one or two large stores with such a person and a large inventory of shoe styles and sizes, so a physician should make himself familiar with such stores in his particular area.

Feet increase in length faster than in width, and the changes occur in spurts at various ages. In a growing foot, it is more important to maintain a balanced position of the leg than to improve muscle control of the foot since the effectiveness of muscle action is dependent upon a balanced position of the foot. Excessive pronation is the primary deformity in the unbalanced foot of childhood. In mild cases, a flat pad or cookie can be placed in the shoe to roll out or elevate the arch. The highest point on the inside will lie well in back of the sustentaculum tali, not forward under the navicular. In this position the support exerts an upward thrust preventing pronation of the calcaneus and depression of the subtalar joint.

Infants are best started out in a high-top shoe but after the age of 2, lower-cut shoes are sufficient if the ankle is stable. Straight-lasted and wide square toe boxes are generally all that are needed in children's shoes. Furthermore, tennis shoes or sneakers of adequate fit are quite acceptable for growing children with normal feet. Although many authorities have an opinion that a firm orthopedic shoe is needed to maintain and develop normal arch, this concept has never been proven. It is also clear that the effect of many shoe corrections in children is minimized because many positions adopted by children never involve walking, and there have never been many long-term control studies proving scientifically that shoe corrections are particularly effective.

When we learn from last and shoe manufacturers that 40% of people with "normal" feet have shoe problems, we can appreciate that those with

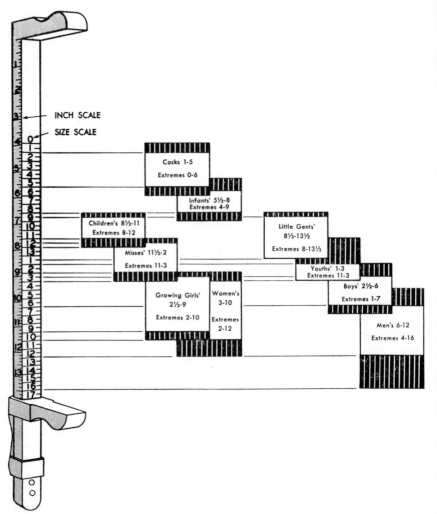

INCH SCALE

SIZE SCALE

Cacks 1-5
Extremes 0-6

Infants' 5½-8
Extremes 4-9

Children's 8½-11
Extremes 8-12

Little Gents'
8½-13½
Extremes 8-13½

Misses' 11½-2
Extremes 11-3

Youths' 1-3
Extremes 11-3

Boys' 2½-6
Extremes 1-7

Growing Girls'
2½-9
Extremes 2-10

Women's
3-10
Extremes
2-12

Men's 6-12
Extremes 4-16

Fig. 11.6. Sketch of simple stick measuring device with shoe size classification. (Reproduced with permission from United Shoe Machinery Corporation of Boston).

abnormal feet must solve the multiple problems of fit, pain, shape, gait, and weight bearing. Shoe modifications are even more important when fitting a person who must wear an orthosis. Such a device will be ineffective if the construction of the shoe is inadequate. Helpful advice concerning types and styles of shoes to fit the newer type of lower extremity orthotic devices has recently been provided by Rubin and associates (21).

The manner in which weight bearing is distributed over the sole remains controversial. There are those who support the three-point pattern shown in Fig. 11.8, that is, weight bearing upon the apex of the plantar surface of

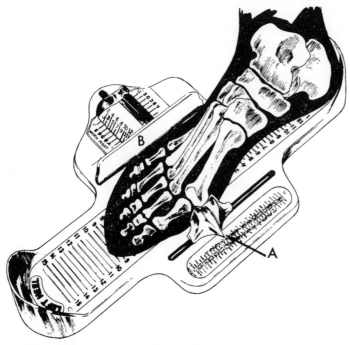

Fig. 11.7. Brannock device for measuring foot size. *A*, movable ball indicator, for length; *B*, movable rail for measuring width. (Courtesy of the Brannock Company of Syracuse.)

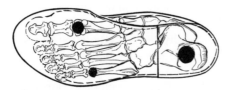

Fig. 11.8. Three-point weight-bearing pattern. Body weight distributed evenly between apex of the calcaneus and the first and fifth metatarsal heads, according to one school of thought.

the calcaneus, the first metatarsal head, and the fifth metatarsal head. Others point to the finding that the second and third metatarsal heads are more anterior than the first and fifth, indicating that they bear more of the weight. This school maintains that there is no actual arch of metatarsal heads during weight bearing. They insist that in pathologic weight bearing, callosities are noted under the metatarsal heads which bear most weight. This is seen over the second and third metatarsal heads quite often. Thus a shoe modification for metatarsal difficulties would distribute the weight as evenly as possible on all five metatarsal heads.

The location, shape, and size of the modifications can be determined by temporarily taping or gluing components to an unmodified stock shoe. Observation of the gait pattern and examination of the shoe bottom for proper tread will indicate the need for any further changes. If extensive changes are necessary, orthopedic shoes should be recommended. Our concern is with modifications that can be made with stock shoes that are available at almost any store.

CHECKING STOCK SHOES

Before prescribing modifications we must check out the stock shoe (Fig. 11.3). The shoe should afford ample width from the metatarsophalangeal joints anteriorly to the ends of the distal phalanges, to allow the greatest amount of toe prehension possible at pushoff. A comfortable but snug fit from the waist of the shoe to its heel is necessary for support and to prevent motion at the quarters during dorsiflexion. The straight inner border, or, as it is sometimes called, the straight innerline combination last, offers these features. By combination is meant a wide or narrow heel with appropriate ball width to achieve proper heel-to-ball conformity; for example, many patients require a very narrow heel with a normal ball width, or vice versa. Because the foot elongates during walking, the front end of the insole should extend ⅝ inch beyond the tip of the great toe.

If there is a clawfoot or hammertoe, the vamp should be raised to provide pressure relief.

The outsole should be made of prime leather, about ¼ inch thick. The heel should be about ¾ inch high and broad enough for stability.

The shoe should include a steel shank that extends from the midheel to the ball of the foot (Fig. 11.5). Proper placement and rigidity of the shoe shank can be determined by holding the shoe in one hand and trying to dorsiflex it with the other. If the shoe bends at the break without too much depression behind that point, the steel shank is correctly placed. With the shoe shank properly placed (¼ to ⅜ inch posterior to the break of the shoe), dorsiflexion of the shoe on the foot will be congruent with that of the metatarsophalangeal joints for rollover. If, however, the shoe shank is placed in front of the break of a low quarter shoe, dorsiflexion will force the quarters distally away from the foot, incurring a great amount of undesirable piston motion in walking. With the more extensive instep and ankle coverage of the chukka or high-quarter shoe, great pressure would be borne at the instep of the foot. If, however, the shoe shank is placed too far behind the break, dorsiflexion will force the longitudinal arches of the foot to depress and the weight-bearing heel surface to shift toward the heel breastline. A foot-slap type of gait in midstance, with possible depression of the medial and lateral longitudinal arches of the foot and ensuing pain, may result from those conditions. Placing the steel shank at the breakline would greatly shorten the life of the shoe since repeated dorsiflexion during ambulation would force the anterior edge of the shank to perforate the outsole.

For metal brace wearers, it is essential that a solid sole be used. If crepe or composition rubber were used, the sole would compress under the vertical load and introduce undesirable pseudoplantar flexion-dorsiflexion and varus-valgus motions. The shoe should also include a steel shank that extends from approximately midheel to the ball of the foot.

For patients with cavus, additional checking will include the height (or depth) of the toe box and the metatarsal region, in addition to the length and width.

Shoe Styles

The stock shoe for men comes in several styles, including the blucher, the bal, the chukka, and the convalescent (bicycle) or postsurgical shoe (Fig. 11.2). The blucher is a laced shoe with a plain toe, the quarters of which, loose at the inner edge, extend forward over the throat of the vamp. The construction affords easy access for the foot, even with limitation in ankle motion.

Although it has front lacing, the bal has less easy access because the vamp is sewn over the quarters at the front of the throat. This shoe is usually prescribed only when there is no problem with the forefoot, for example, in heel elevation where leg shortening exists without foot or ankle deformity.

The convalescent or surgical shoe (Fig. 11.2d), a special variation of the blucher, is prescribed after foot surgery or for the ankylosed foot. The convalescent shoe has lacing to the toes, and the toecap is formed by the extension of the tongue to the front of the outsole. Such a design provides easy entry for the foot that is spastic or cannot be plantar flexed.

Blucher and bal styles are available in low-quarter (1½ inch below the malleoli) and the high-quarter upper (about 2 inches above the malleoli). A shoe with a three-quarter upper that goes to the apices of the malleoli is called a chukka (Fig. 11.9A). The extensive coverage of the foot provided by the chukka and the high-quarter uppers helps to prevent piston motion during walking (which may cause a painful chafing of the calf) and thus is desirable for limited or stiff joints.

The chukka with lacing (Fig. 11.9A) is particularly desirable for a foot with scars that might be abraded by the top edge of a low-quarter shoe. The chukka with strap and buckle (Fig. 11.9B) is often recommended for the patient with poor finger dexterity. A variation that further facilitates donning is the low-quarter with clip fastener tongue (Fig. 11.9C). When the tongue is pushed forward, the patient can put on his shoe with a long shoehorn or by pushing the shoe tip against a wall. With his foot in the shoes he need only tap the clip tongue to close it, in which position it will remain secure until pushed forward for removal. Another variation that achieves the same goal is the low quarter with elastic goring on the medial and lateral sides of the quarters. The use of the elastic laces or Velcro closure on the blucher low-quarter shoe with a long shoehorn will also help

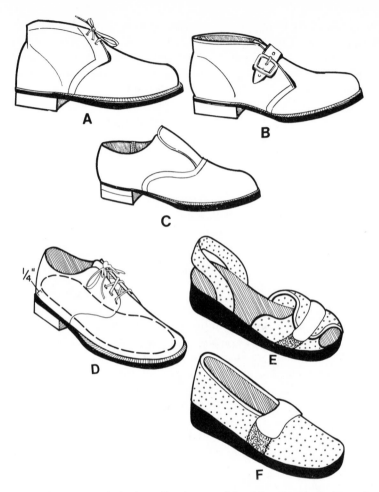

Fig. 11.9. Fasteners. *A*, lacing; *B*, strap and buckle; *C*, clip fastener tongue; special shoes. *D*, extradepth shoe; *E*, Plastazote sandal; *F*, Plastazote shoe.

the patient with poor finger dexterity or lack of hip flexion to put on his shoes.

The extra depth or adjustable insole shoe (Fig. 11.9*D*) available in several men's and women's styles provide the space needed for accommodating abnormalities, particularly in the metatarsal or phalangeal area, as occurs in many arthritics. During the "lasting" procedure of shoe fabrication, an extra insole ¼ inch thick is included. This insole is removable to increase depth ¼ inch in all aspects or can be cut transversely at the waist area of the foot to allow room to treat abnormalities of the forefoot.

Excavation of the surface or preheating the insole with immediate application to the weight-bearing foot may be used to treat sensitive heels, individual callosities, plantar warts, scars, or painful distal ends of the phalanges. In difficult problems the insole can be replaced by a customized insole made from a cast of the patient's foot. This new style of shoe will probably replace many custom made shoes, as it costs little more than a regular shoe.

Extradepth shoes combine the advantages of a stock shoe with those of the custom-made shoe. Some of the advantages are:

1. They come in many styles and are relatively inexpensive.
2. The added depth permits the fitting of a unilateral plastic orthosis, without the need for a mismatched pair of stock shoes.
3. Leg length and foot size discrepancy from such conditions as poliomyelitis can be accommodated readily.
4. These shoes can accommodate or correct gross foot deformities, as shoe modifications are more readily made than in stock shoes.
5. Fluctuating edema of the foot can be accommodated by removing the insole. The same advantage is also available if surgical dressings are required.

Introduction of low temperature foam thermoplastic materials has introduced a new type of custom-made or easily modified shoe. This is the Plastazote shoe and sandal (Fig. 11.9, *E* and *F*), which affords a lightweight adjustable material for the foot with insensitive skin, painful arthritic joints, or postoperative conditions and allergies (10).

Plastazote is a hypoallergenic, inert, nontoxic material described in Chapter 3, Materials for Orthotics. The advantages of Plastazote shoe (Dermaplast shoe, Apex Foot Products, New York, N. Y.) include heat adjustability for a custom fit, easy modification for changes of conditions, and Velcro closures for patients with problems in tying shoes. The shoes are less than 16 ounces in weight and can be hand washed.

The shoe also has two removable ¼-inch-thick insoles to allow space for modifications if needed. The Plastazote insole can be heated and the patient can have a molded insole made for the shoe or molded insole used alone in the sandal. Instructions for making the sandals and how to obtain materials for them have been given by Brand and his associates (5).

TOE DESIGN

The front of the shoe is usually available in one of five designs: plain, straight tip, wing tip, moccasin, or U-tip (Fig. 11.10). The blucher and bal are available in all five styles, but the chukka is made in only the first three. The plain toe is the most practical for all orthopedic shoes since the absence of excessive stitching and overlays allows a smooth inner shoe surface which reduces the possibility of foot abrasions. The other types are not generally recommended for those who need special shoes.

Although the plain toe and moccasin foreparts have no special decoration,

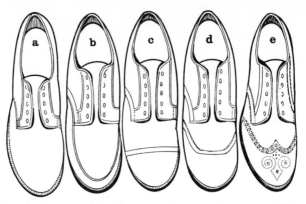

Fig. 11.10. Toe designs. *a*, plain; *b*, moccasin; *c*, straight tip; *d*, U-tip; *e*, wing.

the straight, wing, and U-tips may have pinking, medallions, perforations, or imitation foxing at the quarters. These designs are purely decorative.

Orthotic Attachments

The choice of lower extremity orthotic attachment is affected by the outsole material since the attachment and shoe must be joined to each other rigidly (21). The sole should be of prime leather at least 12 irons thick. If the sole is of rubber, Neolite, Neoprene, or crepe rubber, a rigid union is not possible, even for the simplest attachments (2).

The types of attachments most commonly used are the stirrup, caliper box, and footplate. They may be used as stiff-ankle joints with no motion, with limited motion, with solid or spring-loaded stops, or with free-motion ankle joints. (see Chapter 9).

The stresses applied to the shoe through the orthotic attachment tend to distort the shoe, particularly in the longitudinal arch area. Since the stock shoes purchased by most patients usually contain inferior sole materials and either no shank, a wood shank, or a poor-quality steel shank, proper reinforcement is necessary to prevent depression of the longitudinal arch. Another cause for failure of the longitudinal arch of the shoe is that many prefabricated shoe attachments have narrow tongues with insufficient area for selecting rivet locations (Fig. 11.11). The orthotist is forced to rivet through the center of the steel shank, causing a cross-sectional failure in a short time. If the orthotist cannot influence the manufacturer of such attachments, he can weld or braze a reinforcement plate over the tongue and heel of the regular attachment, shaping the tongue of the plate broadly (Fig. 11.11). The broadened tongue affords sufficient area for selection of rivet locations which will bypass the underlying steel shank and thus eliminate possible perforation and failure of the shank (2).

The effects of shoe distortion caused by poor material or shank failure are obvious. When the longitudinal arch of the shoe depresses sufficiently,

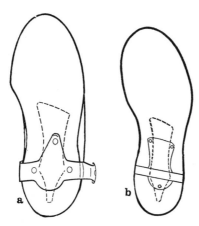

Fig. 11.11. Orthotic attachments. *a*, prefabricated stirrup riveted to shoe (shank perforation); *b*, orthotist-modified caliper box riveted to shoe (shank unperforated at midportion).

the patient may feel pain or discomfort in any or all of the tarsometatarsal and talocalcaneocuboid joints; the subtalar and tibiotalar joints may also be affected. To relieve this discomfort the patient tends to flex his knee, reducing the stress on the brace and shoe but producing an undesirable gait characteristic.

In joining the heelbase and heel to the exposed outsole and brace attachment, holes are generally drilled into the attachment (to assist in nailing) close to the edges of the anterior radii formed by the stirrup uprights and that part of the stirrup in contact with the outsole. These points are normally vulnerable to vertical load and are drastically weakened by the holes. With limited-motion or rigid-stop ankle joints, a cross-sectional failure may be expected at those points after a comparatively short period of wear. To prevent such failures, a cement (such as epoxy or 4110 Laminac Resin) may be used to join the heel and heelbase to the outsole and brace attachment without drilling holes through the latter.

Foot Disabilities

Foot disabilities for which devices for arch support and lateral weight shift are designed include pes planus, pes cavus, and pes valgus. In typical pes planus, the medial longitudinal arch is depressed, causing the navicular bone to become prominent and the forefoot to abduct or pronate. This is a common flaccid flatfoot:—a long slender foot with relaxed tendons and hypermobility of the articular surfaces of all joints. It is often not particularly painful. In adults, most commonly seen is a foot with muscle spasm or ligamentous strain in the lateral longitudinal arch. This may or may not be accompanied by flattening of the long arch or abduction of the forefoot. Physical therapy, including exercises for correct foot posture, should be prescribed. However, a foot support should be prescribed as well because physical therapy alone cannot remove the excessive forces straining the ligaments of the foot.

Pes cavus is characterised by medial and lateral longitudinal arches that are high. This can be congenital or can be a result of shortened extensor tendons of the dorsum with depression of the metatarsus. The flexor tendons may also be involved, and the plantar fascia becomes rigid. Deformity is caused by imbalance of forces in the muscles between the extrinsic and intrinsic muscles which may be congenital or acquired and with or without any recognizable neurological disease. This is typically seen, for example, in a patient with a paralysis of the plantar flexor muscles. Pes cavus may require support to prevent pain in the longitudinal arches.

In pes valgus, the lateral aspect of the plantar surface of the foot is elevated with respect to the medial aspect, i.e., the medial longitudinal arch is depressed, and the subtalar and tibiotalar joints stretch at their medial ligamentous connections, causing the medial malleolus to protrude. Prominence is noted on the medial border of the foot, particularly in the talonavicular region, and this is associated with forefoot abduction. From the posterior view, the calcaneus is in the typical valgus posture, that is, the inferior aspect of the calcaneus is displaced laterally with respect to the proximal part. This condition may be associated with spastic or flaccid muscle states and often requires both support and weight shift.

It should be noted that the key to pes valgus and pes varus is really the posture of the calcaneus and its resulting effect on the whole hind foot. If the calcaneus is in valgus, the foot tends to flatten or assume a planus position; if in varus, the foot arch increases and assumes a cavus position. Furthermore, if the horizontal angle of the subtalar or talocalcaneal joint with respect to the floor decreases (normal is around 45°), pes planus generally results; if it increases, pes cavus occurs.

Motions of the subtalar joint have direct effects on the talonavicular joint (the principal moving component of the midtarsal articulation which is a combination of the talonavicular and calcaneocuboid joints). These joints are intimately linked in function both in normal and abnormal foot posture, as described by Inman (11).

The posture of the calcaneus not only affects the hind foot but may cause the whole forefoot to alter its posture. If the calcaneus is in excessive valgus, the foot excessively pronates, that is, the whole foot everts and the forefoot abducts with respect to the hindfoot. If it is in excessive varus, the foot excessively supinates, that is, the whole foot inverts, and the forefoot adducts with respect to the hindfoot.

Shoe Modifications

The purpose of shoe modifications is to restore foot balance in standing and walking, to achieve a pressure pattern on the sole of the foot in which the weight is distributed between the first and fifth metatarsal heads and

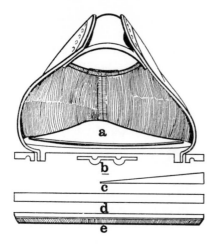

Fig. 11.12. Metatarsal cross-sectional view of shoe and modifications. *a*, metatarsal pad insert; *b*, steel sandwich shank; *c*, lateral sole wedge (sandwich); *d*, outsole; *e*, overlay (rocker bar).

the apex of the plantar surface of the heel. If the foot has a normal calcaneus (not tilted anteriorly or posteriorly), its position in the shoe can generally be used as a reference point for modifications within the shoe, usually located at the midpoint of the heel.

Inserts and sandwich modifications are classed as internal components, and overlays are classified as external components (Fig. 11.12). An insert is placed over the surface of the insole; it may be removable or permanently mounted. A sandwich may be placed between the insole and outsole between the heel seat and the heelbase, or between the heelbase and the heel.

Arch Support and Lateral Weight Shift

The following components are listed in order of the amount of support that they provide to effect medial longitudinal arch support and lateral weight shift:

Internal	External
1. Steel shank in shoe	6. Thomas heel
2. Cookie insole and insert	7. Thomas heel wedge
3. Navicular (scaphoid) pad	8. Medial sole and heel wedge
4. Longitudinal arch support	9. Medial shank filler
5. Long counter on medial side	10. Valgus strap

External arch supports must be considered largely as adjuvants with the possible exception of the valgus strap which, when used with an orthosis is quite effective.

MODIFICATIONS FOR LATERAL WEIGHT SHIFT

Steel Shank in Shoes

Most custom and stock orthopedic or fine stock shoes contain a steel shank to provide adequate arch support on the medial side. If the shank is not positioned as explained under checkout, it will not function properly. If the steel is of poor quality, the longitudinal arch of the shoe will sag with prolonged weight bearing. The posterior end of the steel shank should be at least ½ inch in back of the plantar apex of the calcaneus and extend anteriorly to a point ¼ to ⅜ inch posterior to the break of the shoe. The width of the steel shank is determined by the width of the shoe, weight of the wearer, type of brace, and occupation of the patient. Since the inexpensive shoe rarely includes an adequate steel shank, it is often advisable to remove the original shank and install an adequate support.

Cookie Insert or Insole

If a steel shank does not provide enough support for the longitudinal arch, the addition of a cookie may. The cookie is usually made of rigid shoulder leather and is in the shape of the longitudinal arch with the highest point in the region of the talonavicular joint (Fig. 11.13). It should extend from about 1¼ inches behind the heel breastline to about ½ inch behind the first metatarsal head. The medial edge, which is feathered, should lie against the quarter lining on the medial side of the longitudinal arch. The distal surface of the cookie lies against the insole. It provides a more rigid support when used with a long counter on the medial side. The cookie insole is an integral part of the orthopedic or prescribed shoe. A cookie may be inserted at any time in any shoe. Cookies are available in different sizes and may be cemented in place permanently.

Navicular (Scaphoid) Pad

The navicular pad is also designed to provide additional support for the longitudinal arch on the medial side. It is usually placed in the same part of the shoe as the cookie and has the same contour. It provides better support if used with a long counter on the medial side. To provide a resilient support, the navicular pad is made of compressible material such as sponge rubber of various durometers of hardness; the rubber surfaces are covered with leather for comfort. The navicular pad is generally prescribed for patients who cannot tolerate the rigidity of a cookie.

A *longitudinal arch support* may be prescribed where broader areas of support for the medial longitudinal arch are required. The broad extent of

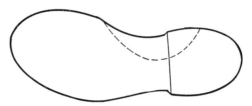

Fig. 11.13. Placement of cookie insert (navicular pad).

the arch support tends to shift the body weight laterally and in some cases may preclude the use of a valgus strap. Longitudinal arch supports are available in metal, plastic, or leather. Sometimes it is necessary to hammer, heat, or bend them for good fit.

Metal longitudinal arch supports, such as the Whitman plate, are not indicated in children and rarely useful in adults as they have been replaced by a newer plastic material. The most widely used and successful introduction in arch supports has been the UCBL laminated insert (11). This is a semirigid plastic-laminated shoe insert based on biomechanical concepts of foot movement and provides not only support for the sole, but also positioning of the heel in the correct posture. This shoe insert must be custom-made from a cast.

Long Counter (Medial)

The medial counter on the stock shoe usually extends to about ⅜ to ½ inch forward of the heel breast (Fig. 11.14). In the stock shoe with orthopedic features, it extends about midway between the heel breast and the break of the shoe, thus providing additional support for the longitudinal arch. Regardless of the shoe type, the counter is usually made of shoulder leather since its function is to provide a rigid wall to retain the foot in the desired alignment. The entire counter is sandwiched between the quarter lining and the quarter of the upper during the lasting step of shoe manufacture. Even with a long medial counter in the stock shoe with orthopedic features, it is sometimes necessary to use a cookie or navicular pad as well. The counter in the custom orthopedic shoe will provide more effective support because of the closer conformity of the longitudinal arches of the foot and shoe.

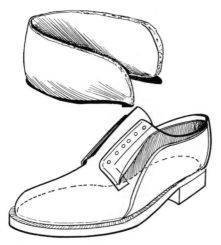

Fig. 11.14. Long medial counter.

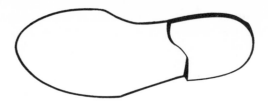

Fig. 11.15. Orthopedic, or Thomas heel.

Orthopedic (Thomas) Heel

The orthopedic (Thomas) heel is similar in appearance and material to a standard heel, except for the extension of the medial heel breastline (Fig. 11.15). In the stock shoe with orthopedic features, the anterior projection of the medial breast of the Thomas heel extends about ½ inch forward of the normal breastline, at which point it is directly under the navicular bone. In the custom orthopedic shoe, it may extend to any desired length, giving more extensive support to the medial longitudinal arch. The Thomas heel provides additional support and stability to the medial longitudinal arch. The Thomas heel is sometimes called an S-shaped or keystone heel. It is available as a half heel in several sizes but can be made in the shop from Neoprene or crepe rubber or from a standard rubber heel which is as long as the projection required.

Orthopedic (Thomas) Heel Wedge

If it is desirable to increase the medial longitudinal support more than provided by the Thomas heel, a medial wedge for the heel may be prescribed. The wedge is made of shoulder leather ¹⁄₁₆ to ⁵⁄₁₆ inch thick, depending upon the weight of the patient and the amount of support desired. Since it augments the function of the orthopedic heel, the wedge is usually sandwiched between the heelbase and outsole over the area of the forward extension of the heel, though it may also be applied between the heel and heelbase.

Medial Wedging

Medial wedging may be prescribed if there is a greater need for shifting the body weight laterally than for support of the medial longitudinal arch alone. Wedges for this purpose may be applied to the sole or the heel, or over the full length of the sole and heel. Medial wedges are generally made of shoulder leather, although other material may be used.

Sole wedges are modifications that are intended to shift the body weight from the medial to the lateral side of the tarsal and metatarsal aspect of the foot. The medial sole wedge is seldom used as a corrective device unless, for some reason, the patient wears off the inner border of the sole in walking so rapidly that it must be resoled too often. For correction of weak feet and flat feet, a lateral sole wedge in conjunction with a medial heel wedge is the most common combination used. This produces a tendency to invert or supinate the heel, and abduct, evert, or pronate the forefoot, the combination of which results in elevation and support of the long arch.

The sole wedge is best placed over the outsole (the overlay) starting midway between the medial heel breastline and the break of the shoe, extending to the front end of the sole. Laterally, the sole wedge extends approximately to the longitudinal midline of the sole. Its lateral expansion depends upon the total elevation of the wedge since the most gradual feathering is used to avoid creating "pockets" on the sole which do not touch the ground. As an overlay, rather than a sandwich, the thinner insole is not distorted, and there is less likelihood of significant pressures being transmitted to the plantar surface of the foot. Another advantage of applying the wedge as an overlay is its ease of adjustment or replacement without damage to the outsole or welt. Walking on the replaceable wedge rather than on the sole also prolongs the shoe life.

Heel wedges are used to shift the weight laterally in the region of the talocalcaneal and talonavicular joints. A heel wedge may also be used to counteract the effect of a lateral sole wedge and prevent an uneven tread pattern (cross wedging). The heel wedge should be sandwiched between the outsole and the brace attachment and the heel; however, if it is placed between the brace attachment and the heel, the effect of the lateral weight shift would cause tilting of the limb and brace. The effect on the gait pattern would be undesirable since there would be a tendency toward adduction of the limb.

Sole-and-heel wedges are prescribed for the foot which bears too much weight on the medial side, as in valgus or in depression of the medial longitudinal arch. The wedges are often used in conjunction with a longitudinal arch support insert to augment the effect of a lateral weight shift along the entire length of the foot. This type of wedge may be applied as a unit which extends the full length of the sole and heel, or it may be applied in two sections, sole and heel (Fig. 11.16).

The heel-and-sole wedges offer more longitudinal support than the separate section. Its effectiveness in shifting body weight laterally is approximately the same. The combined wedge is inserted as a unit overlay of the outsole and laid under the heelbase in the conventional manner. The portion extending over the medial longitudinal area gives longitudinal support by its added substance, which reinforces the outside and, to some extent, the shoe shank.

Medial shank fillers are prescribed where the weight of the patient depresses the longitudinal arch in the shoe. By its characteristic shape, the medial shank filler eliminates the void existing between the ground and the medial plantar surface of the longitudinal arch of the shoe (Fig. 11.17). Increasing the height, elevation, and lateral weight shift can aid a depressed medial longitudinal arch or valgus condition. This component extends from

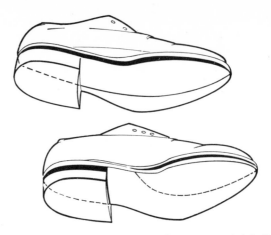

Fig. 11.16. Medial sole-and-heel wedging. *Bottom,* sandwich (in two sections); *above,* as an overlay unit extending the full length of the sole and heel.

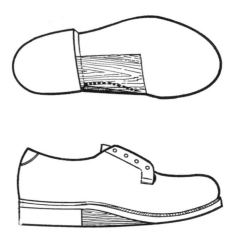

Fig. 11.17. Medial shank filler. *Above,* plantar view; *below,* medial view.

the medial breastline anteriorly to the head of the first metatarsal, at which point the shank filler is feathered and blends into the level of the outsole at the break of the shoe. Laterally, the filler can extend from the breastline to afford adequate longitudinal arch support. This extension would be carried forward to a point at the line of the metatarsal heads where it too would feather and blend into the level of the outsole at the break of the shoe.

The *valgus strap* (*T-strap*) is applied medially in conjunction with an orthosis to prevent the foot and ankle from assuming a valgus attitude (Fig. 11.18). In spasticity or muscle contracture, where the foot, even when unweighted, intermittently or continuously assumes a valgus position, the strap maintains good mediolateral alignment. The strap prevents the foot

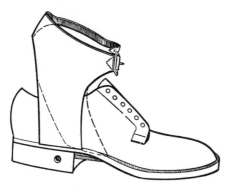

Fig. 11.18. Valgus corrective strap. *Dotted line* indicates more effective placement. Note hole in heel for caliper box attachment.

from going into valgus by opposing the spastic or contracted muscles. It may also be used in mild spasticity and the contracture of flaccidity where the foot assumes a valgus attitude only on bearing weight.

For efficiency, the valgus strap should lift or prevent depression in four areas: (a) the medial anterior aspect of the talocalcaneal joint; (b) the talonavicular joint; (c) the navicular-first-cuneiform joint; and (d) the first cuneiform base of the first metatarsal joint. Therefore, the area of attachment for the distal end of the strap should be from a point ½ inch posterior to the medial breastline (or ½ inch plus the length of the medial projection of a Thomas heel) to a point approximately 60% of the distance between the heel breast and the break of the shoe.

For cosmetic reasons, however, the distal attachment of the strap is frequently placed more posteriorly, extending anteriorly approximately to the breastline of the heel. The reason for this posterior attachment is to position equivalent amounts of material on either side of the brace uprights for shoe attachment. In this position, the force of the strap is applied primarily in the area of the calcaneus and talus, and the effect on the foot is reduced due to the relative motion between the talus and navicular, navicular and first cuneiform, and first cuneiform and base of the first metatarsal.

From its distal attachment, the strap extends proximally to a point about 1½ inches above the apex of the medial malleolus, where it divides into an anterior and a posterior strap encircling the leg and the lateral brace upright and then buckles on the lateral side.

Lateral Longitudinal Arch Support

The following components are listed according to the amount of support they provide to effect lateral longitudinal arch support and medial weight shift.

Internal	External
Long counter on the lateral side	Lateral heel and sole wedge
Lateral heel wedge insert	Reverse orthopedic heel
	Lateral shank filler
	Lateral flaring of sole and heel
	Varus strap

Disabilities of the foot for which the components listed above are used include lateral pes planus, varus, and ankylosis.

In *lateral pes planus,* the lateral longitudinal arch is depressed. This causes the base of the fifth metatarsal and the cuboid bones to protrude at their plantar surfaces. The forefoot will usually adduct. As in medial pes planus, we should give support or elevation for relief.

In *varus,* the medial aspect of the plantar surface of the foot is elevated, and the lateral longitudinal arch is depressed. The subtalar and tibiotalar joints lean and stretch at their lateral ligamentous connections, causing the lateral malleolus to protrude. Support and weight shift are often required for relief and restoration of foot-ankle alignment.

With *ankylosis,* fixation of the articular surfaces of margins of the joints of the lateral longitudinal arch allows only slight passive motion or none at all. Pain, experienced when movements toward varus or valgus occur, is usually relieved by the support of a lateral wall with an extended (flare) base (13).

MODIFICATIONS FOR MEDIAL WEIGHT SHIFT

A *long counter on the lateral side* helps prevent depression of the lateral longitudinal arch by providing a rigid wall which restricts movement of the foot into varus. To provide the most effective support, the anterior extent of the counter should end at a point just behind the fifth metatarsal head. The long counter can be simulated by gluing a prefabricated or preshaped half counter into a stock shoe, but the shoe must be wide enough to allow for this modification. The extended counter can be covered with a thin piece of leather for comfort.

A *lateral heel wedge insert* (Fig. 11.19) may be indicated if the long counter does not provide sufficient lateral support. This modification raises the lateral longitudinal arch and shifts the body weight toward the medial side of the foot. In some flaccid feet it may obviate a varus strap.

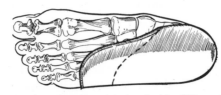

Fig. 11.19. Lateral heel-wedge insert extended to fifth metatarsal head. *Dotted line* indicates position of lateral heel wedge insert to fifth metatarsal base.

The wedge is placed inside the shoe with the thickest section beneath the lateral weight-bearing point of the calcaneus. When properly fabricated and installed, the insert should provide additional support in the area of the base of the fifth metatarsal; this will also give slight support at the plantar protuberance of the cuboid bone. If it does not provide such support, some of its effectiveness is lost through the relative motion between the bones of the midfoot and the forefoot.

Although sponge rubber in varying durometers of hardness is frequently used, other materials, such as leather and cork, are also suitable. The material is covered with thin leather or plastic sheeting, and the insert may be glued permanently or left removable.

Lateral Wedge (Sandwich)

The external lateral *heel* wedge serves the same purpose as the internal insert, but gives less support since it does not conform directly to the foot and extends only to the breast of the heel. If it is sandwiched between the brace attachment and the outsole, it will be somewhat useful in preventing a varus inclination of the talocalcaneal and tibiotalar joints. If, however, the lateral heel wedge is sandwiched between the brace attachment and the heelbase, the weight of the limb is shifted by the tilting of the brace, which causes undesirable pressure points on the thigh and leg. A lateral heel wedge properly applied can relieve or correct a flaccid genu varum with or without a side-pulling kneecap. The angle of the flaccid ankle joint in varus should, during the stance phase of gait, also be reduced and approach normal alignment.

Sole Wedge

A medial longitudinal arch support or a medial heel wedge designed to shift the body weight laterally may require compensation in the form of a lateral sole wedge (cross-wedging). This may also be indicated for depression of the lateral longitudinal arch in the area from the head of the fifth metatarsal to its base, including the anterior third of the cuboid.

As mentioned above, the lateral wedge is more effective as an overlay than as a sandwich. When properly installed, its lateral side extends from a point about 1½ inches behind the break of the shoe to the anterior tip of the sole, with its highest point slightly behind the head of the fifth metatarsal. Its medial extension is governed by the total elevation of the wedge and the need for very gradual feathering. As it slopes medially, however, it provides additional support for the heads of the fourth and fifth metatarsals.

Sole and Heel Wedge

For varus or club feet with residual deformities, where surgical correction is not possible, wedging of the outer border of the heel and sole is indicated, possibly with flaring of the heel and sole. Lateral wedges are relatively ineffective against varus. However, in young children with nonrigid deformities or tendency to toe-in, as in metatarsus varus or pigeon toe, a lateral sole wedge may be helpful. In fixed varus deformity, wedging is ineffective; surgical correction is the treatment of choice, and if this is not possible, bracing.

Reverse Orthopedic (Thomas) Heel

As mentioned above, orthopedic heels are available commercially as half heels in a range of sizes. Their distinguishing feature is the anterior projection of the medial side of the heel breasting. When applied to the heel base, they provide support for the medial longitudinal arch. If it is desirable to support the lateral longitudinal arch, a "left" orthopedic heel is used on the right side and vice versa (Fig. 11.20). This variation is seldom used.

The projection of the reverse orthopedic heel extends from ½ inch anterior to the normal heel breastline and is located beneath the lateral prominence of the base of the fifth metatarsal. It therefore provides support in the areas of the calcaneocuboid and the fifth tarsometatarsal joints.

A *lateral shank filler* is prescribed when the patient's weight requires additional support for the lateral longitudinal arches of the foot and shoe. With the characteristic shape of the medial shank filler, the lateral shank filler eliminates the void existing between the ground and the lateral plantar surface of the longitudinal arch of the shoe (Fig. 11.21). By increasing the height, elevation and medial weight shift can aid a depressed lateral longi-

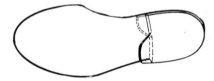

Fig. 11.20. Reverse orthopedic heel. *Dotted line* indicates position of regular orthopedic heel.

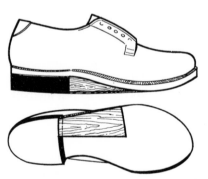

Fig. 11.21. Lateral shank filler. *Above,* lateral view; *below,* plantar view.

tudinal arch and varus condition involving the calcaneocuboid, fifth tarso-metatarsal, and the subtalar and tibiotalar joints. This shank filler extends from the lateral breastline anteriorly to the head of the fifth metatarsal, at which point it is feathered into the level of the outsole at the break of the shoe. Medially, it can extend from the breastline to a point necessary for adequate longitudinal arch support. This extent would be carried anteriorly to a point at the line of the metatarsal heads where it, too, would feather into the level of the outsole at the break of the shoe.

Lateral Flaring of Sole and Heel

In painful ankylosis following unsuccessful arthrodesis of the tibiotalar, subtalar, talonavicular, calcaneocuboid, or tarsometatarsal joints, the tendency of the foot toward varus should be prevented by flaring the heel, sole, or both on the lateral side (Fig. 11.22). The extent of the flare will depend upon the degree of restraint needed and is determined by trial and error. The medial longitudinal arch should be supported adequately at the same time to prevent medial weight shift.

Flaring the heel alone will suffice to discourage varus in the area of the tibiotalar, subtalar, and the calcaneocuboid joints. The heel is removed, and the heelbase and outsole are cut on the bias with the feathered edge on the lateral side. A piece of heelbase and a piece of outsole leather are shaped with their lateral shoulders flared to replace the cutaway portions. A heel is attached to the base, and its lateral wall is flared to match the heelbase and to provide the desired degree of flaring at its plantar surface.

In the custom orthopedic shoe, the outsole can be prepared initially for sufficient flaring. At that point, however, it is important that the broadened plantar surface of the heel not include wedging to any degree since a moment toward valgus or medial longitudinal arch depression should be

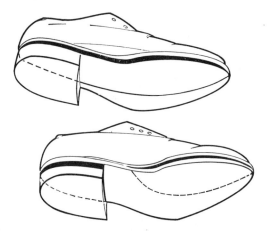

Fig. 11.22. Lateral flaring of sole and heel. *Above,* plantar view; *below,* lateral view.

prevented. To augment the flare further, a thicker more-rigid-than-usual long counter on the lateral side can be simulated as a glue-in over the lateral quarter lining. If this kind of restraint is required over a broader area, extending into the tarsometatarsal region, a reverse orthopedic heel or lateral shank filler may be installed with a flare in the same way.

Flaring the sole can be used for additional support in the area extending from the cuboid to the distal end of the fifth toe. The area of flare should be about 1 to 1½ inches posterior to the base of the fifth metatarsal and extending anteriorly to the toe end of the outsole. In the stock shoe, the outsole must be detached from the welt, and the welt removed from the insole and upper joint, extending from an area ½ inch anterior to the lateral heel breastline up to the lateral anterior end of the toe. Welting, wide enough to afford an adequate flare, spliced at the terminals of the areas mentioned above, should be hand-stitched or McKay machine-stitched to the upper and insole. To apply this modification, the heel and heelbase must first be removed and then replaced. The void existing between the ground and the medial aspect of the sole, from toe to mid-shank, should be filled to allow for the addition of the outsole so that with the proper flare on the lateral aspect of the outsole, a close-to-normal weight-bearing pattern is achieved. Lateral wedging should be excluded to prevent a moment toward valgus, and the medial longitudinal arch should be supported.

A long rigid counter on the lateral side, extending anteriorly to the fifth metatarsophalangeal joint, can be installed to afford a strong retaining wall. The lateral shank filler mentioned earlier can also be used with a flare.

Flaring the sole and heel will prevent varus along the lateral aspect of the foot (Fig. 11.23). This can be accomplished as described for each of the segments individually. If the required lateral flare is so extensive that it distorts under weight bearing, another outsole may be applied over the first for added strength. In this case it is also necessary to add another sole to the sound side to maintain equal leg length. Flaring of the sole and heel are not always acceptable cosmetically.

The *varus strap* applied laterally in conjunction with an orthosis is

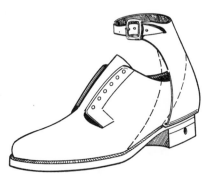

Fig. 11.23. Varus corrective strap. *Dotted line* indicates most effective placement.

designed to discourage a varus attitude. In spasticity or muscle contracture, where the foot, even when unweighted intermittently or continuously, assumes a varus position, the strap maintains correct mediolateral alignment by opposing the action of the spastic or contracted muscles. It may also be used in cases of mild spasticity, contracture, or flaccidity, where the foot assumes a varus attitude only on weight bearing.

The varus strap should lift or prevent depression in the following areas: (a) lateral anterior aspect of the talocalcaneal joint; (b) calcaneocuboid joint; and (c) the cuboid base of the fifth metatarsal joint (Fig. 11.23). The area of attachment for the distal end of the strap should be from a point ½ inch behind the lateral breastline to a point about 60% of the distance between the heelbreast and the break of the shoe. The varus strap is sometimes rejected for cosmetic reasons. In the varus strap narrowing the width would reduce lifting at the talocalcaneal joint and the talocuboid joint. From its distal attachment, the strap extends proximally to a point about 1½ inches above the apex of the lateral malleolus, where it divides into an anterior and posterior strap encircling the leg and the medial brace upright, buckling on the medial side in a convenient position for the patient (Fig. 11.23).

Metatarsal Arch Support

Opinion varies on the number and importance of arches in the foot. For the purposes of this book, we shall discuss the arches in the traditional manner. There are two metatarsal arches, the anterior and the posterior. The anterior metatarsal arch is made up of the heads of the metatarsal bones, and the posterior metatarsal arch is formed by the bases of the metatarsal bones. Most foot disabilities are related to one or both of these arches. Indeed, a list of possible deformities of the metatarsal arches is long and includes pes cavus, fracture, bursitis, hallux valgus, hallux rigidus, Morton's toe, splay foot, plantar warts, and metatarsalgia. To reduce pain and assist in restoring normal gait in these conditions, the following supporting components for the metatarsal arch are used:

Internal	External
Metatarsal pad, dancer pad, or meta-tarsal corset	Metatarsal bar
	Rocker bar
Levy-type inlay, with or without hallux valgus pad	Denver heel or bar
	Long steel spring and rocker bar
Morton's toe extension	Solid ankle cushion heel (SACH) heel

In *pes cavus,* the extensor tendons of the dorsum are shortened, causing the longitudinal arches to become high or "hollow" and also causing the proximal phalanges of each toe to dorsiflex while the middle and distal phalanges plantarflex. The dorsiflexion of the proximal phalanges forces the metatarsal arch to depress so that all of the heads are in contact with the ground. Callosities usually develop on the plantar skin over these heads, and pain ensues. The plantar fascia also shortens and contributes to the cavus deformity.

A combination of a metatarsal bar and pad is frequently helpful in relieving pressure on the unusually depressed and prominent metatarsal heads. The combination of metatarsal elevation and hollowing out under the metatarsal heads as incorporated in a full-length cork sole custom-made from the cavus foot, is often the most helpful device which can be prescribed for pes cavus.

Fractures of the metatarsal bones often result in the formation of callus tissue during healing. When weight is borne upon the plantar tissue that is sandwiched between the thickened bone and the tread area, pain ensues. If the periosteum is penetrated by the fracture, bone tissue may grow in irregular shapes and project beyond the surface of the remaining bone and periosteum. Such a bone projection, called an exostosis, causes pain when pressed against plantar tissue. If securely held by fibrous tissue, a malunion in a metatarsal bone may be comfortably supported by a metatarsal arch support.

If *bursitis* develops at the metatarsophalangeal joints, relief of tenderness is obtained by proper metatarsal support padding.

Morton's toe is a name applied to two different conditions, described by two different Mortons. Dudley Morton, an anatomist, wrote of a congenitally short first metatarsal bone which changed the weight-bearing pattern of the foot, placing so much additional pressure on the second metatarsal as to result in pain, especially in rollover of the stance phase of walking or toe spring at pushoff (18). Support and elevation (Morton insole) offers an extension pad under the first metatarsal head to produce the clinical effect of lengthening the bone. Many orthopedists feel that a simple metatarsal pad behind the second and third metatarsals is at least as effective as the Morton insole.

The other Morton's toe is an acute anterior metatarsalgia or severe neuralgia involving the third and fourth toes arising from a neuroma or pseudoneuroma of the junction of the medial and lateral plantar nerves in the web between the third and fourth toes or third and fourth metatarsal heads. This condition is sometimes helped by a metatarsal pad bar or arch support. The usual treatment is surgical removal.

Plantar warts are rather deep-rooted neoplasms, resulting in a needle sticking type of sensation. These warts commonly grow between and under the heads of the metatarsals; they also grow elsewhere on the plantar surface of the foot. Proper padding will help to relieve this condition.

Hallux valgus is generally associated with a medial displacement of the first metatarsal with a lateral displacement of the phalanges. It would be more appropriate to speak of metatarsus varus for the metatarsal part of the deformity and hallux valgus for the toe part. Inner molds with padding to attempt to realign the great toe do not correct, or even prevent, the progression of the deformity. In mild cases a night splint to hold the toe in marked medial deviation requires many years of faithful application to succeed. Where manipulation is not painful, an innermold with padding to realign the hallux, placed in a straight inner-border last shoe, is indicated.

When surgery is not possible, a shoe with an outflare or straight inner-border should be recommended.

Hallux rigidus is a deformity characterized by a rigid first metatarsophalangeal (MP) joint and by a gait pattern with a heel strike that is more lateral than normal and with a weight shift to the lateral border of the foot and shoe during advance into midstance. At the midstance phase, the ankle is in slight voluntary varus with the midtarsal and forefoot in enough supination to relieve the first MP joint of weight bearing. Hallux rigidus may be congenital or follow trauma or arthritic joint degeneration. The exostosis may develop at the base of the proximal phalanx of the hallux or at the first metatarsal head. As the exostosis grows into a joint stop, movement of the first metatarsophalangeal joint becomes restricted and painful. To relieve the deformity, a medial longitudinal arch, a properly fitted metatarsal support for the first metatarsal head and a long steel spring and rocker board are needed (20).

Splayfoot is a deformity in which the metatarsal bones abduct from each other mediolaterally, at their heads, and compress at the closely mated articular margins of the tarsometatarsal joints, depressing the anterior metatarsal arch. The degree of abduction and depression is dependent upon the laxity of the intrinsic muscles (plantar interossei and the adductor hallucis) of the foot. These muscles and their tendinous connectors normally truss the metatarsal bones so that they form a dome-shaped anterior arch and thus allow compressionless articulation to exist at the tarsometatarsal joints. Bandaging or corseting the foot from the waist level up to the tarsometatarsal joint level is the treatment generally administered this deformity. A metatarsal pad may be included for relief, if necessary (23).

Splayfoot is characterized by a flatfooted-type gait in which the patient carries out heel strike and midstance, but then precludes rollover and toe-off by raising the foot horizontally from the ground. This type gait is a result of pain experienced while trying normal rollover and toe-off. The plantar flexors of the toes cannot be relied upon to perform normally in supplying spring forces. With the malalignment of the metatarsal bones, the spring forces necessary for toe-off would only further depress the anterior metatarsal arch, and pain would ensue. Another common problem with this deformity is that the patient wears a stock shoe that is much too wide at the ball of the foot, yet he will usually complain that his shoe is too tight; the fact is that with proper corseting there is a great amount of space in the shoe. Corseting may be ineffective if it is not checked for its proper position.

MODIFICATIONS FOR FOREFOOT PROBLEMS

Regular *metatarsal pads* are commercially available in many sizes (Fig. 11.24c). They relieve moderate metatarsalgia by elevating the inner sole

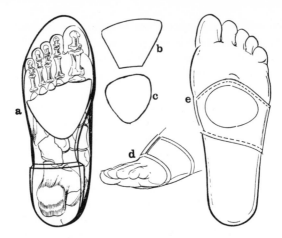

Fig. 11.24. Metatarsal pads. *a*, contoured dancer pad; *b*, noncontoured dancer pad; *c*, regular metatarsal pad; *d*, metatarsal corset (lateral view); *e*, metatarsal corset (plantar view).

behind the metatarsal heads and redistributing weight bearing in that area. For more serious metatarsalgia, the broad shape and thickness of the *dancer pad* (Fig. 11.24, *a* and *b*) is more helpful since it provides more support than the regular metatarsal pad. Dancer pad, sometimes called "buttons," can be shaped to fit directly behind each of the metatarsal heads (Fig. 11.24*a*) so that their feathered edge comes under the surface of the metatarsal heads. This placement is particularly beneficial for the flexible foot. With the rigid foot or pes planus, the pad should be placed slightly more posterior to the metatarsal heads to relieve the pressure on them. The shaping of the dancer pad must conform to the soft tissues that cover the metatarsals, otherwise there will be tissue stretch which counteracts the intended benefits of pressure relief. In fact, tissue stretch increases the sensitivity of prominent callosity areas, even though the callosities are relieved of body-weight pressure. The *metatarsal corset* (Fig. 11.24*d*) allows the patient to change footwear without removing the arch support, thereby avoiding frequent repositioning of the metatarsal pads. The corset incorporates either the regular metatarsal pad or the dancer pad, and it may be fastened with elastic strap or buckle. The metatarsal corset can also be used for splayfoot since its trussing elements are lax enough to permit abduction of the metatarsal heads and depression of the anterior metatarsal arch. The *insole pad* is another type of arch support that may be used as a removable component. It is mounted on an insert which is shaped to conform to the insole of the shoe from the heel to the area of the midmetatarsal heads, where the insert feathers.

Levy inlay is often used when the plantar surface of the metatarsopha-langeal or interphalangeal joints are hypersensitive to pressure. The Levy component is made by cementing a sponge or foam rubber forepart to a combination arch support. Since the inlay is removable it can be adjusted whenever necessary. The full innermold coverage of the Levy inlay is also used to treat hallux valgus. A wedge-shaped pad made of resilient foam rubber should be placed between the hallux and the second toe in order to abduct the great toe and realign the first metatarsophalangeal joint toward a normal attitude (Fig. 11.25). A mittenlike sock with a separate section for the great toe helps to prevent wrinkles from forming between the pad and the toe.

Morton's toe extension toe extension is used to ease the pain which often results from an abnormally short first metatarsal (Fig. 11.26). By raising the level of the first metatarsal bone and the phalanges of the hallux, the extension restores the proper three-point weight distribution pattern, that is, the weight is distributed between the plantar apex of the calcaneus and the first and fifth metatarsal heads. For greatest effectiveness, the Morton insert should extend from the heel to the tip of the hallux, passing and supporting the medial portion of the longitudinal arch. The lateral extent of the insert should be feathered at the medial peripheral line of the second toe, forming a sharp radius between the first and second MP joints. At the lateral end of the radius, the insert should extend to the fifth MP joint. A properly fitted metatarsal support should be installed to relieve the second metatarsal head and any other requiring relief. The orthotist can fabricate

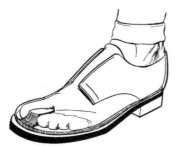

Fig. 11.25. Foot fitted with hallux valgus support on Levy-type insole and mitten-like sock.

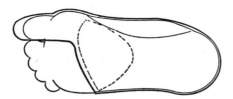

Fig. 11.26. Morton's toe extension (plantar view). *Dotted line* indicates metatarsal support to relieve pressure on metatarsal heads.

such an insert from a semiprefabricated longitudinal arch support and add the hallux extension. The choice of materials depends upon the patient's weight and the sensitivity caused by the deformity.

The *metatarsal bar,* an external support, may be used to relieve pressure from the metatarsal heads (Fig. 11.27, *a* and *b*) when foot sensitivity is too great to tolerate an insert. It may also be used to augment the use of an insert for the nonsensitive foot. In a stock shoe with a thin insole which may be reshaped by perspiration, the metatarsal bar should be applied as an overlay; if the bar were applied as a sandwich it would soon begin to rise in the shoe, reducing foot room and causing pressure against the sensitive metatarsal area. The metatarsal bar should be placed on the outsole, with its thickest point directly behind and parallel to the line between the first and fifth metatarsal heads so that after heel strike in rollover, the weight is borne at the area *behind* the metatarsal heads rather than upon the heads. The anterior extent of the metatarsal bar should taper about 1½ inches; its posterior taper may be short since it serves no function in pressure relief. As an overlay, the metatarsal bar has the added advantage of being easily adjusted or replaced without damage to the outsole and welt, thus prolonging shoe life. Some patients prefer an internal metatarsal bar. It is more cosmetically acceptable and not subject to localized wearing off, as is the external bar. However, the internal metatarsal bar does occupy more space in the shoe and crowds the toes and foot within the shoe.

The *rocker bar* (Fig. 11.27, *c* and *d*) is more extensively used than the metatarsal bar, particularly when improved gait function and a degree of immobilization are desired for the ankle, tarsal, transmetatarsal, metatarsophalangeal, or interphalangeal joints. Like the metatarsal bar, the rocker bar is prescribed to relieve pressure from the metatarsal heads. In stock shoes, the rocker bar should be installed as an overlay, with its apex directly behind and in a line parallel to the first and fifth metatarsal heads. The front of the rocker bar extends farther to the toe end of the shoe than does

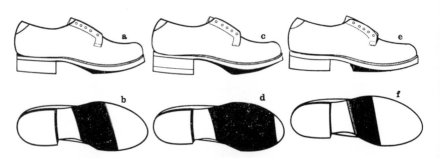

Fig. 11.27. Metatarsal (rocker and Denver bars). *a,* metatarsal bar (lateral view); *b,* metatarsal bar (plantar view); *c,* rocker bar (lateral view); *d,* rocker bar (plantar view); *e,* Denver bar (lateral view; *f,* Denver bar (plantar view).

the metatarsal bar. The exact extent is determined by the height of the apex and the feathering. The extension of the wearline of the sole toward the heel and the placement of the apex of the bar posteriorly reduce the posterior and midfoot weight-bearing force appreciably during the period of rollover and pushoff. Without the rocker bar, the weight-bearing force would normally be applied to the metatarsal area during gait.

The *Denver* bar (also called the Dutchman) is a metatarsal support, usually made of leather and applied as an overlay to the outsole by cementing or nailing (Fig. 11.27, *e* and *f*). The posterior extent of the bar can be increased or decreased depending upon the lesion. Usually, the posterior face of the Denver bar is placed at the plantar surface of the instep, that is, directly beneath the transverse arch of the foot at the tarsometatarsal joints. It is important that the orthotist achieve a balance between the shoe heelbreast and the Denver bar so that during rollover in the stance phase of gait, the transverse arch is raised. As the transverse arch is elevated, the metatarsal bones are pulled back and the weight on the metatarsal heads is relieved. If there is need to support the navicular bone or to effect a lateral weight shift, the orthotist may extend the Denver bar posteriorly or elevate the component.

Figure 11.28 demonstrates a wide variety of bars and wedges which may be prescribed for children's shoes.

Long Steel Spring and Rocker Bar. In conjunction with extended brace attachment tongues and long steel springs, the rocker bar provides firm support for the forefoot until late in the stance phase, thus reducing the support required of the toes (Fig. 11.31, *c* and *e*). When used with a stiff ankle brace or a limiting plantar and dorsiflexion brace, the rocker bar also reduces motion in the tibiotalar and subtalar ankle joints, talonavicular, calcaneocuboid, and tarsometatarsal joints, permitting a relief of pain in some foot disabilities.

SACH Heel. A soft heel stimulating a SACH (Solid Ankle Cushion Heel) foot wedge used in conjunction with the rocker bar provides a more natural gait from heel contact to rollover and pushoff. The SACH foot wedge, which is called a SACH heel, is made of resilient materials such as sponge, pedic, or crepe rubbers of appropriate durometers of hardness with a thin rubber heel on top to provide cushioning at heel contact. The depression occurring at heel contact simulates plantar flexion, thereby offering earlier outsole contact with the ground (Fig. 11.31*d*).

Joint Immobilization

Many foot problems require total immobilization of one or more joints, such as the interphalangeal, metatarsophalangeal, and the tarsometatarsal joints or the talonavicular, calcaneocuboid, talocalcaneal, and tibiotalar joints. A patient may be suffering from arthritis or ankylosis, an unsuccessful arthrodesis, or spastic foot. In many of these instances, the patient needs

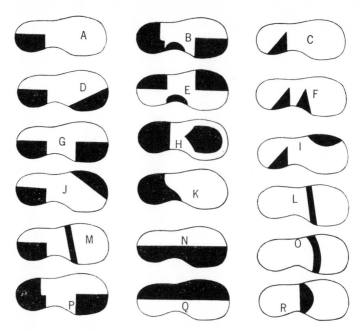

Fig. 11.28. Diagrammatic representation of some of the more common wedges prescribed for children's shoes. *A*, inside heel; *B*, same as *P* but with long counter or cookie; *C*, triangular wedge to relieve strain on longitudinal arch; *D*, inside toe and heel wedge to force toeing in; *E*, inside cookie to assist arch; *F*, twin wedge to relieve pressure on sesamoid area; *G*, inside sole and heel wedge to relieve pressure on longitudinal arch; *H*, Neopolitan tap; *I*, inside triangular and outside sole wedge; *J*, outer toe wedge with inner heel wedge to prevent toeing in; *K*, Thomas heel; *L*, metatarsal bar; *M*, inside heel wedge and metatarsal bar to raise heads of metatarsal bones; *N*, full-length inside wedge; *O*, metatarsal crescent; *P*, inside sole wedge and extension heel; *Q*, outer border wedge; *R*, tarsal raise. (Reproduced with permission from the Wedge Chart of Julius Altschul, Inc., of Brooklyn.)

joint immobilization, along with as normal a gait as possible. This can be achieved with the following components:

Internal	External
Steel shoe shank	Steel-reinforced tongue of brace at-
Long steel spring, if the metatarsal,	tachment
phalangeal, and interphalangeal	Stiff or limited-motion ankle joints
joints are involved	SACH heel and rocker bar
Steel-reinforcing plate on insole	Medial and lateral shank filler

If the foot is deformed or amputated at the level of the interphalangeal, metatarsophalangeal, or the tarsometatarsal joints, ambulation is usually painful, which causes a gait deviation. In order to avoid pain during rollover and pushoff in the stance phase, the patient pivots on his heel and abducts the midtarsal and forefoot by his voluntary outward rotation of the ankle and hip joints. This action eliminates rollover and pushoff entirely.

When ankylosis or arthritic deformities occur, the action of the affected joints and their ligamentous connectors is restricted, impeding flexion and extension. Unchecked moments of force at the affected joint levels will cause tissue stresses to develop. These stresses, if allowed to go unchecked, can cause a corresponding degree of tissue destruction and pain. Components must therefore be used that will prevent moments toward flexion or extension. The combinations of components for such foot disabilities are the same as those used for foot amputations at the various coincident skeletal levels.

MODIFICATIONS TO IMMOBILIZE JOINTS

A *steel shoe shank* of at least 0.05 inch thickness with one or more corrugated ribs and length, width, placement, and function as described above, is the first prerequisite for proper shoe construction.

A *long steel spring* sandwiched into the shoe prevents dorsiflexion to immobilize the interphalangeal and metatarsophalangeal joints. Like the solid steel shank, the steel spring should be at least 0.05-inch thick and at least 1 inch wide. It should be made of spring steel and sandwiched between the insole and outsole. The long steel spring should extend from a point ⅜ inch posterior to the insole rib at the toe end and to a point about ½ inch anterior to the upper edge at the heel. The heel-to-toe extension of the long steel spring prevents any dorsiflexion or plantar flexion from occurring at the break of the shoe. To increase the rocker action in rollover, the steel spring can be made slightly convex, and this internal curvature will lead to a more normal gait pattern. This spring can be installed when resoling of the outsole is necessary; otherwise, the shoemaker must open enough stitches between the welt and the sole at the toe or at the posterior quarter-to-sole joint, where no welt is usually found, to afford adequate passage of the spring. At the time of resoling, a thin leather or cork separator should also be sandwiched between the steel shank and the steel spring to prevent a metallic clicking noise when the wearer walks. Adhesive tape may also be wrapped around the spring to dampen metallic clicking noises.

A *steel reinforcing plate* helps stiffen the heel end. It should be set ¼ to ⅜ inch behind the break of the shoe; it can be made of spring steel or stainless steel of any desired thickness. The plate is attached on the shoe insole, sandwiching the insole and outsole between the brace attachment and itself.

A *steel-reinforced tongue* of the brace attachment to the shoe is made broad enough to bypass the steel shank in riveting, as described above. When welded or brazed to the tongue of the attachment, it strengthens and stiffens the longitudinal arch of the shoe. If the patient's weight warrants it, the insole plate is used in conjunction with the attachment.

Stiff or limited-motion ankle joints prevent plantar flexion or dorsiflexion at the tibiotalar joint or at the metatarsophalangeal joints. Such joints permit dorsiflexion or plantar flexion to a limited degree, which is an asset during gait exercise.

The *SACH heel and rocker bar* used for limited and stiff-ankle joints contribute greatly toward the comfortable restoration of near-normal gait (14, 15). As in the SACH heel of artificial legs, the SACH heel component is very resilient. At heelstrike, it acts as a shock absorber, compressing and bringing the rocker bar into early contact with the ground. The compression of the SACH heel at heelstrike affords the patient a pseudoplantar flexion without forcing his ankle toward plantar flexion. Since early ground contact is made at the apex of the rocker bar, the shoe is ready for rollover and toe-off so rapidly that motion of the tarsometatarsal, talocrural, or subtalar joints is minimized. The use of the SACH heel in immobilizing the tarso-metatarsal joints gives other advantages. The resiliency of the SACH heel helps to relieve the pressures at the brace calfband to prevent disturbance of the brace-to-leg alignment. The brace should have either a limited or a fused-solid ankle joint and also, for the heavy patient, a metal insole plate that rests on top of the leather insole. The stirrup, or other form of shoe attachment, should have a broad tongue to bypass the steel shank.

Medial and lateral shank fillers can be used to prevent longitudinal arch depression and to maintain a rigid heel-to-ball section in cases of excessive obesity or in the base of a Chopart's or Lisfranc's amputation (Figs. 11.17 and 11.21).

Arch Supports

A prescription is not required to purchase arch supports which are sold over the counter of a department or drug store without measurement or fit. If the purchaser prefers to acquire a support in this manner, he may receive some symptomatic relief from the insert. More often than not, he will receive no benefit, and in many cases his disability may be aggravated by new areas of irritation. The sufferer who is willing to obtain advice as well as supports will find many differences of opinion among those who by profession and training or experience are consulted: the shoe salesman, orthotist, podiatrist, orthopedist, or physiatrist.

The functions of arch supports are (a) to relieve areas of pressure which are calloused or scarred; (b) to support weak, flat, or painful feet; or (c) to align areas up to and including the pelvis by elevating the medial or lateral aspect or by increasing the thickness of height of the supports, thus changing the direction, angle, and distribution of body weight to the foot or the affected side of the body. The measurement procedures used for arch supports include the use of prefabricated or partially prefabricated supports, paper impressions, and plaster of Paris casts.

Many prefabricated arch supports are measured by size of the shoe and width of the patient's foot.

Semiprefabricated supports are commercially available according to shoe size and the patient's weight. They afford a simple and accurate way to measure and fit arch supports. The medial or lateral portion of the longitudinal arch support is shaped to conform to the patient's needs, a metatarsal pad is added as prescribed, and the entire unit is covered with vinyl sheeting. This combination of fitting and modifying, along with a preliminary gait study, can usually be completed during the patient's first visit. With such a procedure, much labor in casting and fabrication is saved, excellent fittings are possible, and the number of follow-up visits is kept to a minimum.

Paper impressions are made with phenolphthalein or the ped-o-graph. *Phenolpthalein paper* will activate and develop an impression of a foot, sponged lightly with an alkaline (sodium bicarbonate) aqueous solution. *Ped-o-graph* impressions are made by pressing the foot against an impression paper under an inked pad. Paper impressions show the foot outline, within which darkened areas represent the pressure points which are too often limited in detail to be useful in severe foot disabilities.

Presto-Cast or *Presto-Foam* impressions are made with compressible foamed urethanes in a shoebox-like container. The foot is lowered into the container very gently, with a resultant impression of the plantar and part of the medial and lateral aspects of the foot. Although the definition is not as fine as that rendered by plaster of Paris, it can be used for the unexceptional foot problem. A plaster of Paris mixture is poured into the impression to obtain a positive cast of the foot.

Plaster of Paris casts are made by placing the patient's feet into a mixture of plaster so that the plantar surfaces of the feet are covered. The deepened contours of the resultant negative cast impression indicate the pressure areas. Much more information of foot contouring is possible with form plaster casts than from two-dimensional paper impressions.

The best reproductions of the patient's feet are obtained with plaster of Paris *wraps*. The wrap cast, applied properly, covers the plantar, medial, and lateral aspects of the foot, as well as portions of the dorsum, up to an area just below the medial and lateral malleoli. The positive casts rendered from the negative wrap casts are excellent replicas of the patient's feet. Any indelible pencil markings over or around calloused, scarred, or sensitive areas are transferred from the foot to the negative, then once again to the positive cast. A maximum of information is obtained by this type of fitting impression.

The four types of support in common use are: (a) three-quarter length without flanges; (b) three-quarter length with medial flanges; (c) three-quarter length with medial and lateral flanges; and (d) full-length with or without flanges.

FITTING THE ARCH SUPPORT

In fitting an arch support to the foot, as distinguished from fitting the arch support to the shoe, a basic check for conformity, alignment, and provision for pressure relief at scarred and calloused areas must be made. With the use of metal arch supports, a further check must be made for the absence of sharp or rough edges, which would injure the feet or mutilate the shoes.

To check for proper support length, place the conformed arch support against the patient's foot with the heel edge parallel to, and in a continuous line with, the posterior apex of the patient's heel, where a triangular space occurs because of the natural radial contour of the soft tissue of the heel. With the heel length properly positioned, the medial and lateral longitudinal arches of the foot should be checked. In a rigid pes planus, both longitudinal arches should have support; support and elevation medially will cause a lateral weight shift.

In a semirigid pes planus, support and elevation may be indicated without a shift of body weight. In a flaccid pes planus, both support and elevation are usually necessary to restore a normal longitudinal arch and reduce the effects incurred at the ankle joints.

In rigid pes cavus, the longitudinal arches should be conformed to closely, leaving no voids which would allow movements toward depression and ensuing pain. In semirigid pes cavus, some degree of depression can usually be tolerated without discomfort; however, there are many cases that require as much support as rigid pes cavus. In the flaccid pes cavus, the foot should be supported at the height of a normal longitudinal arch.

With the arch support held in the proper position at the heel, its front end should be contiguous with the midline of the metatarsal heads (Fig. 11.29a). Since dorsiflexion of the toes causes a slight forward movement of all of the metatarsal heads, the edge of the support, if measured for the proper length, will not be felt by the patient as he walks.

After the arch support is checked for proper length, the metatarsal pad is checked for proper positioning.

Forefoot Extension. To provide an insole filler to prevent anterior shift of the arch support during wear, a forefoot extension piece can be made of a thinned or split-belly center leather or equivalent material for the purpose. If the metatarsophalangeal and interphalangeal joint plantar surfaces are calloused, scarred, or sensitive, a soft foam or sponge rubber surface is indicated. Soft forefoot pieces should generally be about ⅛ inch thick and covered with thin skin leather or vinyl sheeting for smoothness and comfort.

Forefoot pieces can be spliced and cemented to commercially available prefabricated or semiprefabricated arch supports. If the orthotist makes a

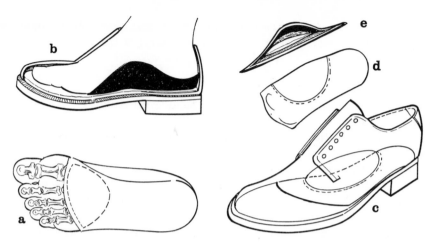

Fig. 11.29. Arch supports. *a*, fitting of arch support to foot (*dotted line* indicates metatarsal pad placement); *b*, fitting of arch support to foot in shoe; *c*, wafer-type medial longitudinal arch support in shoe; *d*, dorsal view of wafer support; *e*, medial cutaway of wafer support showing wafer inserts.

wrap cast or shoe last of the patient, the forefoot, midfoot, and "hindfoot" piece are in one unit, a type of inlay that provides truest conformity to the entire plantar surface of the foot; the inlay also includes the features that have been installed to relieve, support, or elevate specific areas.

Heel pads can be added to any arch support to relieve sensitive plantar surfaces of the calcaneus or to relieve pressure from a calcaneal spur. The sensitive plantar surface can usually be relieved with a sponge rubber pad shaped to fit the heel area of the shoe insole, with feathering toward the midfoot area. The calcaneal spur can be relieved with a similar pad that has a concavity cut to fit directly beneath the spur. To prevent tilting the calcaneus anteriorly, heel pads or cushions should be used with longitudinal arch supports.

FITTING ARCH SUPPORTS TO SHOE

In fitting the arch support to the shoe, the orthotist must place the support in the shoe so that its heel edge rests against the distal posterior aspect of the quarter lining of the shoe (Fig. 11.29*b*). This position must be maintained to ensure replication of the conformity achieved during the support-to-foot fitting phase; otherwise, even a slight anterior shift of the arch support may introduce pain.

There are fitting difficulties that result from poor last and upper styles. Often, a completed arch support has to be thinned out or lengthened to relieve pressure from a tight shoe or widened and thickened to fill up a loosely fitted shoe. Since a metatarsal pad causes some spread and abduction of the toes, a straight inner-border last, rather than a pointed-toe shoe, should be selected. A blucher-style upper or an extra-depth shoe should be used when a metatarsal arch support is necessary, or the patient will find his shoe tight across the lower instep (Fig. 11.29c).

FABRICATION METHODS

Methods of fabricating arch supports include (a) molding, (b) pressing, and (c) hammering.

The molding method can be applied to leather, laminated or sheet plastics, and Celastic. Either the positive foot casts of the patient or shoe-last forms are used as the base over which the materials are molded. The arch shells can be reinforced with steel shanks in the longitudinal area. The pressing method is applied to aluminum or stainless steel which are shaped by a power press over a metallic shoe last. The hammering method which can also be applied to aluminum or stainless steel for fabricating arch supports uses the foot cast as a guide; the materials are hammered against a lead block until they conform to the positive casts. The cementing method is applied to cork, natural or composition wood fiber, and leather lining, rubber, sponge, foam, and latex. The bonding material may be applied to the patient's cast or last.

TYPES OF ARCH SUPPORTS

The word "combination", preceding any of the following terms indicates the use of a metatarsal pad or raise.

Meyer offers metatarsal relief and slight longitudinal arch support. It has no flanges.

Shaffer offers longitudinal arch support and has a centered medial flange.

Shaffer-Meyer offers longitudinal arch support and a medial flange back of center in order to accommodate fashionable women's footgear.

Shaffer with anterior medial flange is used to relieve bunion or hallux valgus.

Shaffer with anterior lateral flange is used to relieve Taylor's bunion, sometimes called bunionette.

Whitman without heel offers medial and lateral calcaneal stability with flanges on each side and longitudinal arch support. With a flat heel, there is somewhat less calcaneal control. With a cupped heel, there is a little less calcaneal control since the extended plantar surface posteriorly prevents the tilting of the mid- and forefoot from the heel. The cupped heel does offer relief to heel sensitivity of bursitis or exostosis.

A *Roberts brace* is similar in function to a Whitman support. It has a flat heel, but its medial flange is lower from the center to the front and where it blends into the apron. In the posterior half, the medial flange develops a sizable projection to cover the medial aspect of the calcaneus.

A *Whitman-Meyer* brace also controls the calcaneus and the tarsal bones without a heel. It has a high and wide medial and lateral flange.

A full innermold insert can be of the Shaffer or Whitman type, with an anterior forefoot extension (Morton's), a hallux valgus toe spreader or toe crest. It may be used in combination with a cork elevation or balancer.

A heel seat or stabilizer controls the calcaneus. It has bilateral flanges which are joined posteriorly at a slightly lower level. The forward extension is immediately anterior to the navicular and just posterior to the cuboid bone. The plantar surface joins the two sides diagonally. These supports are most successful for children.

The UCBL (University of California, Biomechanics Laboratory) insert controls the calcaneus, mid- and forefoot by complete realignment. It has bilateral flanges joined in the back as the heel seat and extends anteriorly on the medial and lateral sides up to the heads of the metatarsals. Trials have shown them best for children (11). In a mature foot, no arch support will realign the bones and joints to change the shape of the adult foot.

Heel Elevation

Heel elevation is sometimes needed to restore horizontal alignment to the pelvic girdle. Leg shortening with or without foot problems or a fixed equinus with no leg shortening may require heel elevation.

Cork Layers. For the patient with a short leg but no foot disorder, the orthotist builds up enough height under the heel to restore pelvic balance. For heel elevations of more than ½ inch, cork sheets of varying thickness are stacked, cemented, and attached as a sandwich component (Fig. 11.30). The highest point should be at the heel, and the elevation should decline gradually at the ball of the foot, leaving the least amount of cork at the toes so that toe spring at pushoff is easier.

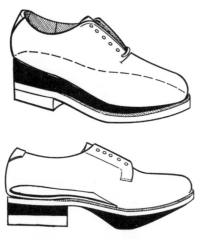

Fig. 11.30. Heel elevations. *Above,* sandwich; *below,* combination insert-sandwich division, with rocker bar installed as integral part of cork elevation to facilitate faster rollover.

To estimate the proper elevation before permanently mounting the cork, the orthotist should stack the cork layers one at a time under the affected leg until pelvic balance is achieved. Taping or gluing the layers temporarily to the shoe will expedite the procedure. After temporarily taping on the elevation, the orthotist should attach a dummy heel to restore the heel-to-sole relationship so that the patient can ambulate and his gait can be studied.

A *metatarsal or rocker bar* can be installed as an integral part of the cork elevation, and rollover can be increased by shifting the apex toward the heel. In a high elevation, the faster rollover facilitates a more normal gait pattern since longer strides can be taken more smoothly.

Flaring. For a fixed equinovarus condition, flaring of the sole or heel may be necessary; it can be installed as part of the elevation. In a stock shoe, the outsole, heel, and welt must first be removed. Skin leather, matching the shoe upper, is then sewn (with the finished side facing and lying against the shoe upper) to the welt, insole, and upper. The cork is cemented in layers to the insole and shaped to the desired height and function. Another insole is shaped to the plantar surface of the cork, and the distal end of the elevation cover is reflected over the circumference and plantar edge of the insole and sewn to a welt. A shoe shank, filler, outsole, and heel are added for completion.

Stock Shoes with Orthopedic Features

In order to offer the patient as much toe prehension as possible, we may recommend a shoe with a straight innerline last, also referred to as a "straight innerborder." This shoe differs from the stock shoe in that the anterior sole perimeter from the first metatarsophalangeal joint to the distal

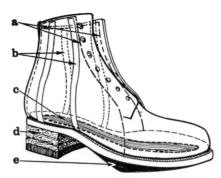

Fig. 11.31. High-quarter shoe with combination of modifications prescribed for a painfully ankylosed ankle or foot. *a*, high bilaterally extended counter; *b*, reinforcing steels; *c*, long steel spring; *d*, SACH heel; *e*, rocker bar. If patient is obese, medial and lateral shank fillers would be used, and the SACH heel would be replaced by a heel of regular hardness to prevent rolling or vaulting over the shank fillers from heelstrike to toe-off.

end of the hallux is a straight line, which permits the hallux to lie in normal alignment.

The "bunion-lasted" shoe also has a straight inner line but is distinguished by the very close conformity of shoe upper to the area behind the first metatarsal head on the medial side (waist level of the foot). The snug conformity puts pressure on the abductor hallucis, with consequent forcing of the proximal phalanx, and thus forces the entire hallux toward the medial line. This function helps to correct and relieve severe hallux valgus, which has a moderately mobile MP joint.

Stock shoes with orthopedic features, such as a long counter on the medial side, should be obtained when a rigid wall is necessary to retain the foot in the desired alignment. The long counter, extending between the heelbreast and the break of the shoe, can assist in longitudinal arch support in correcting a flaccid valgus or in preventing a rigid valgus from becoming more severe.

As previously mentioned, if the patient is to wear arch supports, he should be advised to purchase the straight inner line shoe with blucher-type uppers. Such a combination will give his foot the extra space needed when the toes abduct and extend under weight bearing when a longitudinal arch support is used. If there is need for ankle support or immobilization of the ankle joints, high-quarter shoes should be obtained. Low-quarter shoes, however, can be used if a high-quarter-shaped cuff is sewn onto the upper.

Fig. 11.31 is a diagrammed composite of several modifications incorporated into a high-quarter shoe for the relief of pain resulting from an ankylosed ankle or foot.

There are additional advantages to the SACH heel. When there is a lesion that precludes ankle motion, a hard heel causes the posterior forces at the calfband to be so great that instability at the knee joint results. If the quadriceps is not strong enough to override this force, above-knee braces with locks must be provided. In contrast, the SACH heel not only absorbs shock and reduces posterior calfband pressures, it also allows inversion and eversion, reducing the lateral calfband pressures when the brace-wearer walks on uneven ground. The SACH heel rubbers can be glued to the brace attachment with an epoxy adhesive, one layer of rubber being glued to another, including the thin rubber heel, with Stabond.

Table 11.1 gives an overview of general foot disabilities and the shoe modifications usually prescribed. These suggestions are only a very general guide, as each person must be considered for his or her individual requirements. Requirements for children's shoes, with which we can actually alter growth and development of the foot, are very different from those for adults, for whom alteration of growth and development is impossible. A thorough shoe checkout is most important before applying modifications since the shoe is the foundation of the orthosis, as well as the foot.

TABLE 11.1. Foot Deformities and Shoe Modifications Used for Their Correction Using Stock Shoes

Foot deformity	Suggested shoe components		
	Insert	Sandwich (in addition to solid steel shank)	Overlay
Amputation, ankylosis, arthritis of interphalangeal, metatarsophalangeal, or tarsometatarsal joints (Lisfranc's) talonavicular and calcaneocuboid joints of Chopart's)		Long steel spring Long steel spring & high-quarter uppers with reinforced sides High-quarter uppers with reinforced sides	Rocker bar Medial & lateral shank fillers, a rocker bar, SACH heel SACH heel
Subtalar, (talocrural joints)			
Bursitis	Full-length innermold	Long steel spring	Metatarsal bar or rocker bar SACH heel
Calcaneal spur or pressure-sensitive heel tissue	Longitudinal arch support & heel cushion		
Equinus (fixed)	Heel elevation	Cork heel elevation & heel base elevation of other shoe	Rocker bar
Fractures, exostosis, hallux rigidus, or malunion	Full-length innermold	Long steel spring	Rocker bar
Hallux valgus	Full-length innermold		
Leg shortening	Heel elevation	Cork heel elevation or heel base elevator	Rocker bar or Neapolitan tap
Metatarsal bone (shortening of the first)	Elevator support for hallux & 1st metatarsal		
Metatarsalgia	Regular metarsal pad or dancer pad or metatarsal insole or metatarsal corset		
Metatarsus abductus		Anterior-medial toe & medial heel wedges	
Metatarsus adductus		Anterior-lateral sole & medial heel wedges	
Pes cavus	Regular metatarsal pad or dancer pad or metatarsal insole or metatarsal corset		Metatarsal bar or Denver heel

TABLE 11.1—continued

Pes planus			
Laterally	Long counter on lateral side; lateral heel wedge cookie or navicular pad		Reversed orthopedic heel
Medially	Cookie or navicular pad & longitudinal arch support	Orthopedic heel wedge	Orthopedic heel
Plantar warts	Regular metatarsal pad; dancer pad or metatarsal insole or metatarsal corset or full-length inner mold		
Sesamoiditis		Medial heel & shank twin wedges	
Valgus (flaccid)	Cookie or navicular pad long counter on medial side		Orthopedic heel; medial sole-and-heel wedge
Valgus		Medial triangular heel wedge & lateral sole wedge	
Varus			
Ankylosed	Long counter on lateral side		Lateral flaring of sole, heel, or sole & heel
Flaccid	Cookie or navicular pad; long counter on lateral side; lateral heel wedge; longitudinal arch with lateral heel support		Lateral sole & heel wedges

Some Useful Shoe and Leather Terminology[1]

Anterior Heel—term for a specific type of metatarsal bar.

Backpart—that portion of the last extending from the ball to the back.

Back Seam—posterior seam joining the quarters of the uppers.

Bal—A low front-laced shoe in which the quarters meet and the vamp is stitched over the quarters at the front of the throat. The word is an abbrevation of Balmoral, the Scottish castle where the shoe was introduced in 1853.

Ball—widest part of the sole (at the metatarsal heads).

Ball Girth—the greatest dimension around the last passing through the ball break.

Bar, Comma—a comma-shaped bar wedged laterally and posteriorly, *e.g.,* Hauser type.

Denver (often referred to as Denver Heel)—a metatarsal bar, the apex of this bar coincides with the posterior edge under the posterior half of the metatarsal shafts.

Jones—a metatarsal bar placed between the innersole and outersole of a shoe.

Metatarsal—any bar of rubber, leather, or synthetic material applied transversely across the bottom of the shoe sole, with the apex immediately posterior to the metatarsal heads.

Mayo—a metatarsal bar with the anterior edge curved to approximate the position to the metatarsal heads.

Thomas—a narrow metatarsal bar with abrupt anterior and posterior drop-off.

Bate—to treat unhaired hides or skins with a warm aqueous solution of any enzyme to remove certain undesirable nitrogenous constituents.

Blucher—a front-laced shoe pattern with the tongue as part of the forepart and in which the quarters lap over the vamp or forepart.

---

[1] We are grateful to Lester Weitsen of the Apex-Ensloe Shoe Co. of New York for permission to use some of the definitions of terminology as proposed by the Educational Committee of the Prescription Footwear Association, January 1972.

Boot—high-quarter shoe in which the quarters cover the malleoli to any point up to the hip.

Bottom Filler—material used for filling the cavity between the insole and outsole of shoes. The most widely used materials are made from granulated cork in a resinous binder. Other fillers contain rubber latex, cork sheet, impregnated felt, or man-laminated wood cut to shape.

Box Toe—a stiffener used to maintain the shape of a shoe toe, preserve the toe room, and protect the toes from blows. Rigid box toes are made of leather, thermoplastic, resin-impregnated fiber, or starch-impregnated buckram.

Breast—anterior surface of the heel.

Breastline—an arbitrary line defining the forward boundary of the heel.

Break—the wrinkle or crease formed in the vamp of a shoe when the shoe is flexed at the ball.

Brogue—shoes of rugged construction and usually perforated and pinked with tips, foxing, and medallions on the toe caps.

Buckskin—a general term applied to leather from deer and elk skins. Used for shoes and gloves and, to some extent, in clothing. Leather finished from the split or undercut of deer skin must be described as split buckskin. Only the outer cut of the skin, from which the surface grain has been removed, may be defined correctly as genuine buckskin.

Buffing—a very light cut of grain portion (about one-half), taken from the surface of cattlehide. It is usually produced in the manufacture of upholstery leather and is used for bookbinding and fancy leather goods. Buffing is also used to produce a fine nap on leather with an emery wheel.

Butt—that part of the hide or skin covering the rump or hindpart of an animal, for example, a "horse butt." Belting butt is a whole cattlehide tanned for leather belting after the head, belly, and tail have been trimmed off. Butt end is what remains of a butt after trimming off a double shoulder.

Cack—an infant's shoe under size 5.

Calfskin—tanned calfskins, preferably of mellow heavier weights, which are of finer texture and are very durable.

Capeskin or Cape Leather—a term applied to all glove and garment leather made from sheepskins with the natural grain retained. More accurately, it is leather from South African hair sheep.

Celastic—a pyroxilin material that can be molded and fixed into a rigid form.

Chukka—a ¾ blucher boot pattern, with two or three eyelets or strap with buckle.

Closure—method of inclosing, binding, or confining.

Collar—a band of leather stitched to and encircling the top of a quarter of a shoe.

Cone—the curved upper surface of the backpart of the last, which is divided by a V-cut into a front and back cone.

Cookie—a wafer-shaped piece of leather used in a shoe as a longitudinal arch support.

Cordovan—a leather produced from the butt of a horsehide (a "fascia" between the hair and flesh sides).

Corset—reinforcement of firm leather or stays incorporated in the upper to support or restrict ankle motion.

Counter—reinforcement to preserve the shape of the backpart of the shoe.

Crest—ridge or prominence (as cushion or filling under the cavity under the phalanges).

Cross Wedging—combination wedging (as in medial heel and lateral sole).

Crown—lateral curvature of the bottom of the last.

Cuban Heel—a broad "high" heel.

Cuff—a band of leather stitched to the top of the quarter of a shoe to increase its height.

Doeskin—trade term applied to sheepskins and lambskins, generally fleshers, tanned by the formaldehyde-and-alum process. This creates a soft-finished, supple leather which is produced in a variety of shades but is usually white.

Doubler—an interlining placed between the vamp and vamp lining for additional body and shape reinforcement.

Drop-off—the anterior vertical edge of a metatarsal or rocker bar.

Dutchman—traditional term applied to wedges.

Elk—chrome-tanned cattlehide leather, distinctive for softness and strength. Genuine elk leather is called buckskin.

Embossed Leather—finished by stamping designs on hides or skin with etched, engraved, or electrotyped plates or rollers. It is used extensively on fancy pocketbook leather, upholstery and bag leathers, and splits, as well as on shoe upper leather.

Eyelet—a hole or metal ring used for lacing.

Fatliquor—an emulsion of oils or greases in water, usually with an emulsifying agent, used to lubricate the fibers of leather.

Filler—any material, cork composition, felt, or rubber placed between the innersole and outersole or providing leveling and cushioning.

Flanged—a projected edge.

Forepart—that portion of the last extending from the ball break to the toe.

Foxing—a piece of leather applied to the quarter, or a perforated design in the quarter for decoration.

Full Grain—leather where the top grain has been left intact without correcting.

Ghillie—a shoe that is open from throat to instep.

Girth—dimension measured around the last.

Goring—a woven elastic fabric inserted in the front or sides of a shoe upper, the expansion of which allows a larger opening to insert the foot.

Grain—the outer or hair side of skin where the hide is split into two or more thicknesses or is of unsplit skins that are finished on the grain side.

Heel Base—the part of the heel next to the sole, usually concaved to fit the heel seat.

Heel Breast—the forward face of the heel, often concaved toward the shank.

Heel Elevation—(orthopedic modification)—measured in a vertical line at the posterior of the heel from the treading or plantar surface to the heel point at the heel seat.

Heel Height—(commercial manufacturer's)—measured vertical line from the treading or plantar surface to the heel seat at the breast or anterior surface or the heel—usually denoted in increments of eights of an inch.

Heel Types—(a) spring heel ³⁄₈ to ⁶⁄₈ inch." Heel base lies under the outersole, eliminating a definite heel breast. (b) flat heel, ⁶⁄₈ to ¹⁰⁄₈ inch, broad base. (c) military heel, ¹⁰⁄₈ to ¹³⁄₈ inch, medium base. (d) cuban heel, ¹³⁄₈ to ¹⁴⁄₈ inch, narrower base than military. (e) wedge heel, ⁴⁄₈ to ¹⁴⁄₈ inch—extends from ball break backward to posterior heel surface as a solid wedge.

Heel—(Ashley types)—heel with breast set anteriorly with medial and lateral flares and pitched well forward to obtain additional longitudinal support, as well as medial and lateral stabilization.

Heel Pad—material placed in the shoe over the rough areas of the heel seat.

Heel Pitch—inclination of the heel from the vertical at the posterior surface.

Heel Point—the rearmost point of a last at the heel seat.

Heel seat—(a) place to which the heel is attached and (b) area on which the anatomical heel rests within the shoe.

Heelstrike—posterior heel contact against the treading surface.

Hide—when used to describe tanned leather, it refers to a pelt from one of the larger animals (cattle, horse) in its entirety, containing the superficial area of the source animal.

Horsehide Leather—leather made from the hide of a horse or colt.

Inflare—to spread out or turn medially. Inward swing of shoe forepart.

Inlay—refers to any type of arch support or foot mold inserted in a shoe.

Innersole (also called insole)—a sole of leather, cork, or other material cut to fit the exact size and shape of the last bottom.

Instep—(a) the arched dorsum middle portion of the human foot and (b) that part of the shoe over the anatomical instep.

Iron—a measure of sole thickness—¹⁄₄₈ inch equals 1 iron, *e.g.,* 12 irons equal ¼ inch.

Jimmy—a piece of material of felt, cork composition, or leather, shaped as the forepart of an insole and inserted in a shoe to tighten it.

Kid—chrome-tanned grain glove leather from goatskin or lambskin of wool or hair type. It is not made from kidskin.

Kidskin—a soft, strong leather of tanned baby goatskin.

Lace Leather—rawhide (cowhide) leather for lacing together sections of driving belts. It is usually prepared with combined tannage.

Lace Stay—portion of the upper containing eyelets for lacing.

Lace-To-Toe—low- or high-quarter pattern with eyelets to the toe, usually blucher, for easiest access.

Lamelift—sheet of natural cork used to laminate and shape into shortage elevations.

Length—dimension along the last bottom center line from toe point to the heel point.

Linings—material, usually of canvas, leather, or plastic, covering the inner portions of the shoe in contact with the foot—to provide a smooth surface.

Medallion—perforated design used to decorate the toe of a shoe.

Midsole—a sole placed between innersole and outersole.

Moccasin—(a) shoe of one-piece vamp quarter and sole, stitched back seam, and tongue or (b) a stitched and/or perforated circular design on the vamp of a shoe for decoration.

Monk Pattern—low-quarter blucher with strap and buckle.

Napoleon Tap—a sole placed under the original sole but undercut smaller than the original.

Oak—sole leather produced from hides and vegetable-tanned, with a combination of tanning materials.

Oil Tannage—tanning with fish oils. It is used especially in the manufacturing of certain soft leather, such as chamois and buckskin.

Outflare—to spread out or turn laterally—a swing out of forepart of shoe.

Oxford—low-quarter shoe—quarters extend to just below malleoli.

Patterns—templates of cardboard or fiberboard, brass bound, approximating the last as guide. These are used for cutting components of the uppers and linings to be incorporated in a shoe.

Perforations—a series of punched holes for decoration or ventilation.

Pigskin—leather made from the skin of pigs or hogs but also from the peccary and carpincho. The "pigskin" of footballs is made from cattlehide.

Pinking—edge of material serrated into angles or scallops for decoration.

Plate—a flat piece of material (steel, aluminum, leather, or plastic) moulded to form an arch support.

Platform—a thick midsole usually made of cork to raise the sole.

Pump—any shoe not built above the vamp and quarter lines and held to the foot without fasteners.

Quarter—posterior or backpart of the uppers.

Rawhide—term for cattlehide that has been dehaired, limed, and oiled, but not tanned. It is used for mechanical purposes such as belt lacings and pins, loom pickers, gaskets, pinions, gears, luggage, and trunk binding.

Rocker—curved base causing rocking instead of flexing action.

Saddle—a piece of leather extending from the shank over the throat and up to the top of the quarters.

Shank—area of the shoe between the heel breast and ball.

Shank Piece—reinforcement of shank (spring steel, wood, or plastic).

Shell—unfinished framework or base of an arch or full-length foot mold.

Side or Side-Upper Leather—a term to describe a shoe upper leather consisting of the grain or hair side of cattlehides. The name originated from the practice of slitting a hide along the backbone into two halves or "sides."

Skive—to cut off in thin layers or to a fine edge.

Skiver—a grain-split of a sheepskin, used for hat sweatbands, linings, bindings, and fancy leatherwork. It is also known as "corrected grain."

Slipsole—a half-sole extending from toe to shank between the outer and innersoles.

Sock Lining—a piece of leather or coated fabric pasted over the whole insole on the inside of the shoe to cover stitches and staples.

Split Leather—leather obtained from the underside or flesh portion upon splitting of the original skin to get the desired weight or thickness.

Splint, Dennis Browne—any bar of rigid material used to maintain the position of shoes and/or feet for correction of abnormal conditions of the feet, legs, or hips.

Splint, Counter—a strip of flexible material attached to the counters of a shoe, used to limit internal rotation.

Suede Finish—a finish produced by rubbing the surface of leather on a carborundum or emery wheel to separate the fibers and produce a leather nap. The grain of leather may be suede-finished, but the process is most often applied to the flesh surface.

Support—a reinforcement or arch used to control the stress of weight-bearing areas.

Tanning—process of curing animal or reptile skins into leather.

Tap—a sole placed under the original sole.

Tawing—an Old English term to describe alum tanning.

Throat—the shallow part or entrance of the shoe, normally at the waist or where the vamp and quarters meet at the base of the tongue.

Toe Box—reinforcement used to retain the original contour of the toe and guard against trauma or abrasion.

Toe Cap—an extra piece sewed to the vamp, covering the toe area.

Toe Point—the foremost point of a last at the toe.

Toe Recede—slope of the top surface of the last or shoe from toe point to the point of full-toe thickness.

Toe Spring—space between the outersole and base plane or horizontal treading surface measured vertically at the toe (allows rocker effect for toe off).

Tongue—strip of leather attached to the vamp, lying under the lacing or straps of a shoe.

Toplift—layer of material forming the plantar wearing surface of the heel.

Tread—the weight-bearing surface of a shoe sole between the shank and forepart.

Treadpoint—the point of the bottom forepart of last or shoe in contact with the base plane or treading surface.

Turn Shoe—a single shoe with flexible sole in which the upper and sole are stitched together with a horizontal chain stitch while the wrong side is out on the last (then turned).

Upper—combined upper portions of the shoe, above the sole construction, including the outer surface materials, linings, and closures.

Vamp—anterior or forepart of the upper.

Velcro—nylon hook and loop tape fasteners, which cling together on contact and are easily separated.

Waist—the smallest dimension in girth between the ball and instep.

Wall—medial and lateral perimeter of the forepart of last or shoe—the relatively straight sides around the periphery of the last or shoe.

Wax Finish—a process to finish heavier leathers by working wax into the flesh side. It is used in the manufacture of heavy-duty work shoes.

Wedge—a piece of leather tapered to a thin edge, used to elevate one side of sole or heel.

Well—a hollowed area (hole).

Wellington—a square-tipped boot.

Welt—a narrow strip of leather used to unite the upper, innersole, and outersole of a shoe by means of stitching.

Width—dimension across the ball area of the last or shoe, at its widest point.

Wing Tip—a perforated and pinked design, wing-shaped, decorating the vamp.

REFERENCES

1. ALTSCHUL, J. Altschul Shoe Company of Brooklyn. Personal communication, 1965.
2. AMERICAN ACADEMY OF ORTHOPAEDIC SURGEONS. *Orthopaedic Appliances Atlas.* J. W. Edwards, Ann Arbor, 1952.
3. BORDOLI, E. *The Boot and Shoe Maker.* Gresham Publishing Co., London, 1935.
4. BRAND, P. W., AND BERGTHOLDT, H. T. Thermography: an aid in the management of insensitive feet and stumps. *Arch. Phys. Med. Rehabil., 56:* 205–209, 1975.
5. BRAND, P. W., DRURY, F. A., BUKKE, J. F., JOHNSON, G. A., AND WELCH, D. *Construction of Sandals for Prevention of Injuries to Insensitive Feet.* Rehabilitation Service, United States Public Health Service Hospital, Carville, La.
6. BRITISH STANDARDS INSTITUTION. Method of measurement for surgical footwear. British Standard 3350. London, 1961.
7. CHERNINA, N. P., AND DAVIDOWA, V. P. Changes of sole pressure depending upon the height of the shoe heel. *Ortop. Travmatol. Protez., 2:* 146, 1964.

8. DICKSON, F. D., AND DIVELY, R. L. *Functional Disorders of the Foot.* J. B. Lippincott Co., Philadelphia, 1944.
9. GILL, W. S. *Shoeman's Manual.* Gill Publications, Camden, Maine, 1951.
10. HERTZMAN, C. A. Use of Plastazote in foot disabilities. *Am. J. Phys. Med., 52:* 289–303, 1973.
11. INMAN, V. T. UC-BL Dual-axis ankle control system and UC-BL shoe insert. *Bull. Prosthet. Res.,* 10–11, 1969.
12. LEVINE, H. AND LEVINE, B. Herbert Levine Shoe Company of New York. Personal communication, 1965.
13. LEWIN, P. *The Foot and Ankle.* Lea & Febiger, Philadelphia, 1954.
14. LOWMAN, C. L. The rocker soled shoe. *Orthop. Prosthet. Appl. J., 8:* 40, 1959.
15. MCILMURRAY, W., AND GREENBAUM, W. The application of SACH foot principles to orthotics. *Orthop. Prosthet. Appl. J., 8:* 49, 1959.
16. MCLEAN, R. Jones & Vining Company of Brockton. Personal communication, 1965.
17. MORRISON, R. T. Genesco, Nashville. Personal communication, 1965.
18. MORTON, D. J., AND FULLER, O. D. *Human Locomotion and Body Form.* Williams & Wilkins, Baltimore, 1952.
19. MURRAY, A. E. Murray Space Shoe Company of Bridgeport. Personal communication, 1965.
20. RABL, C. R. H. *Orthopadie des Fusses.* F. Enka, Stuttgart, 1963.
21. RUBIN, G., BONARRIGO, D., DANISI M., AND DIXON, M. The shoe as a component of the orthosis. *Orthotics Prosthet., 30:* 2, 1976.
22. SHENK, F. Veterans Administration Prosthetics Center of New York. Personal communication, 1964.
23. THORNTON, J. H. *Textbook of Footwear Manufacture.* London, 1964.
24. WHITMAN, R. *Orthopedic Surgery.* Philadelphia, 1919.
25. WRIGHT, T. *The Romance of the Shoe.* London, 1922.
26. UNITED SHOE MACHINERY CORPORATION. *How American Shoes Are Made.* Boston, no date.
27. ZAMOSKY, I. Shoe modifications in lower-extremity orthotics. *Bull. Prosthet. Res., 10-2:* 54–95, 1964.

12

Crutches, Canes, and Walkers

GEORGE VARGHESE, M.D.

Holding sticks or staffs in the hand to assist in walking is perhaps as old as the history of mankind. The oldest of the assistive devices is the cane. In early days it was used for support, defense, and the procurement of food. Later, it became the symbol of power and aristocracy. Historically, it has many associations apart from use as a walking aid.

The earliest known documentation of any gait aid is the carving at the tomb of Herkuf of the 6th Egyptian dynasty (2830 B.C.), which depicts a crude staff (1, 4, 5). Graphic recordings on vases from 5th century A.D. Greece show crude forms of crutches with a single upright bar and a crossbar at the top. Many carvings and paintings of the middle ages show ambulation aids; long and short crutches, peg legs, knee pads, etc. (4). Many additions of crutches and canes have been made since the 18th century. Present crutches, canes, and walkers are used to provide support and protection, to reduce pain in the lower extremities, and to improve balance during ambulation. This chapter will review the major types of hand-held ambulation aids used today.

Selection of Gait Aids

Most patients with physical disabilities of the lower limbs will need a walker, crutch, or cane for ambulation. Generally, the more diabled the individual, the more complex the walking device required; the walker supplies the most support, and the cane gives the least. The prime objective is to select a gait aid most suitable for the functional needs of the patient. It is not only important to select an aid but also to determine the most suitable gait pattern. As there are a variety of gait aids and gait patterns, their selection should be made by a physician or a physical therapist. Furthermore, the patient often needs preambulation exercises in addition to training in the use of the gait aid, and these exercises must be prescribed.

432

A successful ambulation training program starts with complete evaluation of the patient. Factors that influence gait training apart from joint range and muscle strength in the lower extremities include range of motion of joints and muscle strength in the upper extremities, coordination and trunk balance, and impairments in sensory perception. Age of the patient, mental status, and physical endurance will help to determine the ambulatory needs of the patient. In training, the patient often starts ambulation between the parallel bars and then progresses to walker, crutch, or cane. Very few patients can perform crutch gaits without practice. Therefore, it is essential that all disabled persons with gait problems have a supervised period of training. Ideally, patients should continue training until their use of walking aids approaches their normal gait as closely as possible.

CONSTRUCTION OF GAIT AIDS

Canes were first made from cuttings of tree branches and have until recently almost always been made of hardwood. Until the 18th century, crutches consisted of a single piece of wood with a crossbar at the top made of wood or cow horn (4). Since then, a variety of designs and materials have been introduced in construction of gait aids. The introduction of tubular aluminum about 60 years ago has made important changes in fabrication. Tubular aluminum is strong and significantly lighter than wood. At the present time, both wood and tubular aluminum are the main materials of use for construction. Hardwoods like birch, hickory, or maple are usually selected for wood construction. Tubular aluminum or steel are exclusively used for walkers. Materials such as plastic, plastic foam, and rubber have also been used as accessories in construction of aids to improve safety and comfort of the users. All devices come in adjustable sizes, and new designs are frequently introduced. However, the standard types of walking aids have remained unchanged for years and still serve their purposes extremely well.

CANES

A cane can transmit 20 to 25% of body weight away from the lower extremities (6). It has only a single point of contact with the body and, so, the support provided is less, compared to other gait aids. In cases where more than partial weight relief or support is needed, a cane will not be the appropriate aid.

When one is walking, the cane is held in the hand opposite the involved side (1, 2). This provides a more physiological gait because in normal walking the opposite leg and arm move together. Moreover, in unilateral lower extremity disorders, this method will widen the base of support and reduce stress on the opposite hip because of the shift in center of gravity produced by the contralateral arm support. Canes of aluminum are adjustable in total length, but wooden canes must be cut to size.

Regular canes generally have a 'hoop' or 'T'-shaped handle but come in many forms (see Fig. 12.1). A small amount of additional stability can be

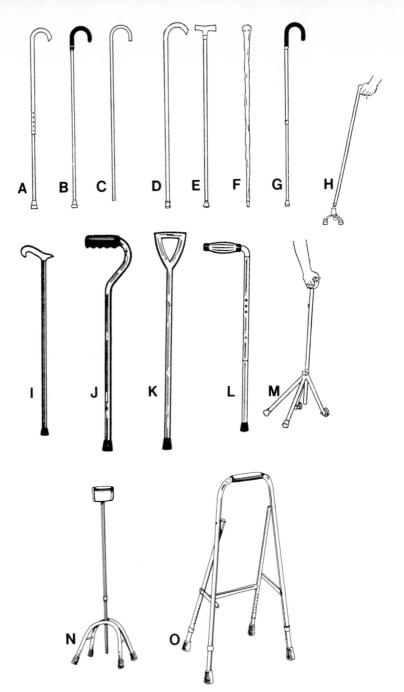

Fig. 12.1. Canes. *A*, adjustable aluminum cane; *B*, aluminum cane with rubber-covered handle; *C*, nonadjustable aluminum cane; *D*, crook-top cane; *E*, T-top cane; *F*, straight or ball-top cane; *G*, adjustable aluminum cane with rubber-covered handle; *H*, crook-top cane with crab foot attachment; *I*, slant-handled cane; *J*, curved-top cane; *K*, shovel-handled cane; *L*, straight-handled cane; *M*, cane glider with wheels; *N*, quad cane; *O*, walk cane.

provided by the four-legged or "quad cane" (see Fig. 12.1). Any four-footed cane makes the gait slow, but the quad cane is particularly useful for hemiplegic patients because of the additional stability that it provides. The disadvantage of slowing the gait is negligible in most hemiplegic persons because their gait is slow anyway.

The walk-cane or "hemi-walker" (see Fig. 12.1) is another design with four feet. This combines the features of a walker and quad cane and is ideal for use in hemiplegics. It has a wider base of support than a quad cane and provides significantly better lateral support. The walk-cane can be used as an intermediate step during ambulation training, that is, as the patient comes out of parallel bars and before he is ready to use the quad cane. It is made of tubular aluminum and is more compact than the quad cane, as it is foldable.

The "Ortho cane" has a plastic palm grip and a curve staff at the top and is supposed to provide better grip and better controlled balance for the patient (see Fig. 12.1).

Other canes are also available with stirrup-like grips and foldable seating. Canes for the blind are generally more flexible, carefully balanced, and very light, compared with those used to shift or support body weight.

Cane length is adjusted so that the highest point of the cane is at the level of the greater trochanter (5). This gives the elbow about 20 to 30° flexion. Incorrectly fitted canes produce an unsightly and inefficient gait pattern. A short cane will tend to hold the elbow in complete extension and reduce support during the stance phase. A long cane will force the elbow into too much flexion, putting excessive demands on the triceps and shoulder muscles, which may increase fatigue.

CRUTCHES

Crutches have two points of contact with the body and thus provide better stability than canes. There are two basic types of crutches—axillary and nonaxillary. A nonaxillary crutch can transfer 40 to 50% of body weight; axillary crutches transfer as much as 80%(6). They also provide better trunk support than nonaxillary or forearm crutches.

Standard axillary crutches have double uprights with a shoulder piece and hand grip or bar. Crutches are available in different sizes. The "extension crutch" is one in which the length can be adjusted. Because of the additional piece of wood, this type is heavier than the regular crutch. However, it is useful with children, for whom the length can be adjusted for growth, and in hospitals, where it can be used for different patients. Adjustable crutches are also made of aluminum.

The 'Ortho crutch' is a single bar aluminum crutch which has a contoured underarm piece and an adjustable hand piece. It is claimed to be more comfortable and lighter than regular crutches. Figs. 12.2 and 12.3 show this and other types of crutches.

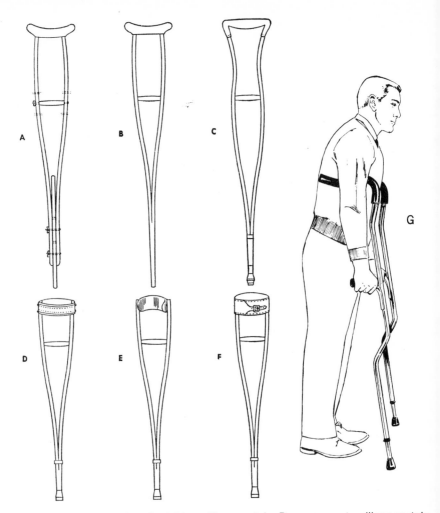

Fig. 12.2. Crutches. *A*, adjustable axillary crutch; *B*, permanent axillary crutch; *C*, spring-top axillary crutch with Whittemore tip; *D*, forearm crutch with closed leather circle cuff; *E*, forearm crutch with U-shaped metal cuff which may be covered with leather; *F*, forearm crutch with open circle cuff, closed by leather strap and buckle; *G*, "Ortho-crutch" (From a photograph supplied by the Lumex Corporation).

Patients using axillary crutches can free their hand for opening doors by leaning on the shoulder piece but should be instructed not to lean the axilla against the shoulder bar for prolonged periods. Pressure against the axilla can cause compression of the radial nerve, which may lead to "crutch palsy" (7). Occasionally, median and ulnar nerves also can be compressed in the upper arm or in the hand and wrist.

Nonaxillary crutches are best suited for patients with good trunk balance

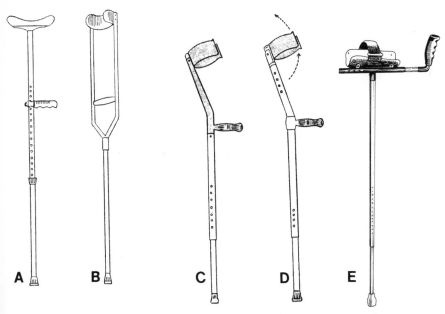

Fig. 12.3. Crutches. *A*, telescopic underarm aluminum crutch; *B*, single-upright arm aluminum crutch with U-shaped cuff; *C*, forearm aluminum crutch with stationary forearm piece; *D*, forearm aluminum crutch with adjustable forearm piece. *E*, platform crutch. [*A* to *D* are from *Therapeutic Exercise* (5).]

and confidence in ambulation. Lofstrand crutches are the most popular nonaxillary type crutches. They are made of tubular aluminum with a padded hand bar and forearm cuff. This cuff helps to stabilize the forearm during weight bearing. It is made of steel or plastic and may be padded for comfort or to reduce noise, as clicking of these crutches can be very annoying. Lofstrand crutches are a most useful substitute for canes because the forearm support stabilizes the wrist during bearing and makes ambulation easier and safer. A person using two canes cannot free his hand to do things like grasp a stair rail, open a door handle, or adjust his clothes. Using a Lofstrand crutch, he can release his hand to perform these tasks without dropping the crutches.

The triceps crutch, often called 'Canadian crutch,' has an extension above the elbow. It has two cuffs, one above and one below the elbow, which support the arm with elbow in extension. This is useful for patients with some triceps weakness.

Platform crutch is often used in patients with arthritis. This has a platform on the top level of the crutch to rest the forearm and a vertical hand grip at the distal end of the platform. It is indicated for patients with flexion contracture of the elbow and also for those with weak grip because of pain and deformities of the hand and wrist. Velcro straps around the forearm may assist in holding the crutch in those with poor grip. The advantage of the platform crutch is that the body weight is borne mostly on the forearm instead of the hand. The hand grip can also be contoured to adapt to the deformities.

Crutch length and the level of hand pieces are the most important considerations when measuring a patient for crutches. There are several ways to measure the length for axillary crutches. One way is to measure with the patient supine, taking the distance from the anterior axillary fold to the heel (without shoes) and adding 2 inches (3). This will be the length from the top of the axillary pad of crutch to the tip. Another method is to measure the patient standing erect with the shoulders relaxed, and crutch length is the distance from anterior axillary fold to a point 6 inches lateral to the fifth toe (3, 8). The hand bars are adjusted in each case to give about 30° of elbow flexion.

Crutch Accessories

Crutch tips are attached to the foot of the crutch. Crutches with absent or inadequate rubber tips are dangerous. All crutches should have safety tips at least 1.5 inches in diameter (see Fig. 12.4). These prevent slippage because of their suction design and also function as shock absorbers. Also available is a retractable metal-spiked tip that can be used on ice, but this is not very comfortable.

Axillary pads are usually made of sponge rubber and prevent undue pressure against the nerve and vessels in the axilla.

Hand grips are also padded with sponge pads to relieve pressure on the hand. This can also reduce the chance for slippage. Hand grips can be built up or contoured as required for special patients.

A triceps band is helpful for patients who have weakness of the triceps and the inability to maintain elbow extension during weight bearing. It is made of metal or stiff leather and is attached to the upper part of the crutch.

A wrist strap of leather or plastic can be used for patients with weak wrist extensors to assist in holding the hand grip. Fig. 12.4 shows a number of these crutches, etc.

WALKERS

Walkers give maximum support during ambulation, as compared to canes and crutches. The main disadvantage in their use is that the gait is very slow and awkward. Dependency on a walker may produce bad posture and walking habits. In most instances a walker is limited to indoor use, and the standard ones cannot be used in climbing stairs. Nevertheless, often, a walker is used in early ambulation training, even in patients who eventually will go to lesser support. As the patient gains more balance and confidence, he can switch to crutches or canes. The walker is best suited for the patients

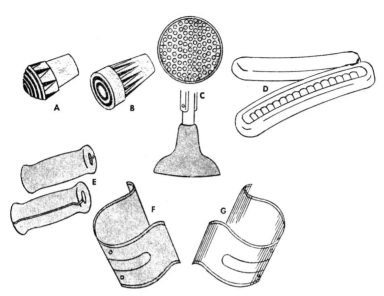

Fig. 12.4. Crutch accessories. *A*, crutch tip, small and unsafe; *B*, suction crutch tip; *C*, Crutshoe large tip with suction bottom; *D*, shoulder pad of latex or sponge rubber; *E*, rubber hand grips; *F*, rubber-covered forearm cuff; *G*, steel forearm. [From *Therapeutic Exercise* (5).]

who are confused or have poor balance, as learning to use it is easy. If safety is a major consideration, it provides good support and a slow safe gait (see Fig. 12.5).

Walkers are made in several sizes, both for pediatric and adult groups. They are all made of tubular aluminum or other tubular metal, with plastic hand grips and rubber-tipped legs. Most are light in weight and very durable. Standard models have telescopic or adjustable legs and, so, the heights of walkers can be adjusted to most individual patients. However, for very tall patients, an especially tall design may need to be ordered. Several additional types and features are available. The "rollators" have wheels on the front legs. To push this walker, the patient has to raise the back legs off the floor. This feature helps patients with incoordination of the upper extremity and trunk, where lifting crutches or walkers and placing them forward may be difficult. However, the instability introduced by the wheels may prove dangerous. Patients with weak upper extremities also may benefit from a rolling walker.

The reciprocal walker has swivel joints allowing reciprocal action as each side of the walker moves alternately. This allows a longer stride and a less awkward gait. Walkers are also available with platform type of forearm support (see Fig. 12.5). This is helpful in patients with flexion contracture of

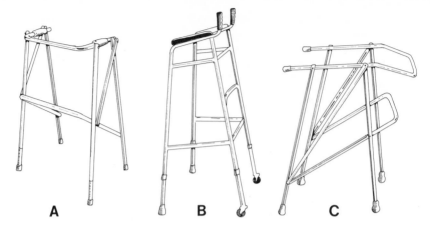

Fig. 12.5. Walkers. *A*, standard walker; *B*, forearm support walker; *C*, stair-climbing walker.

the elbow or pain or deformities of the wrist and hand, but they are generally quite heavy.

Most walkers are too light for patients who have incoordination but good strength in their upper extremities. Therefore, one may wish to try adding weights such as sandbags to the crosspieces of the walker for such cases. A heavy-wheeled walker with foldaway seat and removeable back has been used for years around institutions. It is generally awkward and unsafe and is not particularly useful for most patients.

Finally, there is a stair-climbing walker that is useful primarily in patients with good balance and superior strength in their upper extremities, such as young paraplegics (see Fig. 12.5).

The walker is fitted by placing it about 10 to 12 inches in front of the patient so that it partially surrounds him. The correct height is set with the patient standing straight, shoulders relaxed and elbows flexed to between 15 and 20° (2).

Gait Patterns and Preambulation Exercises

Gait aids are an extension of upper extremities to transmit the weight bearing and to provide support. Therefore, strength and mobility of the upper extremities are prime considerations in gait training of disabled persons. The important muscle groups are shoulder depressors (latissimus dorsi, lower trapezius, pectoralis minor), shoulder flexors, elbow and wrist extensors, and finger flexors (3, 5). Exercises to increase strength and coordination of all these groups can be started while one patient is nonambulatory. In addition, the patient may have to have exercise of the trunk muscles to improve his balance-and-endurance period. As soon as the patient is ready to stand up, he starts balancing exercises between the parallel bars and then balances with appropriate gait aids. Walking should not be started unless standing balances are secure and posture is satisfactory.

Learning the use of crutches needs more skill than other gait aids. Determining which gait aid is the best for the patient depends on the following factors: (a) general functional ability; (b) amount of weight bearing allowable on the lower extremity; (c) balance; and (d) ability to maintain the body erect (3).

There are basically two variations in crutch gaits, the point gaits and the swing gaits. The point gaits are as follows: (a) four-point gait. The sequence of placement of "points" is right crutch, left foot, left crutch, right foot. Because three points are always in contact with the floor, this is a very stable gait and is often used in patients with ataxia. The disadvantages are that it is rather slow and people with limited mental capacity have a problem learning it. (b) Two-point alternate gait. The sequence is right crutch, left foot, left crutch, right foot. This is faster than four-point gait and is fairly stable. It is used in ataxia and to reduce weight bearing. (c) The three-point gait. Both crutches and the weaker or painful leg are together and then the sound leg. This gait is used when one leg is painful or nonweight-bearing and generally requires good balance. (d) There are tripod gaits of two types: tripod alternate gait, in which the crutch sequence is right crutch, left crutch, then drag the body to the crutch level, and tripod simultaneous gait, in which both crutches are advanced simultaneously, then drag the body. Tripod gaits are slow and laborious, but they are stable gaits. Paraplegic patients usually start with the tripod gait, and when they improve their balance, they change to a swing gait.

There are two types of *swing gait*: (a) swing-to gait. In this type, both crutches are moved first, then lift and swing the body to the level of the crutch. Swing to gait is easy to learn, and most paraplegics resort to this gait. (2) swing-through gait. The sequence is that both crutches are advanced simultaneously, the arm pushes down, and the body is lifted and swings beyond the crutch level. Swing-through gaits are very energy demanding and difficult. They require a good trunk balance and good strength in the upper extremities.

With the cane, only point gaits are possible. As discussed earlier, when only one cane is used, it should be held contralateral to the affected lower limb. The cane and affected limb are advanced simultaneously with weight borne through the arm as required. With two canes, the patient resorts to a point gait, just as in the case of crutch walking.

In climbing stairs with crutches or canes, handrails should be used. The safest technique is to advance the unaffected leg first when going up and advance the affected leg first on descending. Gait training is not complete unless the patient has learned not only how to walk on the level but also how to walk around inclines and up and down curbs with gait aids.

REFERENCES

1. BLOUNT, W. Don't throw away the cane. *J. Bone Joint Surg. (Am.) 38:* 695–708, 1956.
2. BURGESS, E., ALEXANDER, A. Mobility Aids. In *Atlas of Orthopedics.* C. V. Mosby Co., 1975.
3. DEAVER, G. G. What every physician should know about the teaching of crutch walking. *J. A. M. A.* 470–472, 1950.
4. EPSTEIN, S. Art, history, and the crutch. *Ann. Med. Hist., 9:* 304–313, 1937.
5. HOEBERMAN, M. Crutches and cane exercises and use. In *Therapeutic Exercise,* Chapter 15. E. Licht, New Haven, 1958.
6. JEBSEN, R. Use and abuse of ambulation aids *J. A. M. A., 199:* 63–68, 1967.
7. RUDIN, L., LEVINE, L. Bilateral compression of Radial Nerve. *Phys. Ther. Rev. 31:* 229–231
8. SINE, R., LISA, S. *Basic Rehabilitation Techniques.* Aspin System Corporation, Germantown, Md., 1977.

13

Wheelchairs and Other Indoor Vehicles for the Disabled[1]

HERMAN L. KAMENETZ, M.D.

History

At all times, as is still the case today, those unable to walk have been carried or helped to walk by others. They have also been helped by various objects, from walking sticks to sedan chairs to vehicles on wheels. The latter, used indoors, are the subject of this chapter. The oldest illustration of a vehicle on wheels is probably that on a Greek vase dated about 530 B.C., now in the Louvre. It shows a bed on small wheels, occupied by a child (49, 84).

We have to advance by more than 1,000 years to find what probably is the oldest representation extant of a wheeled chair. Two specimens of it are beautifully pictured on stone slabs of Chinese funerary couches. Now at the William Rockhill Nelson Gallery of Kansas City, Mo., they date from the 6th century A.D. They show a large, obviously heavy, wooden chair occupied by a man keeping his feet on the seat. The chair has three wheels, the single wheel being in the front. Two short poles protrude to the rear, and the axle protrudes to the sides, most likely so that the chair could be carried, when necessary. It seems that three helpers were needed to carry the chair and at least one to push it (49). There is no indication that either the Ionian bed on rollers or the Chinese chair on wheels were meant for those who could not walk, but we may assume that they served such individuals as well.

We have to proceed to the Middle Ages or later to find proof of wheeled vehicles for the sick and disabled. However, we encounter there, besides the

---

[1] Some passages of text were reproduced from *The Wheelchair Book* (49) with permission of the publisher, Charles C Thomas.

usual all-purpose vehicles such as the horsedrawn carriage and the valuable, if humble, wheelbarrow, only two which could also have been used indoors. The simplest one of all time was a seating board on four small wheels. Low enough for the users to push themselves by using their hands against the ground, it resembled the scooting board of today, used by mechanics to slide under an automobile. Woodcuts dating from the Middle Ages which show such rolling seats, mainly used by individuals without legs, are probably the oldest representations of a wheeled conveyance moved by the disabled himself. A little more elaborate was the slightly higher seating board with sidewalls, resembling an open box with two larger wheels. Hans Burgkmair, early in the 16th century, made several engravings of such a cart, which was to be pulled with the aid of a rope, or pushed (83). Thus, it needed outside help.

For easy moving of the sick inside the house, beds and armchairs were fitted with small wheels or rollers (49). They were certainly of general use and not only for the sick.

From the 16th century on, however, several reports were known (45) on invalid chairs on rollers, made for particular individuals. One example is outstanding for several reasons: it was made for a king, it was described and illustrated in minute detail by its constructor in a book, and it had many features of chairs on wheels built three centuries later (Fig. 13.1). Philip II, King of Spain, had a most devoted Flemish nobleman in his service, Jehan Lhermite, who built this "gout chair" for his sovereign, as he reported in 1595 in his memoirs (59). The chair moved on four small wheels and had a reclining back and an elevating legrest with footboard. Curved metal bars with notches fixed the back and the legrest in various positions. The

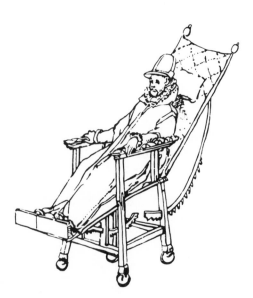

Fig. 13.1. King Philip II of Spain in his rolling chair. After a pen drawing from 1595 (59). (Courtesy of Yale Sterling Library and Russ Chester, Veterans Administration Medical Center, Washington, D. C.)

armrests could be reclined sideward. The chair was covered with a horsehair mattress and, "though it was but of wood, leather, and ordinary iron, it was worth ten times its weight in gold and silver for His Majesty's comfort," in the words of his devoted servant, the maker of the chair.

Yet, there was still one feature that even this ingenious chair was lacking: self-propulsion. With the exception of the primitive scooting board, no vehicle had apparently been reported that could be moved by its user himself until the 17th century. The first of these were chairs moved by two cranks that turned the single frontwheel.

Johann Hautsch in Nuremberg made several such chairs in the 1640's, mostly for patients with gout (21). In nearby Altdorf, about 1655, Stephen Farfler, a paraplegic watchmaker, built a small cart for himself, also with two cranks. Solidary with the frontwheel was a wheel very much resembling that of a watch, only larger, of course. The vehicle, which had been used by his owner even outside his home, could still be seen until it perished during the war in 1945 (21, 67, 73).

Scientifically-minded Prince Rupert of the Palatinate, in about 1675, built an armchair to be used by someone to "drive around easily in his room if he does not feel well enough to walk" (28). Twenty rolling chairs were recorded in the inventory of the Castle of Versailles in 1700, and it was in such a *roulette* that Louis XIV took his last meal in 1715 (45).

Finally, in the 18th century, after other crank-operated chairs (2), there appeared the first chairs moved by directly turning the large wheels, as shown in an Italian catalog of medical instruments (86). From several drawings made between 1792 and 1798 by Thomas Rowlandson (39), we know of bulky heavy wooden wheelchairs which were pushed by a man, but which had wheels, apparently made of one piece of wood, large enough for self-propulsion. A third small wheel was under the footboard. This chair, which figures in several of the caricaturist's indoor and outdoor scenes of the English spa of Bath, seems to be the link between King Philip's chair and the wooden hospital chair of the 20th century.

Many of the rolling chairs used in Bath and other spas were no doubt manufactured by the brothers John and Alfred Carter (14) in London, the creators of many chairs for indoor and outdoor use. In their 1881 catalog, among a great variety of rolling chairs, invalid couches, and beds, there are a folding reclining chair of iron on small rollers and several models of a chair with wheels large enough to be operated by its occupant (13).

In the U.S., wheelchairs were apparently not used until the Civil War, but those of that period show a striking resemblance with the wooden chairs for self-propulsion with a single smaller metal wheel in the rear (70) that can still be seen today, 100 years later. The large wheels were still made of wood. However, by 1880 the great bicycle craze had started, after bicycle wheels had changed from wood to iron, the hollow rubber tire had been added, and their sizes had been standardized. Peter Gendron is probably to be credited with being the first in this country to make wheelchairs with wire-spoked wheels in about 1890 (20, 34).

Wheelstretchers, around the turn of the century, were fitted with the same wheels. Frequently, one of these wheels was placed at the middle of each long side and either a swivel wheel at the middle of each short side or a small roller at each corner. At that time, however, we find the stretcher as it is used today, i.e., with large wheels at one end and small wheels at the other (93), and by about 1911, a wheelstretcher for self-propulsion, although without handrims, was commercially available (17).

Wheelchairs, whose large wheels had been fitted with handrims for self-wheeling as early as the Civil War (49), continued to be seen without handrims far into the 20th century. Wheels were, however, large enough for self-propulsion. Folding chairs on wheels—they folded from back to front—became also available around 1910, according to an American catalog, but there was still no folding wheelchair for self-propulsion, except for one in which only the back was collapsible (17). A chair made commercially available in or before 1914 was fully folding, although still from back to front, and was probably for self-wheeling, because it had bicycle wheels (9). Its shortcoming was its weight: 70 pounds.

The victims of World War I increased the demand for invalid chairs, the automobile stimulated the search for a chair of easy handling that was light and foldable so that it could be put in the car, and technology developed to the point of enabling the founding, in short succession, of two manufactories of the modern lightweight foldable self-propelling wheelchair. In 1933, Herbert A. Everest and Harry C. Jennings, two engineers in Los Angeles, began manufacturing wheelchairs and in 1934, Samuel Duke, who had a rental supply business in Chicago (49), began to do so. Since then, the wheelchair, as well as other indoor vehicles, has markedly improved, and their importance has increased as valuable adjuvants in the medical rehabilitation of the disabled. Wheelchair users have organized in associations for the practice of sports and many other activities. Airplanes and hotels have made possible trips beyond national borders.

It is estimated that in the U.S. and other countries, 1 out of 600 persons is a wheelchair user (36, 96). This ratio is probably steadily increasing because of the increasing older population; the ratio was indeed found to be 1:46 for persons 75 years old, or older (96).

The increase in the number of wheelchairs and their more extensive use are reflected in architectural changes of private homes, public buildings, and streets (5, 12, 18, 41, 69). The wheelchair has become the symbol of the handicapped and the symbol of access for the handicapped (Fig. 13.2), and the possibilities for access are steadily expanding for the motivated wheelchair user (6, 7, 22, 40, 42, 48, 64, 65, 91, 94).

Advances in technology in general and in biomedical engineering are leading to constant improvement in vehicles for the disabled. The U. S. Veterans Administration developed a program of evaluation of vehicles,

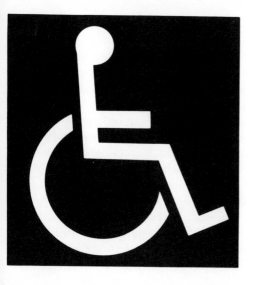

Fig. 13.2. Accessibility Symbol. Emblem used to designate areas accessible to the handicapped.

accessories, and other functional aids in order to provide an intelligent basis for their selection and use, to establish functional standards, and to guide manufacturers and researchers. Findings are reported in the Bulletin for Prosthetics Research (8, 60, 61, 75, 77, 92, 97, 98), which has been published since 1964 by the Prosthetic and Sensory Aids Service of the Veterans Administration. A new Service of Rehabilitative Engineering Research and Development was created in 1977. The results of such an endeavor will no doubt include further progress in the field of indoor vehicles and their appropriate use by the handicapped. To assure such appropriate use is the purpose of this chapter.

Classification of Indoor Vehicles

The following classification may serve as a synopsis of the various devices discussed in this chapter. More detailed definitions are given in the respective sections.

Rolling chairs: chairs on wheels, casters, or rollers. Examples:
   a. wheelchairs—for self-propulsion.
   b. glide-abouts or casterchairs—easily moving, with little pressure.
   c. push chairs—usually needing an attendant.
Rolling walkers: for ambulation—some with seat for resting.
Rolling stands: for the upright occupant whose lower limbs remain stationary.
Rolling stretchers: for the recumbent patient.

Indications and Contraindications for Indoor Vehicles

The great variety of available vehicles and accessories should give the physician a high degree of specification in his selection of a device for his individual patient. General guidelines are given here. Indications, precautions, and contraindications for a particular vehicle, part, or accessory will be discussed, together with the description of the object itself.

Among the indoor vehicles, it is the wheelchair in particular that is not only a means for the transportation of a sick person but also a vehicle in its own right, a functional aid which can spare the heart, support the body, stimulate activities, and afford locomotion while maintaining, immobilized, one or another part of the body. For the disabled, it can be "an extension of his body" (80), can assist him in some of his functions, and can enable him to perform tasks otherwise impossible. The maneuverability of the wheelchair enables many patients to move about without undue effort. In many instances, it means the difference between needing and not needing an attendant, between confinement to a space spanned by the patient's outstretched arms and his freedom of locomotion throughout his apartment, an institution, or even out of doors, allowing the use of a desk, an office, a classroom, or an automobile. Among its psychologic values are that of stimulating greater interest in one's surroundings and a greater desire to keep moving.

Yet, there are disadvantages, limitations, and even contraindications to the use of a vehicle. It is therefore imperative that the physician prescribe its specifications and supervise its proper use. He must assess the patient's remaining capacities, abilities, functions, and potentials, in addition to his disability and loss of function. Indeed, it will not suffice to make an assessment of the patient's morphology and loss of function; it may be necessary to test joint ranges, muscle strength, coordination, and endurance. The cardiovascular system must also be evaluated and, in some cases, pulmonary function tests will help to answer the question as to whether the patient should propel his wheelchair himself or have a push chair and be helped. We must consider the natural history and progress of the disease or disability, along with such elements as growth, the danger of prolonged use, the possibility of amputation of one or both lower limbs—lest a faulty prescription deprive the physician of success and the patient of money. In some instances, final purchase should be deferred until the physician is reasonably sure of the level of permanent disability. Meanwhile, it is advisable to rent a wheelchair from a reliable supply house where rental payments are usually credited toward the purchase price of a chair. Sometimes, a vocational evaluation is also essential.

INDICATIONS

Those who need wheelchairs are those who either should not or cannot walk, which means that walking is either inadvisable or impossible.

Inadvisability of ambulation may be because of contraindications to weight bearing or to dependency of a leg, interference with wound healing, convalescence prior to ambulation, inadequate safety in walking, or a deficiency of the patient's judgment. In all of these conditions, the restriction against walking may be temporary and so is the indication for a rolling chair. After the wound is healed or the cardiac problem has improved, ambulation will probably be desirable. However, until such progress has been achieved, in many instances where ambulation is contraindicated, complete bedrest is not desirable either. Indeed, since the 1950's, much evidence has been collected that for the cardiac patient, the sitting position is preferable to the recumbent (58). If the armchair treatment is the treatment of choice, then the wheelchair is the chair of choice in many instances, but its advantages should be weighed against those of other rolling chairs.

Deficiency in ambulation results usually from the involvement of both lower limbs by one or more of such conditions as: absence of an essential part, paralysis, deformity, pain on weight bearing, or incoordination.

In all of these conditions, other devices such as canes, crutches, braces, prostheses, and walkers should be considered because a chair will not always be required. However, the indication applies when such other means of ambulation are not feasible, or if any of them cannot be used because: (a) a prosthesis or aid needs repair and there is no replacement; (b) application is time consuming (as in an urgent visit to the toilet); (c) use is not practical, as during bathing; (d) use is not advisable when walking on a hazardous surface such as ice; (e) when an additional condition occurs, such as a lesion of the hand or of an amputation stump. In other words, whenever a patient depends on two lower limb appliances or other walking aids, it is advisable that he have a rolling chair at his disposal. At least, he should be familiar with the correct use of such a chair. The physician should procure appropriate wheelchair training for such patients.

A wheelchair is an additional means of locomotion. Each paraplegic should have his own wheelchair, even though many are able to walk with crutches. Abramson (1) is a strong advocate of the combination of crutch-and-brace walking and wheelchair locomotion for those for whom ambulation is excessively costly in terms of energy. There is another large group of patients of all ages and many diseases who are totally unable to walk, even with the help of any device. For them, there is only the bed or the wheelchair. Wheelchairs cannot only open new vistas but also, with proper training, many patients can learn to increase their level of independence by self-propulsion and self-transfer. Even a partial decrease of dependency by the use of a properly prescribed wheelchair can represent an important gain for a patient and for those around him.

Many activities are performed much better or can be performed only with the aid of a wheelchair. It frees the hands that otherwise would hold onto crutches or furniture. It allows more rapid motion from place to place and permits the carrying of objects, or even a baby, safely and independently. Many recreational activities and sports are accessible to bilateral leg amputees or paraplegics only from the wheelchair.

CONTRAINDICATIONS AND LIMITATIONS

Among the contraindications to sitting in general are truncal weakness, postural defects, disc and nerve root compressions, low back pain from other causes such as strains and sprains, ischial decubitus ulcer, other surgical or postoperative conditions of the pelvis, vertebral fractures, and certain fractures of the pelvis or the proximal part of the femur. In all instances in which weakness of the trunk muscles or a postural inadequacy contraindicates sitting or prolonged sitting, a stretcher, possibly for self-propulsion, might be considered.

If there is a danger of development of scoliosis, it may be greater in a chair that is too wide. A kyphosis may develop more readily in a chair with a soft (hammock) seat and back. Much can be done to improve posture with a solid seat, solid back, posture panels or scoliosis pads, bolsters, lapboards, and abduction-adduction wedges. The advantages and disadvantages must be weighed against each other in each case.

Prolonged sitting without any change in position is fraught with the danger of decubitus ulcers around the pelvis and flexion contractures of hips and knees. The ease with which a wheelchair may bring its occupant from one place to another favors this immobility of the pelvis and lower limbs. This hazard must be given consideration before a wheelchair is ordered and should be checked by a program which includes changes of body position and appropriate exercises. The dangers of pressure sores may also be lessened by pads such as alternating-pressure pads, low- or high-density foam cushions, simulated gel cushions, true gel cushions, or air release pressure-controlled cushions (29, 53, 89). Flexion contractures may be lessened by the elevating legrests discussed below.

One of the side effects of a wheelchair is the tendency toward too much dependence upon it, as in the case of patients who do not wish to walk or learn to walk again by themselves. Whenever a wheelchair is given to such a patient, we must teach him to understand that the chair is an auxiliary but that walking is preferred, even if it requires braces, prostheses, crutches, and hard work.

Patients with a hysterical inability to stand or walk (astasia-abasia) may become overdependent upon a wheelchair. Psychiatric guidance is recommended in such cases before prescribing a wheelchair.

Psychologic problems may arise from the use of a wheelchair which does not fit the patient, which is deficient in its functions, or is otherwise not "tailored" to the individual. The aims of this chapter include the prevention of such complications.

Selection of a Wheelchair

All wheelchairs should be prescribed by a physician. In prescribing a wheelchair, the physician should be aware of the differences—varying with the make—between various types and modifications of wheelchairs on the one hand and accessories on the other. The former have to be determined at the time of the prescription; the latter can be ordered and attached later. For the selection of the type and size of wheelchair and its modification, the catalogs of one or more manufacturers should be consulted to ascertain the names, dimensions, and special features which are not the same for all makes. To assist in ordering wheelchairs, the following form might be used

WHEELCHAIR PRESCRIPTION

Name   Weight   Height   Age

Disability and other special conditions

Administrative information

Add the missing items and encircle all that apply

Size: adult   junior (youth)   large child   small child

Type: rearwheel-drive   frontwheel-drive   one-arm-drive: L R   amputee

semireclining   fully reclining   heavy-duty   nonfolding

motorized with control L R

Large Wheels: 20" 24" extra socket **Tires:** regular   pneumatic

Casters: 5" 8" **Caster Tires:** regular   pneumatic **Casterlocks Swivel Locks**

Handrims: ordinary   plastic-covered **Knobs Rods:** radial   horizontal

Brakes: regular   toggle   brake extension L R   push   pull

Seat: hammock   solid   low   elevating

Back: hammock   solid   removable: zipper buckles L R

Arms: fixed   removable   offset   desk   adjustable   retractable

Locks: pin   button   flip (lever)

Armrests: metal   wooden   padded   retractable

Legrests: none   stationary   swingaway   elevating   removable

Footplates: extra large   metal heel rest L R   heel loop L R   toe loop L R

Upholstery:

Other Accessories: headrest   headcushion   crutch-holder L R   overhead sling

lapboard   belt   leg panels   leg guard   legstrap   pocket

Brand   Date   Prescribed by

Ordered   Vendor

Fig. 13.3. Wheelchair prescription form.

Selection will depend not only on the nature of the disability but also on the age, height, and weight of the patient; whether the chair will be used only at home or also out of doors; whether it will be used for propelling with both upper limbs or with a motor. As remaining abilities will determine the prescription of a wheelchair and its accessories, final selection may not be possible until the patient has reached a plateau in his disease. The definitive need for a wheelchair, its type, and accessories can be established only when no additional changes are foreseen. Often, a wheelchair is necessary before that stage has been reached, and frequently a wheelchair is important to delay, as much as possible, progression of a patient's disability. A compromise will then become necessary between immediate and future needs. In some instances, it will be possible to respond to the immediate need and make provision for future modifications. Therefore, it is sometimes advisable to try a chair for a few weeks or months. Supply houses and departments of physical medicine and rehabilitation should have a few demonstration chairs for trial by the prospective purchaser. During the trial period, he should have the chair that fits his needs best. A chair should be selected in relation to the area in which it is to be used, the patient's measurements, his comfort, his abilities, the functions and services expected from the wheelchair, its collapsibility, weight and size, safety, workmanship, appearance, and cost (10, 24, 27, 30, 33, 38, 43, 55, 57, 68, 72, 87, 88).

Operating Areas

We must consider the space in which the chair will be used: indoors, outdoors, obstacles of passage, and thresholds. This leads to a choice among casterchairs, chairs with a rearwheel or frontwheel drive, and other considerations, such as the type of tires. Doorways should be measured in relation to the width of the wheelchair, making allowance for the patient's hands if he is to propel the chair himself. Other measurements to be considered are the height of tables, the height of shelves, and the furniture in his place of employment and home, especially in the kitchen and bathroom.

According to the American Standards Association (5), "The fixed turning radius of a standard wheelchair, wheel to wheel," (that is, the tracking of the small and large wheels when pivoting on the spot) "is 18 inches (46 cm). The fixed turning radius, front structure to rear structure," (that is, the turning radius of a wheelchair, left footplate to right rearwheel, or right footplate to left rearwheel, when pivoting on the spot) "is 31.5 inches (80 cm). The average turning space required is 60 by 60 inches (152 cm). A turning space that is longer than it is wide ... is more workable and desirable. In an area with two open ends, such as might be the case in a corridor, a minimum of 54 inches (137 cm) between two walls would permit a 360-degree turn. A minimum width of 60 inches (152 cm) is required for two individuals in wheelchairs to pass each other." Space and design requirements for household activities of women in wheelchairs have been reported by several authors (36, 48, 65).

Sizes of Rolling Chairs

Certain chairs for the disabled may be manufactured in one single size, others in more than one size. Wheelchairs are usually made in three or four standard sizes, but their dimensions are not standardized (Table 13.1).

The *small child* model is for children from about 2 to 6 years of age. As small as a child is, if he can sit upright in a stroller, he can be put in a wheelchair of the smallest standard size. The seat may be elevated, in which case the overall height of the chair is almost the same as that for larger models, and the back, measured from the seat, may be even higher. The push handles must be placed at a proper height for the pusher. Up to about 4 years old, the child will be in a long sitting position, that is, with knees extended. Later, with knees flexed, the feet rest on a footboard or a pair of footplates. The footboard can be screwed to the uprights at various levels whereas the footplates attached to telescoping struts can be fixed individually at any desired level. As the child grows, the height of the foot support can be adjusted over a range of about 7 inches (18 cm).

Until such time as the child attempts to propel himself, there may be more advantage to a simple baby carriage or stroller than to a wheelchair since a very small child must be secured at times by a safety belt or may have to be made comfortable by some pillows or bolsters on each side or behind the back. As soon as the child is ready for the wheelchair, this becomes an instrument of sport and exploration on the path toward independence.

The next standard size of wheelchairs, *large child*, is for children between about 6 and 12 years old. Allowance for growth is made by adjustment of the footrests over a range of about 5 inches (13 cm) and by adjustment of the height of the seat. Here again, extra pillows, an upholstered wooden box at each side, or other supports may be necessary for a good fit. These are removed as the child grows. We believe that deviations of the spinal column

TABLE 13.1. *Principal dimensions of standard wheelchairs in inches (approximate average measurements compiled from several catalogs)*

	Small child	Larger child	Junior	Adult	Extra large or heavy duty
Seat height	18	20	19	20	20–22
Seat depth	11	11	13	16	16
Seat width	12	14	16	18	18–22
Seat to footrests—minimum-maximum	3–9	7–11	13–18	15–20	15–20
Arm height from seat	6	7	9	10	10
Back height from seat	17	15	16	16	16
Overall height	35	35	35	36	36–38
Overall length	30	33	39	40	41–42
Overall width	19	21	22	24	26–30
Width folded	10	10	10	10	11–12
Weight in pounds	35	41	41	43	46–48

are favored by a chair that is too large. For better trunk support, posture panels and other thoracic supports can be used.

The intermediate size chair, (*junior*) is for still larger children and small adults. The back, arms, and footrests are close to the occupant for better fit. A trial in such a chair may show a striking improvement in operation, as compared with the operation of a chair of regular size. The minimum seat-to-footrest distance (15 inches or 38 cm) of the regular wheelchair may prove too long for a short person. A patient who propels his wheelchair with the help of one or both feet must be close enough to the floor, and a distance of 18 or 19 (46 to 48 cm) rather than 20 inches (51 cm) from the seat may be necessary. The patient may approach closer to furniture and kitchen equipment, which is of particular importance since women usually belong to the group for which a junior model is indicated. In spite of its name, the junior model is often more appropriate for the very old, among whom smaller people outnumber the larger.

The term *adult* size applies more to the dimensions and weight than to age. Just as some older persons do better with a junior chair, certain teenagers may need an adult chair. *Narrow adult* chairs are also available and highly appreciated by a good number of users.

Extra Large or Heavy-duty Wheelchairs. For paraplegic men with vigorous shoulders and others who do not object to handling an extra 5 pounds (2.3 kg), heavy-duty construction wheelchairs are advisable. They are built for a more rugged use with stronger axles and propelling wheels. A very large heavy patient needs a chair that not only corresponds to his measurements (*oversize*), but also is of heavy-duty construction. For an unusually tall person, the wheelchair may be constructed with a higher seat, higher arms, a higher back, and extensible elevating footrests. In some instances, such as in patients with severe spasticity, special reinforcement may be necessary. A simple head extension piece may suffice to accommodate for this or other disabilities.

Measurements

The experienced physician will seldom need to measure the patient. He will readily recognize in which of the above-mentioned groups the patient belongs. The beginner, when in doubt, should take measurements of his patient according to Fig. 13.4 and should compare them with those in Table 13.1, a precaution necessary when dealing with patients with uncommon dimensions.

A patient, when measured for a wheelchair, should be fully dressed, including corset, braces, and prostheses, and should be sitting in a straight chair with a rigid seat and back. A metal tape measure and two boards about 1 by 6 by 20 inches (2.5 by 15 by 51 cm) are also recommended.

Height of the Seat (Distance from the Floor to the Seat). The patient sits in an ordinary chair, his hips in about 80° of flexion, knees at about 90°

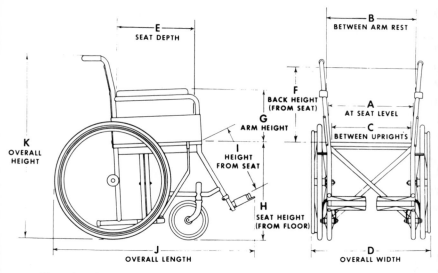

Fig. 13.4. Diagram for wheelchair measurements (Colson Corporation).

of flexion, and ankles in the neutral position, with his legs vertical and soles and heels of the shoes flat on the ground. If this position cannot be assumed because of the unavailability of a fitting chair, either elevate the seat or place a wooden platform of suitable elevation under the feet. The distance to be measured is that between the floor and the upper horizontal rigid surface of the seat. Add 2 inches (5 cm) to compensate for the elevation of the footrests. If one or both feet are to be used for propulsion, 1 inch (2.5 cm) will suffice.

Width of the Seat. The two boards mentioned above are placed parallel to one another and along the outer borders of the thighs of the patient. It is apparent that a pelvic belt or a heavy overcoat may be important. The width of the seat is the inside measurement between the two boards, plus 2 inches (5 cm).

Depth of the Seat (Distance from the Anterior Border of the Seat to the Plane of the Back). The pelvis of the patient should touch the back of the chair or wall. The measurement is taken in the midline. The seat surface should extend not quite as far forward as the back of the knee. It should be possible to put the patient's handbreadth (without the thumb) between the anterior border of the seat and the back of the knee.

Height of the Footrest (Distance from the Seat to the Footplate). In addition to the distance of 4 fingerbreadths, the patient's thigh should be lifted a little so that two fingers (held horizontally) can be slid down between the seat and the thigh. Thus, there will be room for 6 fingerbreadths between the popliteal space and the area of contact between thigh and seat. It is in this position of the thigh that the sole of the shoe marks the plane of the footplate. Where there is particular danger of pressure sores in the region of the ischial tuberosities, the thighs might not be given that extra lift for the additional 2 fingerbreadths or only a minimal amount. With the increased surface of support, the maximal pressure on the ischial tuberosities is decreased. Yet, the legs should not dangle because of the danger of compression of the sciatic nerve and the vessels.

Height of the Armrest (Distance from the Seat to the Upper Border of the Armrest). The patient should lean against the backrest without particular effort, with shoulders relaxed, neither elevated nor retracted, and with the arms hung vertically. The forearms should be at right angles to the arms, that is, in a horizontal position, palms down. One way to measure this is to have a second person hold a board under the pronated forearm and to measure the distance between the seat and the upper surface of the board.

The measurement of the height of the armrest should probably increase by 1 inch (2.5 cm) for better support of the forearm. We must consider the application of a lapboard which will increase the height of the support, as well as various kinds of seats, such as a solid insert seat and cushions which would decrease the height of the support in relation to the seat.

Height of the Chairback. For the adult with ordinary strength in his trunk muscles, the height of the chairback need not extend beyond the lower angle of the scapulae. A simple way to establish this level is to slide one of the mentioned boards between arm and trunk toward the axilla. The upper horizontal border corresponds roughly to the height of the backrest. This same height can be used by people wearing an adequate support. A head support can be added when needed. The height of the chairback will determine the amount of freedom of the shoulders as well as the amount of support needed by the trunk. In quadriplegics with a high cervical lesion, the seat-to-occiput distance should be measured.

Comfort

The first requirement of comfort is "fit"—correct size (4, 52). For children with a chronic illness, there is the problem of good fit *vs.* allowance for growth. Special seat and back supports, inlays, posture panels, wooden boxes at the sides, and adjustment or building up of foot supports (the legs should not dangle) need careful examination; they can add much to comfort. The medical evaluation of current status and prognosis plays an important role in the question of comfort and correct posture.

Patient's Capacities

The present and possible future cardiovascular and pulmonary status are to be considered, as well as the progress of the disease and disability and the possibility of subsequent amputations. We must appraise the absence or the function of one or both of the patient's lower limbs, the use of prostheses, the ability to transfer from and to the chair, the function of his upper limbs, and his power of propulsion.

There are three principal methods of propulsion: (a) attendant propulsion; (b) automotive power; and (c) self-propulsion. When the chair is propelled by another person, it is pushed like a stroller. For this purpose, any chair on wheels may be used, such as a casterchair, which usually offers less comfort and less support. Power may be furnished by an electric battery. In such an instance, the occupant operates a switch by a small movement of some part of his body. If one of the upper limbs has good function, the choice of a power-driven model increases. For self-propulsion, the patient turns the handrims which are part of the large wheels. Other means of self-propulsion include chairs that transmit the motions of one or two handles to the wheels, or pushing the chair along with the feet. An incline of more than 5° cannot be negotiated by every patient, though even a 15° incline can be overcome by a man with good strength of upper limbs and trunk in a well-functioning wheelchair.

Hoberman and coworkers (47) tried to establish a minimum of power for self-propulsion of a wheelchair. They recognized three possibilities, each requiring functional or better muscle groups: for elbow extension, elbow flexion or, if both fail, elevation of shoulder, the elbow being stabilized in extension. For the front propulsion chair, only the two latter possibilities are mentioned. Some investigators studied the force necessary to set three wheelchairs of different makes in motion on a relatively smooth concrete floor. Occupied by a person weighing 140 pounds (65 kg), the wheelchairs required forces between 4½ and 5½ pounds (2 and 2.5 kg) without distinction between forward and backward motion. With an occupant of 200 pounds (91 kg), the registered forces were between 4½ and 7½ pounds (2 and 3.4 kg) for forward and between 5 and 8 pounds (2.3 and 3.6 kg) for backward displacement (71).

Comparative energy expenditures were reported by Gordon (37) in calories per minute as follows: sitting, 1.2; dressing and undressing, 2.3; wheelchair propulsion on a smooth surface at 105 feet (32 m) per minute, 2.4; walking at twice that speed, 3.6. Peizer et al. (8, 77) reported values consistent with those found by these two groups. College students with traumatic cord lesions were tested by Clarke (16) in wheelchair propulsion out of doors. In general, at least for healthy subjects, energy expenditure in wheelchair propulsion is about the same as in walking, but the load on the circulatory system is greater (46). Several studies on energy cost and other physiologic responses of wheelchair propulsion by able-bodied subjects were made by Glaser and his group (35, 54).

A correlation of the ability to operate a wheelchair with the level of lesion of the spinal cord is unsatisfactory. Although the loss of even the lowest trunk muscles (probably even of the thigh muscles) results in some loss of stabilization and, hence, of wheelchair-driving capabilities, and though these in general are lower the higher the lesion, there are many examples of better capabilities in higher lesions. The critical level which separates independence from dependence in wheelchair driving is often placed at the sixth cervical segment. Comparisons between the results of a careful physical examination and the capacities of patients to drive their wheelchairs are at times baffling. There are patients, usually young people, whose performance seems to belie the expected difficulties and does not reflect the result of the manual muscle test. They compensate to a large extent for their muscular weakness by a highly developed kinesthetic sense and trick motions. The physician must, of course, decide whether the patient has passed the stage of motor reeducation and reached that of substitution, where vicarious motions are desired.

There are many ways to increase the efficiency of patients in wheelchair locomotion: a splint applied to a paralyzed hand, a harness for an unstable shoulder, a brace for a weak trunk, or even a simple body strap.

Functions and Services Expected

Ideally, the best chair for a handicapped person is the one that makes him as independent as possible. It should be easily propelled and maneuvered by the occupant and the attendant. It should be versatile and adaptable to various situations and should allow the addition of accessories. It is virtually impossible to combine all the advantages of wheelchairs in one chair since some are mutually exclusive. For some patients, the ideal solution may be the possession of two chairs.

Selection of upholstery will depend upon appearance and function. It distributes pressure more evenly. Naugahyde and other leatherette and plastic materials have great advantages, among which are smooth sliding (on and off the seat) and easy cleaning, but they are not absorbent. When moisture of the skin is a problem, seat and back of porous cloth are better, but they should be lined by a nonstretchable material unless they are of the solid type. Of course, seat and back covers of loose meshes can be added later.

Collapsibility, Weight, and Size

A folding wheelchair should be easily opened and closed with one hand. For self-propulsion, for attendant propulsion, and for transportation in an automobile, especially when the patient must lift the chair in and out of the car by himself, its weight is important; also, there should be room enough between the front and back seats of the car. The lightest safe chair with footrests for an adult weighs about 24 pounds (11 kg). Made of aluminum, it is more expensive and less sturdy than heavier models. Before a chair is purchased, the available space in the car in which it is to be carried should be measured, and a sample of the chair should be tried.

Safety

Safety will depend upon design, workmanship, and the skill and reliability of the patient. The most frequent cause of accidents is slipping of the chair while entering or leaving it, usually because the brakes were not applied. Second in frequency is tipping of the wheelchair when the patient steps on the footrests. There are only a few rolling chairs that support the weight of an adult on the footrests without tipping. A rare but dangerous accident may occur when clothing is caught in a large wheel. A clothing guard may prevent this; otherwise, a patient (usually a woman) can be pulled right out of her chair (80). Unlike ordinary chairs, a wheelchair may be used for an entire day every day of the year and for a great variety of activities. Engineering and design must meet these challenges with a minimum of servicing.

Appearance

The appearance of a wheelchair may be as important to its occupant as that of his clothing or his home. Although it is impossible to make a wheelchair look like a chair on four legs, it should be unobtrusive. There has been a tendency in the U. S. to use chrome finish which, although a protection for the underlying metal, is too shiny for some users. The physician should not disregard the facts that women patients are interested in the appearance of the chair, its beauty, and its color, and that these features may have considerable psychologic importance.

Cost

For many users, cost is a deciding factor, not only in terms of the purchase price but also the expense of maintenance. A casterchair for $125 might give, in certain circumstances, as good service as a wheelchair for $250 or a motorized chair for $1300. The more expensive vehicle is not always the best for a particular patient. The average life-span of a folding wheelchair may be 7 to 10 years. If a device is needed for a few weeks or months only, it may be preferable to rent one.

Types of Wheelchairs

In order to distinguish wheelchairs from other types of chairs on wheels, we define a wheelchair as one that can be propelled by the action of its occupant upon the chair itself. Rolling chairs which are moved by pushing the foot against the floor or which need another person for propulsion are named differently and will be discussed later.

Nonfolding Wheelchairs

The old-fashioned high-backed institutional chair, little changed since the 19th century, is still being used extensively, although not on individual prescription. Its sturdy yet inexpensive construction makes it a good heavy-duty vehicle for the transportation of patients from and to the admitting room and other areas within a hospital and even out of doors. Thus, the chair is commonly used as a push chair. However, the large wheels, particularly when fitted with handrims, can be turned by the occupant, and therefore the chair fits our definition of a wheelchair. The large wheels may be in front (Fig. 13.5) or in the rear.

The chair is usually made of wood, including the legrests and armrests, sometimes with a caned back and seat. The back may be reclining and the legrests elevating (Fig. 13.5). Other modifications are available, such as a commode seat or removable arms. Being usually quite large, the chair admits pillows around the patient, who might appreciate leaving his sickroom for a "change of scenery after a long confinement to bed" (66). Such chairs are, however, manufactured for adults (with wide, standard, or narrow seat), in junior sizes, and for children.

This chair is more cumbersome than the modern foldable wheelchair. To get in and out of it is usually more difficult for the user (the untrained patient steps on the footplate) and to help him is more difficult for the attendant. Some of these chairs are even without brakes which is, of course, a serious fault. A watchful helper is indispensable in many cases.

Nonfolding chairs of modern style are constructed of tubular steel. They take less space and are most frequently used for the transportation of many patients within an institution.

All wheelchairs to be discussed in the following pages are foldable. The few exceptions will be described as such.

Rearwheel-Drive Wheelchairs

This is by far the most frequently used type of wheelchair, the typical modern, folding chair, the most practical vehicle for indoor and outdoor use by the greatest number of wheelchair users. It is typically made of steel tubing with a fabric or plastic seat and back. The rearwheel-drive wheel-

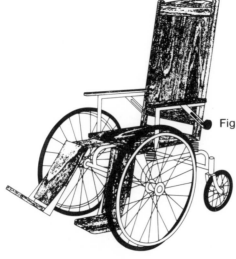

Fig. 13.5. Wooden nonfolding wheelchair.

chair, also known as the conventional or standard wheelchair, has large wheels in the rear, each fitted with a concentric handrim, which is turned by the occupant, and two small swiveling wheels in front (Fig. 13.6*A*).

Leaning against the backrest, an occupant whose upper limbs grade on manual muscle examination *Fair* or *Fair plus* and who has sufficient strength in his handgrip can propel himself on a smooth horizontal surface. He either hyperextends his arms, reaching backward and turning the handrims by flexing the elbows or, grasping the handrims at their highest points (which correspond roughly to his axillary lines), he extends his elbows. A diminished handgrip may be compensated for by handrim projections, or a motor, requiring only pushbutton control, can overcome the weakness in the entire upper limb. By removing one armrest, sideward transfer is possible for many users.

For operation by an attendant, the wheelchair is held by the push handles at the upper part of the back of the frame. Tilting the wheelchair to go up or down curbs or stairs is simplified for the attendant by stepping on a tipping lever, a posterior horizontal bar close to the floor. An adult attendant of normal strength may pull his patient in a rearwheel-drive wheelchair up the stairs, provided that the patient is not too heavy and the stairs are not too steep (Fig. 13.17*E*, *F*).

The rearwheel-drive chair is a vehicle for all purposes. A skilled driver with normal strength in his shoulders and upper limbs can tip such a chair backward, enough to raise the casters to negotiate a street curb. It is the type of wheelchair approved for basketball and other wheelchair competitions. It is the stock model found in shops throughout the U. S. as well as other countries. Although the usual weight of such a chair is about 40 pounds (18 kg) or more, there are also lightweight models which are more expensive but less sturdy (77).

There is also available a type of wheelchair which operates by the forward and backward motion of a lever which requires normal strength of one upper limb. Such a wheelchair can develop good speed, which makes it desirable for outdoor use. In another chair with four small wheels, the circular motion of two handles, one at each side, is transmitted by chains to the frontwheels.

Frontwheel-Drive Wheelchairs

In this chair, typically for indoor use and commonly but unjustifiably also known as the traveler chair, the large (propelling) wheels are in the front. The chief advantage of this chair is that it is 1 to 3 inches (2.5–7.5 cm) shorter and requires less space for turning than the rearwheel-drive chair, which makes it preferred for indoor use, especially in small rooms. It is usually slightly better balanced posteriorly so that there is less risk of tipping backward, as sometimes happens to persons without legs (Fig. 13.6*B*).

In order to propel the wheels or operate the brakes, the occupant must

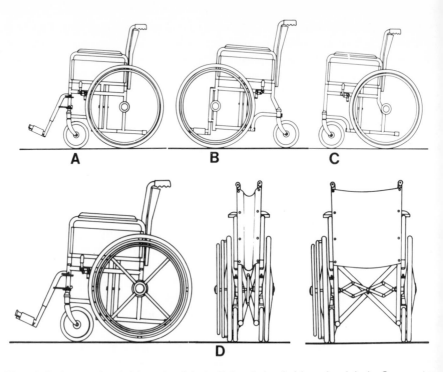

Fig. 13.6. *A*, rearwheel-drive wheelchair; *B*, frontwheel-drive wheelchair; *C*, amputee wheelchair; *D*, left-hand-drive wheelchair (Everest & Jennings).

lean forward slightly, a disadvantage that can be overcome by replacing the regular 24-inch (61 cm) wheels with 26-inch (66 cm) wheels. The slight flexion of the trunk during self-propulsion requires trunk extensors strong enough to prevent falling of the trunk on the thighs. For some patients with strong trunk and shoulders, the work of the upper limbs is made somewhat easier in this chair, an advantage when extension in the shoulder joints is restricted. For most people, frontwheel propulsion is more tiring than rearwheel propulsion.

Whereas with rearwheel propulsion the trunk of the driver is stabilized against the backrest and the upper limbs furnish most of the energy, the occupant of the front-propulsion chair relinquishes the strong fixation of his trunk and there is greater participation of his trunk muscles. A useful "trick" is to bear down on the handrims with stiff elbows and wrists by flexion of the trunk aided by gravity, but here the back extensors have to work harder to bring the trunk back to the upright position. The footplates of this chair are horizontal since they are not pushed forward by the casters, which require a circular space for swiveling. The legs are thus in a vertical position, and the knees are flexed more than in a standard chair. Elevating footrests can be added to this chair. Swinging or removable footrests would be without value for this chair, just as removal of the arms would not facilitate entrance or exit since the large wheels obstruct the passage laterally. This could be obviated by using smaller (20-inch) wheels, but then propulsion would require still greater flexion of the trunk and greater effort.

Though sometimes called an indoor chair, it may also be used outdoors if there are no curbs. The large frontwheels more readily overcome the irregularities of streets and roads, lessen the vibration, and smooth the ride. However, the chair tends to veer from side to side and is much more difficult to maneuver—for its occupant, as well as his attendant—over curbs and particularly over stairs. The attendant cannot tip the wheelchair to go up or down a step: there are no tipping levers. Since a curb can be approached only from the front—lest the patient be dumped out of the chair—a front-propulsion chair must have legrests to clear the curb. The patient will usually need one attendant for curbs and two for stairs.

Amputee Wheelchairs

In order to compensate for the loss of weight in the absence of lower limbs, in the amputee wheelchair, the rear axle and its (large) wheels are set off posteriorly (Fig. 13.6C). The added stability of this type of wheelchair is also appreciated by patients who have a powerful trunk and upper limbs and whose lower limbs are atrophied. When such a patient rolls a rearwheel-drive wheelchair backward, for example, to enter an elevator, he sometimes leans more heavily backward with his trunk in a sudden motion to overcome a doorsill, which may result in tipping backward. The same can occur when the patient operates his wheelchair forward while rising on a steep incline. Such danger is sufficient reason to prescribe an amputee wheelchair, even for patients without amputation. For amputees without prostheses, swinging or removable legrests will allow the wheelchair to be brought closer to a table, bed, sink, tub, toilet, and automobile.

For those patients who have lost both feet and will not wear prostheses, an amputee chair without footrests is best because it is lighter, easier to put in a car and to stow away and, since it is 2 to 5 inches (5 to 13 cm) shorter, it has a small turning circle and can come close to a car, bathtub, or kitchen sink. Whenever a patient without legs has a standard rearwheel-drive wheelchair instead of an amputee wheelchair, it is advisable to use a sandbag of 10 or 15 pounds (4.5 or 6.8 kg) on the footrests to re-establish the lost counterweight or to attach two special axles (amputee attachments) behind the original ones.

Antitipping devices are available on all major brands of wheelchairs.

One-Arm-Drive Wheelchairs (Double Handrim)

When a patient is unable to operate the handrim on one side, as is the case in the absence or paralysis of an upper limb, both wheels may be driven by two handrims mounted on the other side (Fig. 13.6D). The first is the usual handrim close to the wheel with which it is connected directly. The second is mounted outside the first but is connected by an axle to the wheel on the other side. When the need arises, the double handrim can be transferred to the other side. The radius of the outer handrim is about 1½ inches less to avoid hindering operation of the inner handrim alone. Both handrims can be turned together by one hand rolling the wheelchair in a straight line. In older models, the connection of the outer handrim with the wheel on the other side was ɾ steel rod which, upon folding of the chair, projected and had to be dismounted if it presented a problem. Modern chairs are fitted with a folding axle which does not interfere with the folding of the chair. The double handrim can be combined with various types and sizes of chairs, but it always makes the chair slightly wider.

The absence of one upper limb does not always demand a one-arm-drive wheelchair. In many instances, it is possible for a patient to use one or both feet to propel and pilot the wheelchair, in which event one or both footplates are raised to make room for the propelling foot or feet—a good exercise for many. Even patients with hemiplegia are able to operate a regular wheelchair, maneuvering one handrim with the unaffected hand in coordination with the unaffected foot applied to the floor. Many hemiplegics can turn such a chair, even to the unaffected side (which is more difficult), when given a chance to practice. As mentioned by Peszczynski (78), there are three reasons for not recommending chairs with one-arm drive: they are more expensive, they are about 1 inch wider, "and primarily because mildly confused patients do not learn to propel them."

While, however, we might not choose a left one-arm-drive chair for a patient with right hemiplegia or weakness of the right upper limb of another etiology, we might prescribe for him a right one-arm-drive chair in order to stimulate the use of his involved right side, which he might otherwise neglect. It should, of course, be ascertained that the patient is sufficiently alert to use the double handrim correctly. A prescription for the sake of exercise will usually be only for a few weeks or months, until a certain level of strength is reached and the habit of using the involved limb is assured. Outside of an institution, a chair can be rented for such a period of practice.

There are other cases in which, although the patient can use both hands, a one-hand-drive chair might prove useful, that is, when it is important to have one hand free while the other propels the chair. Housewives or workers in various situations might find that this advantage in a one-hand-drive chair outweighs the chair's disadvantages.

Motorized Wheelchairs

A motorized wheelchair driven by a battery can be operated with one finger by a pushbutton or other device anywhere on the chair, usually at the anterior end of an armrest. The arm to which the control box is attached must be stationary, and sideward transfer at this side is not possible. If only the head is able to move, a switch can be installed at the appropriate level. Occasionally, a motor-driven wheelchair is recommended for a patient who is able to maneuver an ordinary wheelchair but whose muscular endurance or cardiac or pulmonary reserve is insufficient for his needs of wheelchair driving. By contrast, for many individuals, the propelling of their wheelchairs can be a very useful exercise which is lost by the addition of a motor. Motors are available that can be attached to almost any make of wheelchair. If at the time of the prescription a motor is not indicated but is contemplated for a later date, this should be discussed with the dealer. A motorized folding wheelchair should be of heavy-duty construction. Such a chair can have handrims for occasional self-propulsion. The combined weight of a 12-volt battery, motor, and transmission equipment will add at least 30 pounds (14 kg) to the weight of a chair which must therefore be constructed for heavy duty. Such a wheelchair is safe, is easily operated, and can be driven indoors or outdoors at slow or full speed, up to about 4.8 miles (8 km) per hour on a smooth surface. This is equivalent to the speed of rapid walking. Depending upon the design, it is possible for a chair to climb an incline with a gradient of about 6°, a slope greater than the maximum recommended by the American Standards Association for buildings (5). For a greater pitch, additional help is necessary either on the part of the driver or an attendant. A fully charged battery provides power for between 10 and 30 miles (16 and 48 km) of progression on level ground. There is a chair powered by a 24-volt battery, which is only 22 inches (56 cm) wide and mounted on three small wheels. The location of the steering column is important. If it is in the center, it must be detached for entry and exit; also, it interferes with the crossing of the legs or wearing of a skirt, and it gets in the way while one is sitting at a table. The steering column may be mounted on either side to obviate these inconveniences.

Motorized chairs for outdoor use are relatively popular in Great Britain but far less so in the U. S. One such chair, known since 1960, was the world's first totally folding portable power-driven wheelchair (A-BEC Halesowen, West Midlands, U. K.). It has, for the first time, allowed power wheelchair users the freedom to travel without the need of a van or large automobile. It has many types of options regarding control, such as a microswitch (or two-speed) proportional control, chin control, and attendant control. It is unique inasmuch as it uses a direct-gear drive which can save up to 30 percent of the energy needed to propel the chair (Fig. 13.7).

Newer models of motorized wheelchairs for indoor and outdoor use and even for stairclimbing are constantly being developed (61, 76, 92).

The most specialized of all power-driven chairs is one which utilizes a *Mulholland* growth guidance chair (L. Mullholland Corp., Los Angeles, Calif.). This chair is the only chair in which the physician can totally create the postural environment which he may deem necessary to correct or check any existing orthopedic deficiencies. The prescription order form allows one

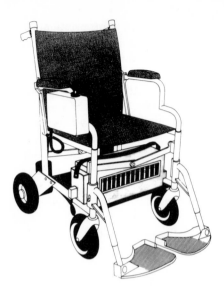

Fig. 13.7. Electrically powered A-BEC wheelchair.

to place a patient in a chair which can control the positioning of the body and provide for future adjustment and growth. A power base with a control (microswitch with auxiliary acceleration speed control) and direct-gear drive is used to propel the chair.

Parts and Accessories of Wheelchairs

The following descriptions and measurements refer to the adult size. Certain of the parts, also called modifications, will determine the type of chair to be selected. Accessories are objects that can be purchased and attached at a later date; a few of them (though correctly called modifications) replace others on the original chair.

THE WHEELS AND THEIR ACCESSORIES

Large (Propelling) Wheels

A wheel combined with a handrim is called a propelling wheel. The wheelchairs of the British National Health Service have propelling wheels of 20, 22, and 24 inches in diameter (51, 56, and 61 cm) (11); the American-made wheels are of diameters of 20, 24, and 26 inches (51, 61, and 66 cm). The 20-inch propelling wheel is about the same height as the seat, and this permits sideward sliding in and out of the chair, provided that the arm of the chair is removable. Many bilateral lower limb amputees and paraplegics have only this means of entering and leaving the chair, which is 2 inches (5 cm) shorter than the standard chair. However, the patient must reach farther down to operate the handrims, and this disadvantage must be weighed against the ease of transfer. For a patient with short or deformed upper limbs, smaller wheels are not indicated. In general, propulsion is a little harder and less rapid than with 24-inch (61 cm) wheels.

The 24-inch propelling wheel is the most practical and by far the most common. For heavy patients or for rugged use of the chair and for motorized chairs, the large wheels should be of the heavy-duty type, with 36 spokes (instead of the usual 28) of 120 gauge (instead of 105) and an axle of $^{10}/_{16}$ of an inch (1.6 cm) instead of $^{7}/_{16}$ of an inch (1.1 cm) in diameter. Such wheels make the chair a little heavier and 1 inch wider.

The 26-inch wheel for a tall person in a chair with a higher seat has handrims which are reached easily and which compensate for the disadvantage of the more difficult reach of frontwheels in the traveler model. Larger wheels not only increase the chair size by 1 inch but also increase the weight slightly and make sideward transfer more difficult. However, there is a gain in the speed factor.

Handrims

Nearly all wheelchairs have handrims attached to the propelling wheels. The diameter of the handrim is about 5 cm shorter than that of the wheel to which it is attached. In one-arm-drive wheelchairs, two handrims are placed on one side; the outer rim, again slightly smaller, is connected with the wheel on the opposite side. In order to obtain a better grip on the rim, it can be wrapped with a friction tape or covered wire. Furthermore, plastic-coated handrims are an accessory available from most major wheelchair manufacturers.

The grip on a smooth handrim can also be much improved by the use of a glove with a rough grasping surface. Gloves protect the hands from dirt on the wheels, from friction burns, callosities, and the rubbing of the knuckles against a doorjamb. The glove may be not more than a piece of cloth or soft leather attached to the heel of the hand, that is, the part likely to be soiled, while leaving the digits free (51). We have found such a miniglove very useful for many wheelchair users who either do not think of avoiding the tire or who need the better purchase afforded by a larger surface of contact.

If the hand cannot grasp the handrim, either because of lack of motion or of power, the handrim can be furnished with projections, also called pegs, which are pushed by the wrist, radial border of the forearm or the hand, or by the hypothenar eminence in supination. Depending upon the most effective way of turning the handrim, these projections can be placed on top of the handrim (capstan type of rim with radial, incorrectly called vertical, projections) or on the side (horizontal or oblique projections). They may be in the form of a short rod or a doorknob. If such projections are required, eight to twelve knobs can easily be screwed into a handrim, depending upon the distance that the rim turns per motion.

Other Means of Self-Propulsion

Among other means of manual self-propulsion, the most important are the lever drive and the chain drive. In the lever-driven chair, there are two long upright levers, one on each side. Each lever is connected with a wheel which is turned by the forward and backward motion of the lever. This requires normal or near normal strength of the upper limb and shoulder and preferably also of the trunk. A lever-driven chair is wider than a conventional chair and requires, therefore, more room for turning. It can develop good speed and is usually more suitable for outdoor use.

A chain-driven chair is operated by two cranks. The larger wheels are usually much smaller than in other wheelchairs. The chair is shorter but heavier. To turn the cranks demands a good grip in each hand, and there is hardly any advantage, as compared to chairs with handrims.

Small Wheels

With the exception of the frontwheel-drive chair, the small swiveling wheels, also called casters, are in the front of almost all chairs and, of course, all rearwheel-drive chairs. In this situation, the footrests are placed sufficiently forward to allow for the circular space needed by the casters to swivel. Casters with a diameter of only 5 inches (12.7 cm) are slightly lighter than the 8-inch (20.3 cm) casters and make the chair slightly shorter, the footrests being closer to the frontposts. A disadvantage of such small casters is that they make operation difficult on rough, soft, and irregular ground, on cracks, stones, sand, lawns, rugs (particularly rug edges), doorsills, and thresholds of elevators. Also, such casters do not have sealed bearings and require more maintenance. The 8-inch caster is almost universally used in modern wheelchairs. Since it is larger, it is slightly heavier and pushes the footrests farther forward than a smaller caster, adding about 3 inches (7.6 cm) to the length of the chair, and it causes the knees to be slightly less flexed with the feet on the footrests.

Tires

Standard Tires are of solid rubber and require no special care during their rather long life. The marring of floors and walls by black rubber tires has been diminished considerably by the use of gray rubber. However, the nonmarking gray tires are less durable than their obsolete black rubber predecessors.

Pneumatic Tires which resemble those used on bicycles must be checked for air pressure and have to be pumped up from time to time. Even with correct air pressure, they require a little more power for propulsion and can be used only with appropriate wheels which make the chair 2 inches (5 cm) wider. However, their shock-absorbing softness is deeply appreciated by patients who suffer from the jolting of wheelchairs with ordinary solid tires. Pneumatic tires do not become stuck easily in small crevices and grooves and do not dig as deeply into sand, soft earth, and thick carpets. On such surfaces, less power is required than with tires of solid rubber. Semipneumatic tires are available for 8-inch casters. They are comparable in all advantages and disadvantages with the pneumatic tires of the propelling wheels, with which they should be combined. They need not be reinflated, but they split occasionally and, in general, their life is shorter. A new shock-absorbing device attaches between the existing rearwheel axle socket and the wheel. The spring then absorbs the shock of the bump and greatly cushions the ride. The device is available at most hospital supply houses.

Brakes

Parking brakes are important for safety. They lock the large wheels, one brake per wheel, securing the wheelchair. They also prevent the chair from rolling when on an incline.

Brakes are commonly applied by a forward motion of the hand, which is usually the easier way: the driver stabilizes his trunk against the backrest. To release a brake requires less effort. Instead of pushbrakes, many patients prefer pullbrakes, depending on the distribution of their muscle weakness or their habits.

When the chair is furnished with removable arms, the brakes should have short handles. Otherwise, they will get in the way on sideward transfers. If necessary, removable extensions may be attached to the short brake handles. In wheelchairs with fixed arms, the brakes have longer handles which are easily reached and can be moved by the wrist or the forearm. Handles can also be angulated for better grasping, but long handles are likely to suffer distortion or break from heavy stress. The toggle brake, attached at a higher level, has a short handle, seems to be better, and can be operated by one finger, if necessary.

Casterlocks (Swivel Locks)

Even when the large wheels are locked by brakes, the small wheels continue to swivel easily, allowing some motion of the corresponding front or rear part of the wheelchair. Locks may hold these small wheels, one per wheel, in a straight position, increasing the stability of the wheelchair. Casterlocks are recommended whenever stability is a problem, especially when the patient is unattended.

THE SUPPORTING PARTS

Seats

The seat in an adult chair is about 16 inches (40 cm) deep, 18 inches (46 cm) wide, and 18 to 20 inches (46 to 51 cm) from the floor. For smaller adults, a junior wheelchair with a slightly smaller seat may be more suitable. With a smaller seat, the passage through narrow doors is easier, but most important for comfort is the depth of the seat, which can be diminished by a firm cushion, a bolster, or a solid insert behind the back. For a short person, for more efficient use of the feet in propelling the chair, the seat should be only 18 inches (46 cm) or less from the floor, instead of the usual height (low-seat wheelchair).

A *Solid Seat* or *Solid Insert* gives stronger support and corrects the sag in the fabric, which may be detrimental to the posture of the patient. A sagging seat tends to adduct the thighs and knees, and this can be prevented by a solid insert. A solid seat insert increases the distance from the floor to the seating surface and also decreases the distance from the seat to the armrests. A hard surface makes transfer easier for those who can only slide on and off the seat. A 2- to 4-inch (5 to 10 cm) sponge rubber pad will compensate for the hardness and help prevent pressure sores. However, this increases the height of the seat still farther, and the advantage of easier sliding is lost, though this loss can be lessened by a very smooth cover. If the chair is to be folded, the solid seat should be easily removable. Some wheelchairs are available with a permanent solid seat to be hinged upward when folding the chair. For better seating control, custom-made abduction wedges are now available in any shape or height. They are made at the same time as the insert seat.

Hydraulic Seat Lift (Elevating Seat)

For patients who do not have enough strength to stand up from the chair or to transfer to a higher chair or bed, a hydraulic lift can raise the seat as much as 9 inches (23 cm) by repeated to-and-fro motions of the handle. This does require some power of one upper limb, but even if this is done by another person, it is still much easier than helping the patient to a standing position. Other types are made with an electric motor seat control. Once the seat is brought to a higher level, it is much easier for the patient to stand up, and for those patients who can walk only after being brought into a near upright position, a rising seat is a boon and graduates them from wheelchair-bound to ambulatory. It is relatively easy to release the lever which lowers the seat. Such a hydraulic lift can be installed on almost any commercially available collapsible chair. When the seat rises, the contact with the footrests is lost, and the support of the armrests diminishes—two reasons for requiring good sitting balance for those who would use a rising seat. There is a model in which the arms elevate at the same time as the seat. A wheelchair with an elevating seat is heavier, and before it can be folded, the seat must be removed. This is not easily performed by a disabled person.

Seat Cushions

Seat cushions, decreasing the danger of pressure sores, are usually made of rubber or plastic foam, of which the latter is preferred because it gives better support and therefore requires a smaller thickness than ordinary foam rubber. The cushion cover should be firm and smooth for easy gliding and may be secured in place by a spring steel clip sewn into a piece of fabric and onto the cushion or simply by using strings at each corner. Almost all commercially produced cushions are now available with washable covers and zippers for easy handling. The addition of a cushion to the seat may bring the armrests too low. In such a case, adjustable armrests are helpful, but in any event the thickness of cushions must be considered in measuring for a wheelchair.

Following rectal surgery, in coccygodynia and other conditions, cushions of special shapes (split or coccygodynia pillows), sparing the involved area, are available or can be made from foam rubber or other material. A cut out seat board may also minimize pressure on the ischial tuberosities. New varieties and types of cushions are constantly being introduced. Air-filled or water-filled cushions have proved particularly valuable in prevention of skin breakdown in spinal cord injury patients. Rogers (85) presents a good review of types of wheelchair cushions and their sources.

Back

The back of the usual wheelchair reaches only to the level of the lower angle of the scapulae but may be extended further by a headrest attached to the uprights. There is a backward slope of the chairback of from 5 to 10° which is usually considered enough (80) for balance and comfort unless the trunk muscles are weak, in which case a safety belt is helpful. Keegan (52), who has studied chairs in relation to low back pain, insists upon a slope of at least 15°, and so do other workers in the field. The back of the chair is made of the same material as the seat for folding. It can, however, be rigid, flat or slightly hollow (contoured), to give additional support to the trunk by a solid insert or a support placed against the back. Contoured backrests for the support of the lumbar curve are strongly recommended by Keegan (52). Additions take up some of the depth of the seat and must be removed before the chair is folded.

A posture panel, made of padded plywood, is attached to the back posts. A pair of lateral supports made of padded curved metal bands can be screwed to the posture panel. These supports have to be tailored to the individual thorax and serve as pressure pads applied to the lateral chest walls at different levels in patients with scoliosis (3). Today, scoliosis pads are available in either adjustable belt-and-foam pads or the more rigid body positioner style. The belt-and-foam style usually has a hard plastic backing and multiple slices in the foam to lessen pressure on the patient.

It is sometimes desirable for the patient to enter or leave the chair through the back rather than the front. This can be achieved either by having a zipper down on one side of the fabric in the back of the chair or by having a detachable back which can be snapped on or off either one of the vertical metal bars. For many quadriplegics, this is the easiest way to transfer from or to the wheelchair, bed, toilet, or other chair. To slide through the open back is often the only way to use a toilet when space in the bathroom does not permit turning the wheelchair. For the opening and closing of the snaps, one upper limb must have some power and skill, though this is easier than closing the zipper back, which demands good coordination.

Semireclining Back

Reclining in a chair takes some pressure off the buttocks, demands less sitting balance, and offers a change in position particularly welcome to those who remain in a chair for many hours. To some patients with insufficient hip flexion who might not otherwise fit into a chair, a reclining back makes the difference between bed and chair. To recline in a wheelchair, a back extension for the head is necessary (see *Headrest*). Though part of the pressure is taken off the ischia, the sacrum must take some of it. Moreover, in the partially reclining patient, there is a shearing force acting upon the posterior sacral tissues which contributes to the development of decubitus ulcers.

Such a wheelchair also has elevating legrests. It is 4 inches (10 cm) higher (not counting the head extension), 6 inches (15 cm) longer, 11 pounds (5 kg) heavier and, of course, more difficult to push and to put in a car than a standard chair. A semireclining back may slope by as much as 30 or 45° and can be locked in any position in between (Fig. 13.8).

Fully Reclining Back

A fully reclining back may be fixed in any position between the vertical and horizontal and therefore permits conversion from a wheelchair to a stretcher. In some models, a few degrees are lacking to the horizontal position, in which case, if the prone position is to be assumed, pillows will be required under the abdomen and pelvis of the patient. In most models, the patient loses his contact with the armrests on reclining. On full reclining,

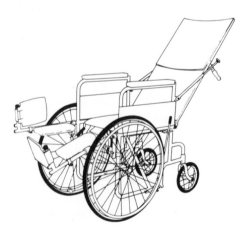

Fig. 13.8 Folding frontwheel-drive wheelchair with semireclining back, headrest, and elevating legrests (Colson Corporation).

the wheelchair loses in stability by displacement of some of the weight of its occupant. To compensate for this loss, one manufacturer has built a chair which lengthens its wheelbase by 4 to 5 inches (10 to 13 cm) on reclining (Fig. 13.9). Otherwise, posterior antitipping devices should be applied, or the headrest must be supported. A wheelchair with fully reclining back is 5 inches (13 cm) higher, 10 inches (25.4 cm) longer, and 13 pounds (6 kg) heavier than a standard adult chair and is, of course, more cumbersome than a chair with a semireclining back.

Back Cushions may increase the patient's comfort, giving a snugger fit of the back and relieving pressure. Combined seat-and-back cushions, as used in automobiles, with and without lumbar pad, are available. Some are made to allow some ventilation in hot weather. Others put more emphasis on contouring. Custom-made cushions can be ordered in virtually any size or shape.

A *Headrest* is an extension to the backrest, is about 14 inches (35.6 cm) high, and is indispensable for any reclining wheelchair (Fig. 13.8). In order to prevent the head from sideward displacement, one type of headrest is constructed with pronounced sag. Headwings, attached at right angles to the headrest, afford still greater protection from such sideward displacement.

Arms

The arms of the chair, at about 9 inches (23 cm) above seat level, give support to the patient's forearms and hands while at rest and in various activities, help to maintain trunk balance, and offer support on standing up, sitting down, and practicing push-ups. They may be bare or covered with a simple thin cover, a wooden or plastic plate or an upholstered pad, the height of which will, of course, increase the height of the armrest. Patients with pulmonary emphysema or asthma prefer slightly higher armrests. Forearms with sensory deficits or those which have to be attached to the armrests because of paralysis require padded armrests because of the danger of pressure sores (50). Adjustable arms, which can be raised or lowered, are

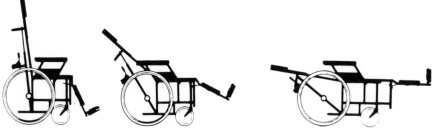

Fig. 13.9. Fully reclining wheelchair with headrest and headcushion. By reclining the back, the wheelbase lengthens and the arms retract (Colson Corporation).

of great advantage: the absence or presence of cushions of various thicknesses or of lapboards of various heights and various activities may call for
armrests of changeable height. For unusually short or tall persons, armrests
of special heights may be necessary.

The side panel or clothing guard, that is, the lower part of the chair arm,
can protect a paralyzed flaccid upper limb from the large wheel by keeping
it inside the chair arm. Similarly, clothing is kept away from the wheel
where it might become soiled or trapped.

Armless Chair

A chair without arms is, of course, lighter and may be wheeled closer to
a table or washbowl. It permits no support for the forearm and hand but
does allow more freedom of movement while sitting or while entering and
leaving the chair sidewards. Good sitting balance is indispensable; otherwise,
the patient may have to be strapped to the chair. A flaccid upper limb not
held back by the arm of the chair is more difficult to protect from the spokes
of the large wheel.

Removable Arms

Removable arms may be lifted out of their sockets, thus permitting
paraplegics and others to enter or leave the chair sidewards, especially when
the propelling wheels of the universal chair are smaller; this is less convenient when wheels are in the front of the chair and are larger. Removable
arms also make it much simpler for attendants to lift the patient in and out
of the chair and avoid the risk of his being hit by the corners of the armrests.
Although a chair with both arms removed has all the advantages of an
armless chair, with the arms in place the chair is slightly heavier than the
standard chair and cannot be lifted by its arms unless the armlocks are
closed. Removable arms are available in different heights. Some can be
reversed, and since the armrest is not centered over the frame, this permits
a choice of two positions of the armrests: either closer to the trunk for
tighter support or farther for freedom of the trunk. The closer position
makes the access to handrims easier, but regardless of these advantages the
chair is 1½ inches (3.8 cm) wider than the standard chair.

Desk Arms

A desk arm (Fig. 13.10) is an arm cut away at its front corner so that the
chair may approach a table 6 inches (15 cm) closer than a standard chair,
thus eliminating the need for a tray. The desk arms allow the patient to
reach his utensils for eating or working easier and in a more erect position,
without obliging him to lean forward. The supporting surface of the armrest
of a desk arm is, of course, shorter. This can be overcome by a specially
built extension to compensate for the cutaway portion or by removable desk
arms which can be reversed so that the cutaway part is posterior. Finally,

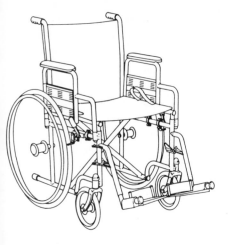

Fig. 13.10. Wheelchair with desk arms (Everest & Jennings).

the chair can be furnished with two pairs of removable arms: one for regular use and one for desk use. When the desk arm is reversed, with the jog at the rear, the handrim on the rearwheel is more easily reached, which is appreciated by some patients.

Fixed or removable offset arms of the regular or the desk type are also available and give an additional 1¾-inch (4.5 cm) width between the armrests without increasing the overall width of the chair.

Armlocks

All removable arms should be furnished with armlocks so that the chair may be lifted by its arms and so that they will not come off on a ramp or stairway. Armlocks are usually either pinlocks, which require a steady hand, or button locks, which require more finger power to operate.

Tray or Lapboard

A tray or lapboard, most frequently attached to the armrests, provides a table-like surface for eating, reading, writing, and other activities. It favors good posture, particularly when the patient would otherwise have to lean forward to reach a working surface. Such a tray is easily applied and removed; as long as it is in place, propulsion is a little more difficult with a frontwheel drive. Patients with poor sitting balance and those with extreme weakness of the upper limbs should have a tray of sufficient height. Some individuals with pulmonary insufficiency breathe more easily when a rather high tray supports their forearms. A tray also provides a means of carrying a baby or objects. For certain activities a tray of variable pitch is preferred, or one with an extra shelf. Some trays are now available in a see-through plastic which enables the patient to see directly ahead. This greatly decreases the possibility of a bruised foot or toe.

Another such tray has a hinged lid which is also transparent. This enables the patient to be taught a lesson or symbols code without fear of a spastic movement to tear or crumple a worksheet. A reading rack can be placed on a tray to hold reading material at an angle more convenient to the eyes. Various portable and stationary work surfaces for wheelchairs were described by several authors (3, 44, 62, 63).

A Forearm Board or *Trough,* usually made of wood or plastic and padded with foam rubber, is fastened to an armrest, at the same or a higher level, in the same direction or obliquely so that the hand points toward the midline. It supports the forearm and hand better than the armrest of the chair, avoids the pull of a flaccid limb by its weight at the shoulder joint, and protects the hand from dropping on the wheel and between the spokes (50). Such a support is particularly useful in hemiplegic patients.

Overhead Slings or Suspension Armslings

In order to protect weak shoulder muscles or to permit exercise and other activities, the forearm can be suspended by a sling embracing the elbow region. If the weakness extends to the forearm and hand, the wrist is supported by a suspension "feeder" or a mobile arm support attached to the wheelchair. Springs connect the slings or the feeder with a curved or angulated rod fixed to the wheelchair back. For a chair with a reclining back, the rod may be attached with a pivoting bracket which allows the rod to maintain a vertical position.

Foot- and Legrests

When the legs are pendant, the feet will rest upon two footplates or a single footboard; if the legs are elevated, they need support for their posterior surface on legrests. A chair without footrests gives much freedom to the feet, which is necessary when the feet are used to propel the chair—an excellent exercise for many. It may be an advantage in certain cardiac and pulmonary patients for propulsion to be done by the lower limbs instead of the upper limbs. Without footrests, the chair is about 5 inches (12.3 cm) or more shorter. This can be important in bathrooms, elevators, and elsewhere. It is about 4 pounds (1.8 kg) lighter, and this makes folding and stowing easier. Such a chair may be wheeled closer to furniture and does not need as large a turning circle, and one is not hindered by footrests in entering or leaving it. It is less well balanced, however, because it has lost some of its length and weight in the anterior portion. It can lose its balance completely and tip over when its occupant tries to jerk it backward over a doorsill or similar elevation on the floor. It is therefore advisable, if footrests are not desired (and particularly without front rigging), to use a wheelchair where the rearwheels are set back, a so-called amputee chair.

The Footrest, Footplate, or Step Plate, attached at a right angle to the strut which springs from the front post, usually forms an angle of a few degrees with the floor. The smaller the front casters, the closer the strut to the vertical position and the smaller the angle of the footrest to the floor. For severe flexion contractures, horizontal footrests can be fixed above the front casters. The height of the footrest can be adjusted over a range of about 6 inches by sliding the telescoping strut up or down according to the leg length. The feet should not dangle. Yet, firm contact of the thighs, except for the distal third where nerves and vessels are more superficial, will take off some of the pressure on the ischial tuberosities. Some footrests consist of a single piece on which both feet rest. This is particularly the case in children's wheelchairs in which the adjustment of their height covers a wide range. In most instances, however, there is a footrest for each foot which can be hinged up into a vertical plane which in the adult allows the feet to reach the floor and thus to participate in the propulsion of the wheelchair.

Swinging Detachable Footrests are of great advantage. They may be swung out of the way like the panels of a double door; their pivot hinge allows complete removal. Whether they are swung out or detached, it is easier to enter and leave such a chair and to approach closer to furniture. After removal of the footrests, the chair has all the advantages and disadvantages of a chair without footrests. Removable footrests are heavier than fixed footrests, but by their removal the chair is made lighter and shorter, which is valuable for stowing a chair in a car as well as for transferring into the car because of its close approach.

Elevating Legrests

For patients with a cast or knee extension contracture, and in other instances, it may be necessary to maintain the leg elevated on an elevating legrest which is usually fixed by a ratchet at any desired height, with the leg up to full extension of the knee and even higher. An elevating legrest requires a leg panel to support the calf. Leg panels that can be raised and lowered are advisable. Elevating foot- and legrests often give comfort to the sitting patient and are strongly recommended in a chair with a reclining back. Contoured leg panels provide particular comfort. The weight and length of the chair are slightly increased by elevating footrests. They are also available as pivoting and removable parts. Usually, ordinary removable footrests can be exchanged for elevating footrests at any time. However, the choice between removable and fixed footrests or, sometimes, no footrests must be made at the time at which the chair is selected. There are, however, leg supports that can be added to chairs at any time, as well as simpler devices, such as a board slid under the pelvis, that can maintain a lower limb in the horizontal position. Adjustable elevating footrests can individually be raised to encourage knee extension or lowered to encourage knee flexion.

In patients with flexion contractures of the knees, panels attached to the struts of the footrests can provide support for the calves and aid against further knee flexion. When a leg is elevated, a support for the calf is required, but it should be padded with foam rubber. An alternate method for gaining support of the calves without rigidity is to stretch a piece of the same material used to form the seat of the wheelchair between the two struts. The two rigid panels can be folded away, opening like a double door. This is not possible with the panel which reaches across; therefore, there is a little less freedom between the struts when getting up or sitting down. With such a device, both legs must be elevated to the same level. Leg panels frequently suffer from the pressure of the leg, especially where there is no heel loop or similar support for the heel. In most cases, the pressure is concentrated on a small region of the calf, which interferes with circulation. The larger one-piece leg panel or leg guard is usually more comfortable. If attached to swinging footrests, it must be attached with clips for easy removal.

Other ways of preventing the legs from sliding backwards are a leg strap or calf strap which connects the struts of the footrests, and individual metal heel clips or webbing heel loops attached to the rear of each footplate. They all help to keep the feet away from the frontwheels, and this is especially valuable when the larger 8-inch (20 cm) casters are used. For patients with whom there is a tendency for the foot to slide forward on the footrest, a toe loop attached to the footplate will be helpful. Frequently, to keep a foot on the footboard, a leg strap or heel loop, together with a toe loop, will be necessary; it is difficult for some patients to get out of the toe loops without help.

If one or both legs are particularly short, a wooden or aluminum box can be secured to the corresponding footplate to support the foot. However, it is advisable at the time of measurement to have these custom-cut to ensure proper fit.

OTHER ACCESSORIES

Narrowing Device

A *Wheelchair Narrower* or *Reducer* fits almost any wheelchair and is easily attached to either side. With a lever or a crank, the wheelchair is squeezed sidewards and narrows by about 3 to 5 inches (7.6 to 13 cm), depending upon the device used. It requires good power in one upper limb and can be operated by the occupant or another person.

Commode Attachment

Unless there is a hydraulic seat or the space below the seat is occupied by a motor, the regular seat can be replaced by a toilet seat with cover above and removable toilet pan below.

Crutch- and Caneholder

Canes and crutches can be held upright by a snap loop attached to the back of the chair and can be supported underneath by a metal cup mounted on a tipping lever. This cup should be at least 2 inches (5 cm) deep.

Antitipping Devices

When both lower limbs are elevated with knees extended, there is much weight in front of the frontwheels. A cast on a lower limb adds further to the weight. A shock such as is experienced on striking a threshold or an attempt to stand up can throw the chair off balance forward. Two curved bars, one at each front post, may be used to act as outriggers by hitting the floor when the chair tilts forward. Depending upon the make of the chair, other antitipping devices exist for the front or the rear of the chair. They are swung away when necessary, for example, when going over a ramp. In some cases, a wheel can be mounted on each tipping lever for indoor use. The front posts that carry the casters may be made longer by caster extensions which lift the front 2 to 3 inches (5 to 7.6 cm) and tilt the chair backward, inclining the seat and back. This position stabilizes the occupant and is an advantage for children and patients with poor sitting balance. However, there is more pressure on the sacrum, some danger of tipping backward, and greater difficulty leaning forward in such a chair.

Reclining Bars attached to the tipping levers give the occupant of a chair without a reclining back a chance to rest his back.

Sliding Board

A very smooth board of polished hardwood, ¾-inch thick (2 cm) (sloping toward both ends), 8 to 12 inches (20 to 30 cm) wide, 2 to 3 feet (61 to 91 cm) long, can be used as sliding board to bridge the gap of transfer between the wheelchair seat and another surface. The development of very hard plastic sliding boards has added another benefit for the patient. These boards have a ridge through the center which, in the case of tub transfers, allows the water to drain. It also decreases the friction of the transfer, thus decreasing the effort somewhat. Furthermore, the sliding board cases attach to some chairs and thus provide an extra convenience for storage.

Miscellaneous

Pockets, Boxes, Cup Holders, Ashtrays, Luggage Racks, and other small accessories are commercially available.

For additional security, a *safety belt* may be applied over the anterior superior iliac spines in the same manner as used in an automobile, at the level of the lower ribs or the axillae. These are available in both auto and velcro styles.

Spastic thighs may be prevented from adduction by lateral *strapping*. If they tend to abduction and outward rotation, a strap around the thighs just above the knees will hold them together.

Other Indoor Vehicles for the Disabled

We have classified indoor vehicles for the disabled in relation to their use in sitting, walking, standing, or lying and have called them accordingly: rolling chairs, rolling walkers, rolling stands, and rolling stretchers.

ROLLING CHAIRS (OTHER THAN WHEELCHAIRS)

Casterchairs

We like to call casterchairs chairs on small swiveling wheels or casters, moving easily in any direction on a slight push or pull. They have also been called gliders, glide-about chairs, roll-about chairs, and mobile chairs (Fig. 13.11). They can be folding or nonfolding.

Most casterchairs are manufactured without brakes and their careless use may lead to falls because of their great mobility. Their stability can be improved by a casterlock, usually a so-called step-on caster brake. The patient can either be pushed in such a chair (some of the chairs have push handles) or he may propel himself by using his feet on the floor or his hands on the walls and furniture and even, occasionally, by using canes in the manner of ski poles. For the patient who needs only occasional transportation, that is, one who is able to take a few steps and is accompanied during a trip, a casterchair may not only suffice but also is considerably less expensive than a wheelchair.

Castercommodes are casterchairs with a toilet pail or pan, thus serving an additional purpose.

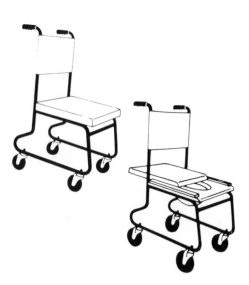

Fig. 13.11. Casterchair and castercommode with push handles (American Wheel Chair).

Occasionally, instead of a rolling chair, one might consider a quadrangular frame or platform with four casters and support for the four legs of any ordinary chair. It is easily made and is also commercially available. Its light weight makes it more transportable than a whole chair, and it can be used with any chair to be found wherever the patient goes.

Push Chairs

In push chairs, two wheels may be larger than casters without being large enough for self-propulsion. Or the frontwheels, while small, might not swivel. Push chairs are available in folding and nonfolding models; some close sideward, as do most wheelchairs, and others fold in the fashion of a baby stroller. A British folding push chair (11) is designed to be carried by two attendants over stairways: there are additional handles at the footrest for the second helper (Fig. 13.12).

A Chair-Table Combination was brought on the market about 1965 and has since then been particularly used in hospitals and nursing homes. It is a nonfolding large push chair with padded seat, back, and armrests, hard plastic tray, and footplate (Fig. 13.13). Called also mobile lounge or geriatric chair, it has four swiveled casters, usually with locks. The table plate or tray, when not needed, is reclined to the side, out of the way and firmly attached to the chair. The footplate slides forward and backward on two horizontal tubes a few inches from the floor and is pushed completely under the chair for standing up and sitting down. The latest adaptation of this chair has been to make it adjustable to six positions, thus also accommodating the dialysis patient.

This type of push chair with table is particularly indicated for persons who do not desire to move around, who do not move around by themselves, or who are little moved by others and only inside the house. It is also advantageous for confused patients who move around—be it walking or in a self-propelled chair—more than is desirable for their own good or the good of others, in an institution, for example. This chair is indeed rather difficult

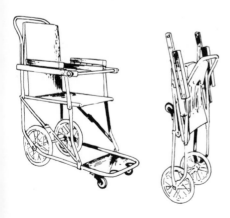

Fig. 13.12. British push chair which folds from front to back. Note handles on footrest. [After a photo supplied by the British Ministry of Health (11).]

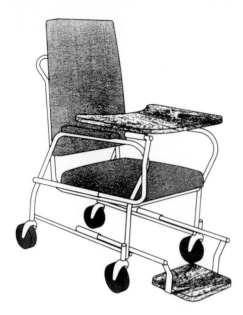

Fig. 13.13. Geriatric chair (after photo from Everest & Jennings).

for its occupant to move, even when the footrest is put out of the way. The chair also restrains the occupant in another way: the tray is locked into place by a mechanism which is simple, yet not managed by the confused patient who thus is kept in the chair. This might be indicated, for instance, when the patient does not realize that he should not walk. Standing on the footplate, when this is pulled out to the usual distance, makes the chair tip forward unless there is a special support under it.

ROLLING WALKERS

Walkers with wheels, usually casters, may be equipped with a foldaway seat so that the user may either stand or sit inside as his feet touch the ground; these walkers may be used for propulsion. Such casterwalkers, also called walking chairs or walking frames, may have a bicycle saddle when designed for children. Many of these walking frames are equipped with hand supports such as those found on canes or crutches, but most of them do not have brakes and may run out of control. For safety, some walkers lock when the patient puts his weight on them. Even so, they may be hazardous unless there is an attendant with the patient. Folding casterwalkers for easy stowing on a trip are available, replacing a push chair.

ROLLING STANDS

A portable collapsible indoor vehicle for propulsion in the upright position, named a "Stand-Alone," became commercially available in about 1961 (Fig. 13.14). About 42 inches (107 cm) high, 40 inches (102 cm) long, 26 inches (66 cm) wide when open, 14 inches (35.5 cm) wide when folded, it weighs 79 pounds (36 kg). It was designed by a paraplegic preacher to permit him his occupational activities in the standing position. The user stands on a platform on four small wheels. Two large propulsion wheels, similar to the handrims of a wheelchair, 19 inches (48 cm) in diameter, reach as high as 40 inches (102 cm) from the floor. Each is connected by a chain with the rearwheel on the same side (74).

To enter the wheelstand, the paraplegic places his feet on the platform, grasps the handles, and brings himself to a standing position by a push-up. An adult with a transection of the cord at the 8th thoracic level will require assistance to transfer between the rolling stand and a wheelchair, but if his remaining musculature is of normal power, he will probably learn to do so without help. For higher lesions, assistance is probably required. By the use of toe loops and three pads, one each against the knees, the abdomen, and the buttocks, the patient stands in this device without braces and without holding on, his upper limbs being free for the desired activity and able to reach objects at the level of a standing person.

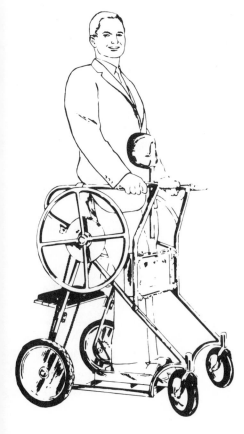

Fig. 13.14. Stand-Alone rolling stand (after a photo supplied by Corporation for Medical Engineering).

A motorized version of the "Stand-Alone" became available in the mid '70s. By use of a battery conversion and adaptation of a hydraulic lift pump, many spinal cord injury patients may rise unassisted into the device. Other devices to assist patients in standing are constantly being proposed or developed.

The standing board or tilt table consists of a firm padded board which can be tilted manually or electrically to any angle up to 90°. A table or tray with an adjustable height top can be set in front of the patient for a working surface. Straps attached to the tilt table secure the patient's trunk and prevent hips and knees from buckling.

Such tables are found in most rehabilitation centers and are used to improve standing tolerance. They can be purchased or made for home use. One such basic homemade board used for handicapped children has been set to wheels and motorized. It utilizes a proportional control mounted on the tray and a direct gear drive for greater efficiency.

A major corporation for mass production made a stand, tested in the late 70's, which resembles a podium on wheels. Like the first-mentioned manual wheelstand, the "Stand-Alone," it has its best application in an office or general work environment. Unlike the motorized wheelstand, it sometimes requires an attendant during initial transfer. (A particularly strong person can pull himself up alone.)

There are physiologic advantages in the erect position on the osseous system, which has a tendency to atrophy, and on the urinary system, which is exposed to stagnation, and the patient may derive a psychologic uplift after a long sedentary period. The wheelstand or standabout can also be used in the preparation of patients for standing and walking with or without braces and crutches. The platform of this upright wheeler is very stable, yet is small enough to be moved about in an apartment, requiring about the same space as a wheelchair. Uneven surfaces and inclines demand particular caution. The secure stabilization of the lower limbs, even without the abdominal pad, allows the patient to exercise his trunk and to stretch the posterior muscles of his lower limbs, an activity deeply appreciated by spastic patients.

All contraindications to the upright position (*e.g.*, orthostatic hypotension) and to weight bearing (certain deformities, fractures and other lesions of weightbearing bones or joints, skin lesions at pressure area) must be ruled out for the use of this rolling stand. It is commonly used only once or twice daily and for not more than 1 or 2 hours per session, but even such a duration is too great in certain vascular insufficiencies. Finally, in all cases, the value and practicability of a rolling stand should be compared with those of stallbars, parallel bars, and other means of maintaining a patient in the upright position. It certainly does not replace walking. It does not replace a wheelchair but might be indicated in addition. The power required for the propulsion of a rolling stand is greater than for that of a wheelchair.

ROLLING STRETCHERS

Many patients who cannot or should not sit but who may lie prone can be given the opportunity to propel themselves by the use of their upper limbs. Some indications are: immobilization of one or both hips, to avoid continuous pressure against the back, to avoid flexion contractures, to exercise the neck and trunk extensors, and to prevent urinary calculi (79).

The opportunity to use a self-propelled litter may be of great psychologic value and may make it more possible to maintain patients recumbent and, in particular, in the prone position.

Self-propelled Stretcher

The usual hospital stretcher is about 30 inches (76 cm) high and 24 inches (61 cm) wide with a length of 5 to 6 feet (1.5 to 1.8 m). Self-propelled stretchers are available with adjustable height from about 24 to 30 inches (61 to 76 cm) (Fig. 13.15). The frontwheels should be large enough—about 24 inches (61 cm) in diameter—to be reached by the prone patient, and should be provided with handrims by which he may operate the stretcher as he would a wheelchair. To propel a stretcher is often more awkward than to drive a wheelchair because of the position of the upper limbs and because the vehicle is much larger, heavier, and more difficult to steer. When a self-propelled stretcher is not available, an ordinary stretcher with smaller wheels may also be propelled by the patient with the aid of a pair of canes with rubber tips, used like ski poles. Since the young people who engage in this sport usually have little regard for walls or even their own bodies, rubber bumpers should be placed at the corners of each of the self-propelled

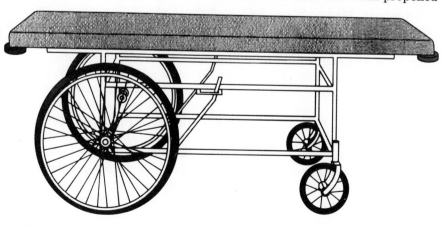

Fig. 13.15. Self-propelled stretcher (after photo from Colson Corporation).

stretchers. On a low stretcher, 21 or 23 inches (53 or 58 cm) high, with wheels 24 inches (61 cm) or more, the patient can propel himself not only while prone but also while supine and sitting, since the wheels are higher than the litter surface.

Prone Scooters and Crawlers

A child in a body cast will gain much in play and exercise from a miniature stretcher on casters, for not only will he maintain mobility but also avoid disuse atrophy of his upper limbs.

The *prone scooter* in its simplest form is comparable to the scooting board, a board with four casters used by automobile mechanics to work under a car. The child, lying prone on it, propels himself with his hands applied to the floor. Such a vehicle can be built by anyone with ordinary mechanical skills from materials which cost but a few dollars. A foam rubber pad will add a little to the cost and much to the comfort. A model is available commercially which consists of a Y-shaped steel frame about 3 feet (90 cm) long, with a centerbar for the trunk and head and a fork which spreads about 32° for the lower limbs. It has safety belts for the trunk and each leg, is upholstered with foam rubber pads to a height of 6 inches from the floor, and rolls on four spherical casters. The leg pads may be elevated or otherwise adjusted according to the size of the child or the amount of abduction of the lower limbs (Fig. 13.16A).

A *crawler* or *creeper* in its simplest form can be likened to a footstool on casters. It is used for children with back muscles too weak to crawl and those who have reached the age, but not the ability, to walk or even to crawl on all fours.

The dimensions of the crawler vary with the size of the child. Its top may be 10 by 12 inches (25 to 30 cm), its height may be 6 inches (15 cm). The child is placed with his chest and abdomen across the platform, his limbs free to move, his hands and toes, sometimes also his knees, reaching the floor to pull and push himself along. Such a device is easily made by a person with some mechanical skill. Instead of the hard board, a hammock sling, wider than long, and held by two lateral bars, may be used.

As the child is stimulated by the quadruped position on the crawler to use his lower limbs for locomotion, his trunk is progressively raised to approach more and more an upright position. This is relatively simple in an adjustable crawler (Fig. 13.16B), which can be raised to 8 or 10 inches (20 to 25 cm). The child may rest with his forearms on the crawler and thus may advance by his feet alone. When he has sufficiently progressed in the use of his lower limbs, and his body is sufficiently raised, he might continue his ambulation with a rolling walker described previously.

A child may also sit on the crawler and propel it with his feet, like a casterchair.

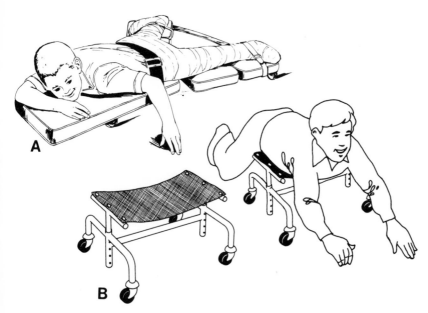

Fig. 13.16. *A*, prone scooter (drawn from an illustration supplied by Everest & Jennings); *B*, crawler of adjustable height (Zimmer Orthopaedic Ltd., Bridgend, Glamorgan, Great Britain).

Wheelchair Training

For the sake of safety, efficiency, and the best possible pleasure and service from a wheelchair, its user should receive instructions from someone highly trained and skilled in this operation, preferably from someone who has required the use of a chair himself. Though some patients understand the management of a wheelchair immediately and would probably have learned to handle it correctly without instruction, others need careful and slowly progressive training. There is always the risk of poor posture, faulty use of the body, substitution during the phase of motor re-education, overwork, unnecessary soiling of the hands by touching the wheels together with the rims, forgetting to apply the brakes or to put the footrests out of the way, and other poor habits. Detailed instructions for the use of chairs are not given in this book, but a series of pictures illustrating some of the primary features will be found on the accompanying pages (see Fig. 13.17). Depending on the disability and their capabilities, patients should learn the use of the brakes, footrests, handrims, forward and backward propulsion, turning, the management of doorsills and rugs, opening and closing of doors, and management of ramps, curbs, stairs, soft ground, and pavement. They must learn transfer from and to other chairs, bed, toilet, bathtub, car, and crutches, as well as the use of the tray and overhead sling. There are many

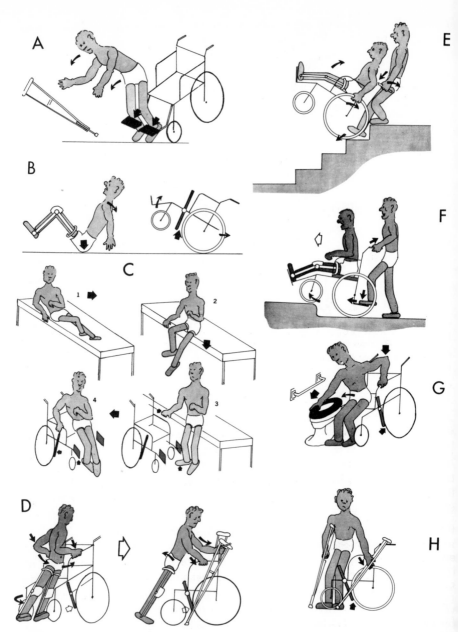

Fig. 13.17. Wheelchair techniques. *A*, before transfer to or from chair, footrests should be raised or swung out of the way; *B*, brakes should be locked during transfer; a movable chair is not secure; *C*, bed-to-wheelchair transfer for the hemiplegic; *1*, patient rises to sitting position with good right hand. Paretic left leg is raised and moved to edge of bed with functional right foot. 2, patient brings body forward by right hand pull, functional right leg used for standing. *3*, chair parallel to bed on good side; brakes locked and footrests raised. *4*, balanced on good right

guides for wheelchair training, of which we recommend, among others, those found in Refs. 23, 25, 31, 32, 47, 49, 56, 81, 87, and 95.

Wheelchair Care and Maintenance

Opening and Closing

A wheelchair articulates in the joints of the cross braces under the seat. To fold or unfold a seat, the wheelchair should be held as close as possible to the cross braces. The farther away the hold, the greater the torque upon the joints. The push handles should never be used to open or close the chair.

To open a folded chair, push down on the lateral seat rails which are part of the cross brace assembly. Another procedure (31) may be used when rough ground increases the resistance to the sideward-gliding wheel and when only one hand is free to open the chair, especially when you have unloaded the folded wheelchair from the car. Face the wheelchair sideward, holding its near armrest, then tilting the chair away from you while pulling the armrest up and toward you. Before closing a chair, make certain that the arms are secure. Move the footrests, solid inserts, and other obstacles out of the way. If there are seat straps, which are located exactly above the seat rails, pull them up. If straps are not furnished with the chair, make a fold in the seat from below. This is done by one or both hands applied under the seat. It suffices to hook one finger under the front part and one under the back part of the seat. After the seat is folded, it may be left either with the fold of the seat raised or with the fold tucked down, narrowing the chair still further. Another method of closing a wheelchair is to tilt it toward you so that its far side is off the ground. By its weight, the far half of the chair

---

foot, patient reaches for farther armrest and with support of right arm sits on chair; *D,* wheels locked, crutches placed on either side of chair where they can be reached by patient. Footrests swung out of way; braces extended and locked. Patient turns in chair facing back of chair, does push-up by grasping left armrest with right hand and right armrest with left hand. Complete turn achieved while standing, hands still on armrests. First, one crutch grasped, then the other. Back arched to prevent jackknifing; *E,* stair ascending-descending. Attendant steps on one of the tipping levers and pulls handles back, tilting chair which rolls on rearwheels. If possible, patient applies backward pull to handrims to retard forward roll in descent or assist backward roll in ascent; *F,* curb climbing. If chair is pushed by an attendant, curb can be scaled if he steps on tipping lever. Downward pressure on levers while pulling back on handle lifts front of chair, which can be moved forward on rearwheels; *G,* chair parallel to toilet; right arm of chair removed. Leaning forward, patient grasps toilet rim and, supported by both arms, swings out upon toilet seat. If there is a wall bar it, rather than seat, may be used for support; *H,* with brakes locked and footrests up, patient faces away from chair and backs into it until posterior surface of his legs touches seat of chair. Left crutch is placed securely against chairback while patient remains supported with one crutch. Left hand takes support on left armrest. Right crutch removed from axilla as right hand grasps handle while sitting (drawings by René Cailliet, M.D., suggested by illustrations in Fowles [31]).

may slide down, closing the chair. Otherwise, either pull the far seat handle or the far armrest toward the near side.

To wheel a folded wheelchair, release the brakes of the large wheels, hold the chair at the push handles, and tilt it so that it rolls only on the large wheels.

General Care

The owner of a wheelchair should follow the instructions and recommendations found in the manual of the manufacturer, which should be furnished with every new wheelchair. If the patient is unable to take care of his own wheelchair, another person should be informed about this need. In a hospital, responsibility for chair maintenance should be documented.

A few points to remember are that any part of the wheelchair when wet should be dried, any part of the wheelchair when dirty should be cleaned with soap and water applied with a cloth or a sponge. After cleaning and drying, suitable protective material such as wax should be applied to wood, leather, and leatherette upholstery; metal parts should receive treatment with oil or glass wax; telescoping metal parts should be coated with paraffin, if required. The crossbars should be lubricated with oil and the axles with grease, and footrest hinges are best left alone since they need friction to operate. Wheelbearings may have to be repacked and greased once a year, depending on the amount of use and dust. Pneumatic tires need frequent checking: they suffer both from too little and too much air pressure. The upper limits are 16 pounds (7.3 kg) for an 8-inch (20 cm) tire and 30 pounds (13.6 kg) for a 24-inch (61 cm) tire. For more detailed instruction, see Refs. 15 and 49 and the manual accompanying every new wheelchair.

REFERENCES

1. ABRAMSON, A. S. Principles of bracing in the rehabilitation of the paraplegic. *Bull. Hosp. Joint Dis. 10:* 175, 1949, and personal communication, 1965.
2. ACKERMANN, R. *The Repository of the Arts, Literature, Commerce, etc.* . . . Vol. 6., No. 34, Pl. 21. London, 1811.
3. AGERHOLM, M. (ed.). *Equipment for the Disabled.* 4 vols, ed. 2. National Fund for Research into Crippling Diseases, London, 1966.
4. AKERBLOM, B. *Standing and Sitting Posture.* Stockholm, 1948.
5. AMERICAN STANDARDS ASSOCIATION. *American Standard Specifications for Making Buildings and Facilities Accessible to, and Usable by, the Physically Handicapped.* New York, 1961.
6. ANNAND, D. R. *The Wheelchair Traveler.* ed. 10. Milford, N. H., 1977.
7. ARTHUR, J. K. *Employment for the Handicapped.* Nashville, Tenn., 1967.
8. BERGSTROM, D. A. (Coordinator). Report on a conference for wheelchair manufacturers. *Bull. Prosthet. Res., 10*(3): 60–89, 1965.
9. BOND, A. R. A folding wheel-chair. *Sci. Am., 110:* 67, Jan 17, 1914.
10. BRENT, S. Z. Basic considerations in the prescribing of wheel chairs. *Am. J. Phys. Med. 39*(2): 47, 1960.
11. BRITISH NATIONAL HEALTH SERVICE. A Handbook of Invalid Chairs and Tricycles. MHM 408. Ministry of Health, Blackpool, Lancashire, 1963.
12. BRITISH STANDARDS INSTITUTION. Code of Practice. London, 1967.
13. CARTER, J. Catalogue. London, 1881.

14. CARTER, J. & A. Personal communication. London, 1965.
15. CICENIA, E. F., SAMPSON, O. C., AND HOBERMAN, M. Maintenance and minor repairs of the wheelchair. *Am. J. Phys. Med. 35*(4): 206, 1956.
16. CLARKE, K. S. Caloric costs of activity in paraplegic persons. *Arch. Phys. Med. Rehabil., 47*(7): 427–435, 1966.
17. THE COLSON Co. Wheel Chairs, Machines for Cripples. Catalog No. 62-E. Elyria, Ohio, c. 1911.
18. DANTONA, R., AND TESSLER, B. Architectural barriers for the handicapped. *Rehabil. Lit. 28*(2): 34–43, 1967.
19. DE CAMP, L. S. *The Ancient Engineers.* Doubleday, New York, 1963.
20. DIEMER, W. H. Personal communication. Perrysburg, Ohio, 1966.
21. DOPPELMAYR, J. G. *Historische Nachricht von den Nürnbergischen Mathematicis und Künstlern.* Nuremberg, 1730.
22. EDGINGTON, E. S. Colleges and universities with special provisions for wheelchair students. *J. Rehabil., 29*(3): 14, 1963.
23. ELLWOOD, P. M., JR. Transfer—method, equipment, and preparation. Prescription of wheelchairs. In *Handbook of Physical Medicine and Rehabilitation,* edited by F. H. Krusen, F. J. Kottke, and P. M. Ellwood, Jr., ed. 2. W. B. Saunders, Philadelphia, 1971.
24. ENGEL, P., BENNEDIK, K., AND HILDEBRANDT, G. DER ROLLSTUHL. Experimentelle Grundlagen zur technischen und ergonomischen Beurteilung handbetriebener Krankenfahrzeuge. (Rehabilitationsforschung 15.) Rheinstetten, 1977.
25. EVEREST & JENNINGS. Wheelchair Prescriptions. Series of booklets for measuring, safety, etc. Los Angeles, 1977.
26. THE EVOLUTION OF THE WHEEL-CHAIR. Sci. Am., *112:* 497 and 502, May 29, 1915.
27. FAHLAND, B., AND GRENDAHL, B. C. *Wheelchair Selection: More than Choosing a Chair with Wheels.* Revised edition. Minneapolis, 1977.
28. FELDHAUS, F. M. Die Technik der Vorzeit, der geschichtlichen Zeit und der Naturvölker. W. Engelmann, Leipzig and Berlin, 1914.
29. FISHER, S. V., SZYMKE, T. E., APTE, S. Y., AND KOSIAK, M. Wheelchair cushion effect on skin temperature. *Arch. Phys. Med. Rehabil., 59*(2): 68–72, 1978.
30. FOWLES, B. H. Evaluation and selection of wheel chairs. *P. T. Rev., 39*(8): 525, 1959.
31. FOWLES, B. H. *Syllabus of Rehabilitation Methods and Techniques.* Stratford Press, Cleveland, 1963.
32. FROST, A. *Handbook for Paraplegics and Quadriplegics.* National Paraplegia Foundation, Chicago, 1964.
33. GARRIS, A. G. Functional Wheels. State of California Health and Welfare Agency, Department of Rehabilitation, Sacramento, Calif., 1974.
34. GENDRON WHEEL Co. Catalog. Toledo, Ohio, c. 1965.
35. GLASER, R. M., *et al.* Wright State University, Dayton, Ohio. Unpublished data, 1978.
36. GOLDSMITH, S. *Designing for the Disabled.* ed. 2. McGraw-Hill, New York, 1967.
37. GORDON, E. E. Energy costs of activities in health and disease. *Arch. Intern. Med. 101*(4): 702, 1958.
38. GRANT, W. R. *Principles of Rehabilitation.* E. & S. Livingstone, Edinburgh, 1963.
39. GREGO, J. *Rowlandson the Caricaturist.* Vol. 1, pp. 309 and 333–349. Chatto and Windus, London, 1880.
40. GUTMAN, E. M. *A Travel Guide for the Disabled.* Charles C Thomas, Springfield, Ill., 1967.
41. GUTMAN, E. M., AND GUTMAN, C. R. *Wheelchair to Independence: Architectural Barriers Eliminated.* Charles C Thomas, Springfield, Ill., 1968.
42. GUTTMANN, L. Sports and the disabled. In *Sports Medicine,* edited by J. G. P. Williams, pp. 367–391. Edward Arnold, London, 1962.
43. GUTTMANN, L. (CHAIRMAN). A symposium on the wheelchair (London, 1963). *Paraplegia, 2*(1): 20–70, 1964.
44. HARTVIKSEN, K., AND KLAVENESS, B. Tekniske Hjelpemidler for Uføre. Oslo, 1956.
45. HAVARD, H. Dictionnaire de l'Ameublement et de la Décoration. Paris, 1887–1890.

46. HILDEBRANDT, G., VOIGT, E-D., et al. Energy costs of propelling wheelchair at various speeds: cardiac response and effect on steering accuracy. Arch. Phys. Med. Rehabil., 51(3): 131-136, 1970.
47. HOBERMAN, M., CICENIA, E. F., AND OFFNER, E. Wheelchairs and wheelchair management. Am. J. Phys. Med., 32(2): 67, 1953.
48. JUDSON, J. S., WAGNER, E., AND ZIMMERMAN, M. E. Homemaking and Housing for the Disabled in the United States of America. New York University Medical Center, New York, 1962.
49. KAMENETZ, H. L. The Wheelchair Book. Mobility for the Disabled. Charles C Thomas, Springfield, Ill., 1969.
50. KAMENETZ, H. L. Wheelchairs for hemiplegics. In Stroke and Its Rehabilitation, edited by S. Licht. Elizabeth Licht, New Haven, Conn., 1975.
51. KAMENETZ, H. L. AND HEDGES, J. P. Miniglove for wheelchair users. Phys. Ther., 48(12): 1396, 1968.
52. KEEGAN, J. J. Evaluation and improvements of seats. Industr. Med. Surg., 31: 137, 1962. 52a. KEEGAN, J. J. The Medical Problem of Lumbar Spine Flattening in Automobile Seats. New York, 1964. 52b. KEEGAN, J. J. Personal communication, 1965. 52c. KEEGAN, J. J. Choosing seating for hospital patients. Hospitals, 40(19):72-73, 1966.
53. KOSIAK, M. Etiology of decubitus ulcers. Arch. Phys. Med. Rehabil., 42(1): 19-29, 1961.
54. LAUBACH, L. L., et al. Wright State University, Dayton, Ohio. Unpublished data, 1978.
55. LAWTON, E. B. Wheelchair prescription. In Arthritis: General Principles, Physical Medicine, Rehabilitation, edited by E. W. Lowman. Little Brown & Co, Boston, 1959.
56. LAWTON, E. B. Activities of Daily Living for Physical Rehabilitation. McGraw-Hill, New York, 1963.
57. LEE, M. H. M., PEZENIK, D. P., AND DACSO, M. M. Wheelchair Prescription. Public Health Service Publication No. 1666. USPHS, Washington, D.C., 1967.
58. LEVINE, S. A. The management of patients with heart failure. J.A.M.A., 115(20): 1715-1719, 1940. 58a. LEVINE, S. A. Chair rest versus bed rest. Hosp. Med., 2(3): 2-5, 1966.
59. LHERMITE, J. Le Passetemps. Vol. I, pp. 257-258 (folio 156-157 of the original manuscript, 1595). J. E. Buschmann, Antwerp, 1890.
60. LIPSKIN, R. Evaluation program for powered wheelchair control systems. Bull. Prosthet. Res., 10(14): 121-129, 1970.
61. LIPSKIN, R. VA Prosthetics Center program for electric wheelchairs and other nonlicensed mobility aids. Bull. Prosthet. Res., 10(22): 326-336, 1974.
62. LOWMAN, E. W., AND KLINGER, J. L. Aids to Independent Living. McGraw-Hill, New York, 1969.
63. LOWMAN, E. W., AND RUSK, H. A. Self-Help Devices. New York University Medical Center. New York, 1965.
64. MAXWELL, G. E. They go to college in wheelchairs. Today's Health, 42(7): 26-29, 63-68, 1964.
65. MAY, E. E., WAGGONER, N. R., AND BOETTKE, E. M. Homemaking for the Handicapped. Dodd, Mead, New York, 1966.
66. MORGAN, E.M. A push anyone? Am. J. Nurs., 58(6): 831, 1958.
67. MUMMENHOFF, E. Der Handwerker in der deutschen Vergangenheit. pp. 36 ff. E. Diederichs, Leipzig, 1901.
68. MURDOCH, G. (ed.) Wheelchairs. In The Advance in Orthotics, Sect. 5, pp. 285-343. Edward Arnold, London, 1976.
69. NATIONAL RESEARCH COUNCIL. Building standards for the handicapped. Associate Committee on the National Building Code, Ottawa, Canada, 1965.
70. NEW HAVEN FOLDING CHAIR Co. Illustrated Catalogue of Folding Chairs. New Haven, Conn., 1871, 1873.
71. NEW YORK TESTING LABORATORIES, Westbury, N.Y. Report of January 25, 1963 (Courtesy Everest & Jennings, Los Angeles).

72. NICHOLS, P. J. R. Prescription of wheelchairs. In *The Advance in Orthotics*, edited by G. Murdoch, pp. 285–293. Edward Arnold, London, 1976.

73. NUREMBERG MUNICIPAL LIBRARY. Personal Communication. Dr. K. Goldmann, Director, Stadtbibliothek Nürnberg, 1966.

74. PEIZER, E. Wheelchairs. In *Atlas of Orthotics*, edited by American Academy of Orthopaedic Surgeons, pp. 431–453. C. V. Mosby, St. Louis, 1975.

75. PEIZER, E., AND WRIGHT, D.W. Five years of wheelchair evaluation. *Bull. Prosthet. Res.* 10(11): 9–37, 1969.

76. PEIZER, E., AND WRIGHT, D.W. Trends in wheelchair design and development. In *The Advance in Orthotics*, edited by G. Murdoch. Edward Arnold, London, 1976.

77. PEIZER, E., WRIGHT, D. W., AND FREIBERGER, H. Bioengineering methods of wheelchair evaluation. *Bull. Prosthet. Res.*, 10(1): 77, 1964.

78. PESZCZYNSKI, M. Exercises for hemiplegia. In *Therapeutic Exercise*, edited by S. Licht, ed. 2. Elizabeth Licht, New Haven, Conn., 1961.

79. PLUM, F. Mineral metabolism following poliomyelitis. *Arch. Phys. Med. Rehabil.* 42: 348, 1961.

80. RAYNER, C. Wheelchairs. *Design* (London), 164: 31, Aug. 1962.

81. REHABILITATIVE NURSING TECHNIQUES IN HEMIPLEGIA, HANDBOOK OF AMERICAN REHABILITATION FOUNDATION. Minneapolis, 1964.

82. J. REYNDERS & Co. Illustrated Catalogue and Price-List of Surgical and Orthopaedical Instruments. ed. 6. New York, 1889.

83. RICHER, P. *L'Art et la Médecine*. pp. 303–304. Gaultier Magnier et Cie, Paris, 1902.

84. RICHTER, G. M. A. Ancient Furniture. Figs. 20, 172. Clarendon Press, Oxford, 1926.

85. ROGERS, J. Wheelchair cushions and related protective devices. In *Atlas of Orthotics*, edited by American Academy of Orthopaedic Surgeons, pp. 454–461. C. V. Mosby, St. Louis, 1975.

86. RONDINELLI, I. Descrizione degl' Instrumenti. . . . Faenza, 1766.

87. RUSK, H. A., AND TAYLOR, E. J. *Rehabilitation Medicine*, ed. 3. C. V. Mosby, St. Louis, 1971.

88. SIMON, P. Systematik der Rollstuhlverordnung. *Medizinisch-Orthopädische Technik*, 96(2): 25–28, 1976.

89. SOUTHER, S. G., CARR, S. D., AND VISTNES, L. M. Wheelchair cushions to reduce pressure under bony prominences. *Arch. Phys. Med. Rehabil.*, 55(10): 460–464, 1974.

90. SPIEGLER, J. H., AND GOLDBERG, M. J. The wheelchair as a permanent mode of mobility: a detailed guide to prescription. *Am. J. Phys. Med.*, 47:(6): 315–326, 1968, and 48(1): 25–37, 1969.

91. SYMPOSIUM ON SPORTS FOR THE DISABLED. Part I. *Physiotherapy* 51(8): 251–269, 1965.

92. STAROS, A., AND PEIZER, E. Veterans Administration Prosthetics Center Research Report. *Bull. Prosthet. Res.*, 10(24): 156–208, 1975.

93. TRUAX, C. *The Mechanics of Surgery*, pp. 83–87, figs. 142–144. W. B. Conkey Co., Chicago, 1899.

94. TUCKER, W. V. (ed). *Higher Education and Handicapped Students*. Kansas State Teachers College, Emporia, Kansas, 1964.

95. UNITED STATES DEPARTMENT OF HEALTH, EDUCATION AND WELFARE. Up and Around. Washington, D.C., 1964.

96. UNITED STATES NATIONAL HEALTH SURVEY. Distribution and Use of Hearing Aids, Wheel Chairs, Braces, and Artificial Limbs, July 1958–June 1959. Health Statistics, Series B 27. Washington, D.C., 1961.

97. UNITED STATES VETERANS ADMINISTRATION PROSTHETICS CENTER. Semiannual report. IV. Orthopedic aids. *Bull. Prosthet. Res.*, 10(3):146–151, 1965.

98. UNITED STATES VETERANS ADMINISTRATION PROSTHETICS CENTER. Annual report of committee on prosthetics research and development. *Bull. Prosthet. Res.*, 10(6): 211, 1966.

14

Beds for Patients

MICHAEL T. F. CARPENDALE, M.D.
JOHN B. REDFORD, M.D.

Look at a patient lying long in bed,
What a pathetic picture he makes!
The blood clotting in his veins,
The lime draining from his bones,
The scybala stacking up in his colon,
The flesh rotting from his seat,
The urine leaking from his distended bladder,
And the spirit evaporating from his soul.
                                    R. A. J. Asher (2)

Bed care, bedrest, bedfast, bedridden: these are common expressions used in medicine. What do they mean to the health care system today?

The word bed is derived from a Welsh word "bedd," meaning "grave." In fact, the earliest use for beds was as a place for bodies of famous men to lie in state. The idea of sleeping in such a structure came much later. It was not until the 14th century that a bed was more than a strong mattress placed on the floor. Today, the hospital bed is a complex arrangement of levers and gears designed for the preservation of life, rather than as a place of death. However, problems remain with beds, particularly for chronically ill patients, as described so graphically by Asher.

In the 30 years since Asher described the problems of the bedfast situation, a great deal of research to elucidate the pathological changes has occurred. Studies on healthy subjects has shown the effects of bedrest uncomplicated by disease (6, 28) and how they may be counteracted (32). This basic information has been used in developing a rational program for management of the bedfast patient (31). A monograph by Browse (3) effectively summarizes this work. More recent studies, in astronauts, have shown many similarities between the effects of bedrest and weightlessness, especially in the engorgement of the intrathoracic circulation (10, 21). They have also emphasized that it is not a matter of many weeks but of only a few days of bedrest—sometimes only one day—that are necessary to produce a major pathological problem.

In all of this research, little attention has been directed to the role of the bed itself in the production of these problems, yet it is clear that the major pathology of bedrest is due to the relative immobility of the patient, the horizontal position, and areas of local pressure, all of which can to a large extent be overcome by modification of bed design. Developments encouraging early ambulation and independence in self-care suggest that older concepts of hospital bed care must be critically re-evaluated.

Ideally, a bed for a sick or disabled person should be designed to:

1. Be at least as comfortable, if not more so, than the bed at home.
2. Hasten, not hinder, the healing process.
3. Prevent and not predispose to other pathology associated with prolonged bedrest or recumbency.
4. Facilitate the performance of necessary nursing needs without inconvenience to the patient.
5. Be economically reasonable, *i.e.*, make good economic sense when one takes all factors into account.

Currently, how many commercially available beds meet these ideals? Consider the following few examples. Vertical sitting helps those with congestive heart failure, as it reduces cardiac work whereas a semireclining position increases cardiac work. Yet, the standard hospital bed does not allow for vertical sitting. A variable height (hi-lo) hospital bed was developed so that in the high position it would facilitate nursing and in the low position would easily allow the patient to get out of bed or transfer to a wheelchair without requiring assistance. An excellent concept, but in practice the majority of hospital beds have only about a 10-inch (25 cm) excursion, usually from a low of 24 inches (60 cm) to a high of 34 inches (85 cm). Twenty-four inches is not low enough to meet the patient's needs, 34 inches is not high enough to facilitate nursing requirements. The development of one bedsore on a patient usually prolongs patient stay from 30 to 60 days, at a cost of at least $5,000 to $10,000. It does not make economic sense to put an elderly paralytic patient on a standard hospital mattress with a plastic cover costing $100, knowing that this predisposes to skin breakdown, when for $200 a mattress proven to significantly reduce liability to bedsores could be given to the patient, not only for his hospital stay but also for use at home.

It would seem, therefore, that few of the criteria for an ideal bed for patients are met in the standard hospital bed of today. Furthermore, there is a lack of concern by hospital staff concerning the dependency produced by bedrest. To the nurse, it is much more convenient to have the patient "tucked in" than to try to encourage him to exercise. To the doctor, it is convenient to have the patient in bed during rounds. There, the bed-bound patient can be easily found, examined conveniently, and treated as a dependent subject. Furthermore, "bedrest" is often the convenient initial order. Medical inertia promotes the triad orders of bedrest, a laxative, and sleeping medication—regardless of the therapeutic indication. This situation may be acceptable on a ward where all patients have acute illnesses but most hospital wards today have a mixture of patients with acute and chronic conditions. Although special rehabilitation in chronic disease units is part of the answer, the promotion of real independence and less time in bed usually can begin in the subacute stages of the illness if physicians and nurses on the acute wards would only encourage them. The thoughtful physician should consider the extent of the need for bedrest, just as he considers the harmful effects of drug allergy and toxicity.

How can we remedy the situation of poor bed design and overutilization of bedrest? First, it is important that physicians, nurses, physical therapists, and family members concerned with bedside care of patients look on the bed as an orthotic device that requires a specific prescription for a specific disorder. Like any other orthotic device, it will increase the comfort of the patient, hasten healing, reduce disability and, in addition, will facilitate care when correctly prescribed. Also, a good bed will make economic good sense. Secondly, few physicians or nurses seem to realize how many of the pathological problems associated with bedrest can be counteracted by features of bed design. As the risk varies for each patient, a specific prescription relative to disease, disability, and age must be considered. Ideally, the prescribed bed should prevent the pathology of bedrest without compromising treatment.

The purposes of this chapter are to:
1. Review briefly the problems of recumbency and indicate how they could be minimized by features of bed design.
2. Critically evaluate currently available commercial beds in supplying these features.
3. Evaluate and compare mattresses and beds for the prevention of bedsores.
4. Describe beds which are designed for special disorders and evaluate how they meet patient needs.

Problems of Recumbency Affected by Features of Bed Design

There are eight groups of problems associated with bedrest that can be reduced or eliminated by six features of bed design. We will review the problems of recumbency in the order presented in this Table 14.1.

Phlebothrombosis and Pulmonary Embolism

Pulmonary embolism is the most severe hazard of bedrest, accounting for 0.5 to 2.0% of all hospital deaths (3). It is the leading cause of death following fractures of hip, cholecystectomy, prostatectomy, hysterectomy, and inguinal herniorrhaphy (23). The importance of prevention rather than treat-

TABLE 14.1. *Problems of Recumbency Counteracted by Features of Bed Design*

Problems of recumbency	Features of bed design					
	Oscilla-tion	Vertical sitting	Compliant porous absorbent supporting medium	Spring-loaded footboard	Patient-operated toilet-opening device	Variable height (hi-lo) (40 in–18 in) mechanism
I. Phlebothrombosis Pulmonary embolism	2*	1	1	2	0	0
II. Syncope Hypotension	3	3	0	0	0	0
III. Atelectasis Hypostatic pneumonia	3	2	0	0	0	0
IV. Muscle atrophy Negative nitrogen balance	2	0	0	1	0	0
V. Osteoporosis Hypercalcuria Genitourinary calculi	3	0	0	0	0	0
VI. Bedsores	3	1	3	0	0	0
VII. Constipation Incontinence	1	1	0	0	2	0
VIII. Transfer and lifting	0	0	0	0	0	3

* 0 = no counteracting effect; 1 = slight counteracting effect; 2 = moderate counteracting effect; 3 = maximum counteracting effect.

ment is emphasized by the fact that half of the cases of fatal embolism occur in subjects with no clinical symptoms (27). In post-mortem studies, Gibbs (14) found that venous thrombosis occurred in 18% of patients after only 7 days in bed and by the 4th week of bedrest, 81% showed evidence of thrombosis. Recent evidence indicates that thrombosis in leg veins often occurs in just the short time that the patient is lying on the operating table (9).

Thrombosis, which most commonly starts in the calf veins, is related to reduced venous flow from compression in the supine position. This is likely to be aggravated by the Fowler or Gatch semireclining position which, by flexing the hip and knee, almost certainly further constricts these vessels (30). Blood flow in leg veins can be increased and so reduces effects of compression by active contraction of the gastrocnemius against a spring-loaded footboard (14) or by increasing peripheral circulation with a rocking bed (24). Local compression of the calf veins can be prevented by avoiding the supine position and can be reduced by lying on a highly compliant medium, e.g., low-density foam or a waterbed.

Syncope and Hypotension

In healthy subjects, circulatory adaptability to the erect position is decreased after 7 days in bed (6, 28). After 21 days of bedrest, it takes 5 to

10 weeks to return to normal. At first, there is a decrease in pulse pressure and, when this reaches 10 to 12 mm, syncope usually occurs. Later, the diastolic pressure decreases. The loss of circulatory adaptability can be prevented by use of a rocking bed or by daily vertical sitting or standing (17).

Atelectasis and Hypostatic Pneumonia

Recumbency increases pooling of blood in the lungs. This results in decreased ventilation associated with decreased vital capacity, minute volume, expiratory reserve, and functional residual capacity (20). Recumbency also causes increased resistance to diaphragmatic movement and, therefore, increased work for the diaphragm and, usually, decreased movement. This results in a lack of aeration of collapsed alveoli, but in healthy subjects this does not usually lead to atelectasis because of active movement in bed and an effective cough reflex. However, in recumbency with generalized weakness or partial paralysis, the reduced body movement produces lack of ventilation. This leads to pooling of mucous on the dependent surfaces of small bronchioles and drying out of the upper surfaces, resulting in decreased ciliary activity, predisposing the patient to atelectasis. Without an effective cough reflex, lack of clearance of secretions, bacterial proliferation in the mucous and, subsequently, hypostatic pneumonia may occur (3, 17).

Pooling of blood in the lungs and increased resistance to movement of the diaphragm can be reduced by vertical sitting and the rocking bed. However, the latter has an additional important advantage in preventing atelectasis by increasing pulmonary ventilation through increased diaphragmatic excursion. Diaphragmatic work is also reduced, and this may be very important for the weak, elderly, or debilitated patient.

Muscle Atrophy and Negative Nitrogen Balance

In a classic study on the effect of bedrest in man, Deitrick et al. (6) showed that in healthy subjects immobilized for 6 weeks, strength and leg muscles secondary to disuse declined an average of 13%. Simultaneously, nitrogen, phosphorus, sulphur, and creatine were excreted in the same equivalent as 5 pounds (2.3 kg) of muscle protein. These losses were more severe in postoperative patients (11).

Muscle atrophy and negative nitrogen balance are significantly reduced using an oscillating bed, and Getzen (12) claims that by increasing the frequency and angle of oscillation, patients can be put into positive nitrogen balance.

Osteoporosis, Hypercalcuria, and Genitourinary Calculi

Measurable loss of calcium from bone accompanied by hypercalcuria can be demonstrated in healthy individuals with less than a week of bed rest (17). Simultaneously, there is an increased excretion of phosphorus predis posing to precipitation of calcium phosphate and the formation of renal and vesical calculi (31). Muscle tension on bone, which is lacking in recumbency, appears to be more important than weight bearing in preventing loss of matrix and demineralization (1). Although use of the oscillating bed reduces excessive calcium and phosphorus excretion and liability to osteoporosis, it appears to be of little or no value if the patient is paralyzed (33).

Bedsores

Because of the importance of this problem, both pathology and prevention are included in a later section on "Special Mattresses and Beds to Prevent Bedsores."

Constipation and Incontinence

The recumbent position, lack of muscle movement, and inhibition associated with the use of the bedpan, if untreated, decrease defecating and voiding reflexes and cause constipation and urinary incontinence (17). Constipation leads to anorexia resulting in lack of bulk of ingested food, which causes decreased peristalsis and further increases constipation. Then scybala form which neither medication nor enemas can evacuate.

Vertical sitting stimulates the orthocolic and voiding reflexes, and a patient-operated toilet-opening mechanism eliminates the dependency on the nurses and bedpan inhibition created partially by unnatural position and hard bedpan surface. Not only do these bed features reduce constipation and incontinence but also they prevent skin abrasions and bedsores.

Transfer and Lifting Problems

In a conference with bed manufacturers sponsored by the American Rehabilitation Foundation in 1965, rehabilitation professionals suggested to manufacturers that ideally a bed should have an excursion of 22 inches (56 cm), from 18 inches (46 cm) low to 40 inches (102 cm) high. Unfortunately, this feature is still not available upon any bed manufactured in the U. S.

Essential Features of Beds to Prevent Problems of Recumbency

Problems of bedrest are more prone to occur in patients who are elderly, debilitated, malnourished, or suffering from vascular or respiratory insufficiency or impaired movement from paralysis or arthritis. To partially or completely prevent these problems, Table 14.1 shows six features considered essential in a hospital bed. Listed in order of importance, they are:
  1. Oscillation
  2. Vertical sitting
  3. Compliant porous supporting membrane and medium
  4. Spring-loaded foot board
  5. Patient-operated toilet-opening device

6. Variable height bed surface, from 18 inches (46 cm) to 40 inches (102 cm)

Let us consider the essential characteristics of each of the features and what is commercially available.

Oscillation

Oscillating beds to counteract the effects of immobility are available in two common types: one is the fore-and-aft motion from head to toe, like a rocking chair—hereafter called a "rocking" bed—and the other is a side-to-side motion—hereafter called a "rolling" bed. Motion in either plane effectively counteracts the immobility of the standard bed. It facilitates the prevention and management not only of bedsores but also of phlebothrombosis, syncope, pulmonary problems, muscle atrophy, and the metabolic problems of negative nitrogen and calcium balance. Furthermore, it is valuable in the treatment of respiratory and cardiac insufficiency and in controlling edema and occlusive vascular disease of the lower extremities (24).

Rocking Beds

The first "rocking" bed was used in 1936 by Sanders (24) in the treatment of cardiovascular and peripheral vascular disease. This was a "slow" oscillation, taking 1½ minutes to tilt the bed at a barely perceptible speed from the horizontal position. This bed should not be confused with the "rapid rocking bed," rocking 10 to 20 times per minute, which has been used for weaning poliomyelitis patients with respiratory involvement from tank respirators (34).

All of the early studies of metabolic effects of the rocking bed were made using the Sander's "slow-rocking bed" but later studies using the "rapid-rocking bed" indicated that more benefit was obtained by the more rapid oscillation through a 30° arc, available only in this bed (11, 12).

Both fast- and slow-rocking beds are still available (J. H. Emerson Co., Cambridge, Mass.) (Fig. 14.1). The main drawback of the available rocking beds is that at present there is no "hi-lo" mechanism. Presently, they are too high even for the nurse to tend a patient without a small platform and much too high for patients to safely arise unaided. The lowest model, named the Motion Bed (J. H. Emerson Co., Cambridge, Mass.), is designed for home use, but still the top surface is 30 inches (75 cm) from the floor. If a hi-lo mechanism were available for the rapid-rocking bed, this would be the most efficacious bed in the treatment of any long-term bedfast patient.

Rolling Beds

The first rolling bed (Kinetic Concepts, San Antonio, Texas). (Fig. 14.2) was designed by Keane (15) for the management of the spinal injured patient. It has a slow motion, taking 4 to 5 minutes to complete a 124° arc

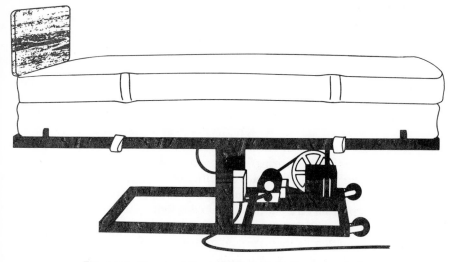

Fig. 14.1. Standard Rocking Bed (J. H. Emerson Co.).

Although, as far as is known, no metabolic or physiological studies have been made on this bed that are comparable to the rocking bed, there has been a considerable amount of clinical experience. The bed has been used in many Spinal Injuries Centers in Europe in the past 10 years. This experience indicates that this oscillating motion has most of the virtues already described for the rocking bed.

Although rocking is probably more valuable for cardiac and respiratory insufficiency, rolling may be more beneficial for pulmonary drainage and in the prevention of atelectasis and hypostatic pneumonia. The bed design permits total skin inspection and care, full range of movement of all extremities, and bedpan placement—all without lifting, turning, or taking the patient out of cervical traction. Not only is it a most valuable bed for spinal injuries, but also for any patient with multiple injuries. It lacks any mechanism for vertical sitting, but if the patient has to remain horizontal and requires vertical traction, it is probably the best bed currently available to prevent problems of recumbency under those conditions.

Vertical Sitting

Vertical sitting is not to be confused with the semireclining Gatch or Fowler position. Vertical sitting is that position adopted when sitting in an upright chair, with thighs horizontal, legs and back vertical, and feet flat, supported at right angles to the legs. To change position in bed from supine to vertical sitting without excessive shearing forces or gaps in the supporting surface presents many mechanical problems. Ideally, the bed should be hinged on an axis which passes through the hips and knees.

Vertical sitting facilitates the prevention and management not only of syncope, but also of atelectasis, hypostatic pneumonia, bedsores, constipation, and incontinence. It reduces both cardiac and respiratory work, as compared with both the semireclining and horizontal position. The vertical sitting position in bed is commercially available in the Burke Home Care Bed (Burke Inc., Mission, Kansas), the Nelson Multi-Purpose Bed (Palo Alto Orthopedic, Palo Alto, Calif.), and in the Circo-lectric Bed (Orthopedic Frame Co., Kalamazoo, Mich.). All of these beds have the advantage of foot boards adjustable for varying leg length. This should be a feature of standard beds to prevent foot drop in the supine position, but it is essential for proper foot support and weight bearing in the sitting position. Fig. 14.3 shows the Circo-lectric Bed, which has great versatility of positioning. The patient can be placed in any prone or supine position and can control these positions himself through an electric motor. This bed is lighter than the conventional hospital bed and requires less actual floor space.

It will go through a 34-inch (86 cm) doorway, so it can be used at home. The tubes can be used for attaching traction devices, slings, and other patient aids. The disadvantages of the Circo-electric Bed are its narrowness and height from the floor, which are a source of apprehension for many patients.

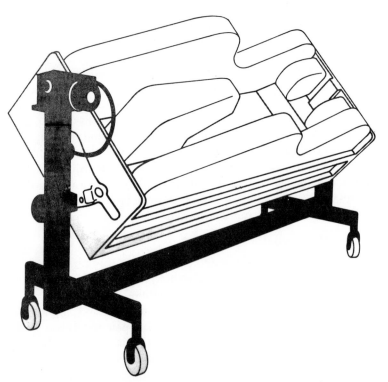

Fig. 14.2. Keane Roto-Rest Bed (Kinetic Concepts).

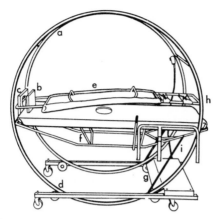

Fig. 14.3. Circo-electric Bed. *a*, top ring section; *b*, permanent footboard; *c*, foot end; *d*, bottom ring section; *e*, anterior frame; *f*, posterior frame; *g*, support bar; *h*, head bar, *i*, balance springs.

Compliant Porous Supporting Membrane and Medium

In bed, a compliant porous supporting membrane and medium will reduce areas of local pressure and help prevent bedsores. Details of this are given later under "Special Mattresses and Beds to Prevent Bedsores."

Spring-loaded Adjustable Footboard

A spring-loaded adjustable footboard facilitates proper positioning of the feet in both lying and sitting, with the possibility of voluntary resistive activity of the leg muscles. This may prevent not only plantar flexion contractures of the ankle, but also phlebothrombosis, muscle atrophy, and negative nitrogen balance. A spring-loaded footboard (Soleus Ergometer, Stanley Cox Ltd., London, U. K.) is available in the United Kingdom but not at present in the U. S. It not only has a variable spring tension to adjust for maximal resistance through full range of plantar flexion but also has a counter which enables the nurse or attendant to record how many contractions the patient has made in a given period.

Patient-operated Toilet Mechanism

Essentials in a patient-controlled toilet opening mechanism should enable the patient to assume vertical sitting and make an opening in the mattress and place under it a container. When the patient has completed his toilet, he should be able to reverse the procedure. This feature is mainly of value in patients confined to bed, either at home or in a nursing home, where help may be unavailable except at certain times of the day—or even in a hospital setting, if the patient has urgency of urination.

No commercially available item like this is known, although one has been fabricated on an experimental bed which has, in addition, all of the other essential features mentioned above (5). The Circo-electric Bed does have a removable section in the mattress which can be replaced with a metal pot by the nurse. As this bed also allows vertical sitting, it is an excellent device for the hospitalized patient with paralytic bowel and bladder, such as a quadriplegic. Nevertheless, a real need exists for the patient-operated toilet mechanism for bedfast patients at home and in nursing homes.

Variable Height Bed Surface (from 18 inches to 40 inches)

A variable height bed from 18 inches to 40 inches (46 to 102 cm) will decrease problems in transfer and lifting, for both patient and nurse but, as previously mentioned, no hospital bed presently meets these specifications. The best available at this time in the U. S. is the Burke "Home Care Bed" which goes from an ideal low of 18 inches to a high of 32 inches, including a 6-inch mattress.

Special Mattresses and Beds to Prevent Bedsores

Bedsores are the most common, obvious, and distressing problem of bedrest. They are not only distressing to the patient and his family but also they are mortifying to a conscientious staff. Good nurses have always insisted that all bedsores are preventable, provided that there are enough nurses to turn the patient regularly every 2 hours and enough pillows to position the patient correctly. Concerned physicians and nurses believe that no mechanical device is a substitute for a good nursing staff. And with the survival of many more seriously injured and diseased patients some experienced nurses consider that in many hospitals staffing is inadequate to ensure prevention of bedsores. Fortunately, in the past few years, a number of new mattresses and beds have been produced which may prove effective in the prevention of bedsores without 2-hourly turning.

It is estimated that more than 3% of patients in acute care hospitals have bedsores (22). This figure is probably higher in nursing homes. The annual cost of healing these sores in the United Kingdom has been estimated to be in excess of $200,000,000 (7).

PATHOGENESIS OF BEDSORES

There are five local factors that predispose to bedsores.

1. Sustained Local Pressure. Sustained local pressure obstructs the local circulation and, if unrelieved, results in arteriolar thrombosis within a few hours. Ischemia and necrosis follow, resulting in gangrene, ulceration, and abcess formation. Local pressure can be reduced in the bedfast patient by distributing pressure more uniformly over a large area by use of a high-compliance medium such as water, air, or low-density foam. An alternative method involves continually reducing the duration of the local pressure below that necessary to produce thrombosis and ischemia. Examples of this are an oscillating bed that continuously alters the body position or an oscillating mattress that continuously changes pressure over the skin. No bedsores have occurred in more than 700 patients treated for a variety of surgical conditions on a rocking bed (12).

2. Friction. Friction on the skin occurs when the patient is dragged rather than lifted across the bed. Friction can be decreased by replacing unnecessary layers such as draw sheet, rubber sheets, mattress cover, etc. with one smooth wrinkle-free surface such as a fitted knit cotton sheet.

3. Shearing Forces. Shearing forces between skin and underlying bone which occur, for example, when gatching the patient to the semireclining position predispose to the formation of a sacral ulcer with a large undermined bursa. Shearing forces can be reduced by maintaining each point of the bed surface opposite the same point on the patient's body in whatever position the bed is placed. In conventional hospital beds, when the patient moves from backlying to sitting, a 6- to 8-inch (15 to 20 cm) shift of the trunk occurs relative to the mattress. This very significant shearing force on the skin and subcutaneous tissue over the sacrum can be reduced by use of a sliding split mattress which moves with the body segments. Shearing forces are also reduced by decreasing stiffness and friction of the surface membrane and medium supporting the patient.

4. Maceration of skin. Maceration of skin associated with excessive perspiration or incontinence is aggravated by nonabsorbent and nonporous materials close to the skin, such as nylon nightdresses and polyester sheets, and impermeable materials, such as rubber seats and plastic mattress covers. Replacing these nonabsorbent waterproof materials with porous absorbent materials such as combed cotton sheeting and reticulated foam mattresses reduces maceration.

5. Infection. Infection producing folliculitis and carbuncles results from nonsterile surfaces and lowered skin resistance secondary to ischemia, maceration, and inflammation. Prevention of infection is assisted by ensuring that all components of the supporting medium, especially the mattress, are bacteriostatic, washable, and autoclavable.

SPECIAL MATTRESSES AND BEDS

In no area of bed design has more work been done than in equipment to prevent bedsores (16). More than 16 different types of mattresses and beds are marketed currently, and for almost every type there are at least two or three manufacturers. Each manufacturer makes special claims for the virtues of his product; we know of only one "study" (4) objectively comparing different types of beds and mattresses in the prevention of tissue ischemia. There are many poorly constructed clinical studies and reports on prevention and healing of bedsores. One interesting study by Fernie and Dornan (8) showed that heightened interest of staff in using a new device hastened the healing of bedsores, even though it was a placebo device and neither staff nor patients knew that it was inoperative!

The two basic types of mattress or bed to prevent bedsores either distribute pressure more uniformly or decrease duration of pressure.

SPECIAL MATTRESSES

A mattress can be considered as a supporting medium ("the core material of the mattress") and an enclosing membrane ("the mattress cover and sheets") which separate the patient's skin from the supporting medium. The ideal supporting medium should have the following characteristics: high compliance, minimum shearing force, high porosity, autoclavability, and lightness. High compliance is essential for uniform pressure distribution but poses a problem for maintaining proper bed positioning that will ensure spinal support, prevent contractures, and permit transfer activities. All of these considerations require a firm, as opposed to a compliant, medium. Therefore, the most effective devices have been made to provide either high compliance or firmness as required in the individual case, *e.g.,* Jobst waterbed or air fluidized bed. Characteristically, the enclosing membrane should include low stiffness, low coefficient of friction, high porosity, and absorbency. For the supporting medium to increase the uniformity of pressure on the skin surface, three materials are commonly used; these are foam, fluid, and air (see Table 14.2).

MATTRESSES THAT PRODUCE UNIFORM PRESSURE

Foam Mattresses

Polyurethane foam provides a medium whose compliance, firmness, and density can be varied over a wide range from supersoft to extra firm. Combinations with soft foam on the top and firm below can provide both high compliance and, yet, good support. As durability depends on density, the greater it is, the greater the weight and the price. Ordinary foam has very little transpiration and, so, may build up a moisture layer whereas open mesh or "reticulated" foam has an exploded air cell which easily allows passage of air and fluids. Unfortunately, "reticulated" foam tends to take a set more quickly than ordinary foam, and it is more expensive.

A 2-inch (5 cm) foam mattress of the usual density can be improved as a resting surface by cutting a square over the pelvic area where the sacrum and trochanters rest. Into this empty square is inserted a water-filled or silica gel-filled wheelchair type pad. We have used this as a measure to prevent bedsores in this area, with good results.

A three-layer foam mattress with knit cotton cover now marketed as The Burke Mattress System is shown in Figure 14.4. This effective supporting medium, meeting virtually all of the desired mattress characteristics, consists of three layers of foam rubber held together by a membrane of knit stretch combed cotton which functions as both mattress cover and sheet. This produces a surface which is wrinkle-free and has a low coefficient of

TABLE 14.2. *Comparison of Features of Mattresses for Prevention of Bedsores*

Mattress*	Medium*						Membrane*			Special features
	Compliance	Firm-ness	Porous	Auto-clavable	Light-weight	Stiffness	Friction	Porous	Absorb-ent	
1. Inner spring (C)†Vinyl	1‡	3	0	0	1	1	3	0	1	1. Standard mattress
2. Firm foam (C) Vinyl	2	2	0	0	2	1	2	0	1	2. Standard mattress
3. 3-Layer foam (C) Knit Cotton (Burke)	3	2	3	3	3	3	2	3	3	3. Knit cotton mattress cover = sheet
4. Egg carton (C) Sheet (Zimmer)	3	1	2	3	3	2	1	3	2	4. Knobbled surface
5. Split firm foam (C) Cotton (Ali Med.)	2	2	2	3	2	2	1	2	2	5. Split mattress
6. Water mattress (C) Vinyl (Sears Roebuck)	3	1	0	0	1	1	1	0	1	6. Inexpensive camping air mattress
7. Modular water bed (C) Vinyl (Rochester)	3	2	1	0	2	2	1	2	1	7. Local water pillows with open-ended manometer
8. Low pressure air bed (C) Vinyl (Simpson)	3	2	0	0	2	2	1	0	1	8. Adjustable pressure. Open air flow system
9. Alternating pressure (C) Vinyl (Lapidus)	1	2	2	0	2	1	1	2	1	9. Variable air pressure + ventilating system

* Mattresses consist of supporting medium enclosed in membrane.
† (C) = Cover + polyester sheet, except for *3.* and *4*, where sheet serves as cover.
‡ 0 = meets no requirements§; 1 = meets some requirements§; 2 = meets most requirements§; 3 = meets all requirements§.
§ Requirements in ideal medium and membrane to prevent bedsores.

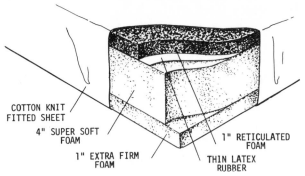

COTTON KNIT
FITTED SHEET

4" SUPER SOFT
FOAM

1" EXTRA FIRM
FOAM

1" RETICULATED
FOAM

THIN LATEX
RUBBER

Fig. 14.4. Layered Foam Mattress (Burke, Inc.).

friction, yet is also porous, absorbent, and soft. This contrasts with the usual combinations of draw sheets and polyester and vinyl mattress covers, which have completely opposite features.

In the Burke mattress, the top layer is 1-inch-thick (2.5 cm) reticulated polyurethane foam. This is 97% air and highly porous, so that any spilled fluid, urine, etc. will quickly drain away from contact with the skin. The middle layer is 4-inch-thick (10 cm) highly compliant foam distributing pressure evenly over as large a body surface as possible. The bottom layer is 1-inch-thick very firm foam, whose main function is to provide a firm, yet compressible, base to absorb shock and prevent bottoming out when the patient suddenly sits on the edge of the bed. The bottom two layers are covered by a very thin, loose, removable envelope of elastic latex rubber. This protects the two base layers of foam from soiling without significantly affecting its compliance or reducing the transpiration of the top layer of reticulated foam. All layers of this supporting medium are machine washable and autoclavable to combat possibility of spread of infection. The highly porous membrane and reticulated foam increases aeration, which reduces temperature and risk of maceration and immensely increases the comfort for the patient. A tendency to mould to the patient's body after prolonged use may create a problem, although theoretically this moulding probably reduces local pressure. The problem of moulding can be eliminated by replacing the middle and bottom layers of foam with one layer of standard, firm, high-density foam, but this will also reduce compliance.

An ingenious use of the versatility of foam is the construction of "egg carton" pads (Zimmer, Warsaw, Ind.). These mattresses, as their name implies, resemble foam egg cartons. They facilitate even distribution of weight, reduction of shearing forces, and improvement of air circulation. They are normally placed under a sheet on top of a standard mattress. The main disadvantage is that their convoluted surface does not provide that smooth flat surface necessary for easy transfer or movement in bed. Also, some patients with thin skin have complained that the egg carton pads leave mottled red spots all over their skin.

Split-Foam Mattress

Foam can be split in parts so that separate sections support the trunk, the thighs, and the legs. In this way, all pressure points from os calcis to sacrum can be positioned in a space between the mattress sections so that they are free from pressure and air circulates freely by them in any lying position. Such a sectioned mattress utilized for initial care of patients in spinal centers in Britian is excellent for patients with bedsores subject to pressure in more than one site. These mattresses are commercially available as a Modular Bed System (Ali Med, Inc., Boston, Mass.).

Water Mattresses

The least expensive water mattress for either hospital or home use is a rib-constructed camping mattress (Ted Williams Brand, Sears Roebuck and Co.) filled with water and air. This can be placed over a standard hospital mattress but is better if placed on 6 inches (15 cm) of medium-firm foam. It should be filled with enough water to ensure flotation but not so much that one reduces the compliance of the containing rubber envelope. Although it is not quite as effective as a good hospital waterbed, its lightness, ease of handling, convenience for patients at home, and especially its low cost make it a first choice for many debilitated malnourished elderly bedsore-prone patients' especially when nursed at home.

Another ingenious solution to the problems of difficulty in positioning patients and the weight and cost of waterbeds is a modular water bed (Rochester Modular Water Beds, Rochester, N. Y.) (29). A small water pad is placed inside a cut out piece of foam at the level of the feet and pelvis, probably the two commonest sites for pressure sores. These foam frames are connected together by solid interlocking blocks of foam. As all the blocks are of standard size, the small 2-gallon (7.6 liters) water pads can be placed at any location. This system enormously reduces weight and cost compared to a waterbed. However, its greatest advantage is ability to grade pressure. Each pad is connected by thin capillary tubing to a reservoir suspended on a pole similar to an intravenous set. The height of the fluid column in the capillary tubing indicates the pressure in the pad. As long as it remains less than 30 cm above the bed, the patient's skin pressure on the pad will be less than capillary pressure. By this means, one can continually monitor pressure-susceptible areas. This fact, along with the ease of positioning and transfer, light weight, ease of use, and economy, make this one of the most important recent additions to our armamentarium in the battle to prevent bedsores.

Low Pressure Air Bed

The low pressure air bed (19) was designed to simplify and reduce the cost of support systems for the prevention of bedsores. The bed consists of two camping air mattresses of box-edge type, placed one above the other on a wooden base. They are connected together by tubing, which in turn is connected to a standard aquarium aeration pump. A further length of tubing is connected by means of a "T" piece to the pump air line. The end of this tubing is immersed in water to a given depth, which sets the pressure inside the mattresses. Within about 15 to 20 minutes after starting the pump, both mattresses become fully inflated. Depending on the depth to which the side tube is immersed in the column of liquid, the mattresses will remain inflated at a given pressure. If a person is now placed on the bed, the consequent rise in pressure will drive air out of the mattresses. Air will bubble out from the end of the tube until the pressure is once more at the preset level. With changes in posture, either excess air will bubble out or air discharge will pause until the pressure has built up once more to the required level. In the steady state condition, the air from the pump passes directly out by bubbling from the tube, with the pump acting as it would in an aquarium.

This bed can be changed from a soft compliant to a firm stiff surface by depressing the exhaust tube to as much as 100 mm of water. It appears to eliminate the need for bedsore-prone patients to be turned every 2 hours.

Although only in use since 1977, reports on this bed from spinal injury units, geriatric centers, and home nursing programs are uniformly good. It is inexpensive and simple to construct, and it may prove as economical as the special foam mattresses, the water mattresses, and the modular waterbed.

MATTRESSES TO REDUCE DURATION OF PRESSURE

Alternating Pressure Point Mattresses. The concept of reducing the duration of pressure on a given area of skin is also incorporated in alternating pressure point mattresses. These usually consist of a series of vinyl tubes or cells which are connected to a pump in such a way that when one cell or tube is inflated, an adjacent cell or tube is deflated. The length of these cycles of aeration varies from 15 seconds to 4 minutes.

The alternating pressure pad is placed on a standard mattress under an ordinary sheet. In theory this mattress should effectively relieve pressure, but in practice it has limitations due to collapse of air cells under high local pressure. Furthermore, lying directly on plastic increases discomfort, body heat, perspiration and, therefore, liability to skin maceration.

To obviate this, one company (Lapidus Airfloat System—American Hospital Supply, McGaw Park, Ill.) has developed a mattress which, in addition to alternately inflating and deflating 40 air tubes, also has 60 to 70 air holes in the tubes producing a continuous flow of air through a foam cushion which separates the patient from the tubes. In our experience, none of these alternating pads has reduced the need for 2-hourly turning to protect the bedsore-prone patient.

Rolling Mattress-Cloud 9. This mattress (J. H. Emerson Co., Cambridge, Mass.) consists essentially of two long interconnected sausage-like air sacs. One sac alternately inflates and deflates so that the other sac responds reciprocally. The patient is rolled from side to side while supported on an air cushion. Early reports indicate that this is a comfortable and effective way of relieving tissue pressure and better than the alternating pressure point mattress.

ROHO Balloon Cushion. This special cushion, consisting of a series of vertical balloons filled with air (ROHO Balloon Cushion, Box 658, Belleville, Ill.) and looking like a tray of wrinkled mushrooms was recently enlarged into a mattress size. This mattress is now available commercially. According to the manufacturer, individual balloon elements conform to the body and thus, the air-filled balloons provide a maximum support area which evenly and comfortably distributes patient weight and thereby lowers peak pressures on the skin. Preliminary clinical experience using the ROHO cushion in wheelchairs has been very satisfactory. Presumably this concept applied to mattresses will be equally effective in preventing pressure sores. The balloons inflate and deflate as the patient shifts in the bed. Therefore, this ROHO mattress can be classed as a mattress reducing duration of pressure with this group of mattresses and its cost is less.

SPECIAL BEDS

There are at least nine beds designed to prevent bedsores:
(1) Rocking Bed + 3 layer foam mattress
(2) Rolling Bed—Roto Rest
(3) Air fluidized Bed
(4) Intermittent fluidized Bed
(5) Jobst Water Bed
(6) Mud Bed
(7) High Air Loss Bed
(8) Low Air Loss Bed
(9) Net Suspension Bed

All of these beds offer significant advantages over the best of the special mattresses in the prevention of bedsores, but usually at a cost of more than $2000. Even this price, however, is much less than the cost of treating one bedsore. Features of each bed are compared in Table 14.3.

Oscillating Beds

Rocking and rolling types of oscillating beds have been described in the previous section. Years of successful nursing experience have shown that as long as the patient's position is changed every 2 hours, bedsores will not occur. Thus, the oscillating bed appears to be the most effective bed in preventing bedsores. In addition to all the advantages already mentioned, the patient sleeps without being awakened by turning, and nurses are freed from the 2-hourly labor and backstrain involved in lifting, turning, and positioning their most immobile patients.

TABLE 14.3. Comparison of Features of Beds for Prevention of Bedsores

Bed + mattress*		Features of								Special features
	Alters pressure periodically	Supporting medium*					Membrane*			
		Compliance	Firmness	Porous	Weight	Stiffness	Friction	Porous	Absorbent	
1. Rocking bed + Burke mattress	3†	3	2	3	2	3	2	3	3	Rocks 1–20×/min 20° head and foot down.
2. Roto-Rest rolling bed	3	1	3	0	2	1	3	0	0	Rolls 70° side to side, every 4 min
3. Air fluidized bed	3	3	3	3	1	3	1	3	2	Floats on continuously air fluidized beads
4. Intermittent fluidized bed	3	3	3	3	1	3	1	3	2	Floats on intermittently air fluidized beads
5. Jobst waterbed	0	3	3	0	2	3	2	0	0	Waterbed with high or low compliance
6. Mud bed	0	2	1	0	1	1	1	0	0	Floats patient higher than on water
7. Low air loss bed	2	3	1	3	1	2	2	3	2	Continuous air flotation
8. Net suspension bed	0	3	1	3	3	3	1	3	2	Low cost net suspension

* Bed includes supporting medium (mattress) + membrane (mattress cover + sheet).
† 0 = meets no requirements‡; 1 = meets some requirements‡; 2 = meets most requirements‡; 3 = meets all requirements.‡
‡ Requirements in ideal combination of bed and mattress to prevent bedsores.

Air Fluidized Bed

In the air-fluidized bed (Support Systems International, Johns Island, S. C.), compressed air is forced through a diffuser into a medium of granular material consisting of glass spheres 75 to 100 μm in diameter (Fig. 14.5). The spheres separate from one another and are suspended in the air flow from the blower. The patient is separated from the glass spheres by a woven polyester sheet with a pore size of 30 μm, which prevents the beads from escaping but permits air to pass easily through it at about 0.6 liters/min. During lying, the sensation resembles that of a waterbed, and it is claimed that no point in the body exceeds a pressure of 20 mm Hg. There is no sensation of moving air, although it will cool the body if the bed temperature is less than 30°C. The temperature of the air is usually kept at 31°C for optimal comfort with minimal perspiration.

This bed has been found effective for treating bedsores, skin grafts, and burns. The lack of maceration is an important factor in hastening wound healing, as compared to the waterbed, where maceration is often seen.

Intermittent Fluidized Bed

A variation of the air fluidized bed is the intermittent fluidized bed, which has the same blower without heaters, heat exchangers, or filter sheet. It has a vinyl cover and is only fluidized for a few seconds every 6 to 10 minutes, recontouring itself to the patient at regular intervals.

This bed has been found of most value when prevention of bedsores and positioning for skeletal fixation are important, such as in orthopedic patients

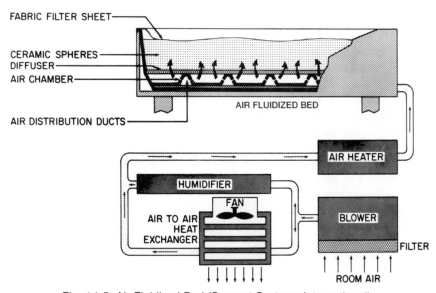

Fig. 14.5. Air Fluidized Bed (Support Systems International).

in casts and traction and in the immobile unconscious patient who needs uniform support to prevent tissue breakdown.

The main disadvantage with both of these beds is expense and weight.

Hospital Water Beds

The main advantage of a waterbed is that point pressures are lower than on a water mattress (18). Its main disadvantage is the nursing problem of moving, lifting, or positioning the patient to prevent contractures as he lies on its jelly-like surface.

One of the few waterbeds that has tackled this problem is the Jobst Hydrofloat (Jobst Institute, Inc., Toledo, Ohio). This has elevating bed sides to which the water cell is attached. Lowering the sides reduces the water in the cell, and the patient rests on a firm surface; elevating the sides floats the patient completely. This bed has proven very useful in the management of plastic surgical patients who require prolonged immobility, e.g., for cross-leg flaps, but has also been useful in managing other conditions requiring prolonged immobility.

Mud Bed

To decrease problems of immersion and instability in waterbeds, in the mud bed (Gaymar Inc., Buffalo, N. Y.), water has been replaced by high-density fluid composed of bentonite clay and barites. This medium floats the patient much higher and resists deformation more than water, facilitating patient positioning. However, this small advantage vs. the great weight (over 1300 pounds or 590 kg) and cost does not seem to justify its use over the more simple methods of flotation.

High Air Loss Bed

The original experimental 'levitation' bed designed by Scales in 1961 (25) has undergone numerous modifications and is now marketed in the United Kingdom as the Mark F6 'Levitation' Bed (26). Basically, the patient is supported on a column of air which escapes between the body and a series of flexible parallel tubular pockets on either side of the body. On this bed, the body can be supported with an air pressure of less than 28 cm of water. It requires nearly 20,000 liters (700 cubic feet) of air per minute. The temperature and humidity of the air can be controlled. It is claimed that this bed has the following desirable features:

(a) Even pressure on the thrust area.

(b) Rapid drying of exudate and accelerated formation of eschar.

(c) Control of body temperature and humidity of the immediate environment.

(d) Isolation of a patient in a sterile environment.

(e) Support of the trunk without touching any surface.

The main indications for this bed are probably for high-risk acute patients and severe burn patients, and it may be a good investment only in burn units. Its main disadvantages are high cost, noise, and the size of the special unit designed to house blowers.

Low Air Loss Bed

To provide a more practical, less expensive, less cumbersome, less noisy bed, Scales and his colleagues (26) developed the Low Air Loss Bed (Watkins & Watson Ltd., Wareham, Dorset, England) in 1971. Unlike with the High Air Loss Bed, the patient is supported on a flexible vapor-permeable film between the skin and the air. Thus, the volume of air required to support the patient is reduced to 2,800 liters (100 cubic feet) per minute, which considerably reduces noise and size of the blower unit and cost.

The patient lies on a number of vapor-permeable air sacs, and the pressures in the groups of sacs under calf, thighs, buttocks, and trunk can each be controlled. As temperature and humidity can be easily regulated, this bed is of special value in the healing of open wounds such as bedsores and burns. It is less noisy and expensive than the high air loss bed but still has these disadvantages.

Net Suspension Bed

The net suspension bed (Mecanaids, Gloucester, England) (13) is essentially a mesh hammock stretched between two parallel bars suspending the net. By rotating the bars, the patient can be raised or lowered over a conventional bed. It appears to offer advantages of high compliance, good pressure distribution, good aeration, and low cost. Its main disadvantage may be the hazard of tearing the net and also proper bed positioning. At present, this device is not widely available, and it was introduced too recently for complete evaluation.

Special Purpose Beds

All of the six features described earlier as essential features in the ideal hospital bed would be of value for any person, sick or well, who has to be confined to bed for more than 2 or 3 days. Many conditions, such as orthopedic and neurosurgical disorders, require small modifications of existing beds, such as overhead suspension or traction apparatus. However, certain disorders present problems in medical nursing care for which special beds are required. Apart from bedsores, these most commonly include cardiac conditions, spinal injuries, and burns.

Cardiac Care Beds

The main requirement in a cardiac care bed is that it can move the patient from the supine position to vertical sitting with no effort on his part. The low position should be no more than 18 inches (46 cm), top surface to floor, so that the patient can easily and safely get out of bed. One bed that at present meets both of these requirements is the Burke Home Care Bed, mentioned earlier. The Nelson Multi-purpose Bed (Kinetic Concepts, San Antonio, Texas) provides good vertical sitting, although its low position of 26 inches (66 cm) is too high for easy and safe patient standing or transfer.

Spinal Injury Care Beds

Essential features in a spinal injury care bed should include the ability to provide: (a) continuous cervical traction, no matter what the body position; (b) turning of the patient from side to side or from supine to prone smoothly; and (c) easy patient accessibility, comfort, and safety. The three beds now available to meet these requirements, in our order of preference, are: The Keane Roto-Rest Bed (Kinetic Concepts, San Antonio, Texas), the Egerton Turning and Tilting Bed (Egerton Hospital Equipment Ltd., Horsham, Sussex, England), and the Circo-lectric Bed (Orthopedic Frame Company, Kalamazoo, Mich.).

Keane Roto-Rest Bed. This bed has been already described (see "Rolling Beds"). It was specifically designed to meet all requirements listed. In the acute stage of cervical spine injury requiring continuous traction, its continuous rolling action prevents bedsores, thrombosis, and hypostatic pneumonia.

Egerton Tilting and Turning Bed. This bed, designed at the national spinal injury center in England, allows one nurse without any strain to turn the patient. The basic bed frame has an interlocking design whereby the patient's spine is supported by two-thirds of the bed's total width during turning in either direction. No matter to what angle or how frequently turning takes place, the patient always remains in the center of the bed. The bed is folded about its longitudinal axis, and the patient lies with his back against one surface and his side against the other. He can thus be safely tilted to 60° sidelying without fear of falling or moving. Although a much less costly bed than the Roto-Rest, it still requires a nurse to operate the turning mechanism, whereas for the Roto-Rest turning is done continuously without any nursing attendants.

Circo-lectric Bed. This bed can provide cervical traction while allowing patient turning from supine to prone through a vertical plane. This can also be done by one nurse without any strain. Its advantage is that it allows for vertical sitting for bowel training and standing to prevent development of postural hypotension. Its main disadvantage is that it is narrow and high, making patients uncomfortable and apprehensive. It probably does not support the spine as effectively as the Roto-Rest or Egerton Beds.

Burn Care Beds

Bed requirements for a severely burned patient include even pressure distribution over the entire skin surface between 10 and 18 mm Hg, no shearing stresses, and a control microclimate of temperature and humidity for the skin. Beds that most nearly meet these requirements are the high air loss and low air loss beds and the air fluidized beds, all of which have been described previously. The high air loss bed appears to be ideal, as it is the only bed in which the patient is actually supported on air, which is not only more comfortable but also permits easier healing of the burn. In practice the low air loss bed appears to provide almost as good results. The air fluidized bed has many advocates in the management of the severely burned patient. Control of the skin pressures between 10 and 18 mm Hg is perhaps most effectively accomplished with this bed. However, as far as is known, no study has been made to compare these three beds in a burn unit; any one of them is superior to support systems, such as waterbeds, which tend to produce maceration.

Conclusion

The bed is a *sine qua non* of clinical (of, or pertaining to the sick bed, Oxford English Dictionary) medicine. However, even today the standard hospital bed predisposes to, rather than prevents, the pathology associated with recumbency. Much of this pathology could be prevented by features of bed construction that are already available. Physicians should take the initiative and responsibility of persuading hospitals to provide the appropriate bed in each situation in which special needs are evident. Unless this is done, the most basic device in our therapeutic armamentarium may continue to be a hindrance rather than a help in the healing of the patient.

REFERENCES

1. ABRAMSON, A. S., AND DELAGI, E. F. Influence of weight bearing and muscle contraction on disuse osteoporosis. *Arch. Phys. Med.*, *42:* 147, 1961.
2. ASHER, R. A. J. Dangers of going to bed. *Brit. Med. J.*, *2:* 967, 1947.
3. BROWSE, N. L. *The Physiology and Pathology of Bed Rest.* Charles C Thomas, Springfield, Ill., 1965.
4. CARPENDALE, M. T. F. A comparison of four beds in the prevention of tissue ischaemia in paraplegic patients. *Paraplegia, 12:* 21, 1974.
5. CARPENDALE, M. T. F., AND FINKELSTEIN, L. A Bed to Counteract the Hazards of Recumbency. Exhibit, AMA Convention, Chicago, Ill., June 1970.
6. DEITRICK, J. E., WHEDON, G. D., AND SHORR, E. Effects of immobilization upon various metabolic and physiologic functions of normal men. *Am. J. Med., 4:* 3, 1948.
7. FERNIE, G. R. Biomechanical Aspects of the Aetiology of Decubitus Ulcers on Human Patients. Ph.D. Thesis, University of Strathclyde, Glasgow, Scotland, 1973.
8. FERNIE, G. R., AND DORNAN, J. The problem of clinical trials with new systems for preventing or healing decubiti. In *Bedsore Biomechanics*, edited by R. M. Kennedi, J. M. Cowden, and J. T. Scales, pp. 315–320. University Park Press, Baltimore, 1976.
9. FLANC, C., KAKKAR, V. V., AND CLARKE, M. D. The detection of venous thrombosis of the legs using 125 I-labelled fibrinogen. *Br. J. Surg., 55:* 742, 1968.
10. GAUER, O. H., HENRY, J. P., AND BEHN, C. The regulation of extra cellular fluid volume. *Annu. Rev. Physiol., 32:* 547, 1970.
11. GETZEN, L. C. Reduction of postoperative nitrogen loss through oscillating motion. *Surg. Gynecol. Obstet., 119:* 1259, 1964.
12. GETZEN, L. C. Personal communication.

13. GIBBS, J. R. Net suspension beds for managing threatened and established bedsores. *Lancet, 1:* 174, 1977.
14. GIBBS, N. R. The prophylaxis of pulmonary embolism. *Br. J. Surg., 47:* 282, 1949.
15. KEANE, F. Roto-Rest. *Paraplegia, 7:* 254, 1970.
16. KENNEDI, R. M., COWDEN, J. M., AND SCALES, J. T. Bedsore Biomechanics. University Park Press, Baltimore, 1976.
17. KOTTKE, F. J. Deterioration of the bedfast patient. *Public Health Rep., 80:* 437, 1965.
18. LILLA, J. A., FRIEDRICHS, R. R., AND VISTNES, L. M. Floatation mattresses for preventing and treating tissue breakdown. *Geriatrics, 30:* 71, 1975.
19. MCCUBBIN, K. J., AND SIMPSON, D. C. A low pressure air bed. *J. Med. Eng. Technol., 1* (2): 98, 1977.
20. OSTLUND, E. Upright positioning: an important aid in the treatment of congestive heart failure in infants. *J. Am. Med. Wom. Assoc., 30:* 743, 1965.
21. PACE, N. Weightlessness: a matter of gravity. *N. Engl. J. Med., 297:* 32, 1977.
22. PETERSON, N. C., AND BITTMAN, S. The Epidemiology of Pressure Sores. *Scand. J. Plast. Reconstr. Surg., 5:* 62, 1971.
23. SALZMAN, E. W., AND SKINNER, D. B. Prevention of Thromboembolism in Surgical Patients by Prophylactic Anticoagulation. Exhibit, AMA, New York, N. Y., July 1969.
24. SANDERS, C. E. Cardiovascular and peripheral vascular diseases: treatment by a motorized bed. *J. A. M. A., 106:* 916, 1936.
25. SCALES, J. T. Levitation. *Lancet, 2:* 1181, 1961.
26. SCALES, J. T., LUNN, H. F., JENEID, P. A., GILLINGHAM, M. E., AND REDFERN, S. J. The prevention and treatment of pressure sores using air support systems. *Paraplegia, 12:* 118, 1974.
27. SEVITT, S. Thromboembolism and its prevention. *Proc. R. Soc. Med., 61:* 143, 1968.
28. TAYLOR, H., HERSCHEL, A., BROZEK, J., AND KEYS, A. Effects of bedrest on cardiovascular function and work performance. *J. Appl. Physiol., 2:* 223, 1949.
29. WEINSTEIN, B. Water bed of modular construction for localized floatation. *Arch. Phys. Med. Rehabil., 54:* 533, 1973.
30. WELLS, C. A. The use and abuse of rest as a therapeutic measure. *Proc. R. Soc. Med., 47:* 177, 1953.
31. WHEDON, G. D. Management of the effects of recumbency. *Med. Clin. North Am., 35:* 545, 1951.
32. WHEDON, G. D., DEITRICK, J. E., AND SHORR, E. Modifications of the effects of immobilization upon metabolic and physiologic functions of normal men by the use of an oscillating bed. *Am. J. Med., 6:* 684, 1949.
33. WHEDON, G. D., AND SHORR, E. Metabolic studies in paralytic acute anterior poliomyelitis. III. Metabolic and circulatory effects of the slowly oscillating bed. *J. Clin. Invest., 36:* 982, 1957.
34. WRIGHT, J. The respir-aid rocking bed in poliomyelitis. *Am. J. Nursing, 47:* 454, 1947.

15

Housing for the Disabled

MARILYN B. WITTMEYER, M.O.T., O.T.R.
MIECZYSLAW PESZCZYNSKI, M.D.

The housing problems of the disabled and elderly are intertwined with the housing concerns of the entire population and must be solved as the concerns of all are solved. Housing problems must be shared by the total population—the family, the neighborhood, the employer, and the community at large. Human needs for security, shelter, privacy, and independence are desired by all, the able-bodied as well as the disabled. In planning for the environment that will not exclude them, consideration should be given to the total needs of the nearly 40 million disabled persons projected to be living in the U. S. by 1985. In the past, there was an attitude of "out of sight, out of mind" toward the disabled; the current attitude, however, places more emphasis upon encouraging the disabled to lead productive lives and to avail themselves of educational and work opportunities.

The progress in rehabilitation in this country is characterized by, among other things, the expansion from predominantly vocational retraining of disabled people to more general rehabilitation services. This includes rehabilitation of those physically handicapped persons who can no longer work but who are expected to be able to live at home either independently or with the least amount of assistance. Another feature of this progress is increasing attention to the more severely involved, especially the aged disabled and the handicapped child. A feature which has also come into the foreground is the growing awareness that the sentimental desire to help the disabled must be bridled by objective assessment of their capabilities and limitations. The relationship between the cost of rehabilitation and the results achieved must be considered.

Current statistics note that approximately 1 of every 10 persons in the U. S. has a permanent disability and that more than a quarter of a million persons are in wheelchairs (6). With the declining birth rate, improved health care and medical advances, and increasing numbers of disabled living a fuller and integrated, rather than segregated, life can be met best through mutual housing concerns. Awareness of the concerns of accessibility for all needs to be built into our educational systems in the immediate future and to become a part of the training for designers, planners, builders, contractors, and realtors, as well as for the consumer. In the past it was the interested individual who was the primary source of assistance to the disabled, but at present the most basic service needed is a source of information with individualized attention from federal, state, or local agencies regarding services and legislation.

U. S. Federal Legislation on Housing

The *Housing Act of 1937* committed the federal government to a general policy of providing for the social welfare of citizens by ensuring "a decent home and a suitable living environment for every American family." The *National Housing Act of 1949* reaffirmed this policy and designated the federal role as one of assisting the private housing industry in providing safe and standard quality housing (18). This assumed increased federal responsibility for meeting the housing needs of the low-income families, and by 1956 the phrase "low-income family" was amended to include the elderly. However, recognition of the housing needs of the disabled was still to come.

In retracing housing problems in the 1950's and early 1960's for the severely disabled, Dr. Landauer, at the *Fourth International Poliomyelitis Conference* in 1957 in Geneva, Switzerland, estimated that the cost of caring for patients at home was one-tenth to one-fourth of what hospital costs would have been (9). This demonstrated the great value of comprehensive rehabilitation and the team approach, resource center and supportive equipment, and home adaptation and attendant care. These were also the years of various forms of institutionalization as a solution to the lack of suitable housing and home services for the elderly and the poliomyelitis-disabled.

With the decrease in cases of poliomyelitis, the respiratory centers became a thing of the past, but another disability group began to grow in number and replaced the poliomyelitis group. This group, the spinal cord injured, was due primarily to automobile and sporting accidents. The rehabilitation need for housing and housing treatment center programs is international; England pioneered the treatment center, followed by Canada. In the U. S., no comprehensive nationwide system approaches the poliomyelitis regional center in programs for attendant care, equipment, home adaptation, and aftercare.

In the early 1960's there was an increased public awareness of the housing problems of the disabled, and legislation began to reflect the concept of normalization, which included community-based living arrangements in home-like settings. The *Housing Act of 1964* concentrated on making suitable housing available and accessible to the physically disabled only. In 1974, the *Housing and Community Development Act* included the developmentally disabled among those who qualified for assistance. During the period from 1964 through 1974, major developments in Federal legislation for housing advancement for the disabled were administered under a variety of programs by the *United States Department of Housing and Urban Development* (HUD).

A reversal of the trend toward institutional living started in the early 1970's, at which time large specialized housing programs went into effect which segregated the disabled from the rest of the community. Special attention was given to developing and implementing legislation on accessibility. Guidelines for removing physical barriers to mobility and making the environment accessible had been developed jointly by the *National Easter Seal Society* and the *President's Committee on Employment of the Handicapped*. Thse guidelines were adopted later by the *American National Standards Institute* (ANSI) (1) as standards for buildings and facilities but not for publicly owned or private residences. These standards, although revised in 1971, are not federally mandated. The states have the option of adopting or not adopting them.

To ensure compliance with accessibility requirements by builders, the *Architectural and Transportation Barriers Compliance Board* was established with the *Rehabilitation Act of 1973*. The Board's first public hearing was held in June of 1975. The responsibility of the Board was to ensure that public buildings met the ANSI standards; it had no authority over residential facilities, except for public housing.

During the 1970's in the U. S., a growing awareness of attitudinal change in respect to human rights and needs became prevalent. This was apparent from the increased legislation for housing, such as the *Rehabilitation Act of 1973* and its amendment of 1974 and the *Developmental Disabilities Act* and the *Social Services Amendments of 1974*. In addition,the *National Center for a Barrier-Free Environment* was established in 1974, which brought together individual representatives of voluntary and governmental agencies concerned with housing for the disabled. Similarly, through the *Rehabilitation Act Amendments of 1974*, the *White House Conference on Handicapped Individuals* was concerned with attitudes toward public civil rights, the elimination of environmental barriers, residential and community-based programs, and educational and recreational opportunities.

In a summary of housing and home services for the disabled in the U. S., Laurie (9) states:

> Housing for the disabled is not merely a place of residence. Housing has become the blanket word for the problems of education, training, employment, transportation, architectural barriers, recreation, attendant care, and living arrangements.

The 1976 *Housing Authorization Act* extended the eligibility for HUD-assisted housing to the nonhandicapped and nonelderly single person. This made it possible to integrate the able-bodied and disabled persons within the same environment and further recognized the importance of involving the disabled in normal community life.

In addition to HUD, three existing federal agencies which administer housing programs were identified by Thompson (18). The *Farmers Home Administration, Department of Agriculture* (FmHA), makes loans for purchase, repair, or rental for the disabled with low-to-moderate incomes. The *Veterans Administration* provides GI home loans for specially adapted housing, and the *Department of Defense* provides housing for military personnel whose family members require adapting or modification. There is no program for general housing accessibility.

Recently, the states have been given much of the responsibility for implementing housing programs. Many are experiencing difficulties in obtaining federal funds. Some of the problems are due to lack of clear federal policies, lack of funds, and appropriation procedures, as well as coordination between agencies. However, Thompson (18) discusses the leadership that many states are taking to devise plans for funding state housing or utilizing joint federal-state funding.

Since 1970 there has been a general acceptance of the normalization principle and of an increasing effort away from institutional living. The trend toward community-based housing instead of institutional housing is apparent. An additional trend is that of individuals and organizations representing disability groups working together for legislation to solve their common concerns and to improve attitudes toward the disabled. Laurie (9) states that attitudes will be changed when people who are disabled are treated as equals and when the environment is modified so that they can function as equals.

Housing for the disabled must reflect an approach that makes provision for the total environment. The goal is to provide a variety of living arrangements that enable the disabled to enjoy options comparable to those available to the rest of the population. The primary principle is to follow normal designs as closely as possible. With this in mind, new housing can be easily and more economically designed to facilitate the needs of all. Living in the community among able-bodied persons should be a choice, not a privilege. The disabled need not be set aside and clustered with others of similar disabilities, even though some may choose to do so, however, because of the mutual bond of support which they find in living with small groups of the disabled. The need for barrier-free design and special services may dictate housing considerations for the severely involved.

Provisions to assure barrier-free site and residence design have been neglected not so much by intent as by lack of knowledge. While environmental planners attempt to make their buildings accessible to the disabled, it is important that these designers be aware of the standards and guidelines of ANSI. Convenient access to a residence frequently is denied because of the manner in which the outside and inside is designed and built. Even an able-bodied person may find that access is limited by the design of a structure, such as a shopper opening a door with an armful of groceries, a pregnant woman unable to cope with steps, or a high counter for a short housewife.

The provisions for accessibility, as defined by ANSI, give specifications for buildings and facilities for the physically handicapped. As pointed out by Small and Allen (16), these ANSI standards have not been fully implemented because they are written in guideline language, using terms such as "may" or "should," rather than "shall," resulting in design, interpretation, and enforcement problems. Updated rules and regulations written in special code language would benefit all concerned designers, builders, administrators, and consumers.

Although ANSI is primarily related to public buildings, the environment consists of paths of travel to and through not only public sites, structures, and facilities but also private ones as well. For this reason, the ANSI standards are a basic guide which should be used to establish regulations for minimum access to all structures.

Building Design for Disabled

Small and Allen (16) feel that certain factors need to be considered when designing for the total population in our man-made environment. Buildings and structures have been designed and built for the average individual, irrespective of that person's size, ability, strength, and mobility. People with ambulatory restrictions usually benefit from the same general considerations as people using a wheelchair; nevertheless, some ambulation-restricted persons who have limited strength still may prefer to use stairs instead of negotiating a more lengthy ramp.

Many ambulant persons finding bending or stooping a problem; thus, there is a need to place controls, and certain items requiring reach, within optimal range of both standing and seated individuals. Ambulation-disabled, and in some cases persons using wheelchairs, need support and balance assists such as handrails and grab bars. For the wheelchair user, two grades of housing arrangements need to be considered, one to accommodate semiambulant wheelchair users and the other to accommodate wheelchair-bound users.

In considering the characteristics of the disabled who are handicapped by building restrictions, Goldsmith (5) clearly distinguishes between the terms *disabled* and *handicapped*. A handicap is the result of obstacles which deter the achievement of certain goals. These obstacles are due to the lack of suitable facilities and cause people with disabilities to be *handicapped* in their use of buildings. He defines a *disability* as a medical condition of physical impairment, which may or may not be handicapping. To clarify this distinction, the architect and builder should be concerned with disabled people who are handicapped by inaccessible structures. For purposes of clarity and conciseness, the terms *disabled* and *disabled persons* will be used in this chapter.

Goldsmith (5) also discusses certain functional criteria that the architect needs to consider when designing for the wheelchair population. These criteria are *mobility, posture, reach, space,* and *strength.* When considering accessibility for the wheelchair user and the ambulant person, *mobility* is defined as the manner in which a person moves from one place to another. Generally, a person ambulates easily in a walking position on levels, steps, and inclines. The person confined to a wheelchair transports himself in the chair with much greater difficulty on levels, restricted inclines and, infrequently, in the use of steps.

An additional problem within the area of mobility is concerned with the surface over which the person moves from place to place. For the ambulant, the floor surface is not critical. For the ambulant disabled, a nonslip surface is important; the wheelchair user needs a smooth and hard finish surface.

There are activities which the ambulant person finds more convenient and more efficient to perform from a standing position, for example, using the kitchen sink or washing the face and hands at the bathroom sink. The wheelchair user is obliged to perform these activities from a seated position. Equipment that is designed for convenient use from a seated position is often less convenient from a standing one. The *posture* which the wheelchair user must adopt often can be resolved by larger doorways, lower window sills, and counter tops.

The *reach* and eye level of a wheelchair user is much lower than that of a standing person when using windows, controls, switches, outlets, and top surface. The comfortable reach for an ambulant person is between 0.68 to 1.75 m (27 to 69 inches) above floor level, with visual range between 1.32 and 1.59 m (52 to 63 inches). The reach of a wheelchair user is approximately 0.61 to 1.22 m (24 to 48 inches) above the floor, with a preferred range between 0.91 to 1.06 m (36 and 42 inches).

A frequent complaint of the disabled, related to reach but further involving *strength*, is the difficulty of opening doors. Since the disabled have problems maneuvering the wheelchair and are not as strong as the able-bodied, the design and type of door handles are important.

In comparing space needs, an ambulant person occupies a standing *space* of 0.46 by 0.30 m (18 by 12 inches); the ambulant disabled person with walking aids requires a space of 0.66 by 0.38 m (26 by 15 inches). A turnabout space with a minimum of discomfort requires about a 50% greater area than that which is occupied when standing. A standard wheelchair occupies a space of about 0.66 by 1.22 m (26 by 48 inches), which is 450% greater than that of the standing ambulant person. In order to turn completely, the wheelchair user requires a space of about 1.52 by 1.52 m (5 feet by 5 feet) or 800% greater than that required by the ambulant person. An ambulant person can negotiate a doorway 0.53 m (21 inches) wide; the wheelchair user needs 0.81 m (32 inches) of width.

Since more than a quarter of a million persons in the U. S. are confined to wheelchairs, the following information describes some of the most frequent and common obstacles that are encountered in and around a place of residence for wheelchair living. Illustrations with specified measurements are given as suggested minimum requirements for access to and within a residence for wheelchair use.

General housing criteria to be discussed include space and reach considerations and both exterior and interior access.

Space and Reach Considerations

An area designed for wheelchair living is also usually more functional and advantageous for the able-bodied person. The space required to easily maneuver a wheelchair will vary considerably and is dependent upon the person's degree of physical and mental function and tolerance, skill, equipment, and devices. The spaces designed to allow for wheelchairs may seem large for the semiambulant person; however, the measurements are intended to reflect basic wheelchair criteria. Most of these specifications for residences are designed for a person using a standard adult wheelchair, primarily for the reason that children become adults and eventually will require an adult-size chair.

In order to allow for variability of wheelchair projections in addition to footrests and projections adapted to wheelchair rims, allowance should be made for the wheelchair length of 1.21 m (48 inches) and a width of 0.81 m (32 inches) (Fig. 15.1). To travel in a straight line, the individual will need 0.91 (3 feet) of width. Straight-on doorway clearance of 0.81 m (32 inches) minimum width should be allowed for passage and arm maneuvering through the openings. A minimum of 0.91 m (36 inches) is required for walkways. In order to make a complete 360° turn in a wheelchair, an area of approximately 1.52 by 1.52 m (5 feet by 5 feet) is necessary (Fig. 15.2). These measurements are important not only on the outside access to the residence but also within the house.

In a wheelchair, a person's standing height is decreased by one-third and

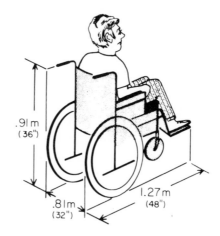

Fig. 15.1 Standard wheelchair measurements. Allowance made for wheelchair rims and footrest projection.

.91 m (36")

.81m (32")

1.27m (48")

his width is doubled (19). Infinite design situations exist that may be restricting to people propelling, pushing, or riding in wheelchairs because even the existing standard wheelchairs vary in size and weight, depending upon the manufacturer. If a person is using a reclining or motorized wheelchair, measurements are increased appropriately.

A person's arm reach from a wheelchair varies considerably, depending on the individual's physical capabilities, size, and the approach configuration. Reaching out from a wheelchair to open a cabinet door or to pick up an item on a shelf not only involves reach which may be restricted by the restraints of range but also by the limitations of dexterity and coordination of the upper extremities. Average arm reach stright out in front of the body is between 0.71 and 0.84 m (28 and 33 inches) (Fig. 15.3). From this frontal reaching position, the actual reach is only a few inches, since a person's knees, legs, and feet extend approximately 0.56 m (22 inches) beyond the wheelchair seat. Those who are able to bend forward from the waist while sitting in the wheelchair will be able to increase this reach somewhat. A person's arm reach is limited by his inability to get his body into close proximity to objects and to the construction of the wheelchair. The most common and efficient use of space is usually a sideward or a diagonal reach

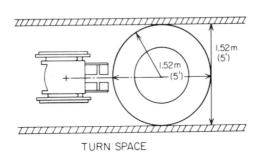

TURN SPACE

Fig. 15.2 Turn space. Minimum turn space required for wheelchair to turn 360°.

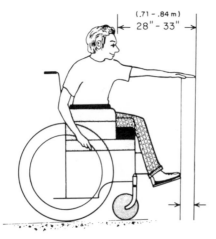

Fig. 15.3 Reach. Horizontal arm reach will vary according to size, strength, and involvement of the individual. May restrict ability to bend, thus limiting range of motion.

(Fig. 15.4). Visual perspective of the wheelchair user is greatly diminished due to his restricted height. A standing person looks down and across; from the chair an individual looks up and across. Usually, whatever is above the height of the raised arm is not within reach, and, in many cases, is invisible.

Exterior Access

The area around and leading to the residence is extremely important to the disabled since it includes elements that can be modified only with difficulty and at great expense. The most picturesque setting is worthless to the disabled unless it is accessible.

Approach Site

The grade level and the slope of the land should be carefully planned for as level an approach as possible. Steps and extended travel distances create additional problems. If an accessible path to the entrance of the residence intersects with walks, ramps, landings, curb cuts, roads, or parking areas, both surfaces should meet and continue at the same level for the intersection.

Walks

Walks must allow a continuous unobstructed movement along an access route. Where the sidewalk approaches the residence and pedestrians pass, the walk should be at least 1.22 m (48 inches) wide. The maximum slope of walks is a 0.025 (1-inch) rise in 0.51 m (20 inches) of run (1 to 20), which is a 5% grade (Fig. 15.5). Any grade greater than that is considered a ramp, and a handrail is required. Also, if the cross-slope is no more than 1 to 50,

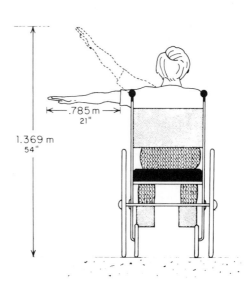

Fig. 15.4 Reach. Lateral or sideward reach is the most common and effective arm reach for individuals in a wheelchair.

.785 m
21"

1.369 m
54"

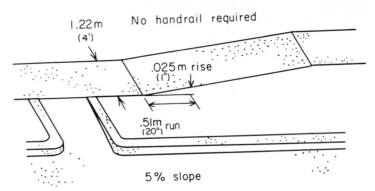

Fig. 15.5. Walks. Slope of a walk should not exceed 5% grade or 0.025 m (1 inch) rise in 0.51 m (20 inches) of run.

surface drainage is possible without upsetting equilibrium. Construction materials should be firm, relatively smooth, and slip resistant. Concrete and macadam are usually preferred to dirt, gravel, or brick.

Curb Cuts

Requirements for curb cuts are the same as for walks and ramps. By cutting into the curb and grading a section of the walk, a direct access to traffic paths is accomplished. In no case should the incline of a curb cutout exceed the slope of 1 to 12, which is 8.33% (Fig. 15.6). The walking surface must be at least 0.91 m (3 feet) wide in addition to the width created by the maximum 1 to 6 slope at the sides of the cut. These curb cuts serve as short ramps between walkways. Curb ramps that project into the roadway are in many instances severe hazards if surfaces are not even. Any obstruction existing in surfaces due to cracking, settling, and rising will impede travel and cause accidents if the surface change is greater than 0.013 m (½ inch) (Fig. 15.7).

Ramps

For everyone's safety, including that of the disabled, ramps are an alternate route for those who are not able to negotiate stairs or unusual site conditions. Where the slope of any walk exceeds 5% (1 to 20), it should be classified as a ramp. The following requirements must be met where the slope exceeds the maximum, when considering the effective and physical construction of a ramp.

Ramps shall not have a slope that exceeds 1 to 12, a grade of 8.33% (Fig. 15.8). The grade of 8.33% is arrived at by dividing the rise of 0.0253 m (1 inch) by the run of 0.304 m (12 inches).

Ramp width must be at least 1.22 m (4 feet) in order to accommodate pedestrian traffic and the wheelchair person.

The incline section of a ramp should not exceed 9.14 m (30 feet) in length.

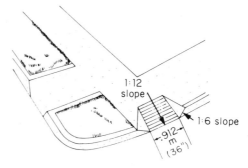

Fig. 15.6 Curb cuts. Curb cuts should not have a slope of more than 1 in 12, with the sides of the curb cuts not more than 1 in 6.

1:12 slope

1:6 slope

.912 m (36")

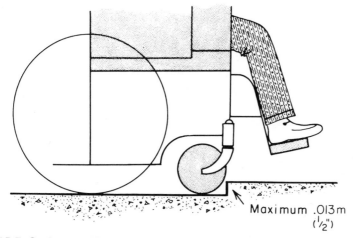

Maximum .013 m (½")

Fig. 15.7. Surface obstructions. Any change in elevation of surfaces is a hazard and a vertical change of 0.013 m (½ inch) is maximum.

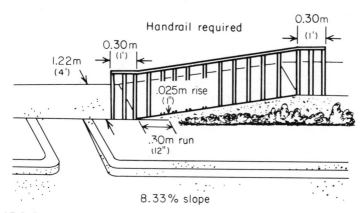

Handrail required

0.30m (1')

0.30m (1')

1.22m (4')

.025m rise (1")

.30m run (12")

8.33% slope

Fig. 15.8. Ramps. A ramp should not have a slope greater than 1 to 12, or 8.33%.

At both ends of each 9.14 m (30 feet) or smaller section, and at each turning point, there should be a straight level area of at least 1.52 m (5 feet) to allow stopping distance for the wheelchair (2). At least one intermediate landing not less than 1.52 m (5 feet) long should be provided for every 0.76 m (30 inches) of rise (10). Surfaces should be of nonslip materials.

Ramps with intermediate switchback platforms can be used when ramping many steps or when there is an inadequate space to accommodate straight-on travel. Fig. 15.9 illustrates a switchback ramp constructed to rise 0.46 m (18 inches). In this situation, adequate space was not available for a maximum slope of 8.33°. One single level was 5.5 m (18 feet) long and, by dividing the areas into three levels and two platforms, the ramp was shortened considerably.

The following problem in ramping is presented in order to visualize a common difficulty. In a hypothetical situation (20) there are three steps, each 0.152 m (6 inches) high or a total rise of 0.46 m (18 inches). The first step is within 3.04 m (10 feet) of the front sidewalk. How wide and how long should a ramp be if the desirable incline is not greater than 0.025 m (1 inch) for 0.304 m (12 inches) of ramp? In this situation, the ramp should be at least 1.22 m (4 feet) wide and 5.5 m (18 feet) long. If there is insufficient room at the front of the house, a switchback ramp, as shown in Fig. 15.9, would be a solution.

Surfaces

The pathway or walk should be firm and relatively smooth in texture and should have a nonslip surface (Fig. 15.10). Where a walk intersects with

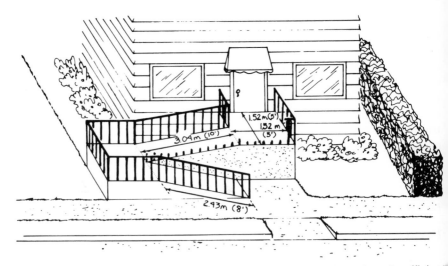

Fig. 15.9. Switch Back Ramp. This may be used when there is not sufficient length to accommodate a ramp.

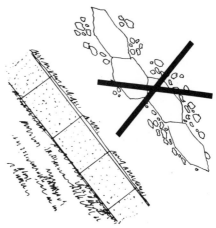

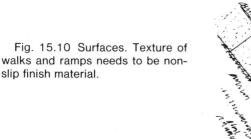

Fig. 15.10 Surfaces. Texture of walks and ramps needs to be non-slip finish material.

other walks or roads, the surface should be made to blend by means of a ramp for wheelchair users or semiambulant persons. This is not only a safety feature for all but also a safety measure for the blind. Any change of elevation at the edge of an accessible route is a hazard. However, since an exterior ramp is more exposed to weather, greater care should te taken for proper drainage, railings, and nonslip surfaces such as a broom-finished concrete, rubber, or carborundum grit. Wheelchair, crutch tip, and a person's foot are impeded by any surface obstruction greater than 0.013 m (½ inch). Many obstructions are due to settling or rising of the ground (Fig. 15.6).

Handrails

Handrails provide support for people who are ascending or descending stairs and ramps to prevent them from falling. If the slope of the walk is 5% or less, no handrail is required (Fig. 15.5). Ramps which have a slope of more than 5%, that is, 1 to 20, should have handrails placed on both sides at a minimum height of 0.81 m (32 inches) and a maximum of 0.91 (36 inches) from the floor. The handrails should be continuous and smooth and should extend at least 0.304 m (1 foot) beyond the top and bottom of the slope of the ramp (Fig. 15.8). The gripping portion of the handrail should be round or oval, smooth, and 0.035 m (1½ inches) to 0.051 m (2 inches) in diameter. A lower rail is advantageous to children and the disabled. This lower rail should be placed at approximately 0.71 m (28 inches) height. A handrail should be designed to support at least 250 pounds and should be securely fastened at all times (19).

Parking Garage

Special driving and parking privileges are increasing for the disabled in business and school areas, but there is a continuing need for better planning to provide these privileges for the residential population. In order to minimize travel distance for the disabled, parking spaces should be located as close to the entrance of a home as is possible. A wider walkway is essential for transfer of persons from a wheelchair to an automobile or a van. Because of their limited physical function, they should be provided a firm, stable, smooth, nonslip, and fairly level surface. The required space to the car for accessible parking requires not less than 3.81 m (12 feet, 6 inches) width (Fig. 15.11). If there is sufficient room to open an average car door all of the way, the space will be adequate.

Assuming that the grade of the site is level and the parking area is fairly level with a hard nonslip surface, the type of parking area should be considered. If the parking area is covered and has a garage door, it should be of the type that can be operated by a remote control device inside the car. Hinged garage double doors should be avoided.

Stairs

Stairs generally represent an absolute barrier to a person in a wheelchair, and ramps and elevators are usually installed to replace them. Some individuals, however, can negotiate a limited number of steps if they are properly designed. Steps should be less than 0.177 m (7 inches) high (Fig. 15.12). Slanted risers are acceptable because risers that extend out at the top of the tread often become a hazard to the person wearing leg braces. Open risers are potential hazards to all persons. The top of the tread should be no less than 0.25 m (10 inches) in width. It is extremely important that the stairs have at least one continuous handrail and preferably two that are placed 0.81 m (32 inches) above the surface of the steps. It is very helpful for the handrail to continue at least 0.46 m (18 inches) beyond the top and bottom of the stairs to guide the person onto a level surface (Fig. 15.13).

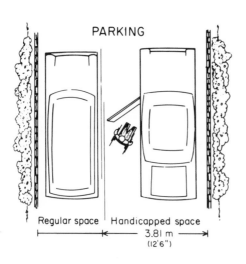

PARKING

Regular space | Handicapped space
3.81 m (12'6")

Fig. 15.11 Parking space. Parking should be located as near as possible to the entrances and should allow at least sufficient room to open a car door all of the way.

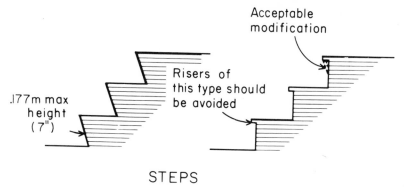

STEPS

Fig. 15.12. Steps. Acceptable stairs have vertical or slanted risers.

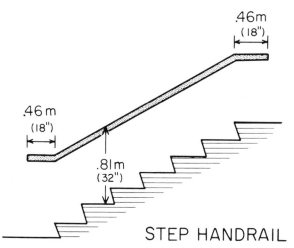

STEP HANDRAIL

Fig. 15.13. Handrails. Continuous handrails which extend 0.46 m (18 inches) beyond stairs help guide the individual past the steps.

Elevators

Most of the elevators on the market have been developed by disabled persons who wanted to transfer in their wheelchair without changing from chair to chair. Elevators should be located as close as possible to the primary accessible entrance. While the cab size will vary, it is desirable that the interior be of a size which will allow a wheelchair user to turn around. This requires 1.52 by 1.52 m (5 feet by 5 feet) of floor space in the elevator. Control buttons must be within reach of a person in a wheelchair, with the top of the control panel not higher than 1.22 m (4 feet) (Fig. 15.14). Horizontal controls located on the side walls are more convenient than those on a panel beside the door. Whenever possible, elevators should

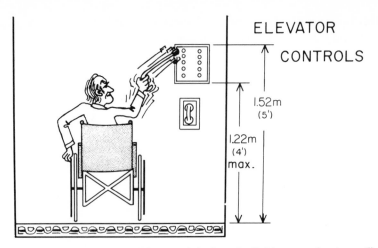

Fig. 15.14. Elevator controls. All control devices for light power, heat, ventilation, windows, doors, and elevators need to be mounted no higher than 1.22 m (4 feet) from the floor.

operate automatically, have a self-leveling device, and be fitted with a sensitive safety light. Doors should be timed to remain open for at least 8 seconds and to close slowly from 3 to 3½ seconds. Personal vertical lifts (Fig. 15.15) usually require major modification or installation but can be the answer to full utilization of a multilevel residence.

Entrance Approach and Platforms

The primary entrance to the home can be easily accessible if planning is done early. The entry level often can be made closer to ground level or an integral part of the design of the building. In existing residences, if the change of the main level is less than 1 to 50 in 0.91 m (3 feet) and if there is sufficient space, a ramp can be constructed. When the change is greater than 0.91 m (3 feet), a secondary entrance or lift system should be considered. This would avoid an excessively long ramp. The designated entrance to the residence must have a platform on both sides of the entrance doorway. A platform large enough to allow a wheelchair to pass through the door without reversing is required. This platform must be at least 1.52 by 1.52 m (5 feet by 5 feet). If the door opens out, a 0.30 m (1 foot) platform is necessary on the side from which the door opens in order to allow the person to open the door (Fig. 15.16).

Doors and Doorways

Doors are all-important to those using wheelchairs or walking aids, as well as to the blind. Both side-hung and sliding doors are useable by the disabled if properly located and provided with the correct hardware. All doors to be used by the disabled should provide a minimum opening of 0.81 m (32 inches) to allow room not only for the wheelchair but also for clearance for hand propulsion. If the location of the door requires an oblique approach, then the opening needs to be increased to approximately 0.91 m (36 inches) wide.

Since doors will be operated by persons with limited manipulative ability and strength, they should open easily with a push or pull of one hand to clear the entrance opening to 0.81 m (32 inches). Door handles should be positioned not more than 0.91m (36 inches) from the floor, and the horizontal lever-type handles or pull knobs are preferred. Pressure required to open a door should not exceed 8 pounds, and when automatic door closers are necessary, such as in apartment buildings, an adequate time delay before closing is also needed. Kick plates or rubber bumpers, located approximately 0.304 m (12 inches) from the bottom of the door, are used to protect the surface of the door from damage from wheelchair footrests and walking aids.

Similar to walks, raised thresholds should be avoided since wheelchair users cannot negotiate a surface rise higher than 0.013 (½ inch).

Fig. 15.15 Vertical lifts. Intermedial lift systems may be more efficient if adequate space is unavailable for a ramp.

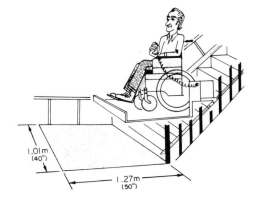

Fig. 15.16 Doors. The floor on the inside and outside of each doorway should be level and clear for a distance of 1.52 m (5 feet) from the door and extend 0.30 m (1 foot) to the side of the door on the side opposite the hinges.

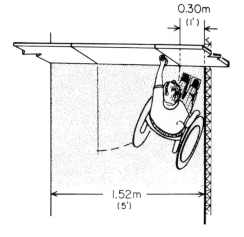

When there are two connecting doors, especially in an entry or a hallway, there must be a space of 1.83 by 1.83 m (6 feet by 6 feet) between the doors for backing and turning the wheelchair (Fig. 15.17). If one of the doors swings into the hall, a 0.30-m (1-foot) space is needed on the side opposite the hinge (10).

Interior Access

Doors, Halls, and Floors

In considering the interior of a residence, doorways become a major consideration for access within the home because the individual travels from room to room and opens and closes doors. Similar to the exterior access, all doorways should provide a minimum of 0.81 m (32 inches) width, and the ease of access from room to room is dependent on the direction of swing of the door. Most interior doors will swing into a room, and this space will be utilized primarily for travel and access in and out of the room. Where there are two doors in close proximity, such as a hallway, there must be at least 1.9 m (6 feet, 6 inches) of space between them, and the minimum width of the hallway should be 1.07 m (42 inches). If the door swings out into a hall, the hallway still must be at least 1.07 m (42 inches) wide. Throughout the residence, the surface of the floors should be a hard nonslip surface. Carpeting, if present, should be short pile for less wheelchair friction.

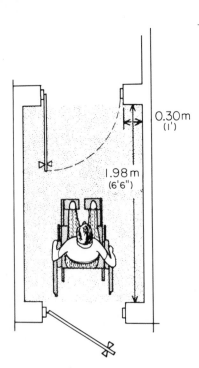

Fig. 15.17 Connective doors. The distance between two consecutive doors must be at least 1.83 m (6 feet by 6 feet).

Controls

Special consideration should be given to the layout of rooms in the residence and especially to the arrangement, location, and space needs for function, use, and accessibility. Some of the common obstacles may involve turn space, floor level, placement of furniture, cabinets, and the height of controls. In checking the location of the utility controls, such as for light, water, fuses, fire alarm, and thermostat, these items should be placed at a maximum height of 1.22 m (4 feet) above the floor or within easy arm's reach while one is seated in a wheelchair. No more than two switches should be located on a single plate. The action of a switch should be simple and positive, such as a pushpad or a large pushbutton. Outlets should be placed at least 0.051 m (2 feet) above the floor. Faucet or electrical controls and spouts should be near the front of fixtures and appliances and should be operable by one hand alone.

Space

It is not always a matter of the size of an open floor space, but rather the placement of the utilities and cabinets, which determines maneuverability and access from a wheelchair. The bathroom frequently presents major barriers and difficulties for access by the disabled. For this reason, this room has been selected to describe in more detail problems of access for wheelchair living. In the bathroom, prime consideration should be given to the placement of the fixtures, for these will affect the type of approach that is necessary in order to transfer from a wheelchair to a toilet, tub, or shower. Of the three transfer methods (Fig. 15.18), side, forward or backward, the side approach is generally preferred but requires adequate space for the wheelchair adjacent to the fixture. When the toilet facilities are stall-like, a 0.91-m (3 foot) width and 1.52 to 1.82 m (5 to 6 foot) depth are required. Stainless steel grab bars extending 0.038 m (1½ inches) from the wall should be placed approximately 0.81 m (32 inches) above the floor (Fig. 15.19).

For greatest convenience in making a transfer, the toilet seat should be nearly the same height as the seat of the wheelchair. A wall-hung toilet allows toe space for the wheelchair footrest to approach the seat. The recommended height is 0.41 to 0.46 m (16 to 18 inches), as in Fig. 15.20. If the bathroom is equipped with a floor-mounted toilet, its front surface should recede quickly to permit part of the wheelchair to go under the toilet bowl for close transfer.

While an open floor space of at least 1.52 by 1.52 (5 feet by 5 feet) is considered minimum in a bathroom (Fig. 15.21), a 1.2 by 1.2 m (4 foot by 4 foot) area would be adequate if toe space were allotted for the wheelchair to pass under the cabinet (Fig. 15.22). Persons with bowel and bladder problems often require special bathroom equipment which is stored in this room.

In order to avoid interference with the wheelchair, washbasins should be

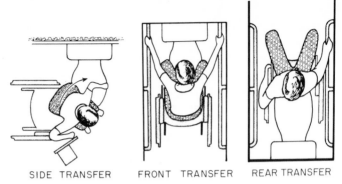

SIDE TRANSFER   FRONT TRANSFER   REAR TRANSFER

Fig. 15.18. Transfers. Three technique methods to transfer onto a toilet: side, front, back-on.

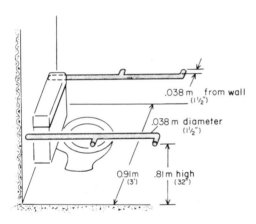

.038 m from wall
(1½")

.038 m diameter
(1½")

0.91m   .81 m high
(3')   (32")

Fig. 15.19 Grab bars. Stainless or chrome-plated steel grab bars need to be mounted on both ends of a wall to support at least a 250-pound load.

wall-mounted on a bracket or in a counter top not more than 0.81 to 0.86 m (32 to 34 inches) high. Additional floor space will be gained, but the exposed hot water pipes must be insulated against hazardous accidental contact. Lever-type faucets are preferred. Like controls and switches, all handles should clear the wall by 0.038 m (1½ inches). The maximum height above the floor for mirrors, shelves, towel racks, and light switches is 1.01 m (40 inches).

Shower compartments should accommodate a person in either the standing or sitting position. Showers should be at least 0.91 by 0.91 m (3 feet by 3 feet), with a slip resistant floor surface having a slope of no more than 0.051 m (2 inches), and a threshold with an edge height of at least 0.013 (½ inch). This curb will confine the water splash, yet is low enough to allow the footrest to pass over it and thus bring the chair close to the stall (Fig. 15.23). Grab bars are attached horizontally from 0.84 to 0.91 m (33 to 36 inches)

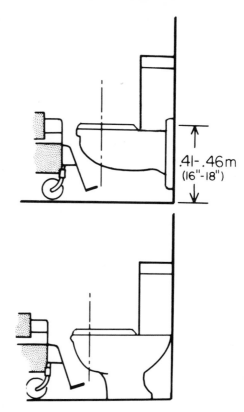

Fig. 15.20 Toilet fixture. Wall hung toilet allows toe space for wheelchair footrest placement, and floor-mounted toilet should have a deep recessed base for footrest placement.

.41-.46 m
(16"-18")

MIN. BATHROOM SIZE

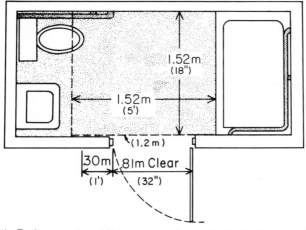

1.52 m
(18")

1.52 m
(5')

(1.2 m)

30 m
(1')

.81 m Clear
(32")

Fig. 15.21. Bathroom size. Minimum requirements for bathroom should have a clear floor space of 1.52 m by 1.52 m (5 feet by 5 feet).

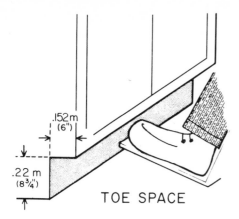

.152m
(6")

.22 m
(8¾")

TOE SPACE

Fig. 15.22 Counter toe space. Additional floor space can be gained if toe space under counters are allotted.

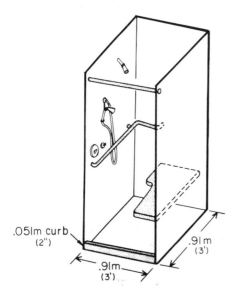

.05lm curb
(2")

.9lm
(3')

.9lm
(3')

Fig. 15.23 Shower stall. Transfers from chair to shower seat allows person to sit in corner using grab bar for lateral support and reach controls on opposite wall.

above the floor, opposite the seat and around the side walls. Single lever handles for water control are used, along with a flexible shower spray that can be controlled with a water thermostat to prevent scalding. A recessed soap tray should be placed at a height of 1.02 m (40 inches).

Adapting Housing

The preceding section has outlined the most suitable measures to adapt and develop housing for persons confined to a wheelchair. When it comes to the actual situation faced by disabled persons upon hospital discharge, there are other considerations that are vitally important. The principles of safety, built-in flexibility, and cost consciousness are the backbone of any advice regarding housing for the disabled. However, the clinical and social maturity of the physician who is in charge of care for the disabled person is also a major factor. His experience with the chronically ill and disabled, his knowledge of the natural history of these disorders, and his ability to predict, to some degree, the future development and to consider possible variations in the prognosis of the particular disability are all invaluable.

It is true that the physican is not expected to be the working hand in developing detailed plans for adapting living quarters to a patient's needs, but his guidance may be crucial to the staff who work out the details.

The recommendations for modifying the environment may differ depending on whether the patient has a progressive disability or a static one. Even in static disabilities, some changes have to be expected. The needs of the disabled child change gradually as he becomes heavier and as his parents, as they grow older, become physically less fit to care for the child at home. A large number of older adults who have sustained such major disabilities as stroke, complex fractures, or amputations may gradually deteriorate due to superimposed general cerebral arteriosclerotic changes. Often, their home has to be periodically readjusted to the organic deterioration. On the other hand, some people with static disability still continue to improve somewhat. For instance, many hemiplegic patients may learn to climb stairs independently within 6 months or so after their discharge from a Rehabilitation Center. The most touchy problem in considering housing is the physician's realistic assessment of the difference between the maximum limits of patient's capability and his actual performance at home. In many instances the equipment and adaptations which are difficult for the patient to use, but which he conforms to under pressure in the hospital, will be discarded when he is at home.

The recommendations for adaptation of the home to the needs of the disabled person will be markedly influenced by changes in the social role that the patient plays in his own family. For instance, having had a parent living with her married son may have been barely tolerated by the son's family prior to the parent's stroke. If the parent is no longer able to climb the stairs to get to the bathroom and bedroom, any suggestions about converting the first floor into a bedroom and providing toilet facilities there, such as a commode, will be resisted by the family. They would prefer to "exile" her to a nursing home.

As another example, the main breadwinner's role in the family may change if he is no longer able to earn at a level to which the family has been accustomed. His previous role may also be displaced by reversal of intrafamily relationships, such as making major decisions or controlling family finances. Thus, his eventual position in the family may affect the degree to which suggested changes in the physical structure of the house will be accepted by the family.

General principles of adapting housing for wheelchair patients have already been considered. The remainder of this chapter will outline details of adapting housing to more common types of disability, with some cases to illustrate these problems. At the end of the chapter, a checklist is given and should be used in conjunction with the measurements given earlier for adapting homes for the disabled.

The usual examples of home problems of the blind and of the respirator patient will be reviewed first. These two groups represent opposite poles. One is trained and able to live with almost no adaptive changes in his environment, while the other needs extensive readjustments and complex equipment to be able to function at all at home.

The Blind

The basic principle of training a blind person to get about in his own home, as well as at work, is to teach him to be systematic and orderly. He has to learn to rely heavily on his memory, and he is dependent on the cooperation of the other members of his family to notify him about any, even small, rearrangement of objects and furniture in his home. The few safety and convenience adaptations which should be taken into account in organizing the daily life of a blind person are as follows.

Outside staircases and steps must have bannisters or some similar protection against the hazard of the blind person falling from them. Where there are blind children, the front lawn, as well as the back yard, should be fenced in to prevent the child from wandering into the street. Similarly, gates must be installed at the entrance and exits of the front or back porch, as well as at the head of the staircases to the second floor and the one to the basement. The newly blind may wish to have a plastic line in the back yard as a guide to the house. Returning to the previously mentioned principle of orderliness, the family should develop a habit of leaving any door either wide open or completely closed to avoid the possibility that the blind person will run into a half-open door.

A knob may be mounted on the telephone dial between the numbers 5 and 6, or a string may be bound on the dial between these numbers, for easier recognition of the two halves of the dial.

Electric stoves are preferable to gas stoves. If a gas stove has to be used, it should have a pilot light. A compact fire extinguisher should hang within easy reach of the stove. Dials on stoves, dishwashers, washers, and dryers should all click during changes of cycles or intensity of activity. Dryers are preferable to wringer-style washers. The newly blind may want to have Braille letters embossed on selected cupboards and cannisters. For detailed information about specific homemaking techniques for the blind, especially kitchen activities, the reader is referred to the literature (22) and to The American Foundation for the Blind, 15 West 16th Street, New York City, N. Y. Their Technical Research department is the only source of supply of cooking aids for the blind and also carries appropriate fire extinguishers. The foundation has an excellent catalogue for any information for the blind.

This selected list of adaptations proves how surprisingly few changes are required in the home of a blind person and how his comfortable daily living is based on systems and techniques, rather than on devices.

Respirator Patients

Contrary to the relatively inexpensive simple problems of the blind patient, most quadriplegic patients will need multiple and complex adaptations at home. Respirator patients are a special example of the quadriplegic patients with unique problems. All artificial respirator aids are powered with energy derived from electrical currents. Respiratory aids are discussed in chapter 21. The average respirator patient usually has two additional safety arrangements in case of power failure at home. Some respirators can be driven by hand during emergency periods whereas all other respirators can be run for several hours with a battery power supply, except for the rocking bed. If they are kept up to date on addressees of respirator patients, electric companies routinely provide priority checkups of these patients' dwellings during electrical storms. The public relations department of local utility companies will provide the family of every respirator patient with special telephone numbers and extensions to secure immediate assistance in case of a power failure. Respirator patients will need extensive help with environmental control systems if they are to have any degree of independence. Such systems are reviewed in Chapter 20.

A long-range survey of respiratory and severe postpolio patients published by The Ohio Rehabilitation Center (13) stressed that one-third of those patients who converted their living rooms or dining rooms into bedrooms expressed dissatisfaction with these arrangements. On the other hand, adaptations of sun porches as permanent bedrooms for respirator polio patients were usually accepted favorably. Such experiences may be valuable when home adaptations or other treatment are developed for these patients and for patients with other artificial organs, such as the renal dialysis patients.

Transporting respiratory patients, as with any severely disabled patient, from one floor, or level, to another is a major problem. Outdoor elevators (Toce Bros. Manufacturing, Box 489, Broussard, La.), enclosed wheelchair elevators, power chair lifts (The American Pulley Co., Philadelphia, Pa.), and stair chair lifts (The American Stairglide Co., Grandview, Mo.) are all variations that are widely used. The selection of one of these depends on such factors as the mode of transportation—bed, standard wheelchair, electric wheelchair, the structural characteristics of the house, finances, and the esthetic sensitivities of the patient or his family. Often, regular doors may have to be replaced with delayed-action doors. Pushbuttons in self-service elevators should be placed low enough to be easily reached by a person in a wheelchair or by a disabled child. A "hold" button is often necessary. Handrails may be advisable. Occasionally, a telephone may be desired inside the elevator.

The installation of an I-beam and overhead tracks for lifts, similar to those in the ceilings of hydrotherapy areas, has been accepted by a number of respirator patients to facilitate their transfer from bed to respirator to the bathroom. Other adaptations for the bathroom have been described earlier.

Paraplegic and Quadriplegic Patients

Modifications of housing for wheelchair living have already been discussed. In addition to the information quoted and illustrated, Goldsmith (5) has given more detail to his fellow architects by offering extensive pertinent measurements on men and women in wheelchairs. Fowles and coworkers (14) have suggested a blueprint of a home for wheelchair living (Fig. 15.24). In a more recent publication, Fay (3) has outlined housing alternatives for the spinal cord injured.

Many of the details about home adaptations for quadriplegic and paraplegic persons are best described by giving a sample of a "home evaluation" letter. Such letters of instructions to the patient and his family, with copies to the family physician and appropriate social agencies, are the result of multiprofessional planning with the patient while he is undergoing rehabilitation and are often preceded by an actual visit to the patient's home. Each case has to be evaluated individually, according to the patient's capabilities and limitations and financial considerations.

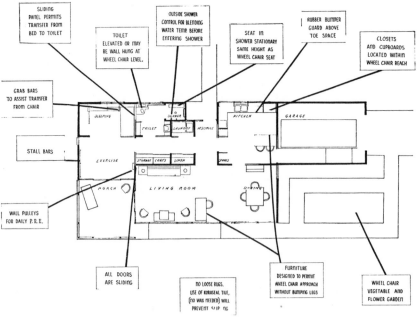

Fig. 15.24. Floor plan from a home for wheelchair living (Reproduced with permission from M. Peszczynski, M.D., and B. H. Fowles, Ph.D. (14), from their mimeographed publication, "Home Evaluations," published by the Highland View Hospital, Cleveland, Ohio, in 1957.)

The following are examples of written advice for two patients: one (R. L.) who was building a new home, the other (A. U.) who was adapting existing housing.

Case R. L.

Patient R. L. is primarily a T-1 spinal cord injured young woman with mild involvement of C-8. All her hand and finger movements are present and functional but are weak and clumsy. The purposes of her recent hospitalization were to teach her (a) to turn over in bed without assistance, (b) to improve her trunk balance while sitting, and (c) to enable her to transfer independently from bed to wheelchair or from wheelchair to toilet. The patient was using a junior "paraplegic" wheelchair and had gained her own experience in limited homemaking from her wheelchair prior to this hospitalization. The following recommendations were made in light of the fact that her husband had decided to build a new home particularly suited to her disability.

GENERAL CONSIDERATIONS FOR THE ENTIRE HOUSE

1. *Windows.* Windows throughout the house should be at an adequate height for Mrs. L. to see outside. Window openings and ventilator controls must be accessible and easy to manipulate from the wheelchair level. Example: winding-type windows.
2. *Floors.* Linoleum floors are recommended for their easy cleaning. The floors should not be waxed or decorated with scatter rugs to ensure safe and easy management of the wheelchair. Wall finishes or baseboards should also be designed for easy cleaning and maintenance.
3. *Heating.* Hot water heat is recommended, particularly for the person with immobilized legs. It is never drafty and does not give areas of sudden blasts of hot air such as in forced air heating. Radiators should be well covered or vents should be installed.
4. *Lights and Electrical Outlets.* Light switches must be located low enough on the wall to be reached from the sitting position. The switches must be so located that a wheelchair can be maneuvered close enough to manipulate them. Master switches with selected fitting controls may even be considered. An adequate supply of socket outlets is necessary. The outlets should be placed approximately 12 to 18 inches from the floor.
5. *Telephone and Intercommunication System.* Since you have planned for plug-in telephones, the telephone outlets should, of course, be located at the same level as the electrical outlets. Your planning for an intercommunication system between main rooms and the entrance door is very good.
6. *Water Temperature Regulation.* A thermostatic valve controlling the temperature of water drawn from the hot water cylinder is

recommended for the kitchen and for the bathroom, particularly in the shower.

7. *Furniture Placement.* Placement of furniture throughout the house should be planned to ensure that adequate space is available to maneuver a wheelchair.

8. *Doorways.* All doorways should be of adequate width for wheelchair passage. A sidewalk ramp is being planned for the front entrance. The base of the incline is 11 feet long, with a maximal elevation of 4 inches at the doorway level. The angle of incline is less than 1°, enabling Mrs. L. to move up or down the ramp without help.

BATHROOM

1. A wall-hung elongated-basin water closet is preferred to a pedestal closet. This type will be easier for Mrs. L. to use.

2. The height of the toilet should be the same as that of the wheelchair seat. A horizontal grab bar, installed on the wall beside the toilet, is also advised to provide a fixed support for stabilization when transferring onto the toilet with the pivoting trapeze. A pivoting transfer bar can be ordered for attachment to a bed. The trapeze may possibly be adapted for installation over the toilet.

3. A bathtub seat with canvas safety back may be used as a shower seat as well.

BEDROOM

1. All bedrooms should be accessible and usable for Mrs. L.

2. Mrs. L.'s bedroom, located adjacent to the bathroom, could perhaps be made even more accessible by installing sliding doors between the bedroom and bathroom.

3. A light, located close to the bed, is recommended.

4. When choosing a bed, remember that it must be sturdy enough to support a trapeze for transfers. Placing the bed in a corner or fitting the legs of the bed with rubber coasters is advised to ensure adequate stabilization of the bed during transfers.

5. All closets should be completely usable and should give access to the full closet space without leaving any corners or pockets. Shoe bags would help to keep one from bending down into corners.

6. Mirrors should be tilted slightly forward to allow for better vision for the seated person while at the same time permitting adequate vision for the standing person.

7. All drawers should be located at a convenient level for Mrs. L. to reach.

DINING ROOM

1. A round, or oval, pedestal table (spider-type base) is suggested for the dining room since it allows the wheelchair more freedom in location.

2. The installation of a windbreak is advised for the planned window door in the dining room. This will prevent unnecessary cooling of

the house when using the window door for a wheelchair entrance on chilly days.

KITCHEN

1. A free passageway from the dining room through the kitchen to the utility room should be planned. This will allow for unobstructed passage through the kitchen.
2. Circular corner cupboards are advised since a seated person cannot reach into far corners. The shelves can then be rotated for easy reaching.
3. All cooking equipment and supplies should be stored in a cupboard near the food preparation center. For this reason, a 30-inch counter mix area, as illustrated in "Kitchens for Women in Wheelchairs" (11), is recommended.
4. The oven should be separated from the burners since it must be high enough for the seated individual to reach with ease.
5. All stove burners should be placed to the rear, rather than two in the front and two to the rear. This will avoid the necessity of reaching over hot front burners to reach the back ones.
6. The controls for both the oven and the burners should be placed in the front of the units for easy reach.
7. A garbage disposal unit, to be installed in the sink, should be a type which will not block free passage under the sink.
8. A refrigerator of average size with revolving shelves and pull-out freezer unit at the bottom is recommended.
9. Overhead storage units may be located above the kitchen bar, keeping in mind Mrs. L.'s highest reach.
10. The double sink should be fairly shallow. It is difficult for a seated person to reach the bottom of the average sink.

UTILITY ROOM

1. A pull-out ironing board closet is recommended so that Mrs. L. can operate it alone and will not need to rely on assistance.
2. A full-length cabinet should be installed to provide storage for long-handled items, for example, for mops.
3. Revolving-shelf cupboards are again recommended.
4. The washer and dryer should be front-loading, with controls located at the front.
5. Two low tubs are advised for convenience in easy rinsing or dampening.
6. A sorting center should be provided, or a double compartment cart can be moved to the machine. This is a counter with a bin on each side and space for a wheelchair between the bins. One bin can be used for dirty clothes and the other for clothes to be ironed.
7. A small rack would be convenient for hanging ironed items while ironing.

Case A. U.

Mrs. A. U. is a 26-year-old married woman of poor socioeconomic background. She suffered a neurologic disorder of unknown etiology, resulting in quadriparesis. At the time she was discharged to go home, she was independent in all wheelchair activities except bathtub transfers, for which she needed the assistance of one person. She was able to dress herself using special devices and techniques. Prior to her discharge from the hospital, Mrs. U. was trained in kitchen activities and demonstrated her awareness of safety factors and planning to conserve energy. A home evaluation visit was made to the patient's home, and excerpts from the written report follow.

ENTRANCE

A wheelchair ramp (Fig. 15.8) at your front door to provide easy access into and out of the corner of the house onto the driveway to allow for a more gradual decline. The angle with the ground (horizontal) should not be any greater than 8 degrees. For greater safety, small tracks may be built for the wheels of the wheelchair on the ramp. This may be done by placing small boards just far enough apart on either side so that the wheels can slide between them.

BATHROOM

Mrs. U. is able to get on and off of the toilet by herself if the toilet seat is the same height as the wheelchair seat plus cushion. It is therefore necessary that an elevated toilet seat be constructed. Transfers to and from the bathtub will require the assistance of one person and should be done in the following manner:

1. A bath chair of the same height as the wheelchair, when one is in the tub, should be in the tub.
2. A strong and securely founded grabber should be installed over the soap dish.
3. Mrs. U. could use either the shower or a spray hose connected to the faucet. For greater safety it is advised that the spray hose be used to prevent any possibility of burning when the water is too hot. A spray hose can be obtained from any department store.

MASTER BEDROOM

It is advised that a nightstand large enough to carry both radio and telephone be put in place of the present one, or that the top of this one be reconstructed. This way the phone will be more easily accessible to Mrs. U. not only from the bed but also from the wheelchair. When transferring to and from the bed, the bed should be stabilized either by moving it against the wall underneath the window, or by placing rubber suction cups under each of the four legs of the bed.

BASEMENT

Mrs. U. should not spend any length of time in the downstairs rooms unless they can be properly heated.

HOMEMAKING

Vacuum cleaner—Purchase or construct dolly or platform with wheels to carry the vacuum cleaner.

Laundry Area—If area in the basement is to be used for short periods of time, it should be properly arranged to enable easy use.

a. Repair washer and dryer if possible or consider taking clothes to laundromat.

b. Place washer and dryer next to each other.

c. Purchase wooden drying rack to be used for all clothing which is not put in the dryer. This will serve in place of a clothes-line.

d. Hand laundry should be done in bathroom or kitchen as much as possible instead of going to the basement.

e. The ironing board should be moved to the main floor, in either the spare bedroom or kitchen area. If possible, an adjustable one would be advantageous.

General Storage

a. Storage of all items should be reviewed and revised so that each item is kept at its most convenient spot. Move more frequently used items to areas that are more easily reached (for example, upper shelves of lower cupboard, lower shelves of upper cupboards, and counter surfaces).

b. Items should be stored at point of first use (for example, pots and pans near stove) or left at the point of last use (as dishes drain dry they are left in the drainer until the next meal).

c. Store all things so they can be seen at a glance and reached without reaching tongs—one layer deep, with handles pointing out so that they can be easily grasped.

Storage of Clothing

a. A central brace is suggested for clothes rod support.

b. Half of the closet should have a low rod for skirts and blouses, the other half a higher rod for dresses. A suspension pole which fits on a regular clothes pole is available.

c. Most frequently used items, such as underwear, should be kept in top of dresser drawers.

d. A shoe rack or bag may make reaching shoes less difficult.

Homemaking Application

a. Mrs. U. should apply work simplification methods to all tasks for which she has a reference list.

b. Strenuous or time-consuming tasks, such as excess ironing, heavy laundry, heavy cleaning, changing beds, and washing floors or windows would be difficult for Mrs. U. to do at present.

c. Mrs. U. can do the following: ironing, vacuuming, hand laundry, washing dishes, straightening a bed, simple meal preparation and serving.

d. We would stress the use of her lapboard and slings for the above activities.

e. Frequent rest periods and working at a moderate pace will be necessary at present.

GENERAL CONSIDERATIONS

a. Take up scatter rugs.

b. Tack down living room rug.

c. Clothing shold be rearranged so that clothing which is used every day is at accessible height and is in the bedroom in which she is sleeping.

d. A mirror, preferably a full-length one, would be advisable on the back of her bedroom door.

e. The wheelchair should be kept (at the bedside), where it is left upon transfer, with clothing to be worn the next morning.

f. Mrs. U.'s wheelchair has a full-year's guarantee against faulty parts. Routine 6-month cleaning is advisable as described in the booklet which accompanied the wheelchair.

The Disabled Child

Adaptations in housing for severely disabled children are not basically different from those suggested for adults or for the aged except that attention is given to the children's smaller size and their limited ability to grasp and avoid dangers inherent in modern living, as well as their special needs for tutoring or therapeutic exercise programs at home. Recommendations for adaptations have to be individualized, just as for the adult.

The outdoor play area should be located where there is both sunshine and shade and usually should be fenced in. As with blind children, the front lawn should also be fenced in to keep the disabled child out of the street.

Slope and size of ramps for children are comparable to those for adults, but where space is available, an ideal angle of elevation is 5°. Wood is often selected for constructing the ramp because of economy, but wood flooring tends to become slick. To avoid this hazard, rubber matting should be firmly cemented to the floor of the ramp. To protect the disabled from the exposure to the elements, the loading area should be at least roofed, if it cannot be entirely closed.

Sliding doors are spacesavers but are good only for persons with good hands. The ordinary type of door may be best for disabled children. Door knobs may be replaced with longer grab bars or rubber sleeve with lever placed over the knobs. The widths of doors should be adjusted as previously described to enable a bed or wheelchair to pass easily. Often, wheelchair narrowing bars are a better solution, especially where narrow bathroom doors cannot be changed.

Large low windows should be considered if a family is building a new home. However, some means of protection, such as a railing, should be provided inside the room to prevent the child from falling through the open windows, even when they are screened. Flooring should be nonslippery, whether wet or dry, and durable but not too hard. Rubber tiles or, in selected instances, wall-to-wall carpeting may be the most satisfactory. In furniture, some tables and chairs should be a child's size.

In the bathroom, washbowls should be sturdy enough to support during toilet transfer and low enough for a child to reach them in a wheelchair. Slanting mirrors are often preferred, as are lever-type faucets. Other bathroom adaptations have been discussed earlier and apply to children as well as adults.

The Elderly Disabled

In many rehabilitation centers the majority of referrals are disabled elderly persons who are expected to be trained to return home. Many low-income community apartment buildings are being erected near golden age centers, and include a limited number of apartments designed especially for wheelchair-bound persons or for elderly couples with one partner who is physically disabled. Whenever possible, especially in these new apartment buildings, good soundproofing is indicated in the living quarters of the aged because elderly people often have to turn up their radios and television sets, and this can be disturbing to their neighbors.

Some guidelines have been formulated from experience in discharging elderly disabled patients from rehabilitation centers to their own homes.

1. Be conservative. Most arteriosclerotic brain-injured persons do not like major changes in the environment to which they have become accustomed.
2. Be slightly optimistic about patients' further, though limited, functional improvement within 6 months after their discharge from the rehabilitation center. For instance, let the elderly disabled try getting along without elevated toilet seats at home for several weeks even if the patient initially needs assistance in standing up. It is more economical to install an elevated toilet seat several weeks after the patient's discharge from the center than to have an installed one discarded. Many hemiplegic or fractured-hip patients who needed assistance to climb stairs while in the hospital learn to do it without assistance a few months after they are back home.
3. Encourage homemaking, even if limited and requiring assistance.
4. The geriatric disabled need good lighting, especially at night, more than anyone else. Dim night lights in the bathroom should definitely be discouraged.
5. Use follow-up community resources such as the Visiting Nurse Association.

Reference Sources

A sample checklist (21) of some of the primary areas found in an average residence is included below. While this list is certainly not complete and should be used only as guide, specific items have been established to familiarize the reader with accessibility barriers.

Anyone planning to develop his knowledge and experience in guiding the disabled and their families in adapting living areas to the best and most economical requirements of daily life will have to acquaint himself with the existing literature and basic reference sources. These basic reference sources are briefly as follows.

The Excerpta Medica reviews current literature on this subject under Section XIX (Rehabilitation), Part 6 (Social Aspects), Number 11 (Homes for the Disabled).

The Technical Information Service of the Royal Institute of British Architects published a book, *Designing for the Disabled* (5). This book provides detailed information and background data on housing for the disabled in the technical language of architects. The American Standard Specifications for Making Buildings and Facilities Accessible to, and Usable by, the Physically Handicapped (1) is a less-detailed, but still basic, publication dealing primarily with public buildings. A great deal of information along the same lines, but aimed at educating the public and trying to influence legislation and municipal building codes, is available in the Semi-annual Progress Reports on Architectural Barriers (17), edited by the National Society for Crippled Children and Adults, Inc.

Planning and Operating Facilities for Crippled Children (15) is a practical book of information accumulated for people who are concerned with housing and schools for disabled children.

Aging, the other end of the human life span, is gaining more and more attention from persons and agencies dealing with the socioeconomic development of our society. Although principally a textbook on the "physiological" disablement of the elderly, *Buildings for the Elderly* (12) also covers primary problems which have to be considered in any long-range planning for a physically handicapped population.

Along with this, Gelwicks and Newcomer (4) discuss various aspects of aging such as competency and capabilities and needs and satisfactions in order to derive planning guidelines for future housing for elderly person.

A fairly complete list of references in the area of Homemaking and Housing for the Disabled in the United States (7) has been made available by the New York Institute of Physical Medicine and Rehabilitation in their Rehabilitation Monograph series. Among a number of publications concentrating on the problem of adapting the home to the needs of specific types of disabled homemakers, two will be mentioned here: Kitchens for Women in Wheelchairs (11) and Home Evaluations (14). The latter discusses the adjustment of the home to the needs of the more severely disabled.

The architectural and transportation compliance board has recognized the need for a Resource Guide (8) to the state-of-the-art knowledge and literature on barriers and barrier-free design. The guide is revised periodically in order to update new literature sources.

REFERENCES

1. AMERICAN NATIONAL STANDARDS INSTITUTE, INC. American National Specifications for Making Buildings and Facilities Accessible to and Useable by the Physically Handicapped. New York, N.Y., 1961 (R1971).
2. COTLER, R. A., AND DeGRAFF, R. A. Architectural Accessibility for the Disabled of College Campuses (annual): State University Construction Fund. Albany, N.Y., 1976.
3. FAY, F. A. Housing Alternatives for Individuals with Spinal Cord Injury. Boston, Tufts University, 1975.
4. GELWICKS, L. E., AND NEWCOMER, R. Planning Housing Environments for the Elderly. National Council on Aging, Washington, D. C. 1974.
5. GOLDSMITH, S. Design for the Disabled. ed. 3. London, Royal Institute of British Architects, 1976.
6. JEFFREY, D. A. A Living Environment for the Physically Disabled. Rehabil. Lit., 34(4): 98–103, 1973.
7. JUDSON, J. S., WAGNER, E., AND ZIMMERMAN, M. E. Homemaking and Housing for the Disabled in the United States of America. Rehabilitation Monograph XX. New York, 1962.
8. JUDSON, J. S. Resource Guide to Literature on Barrier-free Environments. Architectural and Transportation Barriers Compliance Board, Washington, D. C., 1977.
9. LAURIE, G. Housing and Home Services for the Disabled: Guidelines and Experiences in Independent Living. Hagerstown, Md., 1977.
10. MACE, R. L., AND LASLETT, B. (ed.). An Illustrated Handbook of the Handicapped Section of the North Carolina Building Code. Raleigh, Governor's Study Committee on Architectural Barriers, 1974.
11. McCULLOUGH, H. E., AND FARNHAM, M. B. Kitchens for Women in Wheelchairs. Urbana, Ill., 1961.
12. MUSSON, N., AND HEUSINKVELD, H. Buildings for the Elderly. Reinhold Publishing Corp., New York, 1963.
13. NAGI, S. A., BURK, R. D., AND CLARK, D. L. Report on a Survey of Respiratory and Severe Post-Polios. Research Monograph 2. Columbus, Ohio, 1962.
14. PESZCZYNSKI, M., AND FOWLES, B. H. Home Evaluations. Highland View Hospital Publication, Cleveland, 1957.
15. SCHOENBOHM, W. B. Planning and Operating Facilities for Crippled Children. Charles C Thomas, Springfield, Ill., 1962.
16. SMALL, R., AND ALLEN, B. An Illustrated Handbook for Barrier-free Design, Washington State Rules and Regulations. Seattle, Easter Seal Society for Crippled Children and Adults of Washington, Access-Abilities Unit, 1978.
17. STEIN, T. A., FEARN, D. E., AND LAKE, L. J. Architectural Barriers. National Society for Crippled Children and Adults. Chicago, Semi-Annual Progress Report.
18. THOMPSON, M. M. Housing and Handicapped People. The President's Committee on Employment of the Handicapped, Washington, D. C., 1976.
19. UNITED STATES DEPARTMENT OF HOUSING AND URBAN DEVELOPMENT. Barrier-free Site Design. Government Printing Office, Washington, D. C., 1976.
20. WITTMEYER, M., AND BARRETT, J. Wheelchair Accessibility: Opening the Door to Housing (an illustrated manual and slide tape presentation.) Seattle, University of Washington Health Sciences Learning Resources Center, 1975. (Figs. 15.1–15.23 are from this text.)

21. WITTMEYER, M., AND STOLOV, W. Wheelchairs Home Architectural Barriers, *Am. J. Occup. Ther. 32*(9): 557–564, 1978.
22. ZAHL, P. *Blindness: Modern Approach to the Unseen Environment.* Hafner Publishing Co., New York, 1962.

OTHER REFERENCE SOURCES

Barrier-Free Site Design. HUD Publication. U. S. Government Printing Office, Washington, D. C., 1974. (Available from Superintendent of Documents)

KLIMENT, S. A. Into the Mainstream: A Syllabus for a Barrier-Free Environment. Prepared under a grant to the American Institute of Architects by the Rehabilitation Services Administration of the Department of Health, Education and Welfare, June 1975.

HARKNESS, S. P., AND GROOM, J. N., JR. Building without Barriers for the Disabled. The Architect Collaborative Inc. Whitney Library of Design, Cambridge, Mass., 1976.

MAKING FACILITIES ACCESSIBLE TO THE PHYSICALLY HANDICAPPED. New York State University Construction Fund, Albany, N. Y., 1974.

MAY, E. E., WAGGONER, N. R., AND HOTTE, E. B. *Independent Living for the Handicapped and the Elderly.* Boston, Houghton Mifflin Co., 1974.

MORGAN, M. Beyond disability: a broader definition of architectural barriers. *Am. Inst. Architects J., 65:* 50–54, 1976.

OLSON, S. C., AND MEREDITH, D. K. *Wheelchair Interiors.* National Easter Seal Society for Crippled Children and Adults. Chicago, 1973.

appendix
1

Residence Checklist[1]

Key: √ (appropriate item)

Name:
Date:

Area: Approach Site	Accessible		Comments
	Yes	No	
Exterior Surroundings			
Site/Approach			
level/incline			
smooth			
hard			
nonslip			
Parking			
curb			
alternate parking			
location			
Garage			
location			
wheelchair space			
door type/size			
door control/handle			
driveway			
Entrances			
front door			
alternate door			
Other			

Area: Outside Entrance—Front/ Back/Alternate			
Exterior Surroundings			
Walkway			
width			
level/incline			
uncluttered			

[1] From ref. 13.

Appendix 1—*Continued*	Accessible		Comments
	Yes	No	
Surfaces			
hard			
soft			
smooth			
nonslip			
Steps			
ramp (needed)			
Entrances			
Platform			
turning space			
maneuverability			
Screen Door			
width			
knob			
swing/direction			
pressure/weight			
Entry Door			
width			
knob			
swing/direction			
pressure/weight			
lock			
sill			
Gate			
width			
Electrical Features			
porch light			
switch			
Other			
mailbox			
doorbell			
milkbox			
Area:Inside Entry			
Entrance			
Door			
width			
knob			
swing/direction			
pressure/weight			
lock			
doorless access			
Room Space			
Room Size			
turning space			
maneuverability			

Appendix 1—Continued

	Accessible		Comments
	Yes	No	
Windows			
height			
openable (ventilation)			
curtain (or blind) control			
Floor Coverings			
Floor Surface			
hardwood/linoleum/other			
soft carpet			
scatter rug(s)			
Electrical Features			
Light switches			
light(s)			
Outlets (power)			
Telephone			
Heat Vents			
Room Furnishings			
Furniture			
arrangement			
reachable surfaces			
height			
shelves			
Closets/Storage			
Clothes rod			
Mirror			
Door type/handle			
Drawer space			
Fire Safety Features			
Other			
Area: Kitchen			
Entrance			
Doorway			
width			
doorless access			
Room Space			
Room Size			
turning space			
toe space			
maneuverability			
Windows			
height			
openable—sink only (ventilation)			
curtain (or blind) control			

Appendix 1—*Continued*	Accessible Yes	No	Comments
Floor surface			
hardwood/linoleum/other			
scatter rug(s)			
Electrical Features			
light switches			
outlet—no. (power)			
telephone			
Appliances			
Stove			
elements			
oven			
height			
controls			
fan			
microwave			
Refrigerator			
door swing			
door handle			
height			
freezer			
food storage			
Heat			
Room Furnishings			
Furniture—Fixtures			
arrangement			
reachable surfaces			
height			
counters			
table			
work surface(s)			
breadboard			
Sink			
faucets			
garbage disposal			
Cupboards/Storage			
shelves			
upper			
lower			
alternate storage			
drawers			
Paper Towel Dispenser			
Fire Safety Features			
Other			
small appliances			
Area: Living-Dining Room			
Entrance			
Doorway			

Appendix 1—Continued	Accessible		Comments
	Yes	No	
doorless access			
Room Space			
Room Size			
turning space			
maneuverability			
Windows			
openable (ventilation			
height			
curtain controls			
Floor Covering			
Floor Surface			
hardwood/linoleum/other			
soft carpet/scatter rug			
Electrical Features			
Light Switches			
wall			
lamp			
Lights/Lamps			
Outlets (power)			
Thermostat			
TV/Radio/Stereo			
Heat Vents			
Room Furnishings			
Furniture			
arrangement			
reachable surfaces			
height			
storage			
shelves			
dining table			
height			
Fire Safety Features			
Other			
Fireplace			
Area: Hallway			
Entrances			
Doors and Doorways			
width			
knob			
swing/direction			
pressure/weight			
lock(s)			
arrangement			
Room Space			
Room Size			
width			

Appendix 1—Continued

	Accessible		Comments
	Yes	No	
turning space			
maneuverability			
Windows			
height			
openable (ventilation)			
curtain (or blind)			
controls			
Floor Covering			
Floor Surface			
hardwood/linoleum/other			
soft scatter rug(s)			
Electrical Features			
Light Switches			
light(s)			
Room Furnishings			
Furniture			
arrangement			
reachable surfaces			
storage (drawers)			
shelves			
Closets/Dresser			
height			
storage			
portability			
Fire Safety Features			
Other			
Area: Bedroom			
Entrance			
Door			
width			
knob			
swing/direction			
pressure/weight			
lock			
Room Space			
Room Size			
turning space			
maneuverability			
Windows			
height			
openable (ventilation)			
curtain (or blind) controls			
Floor Covering			
Floor Surface			
hardwood/linoleum/other			

Appendix 1—Continued	Accessible		Comments
	Yes	No	
soft carpet			
scatter rug(s)			
Electrical Features			
Light Switches			
wall			
lamp			
Lights/Lamps			
Outlets (power)			
Telephone			
Heat Vents			
Room Furnishings			
Furniture			
arrangement			
reachable surfaces			
height			
storage (drawers)			
shelves			
Mirror			
height			
Bed Mattress			
transfer space			
size			
firmness			
height			
Closets			
door type			
location			
clothes rod			
Fire Safety Features			
Other (commode, electric bed, etc.)			
Special equipment			
Area: Bathroom			
Entrance			
Door			
location			
width			
knob			
swing/direction			
pressure/weight			
lock			
Room Space			
Room Size			
turning space			

Appendix 1—Continued

	Accessible		Comments
	Yes	No	
toe space			
maneuverability			
Windows			
height			
openable (ventilation)			
curtain (or blind)			
controls			
Floor Covering			
hardwood/linoleum/other			
soft carpet			
scatter rug(s)			
Electrical Features			
Light Switches			
light(s)			
Outlets (power)			
Room Furnishings			
Fixtures—Furniture			
arrangement			
reachable surfaces			
height			
storage			
shelves			
Tub/Shower			
transfer space			
shower			
shower doors			
faucets			
Sink			
height			
knee space			
faucets			
Toilet			
transfer space			
toe space			
height			
dispenser (toilet paper)			
Medicine Cabinet			
Mirror			
height			
Towel Rack			
height			
Fire Safety Features			
Other (commode, grab bars, etc.)			
precautions			

16

Respirators and Respiratory Aids

HENRY H. STONNINGTON, M.B., B.S., M.Sc., F.R.C.P. (Edin.)

Respirators are mechanical ventilators used to treat ventilatory failure. Respiratory aids are one of the means of treating ventilatory insufficiency. A working knowledge of both of these groups of assistive devices is of vital importance to anyone looking after patients with catastrophic disabilities. Many such devices are portable, giving patients some degree of independence. Thus, vocational rehabilitation goals for these patients have become realistic.

In this chapter, we will confine discussion mostly to the problems of chronic patients and will discuss neither respiratory emergencies nor the details of inhalation therapy. Years ago, bulbar poliomyelitis was the most frequent cause of prolonged respiratory deficiencies, but today the most frequent cause is spinal cord trauma. Brain stem trauma and disease, poisoning, lung diseases, and muscle diseases are conditions that not infrequently require the use of respirators and respiratory aids.

Basic Respiratory Concepts (2–4)

To provide artificial respiration successfully, we have to know the basic principles of the respiratory process and understand the interdependence of the metabolic processes and mental and physical activities and the gaseous needs of the body. Because of this interdependence, modifications of the mechanical respiratory process not only alter the gaseous interchanges but also may have far-reaching effects on metabolism.

REGULATION OF RESPIRATION

Receptors: Peripheral and Central Chemoreceptors

The peripheral chemoreceptors are located in the carotid bodies at the bifurcation of the common carotid arteries and in the aortic bodies scattered along the ascending arch of the aorta and its branches. They have afferent nerves by which the results of transduction of chemical stimuli to nerve action potentials are carried to the medulla oblongata. These chemoreceptors are influenced by increases of arterial partial pressure of carbon dioxide (Pa_{CO_2}) and pH, but they are unique in their exquisite sensitivity to decreases of arterial partial pressure of oxygen (Pa_{O_2}). They initiate the immediate increase of breathing in response to oxygen lack.

The central chemoreceptors are located near the ventral surface of the medulla. They respond to CO_2 changes much more slowly than their peripheral counterparts do to changes of oxygen and CO_2. They respond through the acidification of brain extracellular fluid by carbon dioxide.

Upper Airway and Lung Receptors

These are receptors scattered from the nose, epipharynx, and larynx to the trachea, and, mostly, they are mechanoreceptors. In the lung itself, there are three classes of receptors: the pulmonary stretch receptors, whose afferents run in the vagus and are the mediators of the classic Hering-Breuer inspiratory inhibitory reflex; the receptors that respond to chemical irritants; and, lastly, the J receptors, which are thought to respond to congestion and edema.

CENTRAL NERVOUS SYSTEM CONTROL OF RESPIRATION

Voluntary respiration is controlled by the cerebral cortex, automatic respiration by various areas within the brain stem. Within the medullary nuclei is generated that respiratory rhythm that helps to delineate expiration and inspiration. Different nuclei drive either the primary respiratory motor neurons or the accessory ones supplied by the vagus. Their automatic centers are in the medulla, as well as in the pons, and their tracts descend to the spinal motor neurons in the ventral and lateral columns of the cord. The voluntary system descends from the cortex, via the corticobulbar and corticospinal tracts, to the reticular formation and spinal cord. Sleep and wakefulness utilize different systems. Furthermore, the anesthetized patient does not necessarily use the same mechanism as sleep. Control during sleep varies according to the stage of sleep (9). During the rapid eye movement (REM) stage, breathing is irregular—in contrast to the regular breathing of the nonrapid eye movement (NREM) stage. During the NREM stage, respiration is entirely dependent on the automatic system whereas during the REM stage the breathing appears to be independent of the automatic system.

Pathways from the cortex and the various brain stem nuclei descend in the spinal white matter and project onto the anterior motor neurons that activate the phrenic, intercostal, and abdominal muscles. In turn, ascending pathways from those muscles influence respiration. Therefore, at the spinal level, all of the central nervous system control is integrated. It can be seen that trauma and disease in any one of these areas will have profound effects. High spinal cord trauma involves both lower and upper motor neurons and may affect either the automatic or the voluntary pathway, or both. Brain stem disease or trauma can affect the automatic centers, leaving the voluntary tract intact. Thus, we get conditions such as Ondine's curse (10), in which sleep is accompanied by apnea.

Mechanics of Respiration

The actual gas exchange between the lung and the cell depends on the movement of gases in and out of the body, on the effectiveness of the circulation, and on the processes of transport and diffusion across the alveolar and capillary membranes.

LUNG VOLUMES (FIG. 16.1)

The amount of air that is inspired at each breath of normal quiet breathing is called the "tidal volume." This volume is influenced by physical and mental activities, metabolic processes, and the various factors discussed previously. The total lung capacity depends roughly on body size and is about 6 liters in the adult male. It is subdivided into the functional reserve capacity and inspiratory capacity. The functional reserve capacity is the volume of gas contained in the lungs at the end of a normal expiration. It contains one-third of the total store of oxygen in the body, and so permits apnea for several minutes. When the person stands, this reserve capacity is

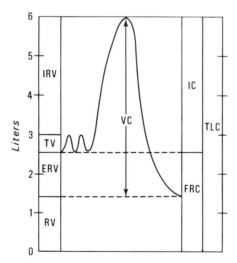

Fig. 16.1. Lung volumes. *IRV*, inspiratory reserve volume; *VC*, vital capacity; *TV*, tidal volume; *IC*, inspiratory capacity; *ERV*, expiratory reserve volume; *FRC*, functional residual capacity; *RV*, residual volume; *TLC*, total lung capacity. Tracing records vital capacity maneuver after tidal volumes.

about equally distributed between the expiratory reserve volume and the residual volume. The residual volume is the volume of air remaining in the lungs after maximal expiration. When the person is supine, however—and in cases of obesity or abdominal disorders, loss of lung compliance, and obstructive lung disease—the expiratory reserve volume is decreased considerably, and the residual volume is increased correspondingly.

The vital capacity is the amount of air that can be expelled with maximal force after maximal inspiration. It is made up of three volumes: inspiratory reserve, expiratory reserve, and tidal volume.

When these various lung volumes are measured, they are usually expressed as percentages of the normal values predicted by use of nomograms. In addition to measuring these static volumes, we can measure dynamic volumes such as the forced expiratory volume per unit time.

Abnormalities often are due to changes in the elastic properties of the chest wall and the lung, which vary with the "chest wall compliance" and the "lung compliance," respectively. Lung compliance depends on the elastic recoil of the lung, as well as on the surface tension of fluid lining the alveoli. The surface tension is due to a monomolecular layer of lipoprotein—the pulmonary surfactant. It is these lung properties that give the alveoli their stability.

Pulmonary ventilation is produced by the rhythmic contraction of the inspiratory muscles. These muscles, therefore, have to overcome the lung compliance (elastic recoil), producing a negative pressure in the potential pleural space. In addition they must overcome the airway resistance, which depends on the size and other characteristics of the airways. If we calculate the total pressure required to force a known volume of air into the thorax, we can calculate the work of breathing, which depends on the multiplicity of factors which we have discussed.

GAS EXCHANGE

Although the tidal volume is around 500 ml at the end of inspiration, 150 ml remains in the airways. This air, which does not participate in the gas exchange, is called anatomic dead space ventilation (Fig. 16.2A). The other 350 ml participates in alveolar ventilation. The whole of the gas exchange takes place in the alveoli. The magnitude of the alveolar dead space depends on the distribution of the pulmonary blood flow. The carbon dioxide tension is governed by the metabolic rate and alveolar ventilation. Oxygen tension is also dependent on these factors, as well as on failure of gas exchange by collapsed alveoli (Fig. 16.2B). Thus, measurement of arterial gas tension is important for learning about the balance between tissue requirements and lung gas exchanges. These tensions tell about the severity of carbon dioxide accumulation, degree of hypoxia, or the presence of overbreathing. Knowledge of these factors helps in determining the indications for artificial respiration and in setting its amount. The principle of partial tension can be

DEAD SPACE

GAS

ALVEOLAR
GAS

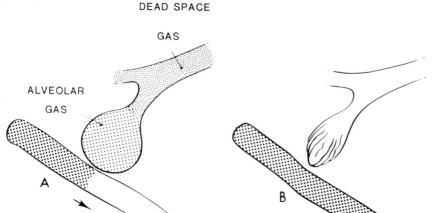

A

B

Fig. 16.2. Gas exchange. *A*, passage of oxygen from capillary to alveolus; *B*, failure when alveolus is collapsed.

appreciated if we consider that the atmospheric pressure at sea level is 760 mm Hg. The amount of oxygen is approximately 21% in the atmosphere. The partial tension of oxygen or of any other gas in the mixture is proportional to the relative concentration. The partial tension of oxygen at sea level, therefore, is about 158 mm Hg and the partial tension of carbon dioxide is about 0.3 mm Hg.

Any liquid, such as water or blood, into which these gases will dissolve becomes saturated to the degree matching the partial tensions of these gases in the air (or gas mixture) that is in contact, provided there is sufficient time for the exchange. The time for this exchange depends on the area of contact and the permeability of any intervening tissues. In other words, the partial tensions are the same in the liquid as in the gas mixture. Exchange of gases takes place, likewise, between different tissues that are separated by semipermeable membranes.

In the body there is an extremely large contact area between blood and alveolar air and another between the solution in the blood and the solution in the tissues. Transfer or diffusion is rapid in the alveoli. The normal range of blood gas tension in the arterial blood is 36 to 44 mm Hg for Pa_{CO_2} and 85 to 100 for Pa_{O_2}

The metabolic processes produce carbon dioxide, so that its tension in tissue fluid is slightly above 44. The venous blood carries the gas away at an average tension of 44. When the blood reaches the lungs, it quickly loses a portion of its carbon dioxide to the alveoli, so that the arterial blood has a Pa_{CO_2} of 40. Thus, the arterial blood is ready for another load of CO_2 from the tissues. In the meantime, the Pa_{CO_2} in the alveoli is maintained at 40 by ventilation so that the alveolar air is constantly able to take carbon dioxide from the venous blood. As noted previously, changes in the values of carbon dioxide, oxygen, and pH affect the receptors and produce hyperventilation or hypoventilation. The body can adapt somewhat to changes in gas tensions and to hyperventilation. The fact that the body can adapt to hyperventilation is important in artificial respiration because the adaptation makes it more difficult to wean the patient from the respirator.

Regarding oxygen, we have (a) transport of oxygen to the alveoli, (b) gas exchange between alveoli and blood, (c) transport by the blood to the tissues, and (d) diffusion from tissue capillaries to the inside of the cells. The uptake of oxygen is affected by both alveolar oxygen tension (PA_{O_2}) and by the factors that cause the arterial oxygen tension (Pa_{O_2}) to be lower than the PA_{O_2} and so give rise to the alveolar-arterial oxygen tension difference ($A - aP_{O_2}$). The volume of oxygen transported by the blood depends on the arterial content and the cardiac output. The oxygen delivery and the volume of oxygen extracted by the tissue govern the mixed venous P_{O_2}.

In conclusion, the arterial blood-gas tensions provide a good indication of the balance between requirements of the tissues and the process of gas exchange in the lung. Whereas carbon dioxide tension is governed by the metabolic rate and alveolar ventilation, oxygen tension is influenced not only by those factors but also by the relation of ventilation to blood flow in the lung and, thus, by the presence of right-to-left shunts (Fig. 16.2).

ACID-BASE BALANCE

The body produces an acid load at a fairly even rate throughout the 24 hours. The respiratory acid load is the carbon dioxide that is excreted through the lungs each day. The metabolic or nonrespiratory acid load is the carbon dioxide that is excreted through the kidneys.

When the rate of production exceeds the rate of excretion, the excess hydrogen ions are buffered by the bicarbonate, the hemoglobin, and plasma proteins in the blood. Additionally, respiratory compensation by hyperventilation or hypoventilation is quickly brought into play. Lastly, renal responses are activated. The pH normally remains around 7.4. If this changes, we get the following conditions:

1. Respiratory acidosis, which can occur in any form of respiratory failure, but particularly in acute and chronic lung disease.
2. Respiratory alkalosis, often due to mechanical or manual hyperventilation or to hyperventilation induced by fear or pain.
3. Nonrespiratory acidosis, in conditions such as starvation, diabetes, or severe diarrhea.
4. Nonrespiratory alkalosis, due to excessive intake or excessive intravenous administration of sodium bicarbonate, or to repeated vomiting.

CONCLUSION

It is difficult to recognize minor degrees of respiratory failure clinically and equally difficult to follow the response to treatment by clinical signs alone. Therefore, it is essential to have the facilities for tests such as measurements of Pa_{CO_2} and P_{O_2} and pH. To allow for errors in sampling and in blood gas measurement, respiratory failure usually is defined as P_{CO_2} above 50 or P_{O_2} below 60 (when the patient is at rest at sea level and there is no primary metabolic acidosis). Values outside these limits should alert the physician to the need for respiratory aids and for some sophisticated respiratory testing. It should be remembered that shortness of breath does not mean respiratory failure. The reverse is also true and even more important: patients in respiratory failure often are not breathless. A thorough awareness of the complexity and the interdependence of various body processes will enable the physician to use respiratory aids early and thus save lives.

Respirators and Their Use

INDICATIONS

Generally, it can be said that mechanical respiration is indicated when there is ventilatory failure, as indicated by raised P_{CO_2}. A statement such as this, however, needs modification. An asthmatic who is exhausted and has a P_{CO_2} of 50 mm Hg may well need this help. However, a patient with chronic obstructive lung disease does not need mechanical ventilation at this level and perhaps needs it only when the P_{CO_2} exceeds 80 because he has adapted to a high P_{CO_2} level and functions well until an exacerbation elevates the P_{CO_2} beyond 80 mm Hg, which is incompatible with life. Of course, the patient who has sustained a C-2 spinal cord injury and has required cardiopulmonary resuscitation at the place of the accident will have to be maintained by mechanical respiration immediately.

The following is a list of several categories of possible situations requiring mechanical respiration:

1. Nervous system pathology
   a. Trauma: high spinal cord injury, head injury
   b. Vascular accident: stroke, particularly with brain stem involvement
   c. Intoxication: drugs such as barbiturates
   d. Infection: encephalomyelitis, poliomyelitis
   e. Neuropathy—such as Guillain-Barré syndrome
   f. Degenerative diseases: amyotrophic lateral sclerosis, multiple sclerosis, sleep disorders—Ondine's curse, Shy-Drager syndrome
   g. Status epilepticus
2. Pulmonary pathology
   a. Any condition with limited vital capacity or diminished tidal volume—to prevent continued deterioration

  b. Obstructive lung disease: asthma, emphysema
  c. Restrictive lung disease: pulmonary fibrosis, pneumothorax, pleural effusion, skeletal abnormalities
  d. Infection—such as nonresponsive pneumonia
  e. Intractable pulmonary edema
  f. Various surgical complications: atelectasis, pulmonary emboli, etc.
3. Muscle pathology
  a. Muscular dystrophy—such as end stage of Duchenne muscular dystrophy
  b. Myasthenia gravis
  c. Muscle spasm—as in tetanus
  d. General debility—as in metastatic disease
4. Pediatric disorders
  a. Neonatal asphyxia due to drugs, cerebral damage, airway obstruction, aspiration syndrome
  b. Respiratory distress syndrome: hyaline lung disease
  c. In infants and children: bronchopneumonia, upper airway obstruction, congenital heart disease, asthma, septicemia, bronchiolitis, cystic fibrosis

TRACHEOSTOMY AND ENDOTRACHEAL INTUBATION

Many of the disabilities discussed in this chapter require a respirator for several days at best and for the rest of the patient's life at worst. In certain cases it is necessary to intubate the patient to control the airways. In that circumstance, endotracheal intubation with a cuffed tube is used as the initial method in the majority of cases. This can be performed quickly, and it avoids some of the complications of tracheostomy. However, if it becomes obvious that artificial respiration will be required for a prolonged time—more than 1 or 2 weeks—tracheostomy will have to be performed.

RESPIRATORS

Modern respirators may be extremely complex, and they usually are referred to now as "ventilators," rather than as respirators. The physician needs to understand some of their functional characteristics and to have trained staff available. For further details he should consult monographs (7, 8, 11) as well as operating instructions of the instrument that is to be used.
  The major groups of ventilators are:
1. Pressure preset: A constant flow of gas is delivered from the ventilator until the predetermined pressure is reached.
2. Volume preset: A predetermined volume of gas is delivered from the ventilator, the pressure being measured.
3. Ventilators that act by producing subatmospheric pressure outside the lungs, such as the tank and cuirass ventilators and rocking bed.
4. Electrophrenic stimulation.
Modern ventilators usually have both volume preset and pressure preset

capabilities. For prolonged artificial respiration, volume preset operation is more often used. The problem with pressure preset ventilation—particularly if the lungs are not maximally inflated periodically—is that alveolar closure occurs, decreasing the functional respiratory capacity and lung compliance. Then the preset pressure is reached with a lesser volume, which is not adequate for ventilation. However, a preset volume ventilator guarantees the necessary delivery of the preset volume of gas.

To overcome the problem of alveolar collapse, modern ventilators have a built-in mechanism for giving a large volume inspiration—a sigh—at regular intervals, say one sigh per 100 cycles.

Modern ventilators can be used in three modes.

1. The inspiratory flow is delivered at a definite time interval (automatic mechanical ventilation).
2. The inspiratory flow is delivered in response to negative pressure—that is, when the patient initiates a breath (demand mechanical ventilation).
3. The patient initiates the inspiratory flow unless there is a period of apnea, at which time the ventilator automatically starts the next cycle (demand mechanical ventilation with automatic standby). With demand-type systems, less change of settings is needed, and this helps to avoid wide shifts of P_{CO_2} and pH.

Tank and cuirass ventilators have fallen into general disuse, but they do have some advantages. Most importantly, they allow the patients to communicate easily: not having to be intubated, they are able to speak. At the moment, however, the technical advantages of the modern intermittent positive-pressure ventilators are much greater, so the tank and cuirass machines are hardly used at all now, and they will not be dealt with in this chapter.

During mechanical ventilation, the changes in transpulmonary pressure are much the same as those of spontaneous respiration. However, as regards intrapleural pressure, there is a difference. Instead of the intrapleural pressure being negative during inspiration, it becomes positive in respect to atmospheric pressure, and this tends to reduce the cardiac output because of its effect on the gradient for venous return. This is the case, not only with positive-pressure respirators but also with the tank type, although with the cuirass type, the effect is minimal. The reduction of cardiac output during inspiration is compensated for in late inspiration and expiration by reflex effects from the baroreceptors, and thus overall cardiac output is maintained. To minimize these effects, the respiratory rate is kept at between 12 and 15 breaths per minute with an inspiratory to expiratory ratio of 1 to 2. On the whole, gas exchange is not badly affected, as the slowing of respiration will ease and equalize gas distribution. Yet, in some conditions, as when functional residual capacity is reduced, special techniques such as application of end-expiratory pressure may have to be used.

MECHANICAL VENTILATORS

There are more than 50 models of ventilator in use. We have chosen a few as examples, but this does not mean they are necessarily better than others. The reader should consult recommended monographs (7, 8, 11) to learn of the many devices available. The accompanying figures do not convey the simplicity or complexity of the machines, but studying them together should give the reader a feel for the ideas incorporated into ventilators.

Bird Mark 7 Ventilator (Fig. 16.3)

Although the Bird ventilators were designed originally to deliver bronchodilator drugs during intermittent positive-pressure breathing (IPPB) therapy, they have been modified so that they can be used for long-term ventilation as well. Thus, the Mark 7 is a pressure- and time-cycled machine. It is driven by a compressed gas source. The inspiratory flow can be varied to between 5 and 40 liters per minute. Part of the flow activates a nebulizer humidifier and at the same time pressurizes a diaphragm that closes the expiratory valve. The rest of the gas goes to the main chamber and then to the patient. Part of this gas flow can be diverted, by opening an air mix control, to pass through a Venturi valve and entrap air in order to dilute the oxygen to about 40%. When the gas passes from the main chamber to the lungs, the coincident increase of pressure moves the diaphragm. However, this movement is opposed by magnet A. The position of this magnet can be adjusted to set cycling pressures between 5 and 60 cm H_2O. Inspiration ends when the pressure on the diaphragm overcomes the magnet pull. This permits a valve to move and stop the supply of gas. Magnet B then holds the valve in an expiratory position. The gas that holds the expiratory valve leaks into the main chamber after passing through the nebulizer, and expiration is allowed to commence. A pneumatic timing device controls the

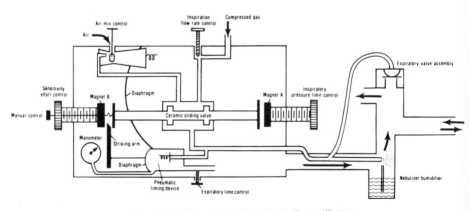

Fig. 16.3. Circuit of Bird Mark 7 ventilator.

length of expiration. A controlled leak, during expiration from this chamber into the main chamber, allows a lever to move the valve rod back to the inspiratory position. Varying the position of magnet B adjusts the sensitivity of the trigger mechanism, with which the patient triggers inspiration.

Bennett MA-1 Ventilator (Fig. 16.4)

This is a versatile and complex ventilator—one that can be pressure-cycled or volume-cycled. It is electrically powered. The principal gas is room air drawn into the unit in expiration and delivered to the patient in inspiration. The room air may be enriched with oxygen to an adjustable calibrated percentage, and 100% oxygen can be delivered when needed. The unit can deliver automatic mechanical ventilation or demand mechanical ventilation or demand mechanical ventilation with automatic standby.

During inspiration, gas is passed through the main flow bacteria filter and through the humidifier, but if the nebulizer is switched on, it passes through that and its bacterial filter instead. The temperature of the gas is adjusted. The flow control adjusts the rate of flow, and the pressure gauge indicates the pressure in the tube system. The ratio warning lamps light up if the inspiration does not end before the midtime of an automatic breathing cycle

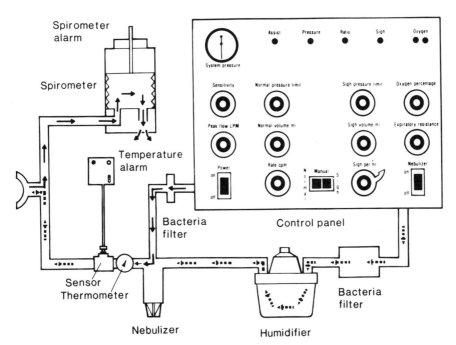

Fig. 16.4. Circuit and control panel of Bennett MA-1 ventilator. Patient on left. *Solid arrows,* expiratory flow; *dashed arrows,* inspiratory flow. *LPM,* liters per minute.

is reached. Inspiration ends and expiration is begun if the unit reaches either the volume or pressure limit or a sigh volume limit. To start expiration, the expiration valve opens for filling of the spirometer. (An expiratory resistance control may retard expiration.) While this goes on, the unit draws in room air and oxygen in preparation for the next inspiration.

Siemens Servo Ventilator 900 (Fig. 16.5)

This is a volume ventilator in which a precision pneumotachograph measures inspiratory flow rates and controls the inspiratory valve.

Spring tension on a bellows filled with gas at the proper oxygen concentration provides the force for inspiration.

Controls on the face of the unit allow the operator to select breathing rate, minute volume (thus tidal volume), inspiratory flow rate, and inspiratory pause. Signals from the inspiratory flow sensor are compared with the settings on the ventilator to close the servo loop and control ventilation.

A parallel flow probe on the expiratory side measures actual patient-exhaled gas and functions during spontaneous ventilation, as well as during assisted ventilation.

Measurement of positive end-expiratory pressure (PEEP) is simple with this ventilator, and patient sensitivity can be adjusted to provide assisted ventilation with PEEP, as well as controlled ventilation.

Thompson Minilung Volume Ventilator (Fig. 16.6)

This small ventilator is ideal for high-level quadriplegic patients, as it is portable and can be placed on a wheelchair. It operates for 16 hours on a 12-

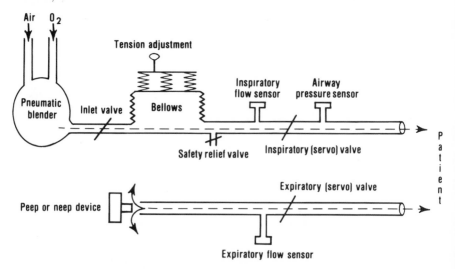

Fig. 16.5. Circuit of Siemens Servo ventilator 900. *PEEP*, positive end-expiratory pressure; *NEEP*, negative end-respiratory pressure.

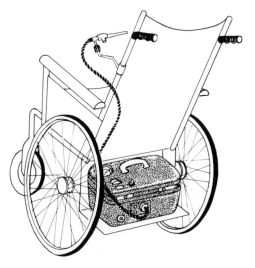

Fig. 16.6. Thompson Minilung Volume ventilator, in place on wheelchair (could be in front of patient, on wheelchair tray). Usually connected to tracheal stoma.

volt battery and for up to 1 hour on its internal rechargeable battery. It will also operate on 110-volt 60-Herz-alternating current. It is volume-adjustable from 300 to 1,500 milliliters and pressure-adjustable from 0 to 100 cm H_2O. The rate is adjustable between 8 and 30 breaths per minute. There are alarms for power failure, low and high pressure, and low battery voltage.

This ventilator gives a measure of freedom to a high-level quadriplegic patient (5), especially if he uses a head-controlled electric wheelchair.

ASPECTS OF PATIENT MANAGEMENT

With mechanical ventilation, there is need of the support of a well-trained respiratory unit staff. An effort should be made to transport patients to such a unit early. This will relieve a tremendous burden on an untrained facility and also may prevent respiratory and other complications from developing.

The patient's position and posture should be changed hourly. Tracheal secretions should be aspirated every half hour, and postural drainage and respiratory therapy should be performed at least every 4 hours. Routine mouth care, aspiration of all nasal secretions, and care of the lips and skin about the mouth should be performed regularly. The physician should examine the lungs thoroughly every day and should be aware of possible cardiac problems such as arrhythmias. He should also look for venous thrombosis and be alert for pulmonary embolism. The patient who is paralyzed or unconscious is particularly subject to such complications. A range-of-motion exercise program for all the limbs is helpful in this regard.

Bladder function should be checked, and a plan should be ready for malfunction. Oral feeding is best, if it is at all possible. However, gut motility is often compromised, and abdominal distention should be looked for. A gastric tube may have to be used. Adequate nutrition should be provided, even if the intravenous route must be employed. A regular bowel program will need to be instituted.

Throughout, the patient needs much psychological support and help with communication. Many a patient is unable to speak because of the tracheostomy or the intubation and therefore will have to have special devices to enable him to communicate and have easy access to the television. If possible, he should also engage in other avocational activities. The occupational therapist is invaluable here.

Weaning the Patient

The patient eventually becomes quite dependent on the ventilator, both physiologically and psychologically, and a weaning process will have to be instituted. If the patient has been hyperventilated for a time, the respiratory center will have to be adjusted to low carbon dioxide tension and increased chest wall movement, so when the respirator is removed, the patient will become dyspneic. One can insert increasing volumes of dead space into the ventilator circuit and thus reverse the respiratory center sensitivity.

On the whole, the patient's response to respiratory therapy will give a good indication of whether he still needs the ventilator. The therapist will note that the patient does his breathing exercises unaided. It is important to check the arterial oxygen tension while ventilating the patient with air: it should remain normal. Some lung abnormalities allow stopping of the ventilator and maintenance of arterial oxygen tension by means of supplemental oxygen, and in that circumstance the patient can then be weaned off of the ventilator while still receiving oxygen. Supervision of the weaning process needs to be close, and use of the ventilator at night should not be stopped until the patient has been breathing on his own for 2 or 3 days.

ELECTROPHRENIC STIMULATION (FIG. 16.7)

The modern methodology for this type of artificial respiration was perfected by Glenn and associates (6). Basically, it uses an external power source—the transmitter—which is battery-powered and transmits trains of pulse-modulated radiofrequency energy to a loop antenna. This antenna is placed over one of two subcutaneous receivers, each of which is connected to a bipolar platinum electrode that surrounds a phrenic nerve (right or left). The pulse train from the transmitter is fixed to give 34 square impulses in 1.35 seconds. This is the inspiratory part of the cycle. There follows a period of 2.65 seconds without stimulation, during which expiration is allowed to occur. This respiratory cycle lasts 4 seconds, making a rate of 15 breaths per minute. The amplitude of the current delivered to the nerve is

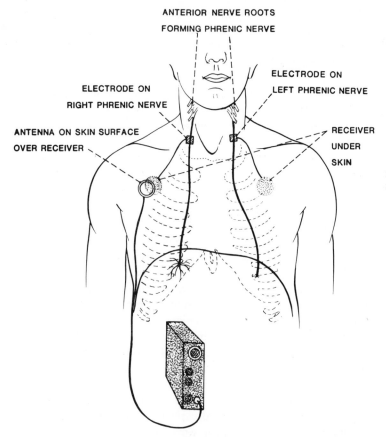

ANTERIOR NERVE ROOTS
FORMING PHRENIC NERVE

ELECTRODE ON
LEFT PHRENIC NERVE

ELECTRODE ON
RIGHT PHRENIC NERVE

ANTENNA ON SKIN SURFACE
OVER RECEIVER

RECEIVER
UNDER
SKIN

Fig. 16.7. Electrophrenic stimulation. Antenna is placed over right or left receiver, to pace breathing via right and left phrenic nerves for alternating periods.

controlled by the pulse width. One regulates it in such a way as to start the diaphragmatic contraction with a minimal current that gradually builds up over the inspiratory part of the cycle, giving the muscle a smooth contraction and not a sudden hiccough. The ventilator is not used until about 2 weeks after implantation of bilateral stimulators. Then stimulation is started, at first for only a few minutes, and gradually extended by increases on each side alternately. Thus, the diaphragmatic muscle is gradually retrained until it can take 24 hours of stimulation.

One of the main indications for this method of artificial respiration is a cervical cord injury around or above C-2. If the injury were at C-4, electrophrenic stimulation would not work because the injury would cause a lower motor neuron lesion of the phrenic nerve, which then could not carry the impulses. With a spinal cord injury, there must be a wait of several months before the pacemaker can be implanted. The chest wall should be fairly noncompliant, for otherwise a flail chest syndrome may result—the chest wall moving as well as the diaphragm and negating the desired effect of diaphragmatic excursion.

Another indication for this procedure is brain stem damage due to degenerative disease, stroke, or injury. Electrophrenic stimulation has been particularly effective in cases of Ondine's curse (wherein the voluntary respiratory pathway is intact but the automatic pathway is damaged, and the patient becomes apneic during sleep) (10).

The most attractive advantage of this kind of ventilator is that it allows the patient to move with much less encumbrance and to speak, even if a tracheal stoma must remain for suction of secretions.

Respiratory Aids

Lung complications are one of the most frequent problems following surgery, as well as serious injury or disease. Devices are available to improve lung function and help prevent complications after serious trauma or surgery. Spinal cord injuries involving thoracic and cervical segments interfere with costal movement. Brain injuries interfere with breathing patterns. Abdominal injuries or disease, particularly when pain is associated, cause breathing to be shallow. Narcotics further decrease ventilation. Collapse of individual alveoli can be a problem with all these conditions. As more and more alveoli collapse, there will be a significant amount of right-to-left shunting because the blood vessels are unable to pick up oxygen from collapsed alveoli and eventually Pa_{O_2} will decline (Fig. 16.2). Also, there will be a decrease of functional residual capacity, with consequent decrease of lung compliance and increase in the work of breathing. Unfortunately, this may not be obvious, even to a careful clinical observer, because the tidal volume may remain constant. Restriction of the functional residual volume does not necessarily affect the tidal volume (Fig. 16.1).

The normal person prevents alveolar collapse with occasional yawns and deep breaths. Therapeutically and prophylactically, there is a need for a maneuver that is highly effective in producing maximal lung inflation without adverse hemodynamic change. This maneuver must achieve the largest possible inhaled volume and high alveolus-inflating pressure for the longest period and yet must simultaneously have a negative intrathoracic pressure. It seems obvious that old methods employing expiratory maneuvers, such as use of blow bottles, are largely self-defeating because they do not open up the alveoli. Of course, one can use ventilator machines for passive production of breathing by intermittent positive pressure. Indeed, that is a common application of some of the ventilators (such as the Bird) described in the preceding section; however, that method is quite expensive. It has been shown that voluntary maximal inspiration, supplemented by use of an incentive inspiratory spirometer, can achieve better results than therapeutic IPPB (1).

The simplest and cheapest of these incentive spirometers is one marketed as "Triflo" (Chesebrough-Pond's, Inc., Greenwich, Conn.) (Fig. 16.8). It has three chambers with a ball in each, and the balls can be raised by inspiration only. To raise the first ball to the top, the patient must inspire at the rate of 600 milliliters per second, and to raise all three, he must inspire at 1,200 milliliters per second. He is told how many times per hour to raise all three and is asked to hold them at the top for 5 to 10 seconds each time that he raises them.

There are a number of more sophisticated incentive spirometers on the market. The most versatile is the Spirocare (Marion Laboratories, Inc., Pharmaceutical Division, Kansas City, Mo.), which has a far larger range, being able to measure inspiratory volume of up to 5,500 milliliters. It provides feedback through a system of lights and a digital display. The Bartlett-Edwards incentive spirometer (McGaw Respiratory Therapy, Division of American Hospital Supply Corporation, Irvine, Calif.) works by a

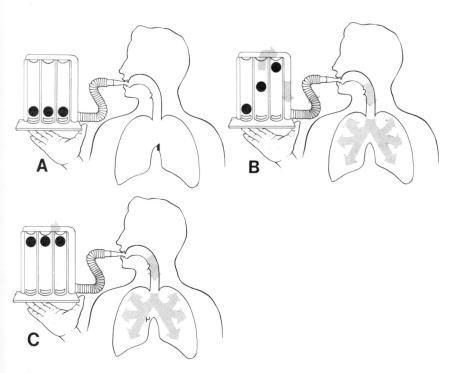

Fig. 16.8. Triflo incentive inspiratory spirometer. A, before inspiratory maneuver, all three balls rest at bottom; B, inspiration not strong enough to lift second ball to top; C, inspiration lifting all three balls to top—at least 1,200 milliliters per second.

system of piston bellows, and the subject keeps a light on if he achieves the present volume.

Conclusion

Respiratory failure is not restricted to diseases that primarily involve the lungs but occurs also in diseases that primarily involve many other systems. Hence, there are indications for using respirators in patients with normal lungs—for example, with overdoses of drugs such as barbiturates, opiates, and salicylates and with carbon monoxide and strychnine poisoning. We use respirators in cases of spinal cord and head injuries, as well as with other neurologic lesions such as bulbar poliomyelitis and Guillain-Barré syndrome. There are disorders that cause muscle spasms, such as status epilepticus and tetanus, and disorders that make muscles weak, such as myasthenia gravis and muscular dystrophy. Of course, there are actual lung diseases that may cause a need for a ventilator, such as severe asthma, pneumonia, and pulmonary edema. We have also discussed the use of other respiratory aids such as incentive spirometers for the prevention and treatment of alveolar collapse. There is evidence that use of these simple devices is preferable to use of IPPB devices.

The progress of respiratory failure should be monitored by means of arterial gas analysis and sophisticated respiratory function tests; clinical evaluation is not good enough. There is far more to managing these patients than managing the lung ventilatory equipment. Always there must be a carefully thought out program of breathing exercises given by a respiratory therapist, who also (together with the nurses) must carefully maintain the tracheostomy and oral passages. The physician not only must have a detailed knowledge of the capabilities of the gadgetry and the therapists but also must know details of inhalation therapy, methods of oxygen delivery, and electrolyte and fluid balance. It is important to realize that we are dealing with individual patients and individual problems.

Yet, there are common features: these patients are very ill and very frightened, and they need a great deal of support. We must explain the machines, as well as the therapy, carefully. This personal contact will give confidence to the patients and will make the use of the equipment, the therapy, and all of the program more effective.

Finally, the physician who undertakes the management of these complicated problems must be a physician who has specialized in this field. It is often advantageous to be an anesthesiologist. This chapter does not pretend to do more for the reader than to orient him towards the needs of these patients and make him aware of the possibilities of respiratory rehabilitation.

REFERENCES

1. BARTLETT, R. H., BRENNAN, M. L., GAZZANIGA, A. B., AND HANSON, E. L. Studies on the pathogenesis and prevention of postoperative pulmonary complications. *Surg. Gynecol. Obstet., 137:* 925, 1973.

2. BERGER, A. J., MITCHELL, R. A., AND SEVERINGHAUS, J. W. Regulation of respiration (first of three parts). *N. Engl. J. Med., 297:* 92, 1977.
3. BERGER, A. J., MITCHELL, R. A., AND SEVERINGHAUS, J. W. Regulation of respiration (second of three parts). *N. Engl. J. Med., 297:* 138, 1977.
4. BERGER, A. J., MITCHELL, R. A., AND SEVERINGHAUS, J. W. Regulation of respiration (third of three parts). *N. Engl. J. Med., 297:* 194, 1977.
5. BURNHAM, L., AND WERNER, G. The high-level tetraplegic: psychological survival and adjustment. *Paraplegia, 16:* 184, 1978.
6. GLENN, W. W. L., HOLCOMB, W. G., SHAW, R. K., HOGAN, J. F., AND HOLSCHUH, K. R. Long-term ventilatory support by diaphragm pacing in quadriplegia. *Ann. Surg., 183:* 566, 1976.
7. MACDONNELL, K. F., AND SEGAL, M. S. *Current Respiratory Care.* Little, Brown & Company, Boston, 1977.
8. MUSHIN, W. W., RENDELL-BAKER, L., THOMPSON, P. W., AND MAPELSON, W. W. *Automatic Ventilation of the Lungs,* ed. 3. Blackwell Scientific Publications, Oxford, 1978.
9. PHILLIPSON, E. A. Respiratory adaptations in sleep. *Ann. Rev. Physiol., 40:* 133, 1978.
10. SEVERINGHAUS, J. W., AND MITCHELL, R. A. Ondine's curse—failure of respiratory center automaticity while awake (abstract). *Clin. Res., 10:* 122, 1962.
11. SYKES, M. K., McNICOL, M. W., AND CAMPBELL, E. J. M. *Respiratory Failure,* ed. 2. Blackwell Scientific Publications, Oxford, 1976.

17

Automobile Modifications for the Disabled

HERBERT KENT, M.D.

This chapter has been designed to inform physicians and health professionals of necessary automotive driving aids frequently recommended to assist the disabled. An unimpaired driver operating a car with manual controls requires continuous coordination of the upper and lower limbs; the hands and feet are used to shift gears, steer, and apply brakes. During operation of the vehicle, it may become necessary to turn on the headlights, switch from low to high beam, operate the windshield wipers and, at times, adjust the heater or air conditioner. Most of the operations of driving are done routinely. The left hand normally steers, the right hand shifts gears; the left foot operates the clutch and the right foot depresses the accelerator. Thus, driving a vehicle is a complex task, particularly when one has to concentrate on the roadway, view the dashboard dials, and operate the automobile safely.

A disability of visual, emotional, or cerebral origin may affect driving skills. Automatic improvements, such as transmissions, have made it easier for someone who has lost a limb to drive. A left below-knee amputee generally operates both accelerator and brakes with the right leg. When a hand is lost, shifting is less frequent, and the steering wheel can be controlled by new skills. Light switches, usually placed on the left, can be modified or changed. Other similar requirements are possible for assisting the driver.

Paraplegics or bilateral amputees cannot always depend on simple modifications. Many others with multiple handicaps require evaluation and selective prescription of optimal driving aid systems. We must therefore match driver assistive aids with the handicapped individual's capacity to drive safely.

Motorized vehicles (automobile, van) and the disabled have been slow in evolving until recent years. Many types of mechanized bicycle-tricycles were developed. Later, these vehicles were motorized, particularly in Great Britain and Europe. A few were safe enought to serve as transports on the public streets and highways. With the coming of the modern automobile and later vans, innovations for the shut-ins and the wheelchair-bound became relatively spectacular.

When specific data is sought concerning the number of physically impaired who drive automobiles, little information can be found. Waller's California study (6) of 2,672 patients and Crancer's Washington review (2) of 39,242 patients were concerned only with chronic medical conditions (epilepsy, cardiovascular disease, diabetes, etc.). Blohmke (1) and Heipertz (3) in Germany discussed amputees and other disabled who drive in road traffic. Long (5) gave a report to a national symposium of his findings on 550 handicapped drivers by diagnosis and their road test ability.

Following World War II, the automobile became a popular mode of transport for the spinal cord injured. Funds from congressional legislation in 1945 encouraged eligible veterans to purchase automobiles and adaptive equipment. Prior to this, hand control aids were in their infancy, but this legislation spurred inventiveness to meet the demand for improvement in driving equipment.

With advances in technology, the van or vanmobile became extremely popular because it was more practical than the automobile. It enabled the disabled person to enter or leave his vehicle without great physical effort and transfer skills. This applied particularly to those in wheelchairs and the more severely disabled, such as bilateral amputees and paraplegics. Van preference was also desirable with the newer additions of so-called "modifiers."

Finally, to protect the patient and public, systematic effort by those in government is being voiced to require that vehicles and adaptive equipment conform to minimum standards of safety and quality. Also, it is recognized that national requirements for licensure of the handicapped will eventually be necessary. Governmental standards setting minimum levels of acceptable safety and quality for automobile driving aids have recently been published in the Federal Register (Vol. 40, No. 65, p. 15017, April 3, 1975).

Meeting Special Needs of the Handicapped Driver

Whether modifications are required for those drivers who have little or no use of their lower limbs or impaired function of the upper limbs, the essential requirement is to match the available equipment with the disability.

A classification of automotive "modifiers" is summarized in Table 17.1. "Modifiers" (automobile, van) can be defined as various automotive and driving aids designed to assist vehicle control, to provide entrance or exit mechanisms, or to provide convenience and safety features for the driver.

TABLE 17.1. *Classification of Automotive Modifiers*

Hand controls	Steering Aids	Gearshift
Push-pull	Knob	Extension bar (R or L)
Push-twist	Yoke	Push-button
Push-right angle pull	Open-face	Switch
	Wrist splint	
	Latch	
	Spinner ring	

Switches	Brakes	Accelerator
Quad key ignition holder	Power (extension, R or L)	Foot (R or L)
Turn signal extension (R or L)	Parking (electric)	Through control location
Light or dimmer switch		Other control location
Horn button location		
Electric windows	Floor (vanmobile)	Other
Cruise control		
Outside dome light	Leveling for wheelchair use	Bubble van top (11 inches or 24 inches)
Automatic wheelchair lift	Channeling for wheelchair driver	Mirror: special design, location, etc.
Door	Seat: tie-down (manual, electric)	Rear or side van entrance
Windshield wiper		Extended doorway widths
		Modified shoulder harness, chest strap, waist belt, etc.
		Steering wheel—small diameter, deep dish
		Air conditioning
		2-way radio communication
		Distress signal flag

A list of adaptive automotive manufacturers can be found at the end of the chapter.

HAND CONTROLS

The conventional method for hand controlling the gear shift lever, accelerator, brakes, and steering wheel generally must be altered. The hand control usually consists of a lever attached to a bracket on the steering column with two rods connected to the brake and accelerator pedal. A cam or gear is added to the lever so that the operating force can be changed from the accelerator to the brake pedal. There is a mechanical advantage built into the system. The ratio is 1:3 as a rule. These hand control systems may be a straight bar type, knob, or yoke end.

At the present time, there are three types of hand control available.

1. *Push-Pull (Fig. 17.1)*

Brake actuation is achieved by pushing the horizontal hand lever *away* from the driver and parallel to the steering column. Accelerator control is achieved by pulling the hand lever *towards* the driver. Generally, the push-pull system is operated with a left hand.

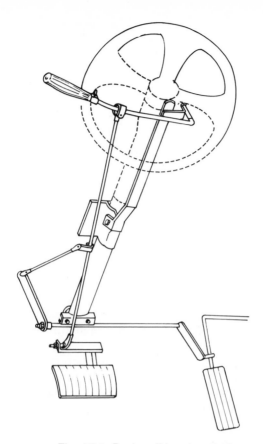

Fig. 17.1. Push-pull hand control.

Advantages
a. Two opposite directional movements are used for braking and accelerating the vehicle.
b. Relatively less costly than others.
c. Often commonly used by car rental companies.
d. Available by mail order.

Disadvantages
a. A functional hand (fingers) and wrist are necessary for the acceleration movement.
b. When stopped on a hill, one cannot use the brake and accelerator at the same time to keep from rolling back.
c. Braking time may be delayed.

2. *Push-Twist (Fig. 17.2)*
Brake actuation is achieved by pushing the horizontal hand lever *away* from the driver and parallel to the steering column.

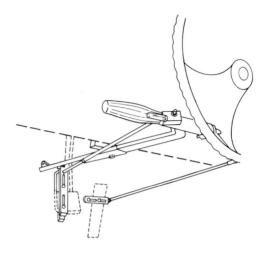

Fig. 17.2. Push-twist hand control.

Accelerator control is achieved by clockwise (forward twisting) rotation of the handgrip similar to motorcycle operation.

Advantages

a. Braking and control of acceleration can be carried out simultaneously.

b. Two distinct motions are readily possible in certain driving circumstances, such as hill stopping and starting, without rolling back.

Disadvantges

Normal grip, pronation, and supination movement are absolutely necessary. Therefore, they cannot be prescribed for bilateral upper limb amputees, median, ulnar, and radial nerve paralysis, quadriplegics, etc.

3. *Push-Right Angle Pull (Fig. 17.3)*

Brake actuation is achieved by pushing the horizontal hand lever *away* from the driver and parallel to the steering column. Accelerator control is achieved by pulling the hand lever in a direction *perpendicular* (at right angle) to the steering column and down toward the driver's lap.

Advantages

a. Used widely by most of the handicapped.

b. Useful for nonfunctional wrists with wrist splint.

c. Acceleration and braking can be done together, as on a hill, without rolling back.

Disadvantages

a. The right angle push control can cause accidents if the accel-

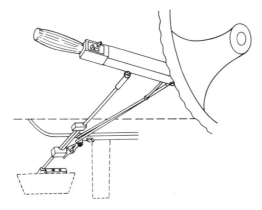

Fig. 17.3. Push-right angle pull hand control.

erator and brake are used simultaneously since these are not on the same plane of movement

b. An unfamiliar nondisabled individual attempting to drive the car can produce an accident readily, *e.g.*, parking lot attendant.

All three types of hand control have the same braking action, *i.e.*, forwards, by a pushing motion. If the car stops suddenly, the driver is thrown forward, transferring his weight to the hand control lever which activates the brakes.

Most hand controls are usually installed on the left side because most of the handicapped, as with normal people, are right handed and shift gears with this hand. Furthermore, the driver can use the left arm rest on the door as a resting or stabilizing device. Finally, this position keeps the hand controls out of the way of other equipment and allows easier transfer, etc.

STEERING AIDS (FIGS. 17.4 and 17.5)

To assist in the steering, there are add-on devices for use with standard steering wheels.

1. A *knob* which can rotate is commonly used as a spinner (Fig. 17.4*A* and 17.5*A*).
2. The *yoke* is shaped like the letter "V." The palmar aspect of the fingers is slipped through the opening and then held in a vertical position by the uprights of the "V" (Fig. 17.4*B* and 17.5*D*).
3. The *open-face* type permits the palm and fingers to be secured palm facing downwards (Fig. 17.4*C*).
4. The *wrist splint* type is a moulded splint permitting a flaccid wrist and fingers to be retained securely by Velcro straps (Fig. 17.5*F*).
5. The *latch* type is similar to the open face with a latch closure device on the extensor aspect of the fingers which then holds the hand snugly in place.

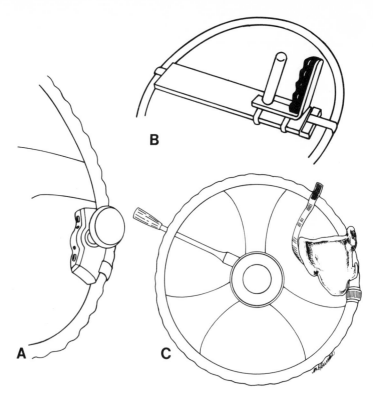

Fig. 17.4. A, Knob—spinner hand control; B, V-yoke hand control; C, open-face hand control.

6. The *spinner ring* is helpful for amputees using a hook (Fig. 17.5C). The point of the hook is inserted into the hole, and the wheel can be maneuvered in any direction.

These aids are useful for paralyzed fingers or wrists, as well as for quadriplegic patients and upper extremity amputees.

GEARSHIFT

1. A *gearshift extension* bar is useful where motions are limited, as in the shoulder or elbow (Fig. 17.5B).
2. *Push-button shifting* is available but rather limited in its usefulness.
3. *Switch shifting* is more experimental and limited in scope.

SWITCHES

The placement of control switches or extension is dependent on the individual needs of the disabled (See list, Tables 17.1–17.4).

An ignition key holder is shown in Fig. 17.5E.

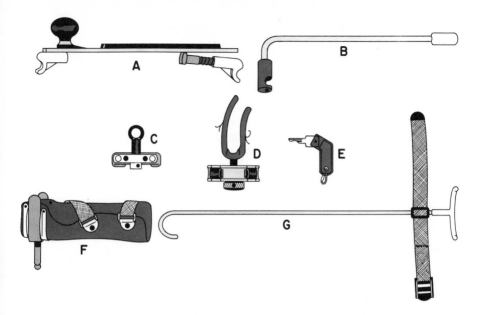

Fig. 17.5. Various steering aids and other devices. A, knob—spinner hand control; B, gear shift extension bar; C, spinner ring hand control; D, yoke hand control; E, quad-key ignition key holder; F, wrist splint; G, hook reacher.

BRAKES

Power brakes are practically a necessity for most disabled drivers. Pedals can be elevated or locations changed. Standard parking brakes are manually controlled but for the handicapped should be made electric so that they can be operated by switch or other controls.

ACCELERATOR

Frequently, the accelerator pedal has to be altered. Where the right foot and leg are amputated or impaired, a left foot accelerator is then installed and is provided in two types—one which is bolted to the floor and one which is attached to the right foot accelerator with a bar extending to the left. Hand-controlled accelerators are mounted on the steering column as described under "Hand Controls."

FLOOR (VANS—SEE FIG. 17.6)

The van is a recent innovation for patients with paralysis of the limbs, bilateral amputees, and those with severe neuromuscular diseases requiring the use of a wheelchair. Modifications to the floor of a van are usually necessary. Many have irregularities, protrusions, bolt heads, etc. which make propelling a wheelchair difficult. Special noteworthy points are:

1. Leveling of the floor is usually indicated with all vans.

2. Channeling permits the entry of the wheelchair into a grooved area leading to the driver's position.
3. Seat tie-downs to fasten the patient and seat to the floor are an absolute necessity. Sudden stops, acceleration, etc. can result in the driver becoming unstable and his chair moving about, imposing a safety hazard. Manually operated or electric tie-downs are available.
4. Vans modified for the handicapped have regular car seats which can be quickly disconnected if desired, and a wheelchair can be used instead.
5. The seat can also be of an electric transfer variety to facilitate changeover from a wheelchair.

OTHER MODIFICATIONS

Obviously, all sorts of changes in vehicular additions may be added and may be essential.

1. Bubble van top raising may be required, as the elevated seat height of a person in a wheelchair makes the head come close or in contact with the roof. In addition, the visual range may become obscured, as the driver may have to crouch forward to see ahead. There are two common size changes (11 inches and 24 inches) available.
2. Mirrors, of special design or changed in placement, are sometimes needed for rear or side vision.

TABLE 17.2 *Automotive Modifier Guide*

Disability	Hand controls	Steering aids	Gear-shift	Switches	Brakes	Accelerator	Floor	Other
Spinal cord disease/injury								
C5,6	+	+	+	+	+	+	+	+
T1,2	+	+			+	+	+	+
T10	+	+		+	+	+	+	+
L4,5	+	+			+	+	+	+
S1,2	+	+			+	+		
Brain disease/injury								
L hemiplegia		+	+	+		+		
R hemiplegia		+	+	+		+		
Cerebral palsy		+	+	+		+		
Amputee								
Upper right or upper left		+						
Lower right or lower left					+	+		
Bilateral upper	+	+			+		+	+
Bilateral lower	+	+			+	+		
AK					+	+		
BK	+	+			+	+		
Multiple sclerosis	+	+	+	+	+	+	+	+
Muscular dystrophy	+	+	+	+	+	+	+	+
Poliomyelitis	+	+	+	+	+	+	+	+

3. With vans, rear or side entrance loading are the options to be considered. Side entry needs wider parking space but rear entry may need more road space.
4. Expanded doorway widths are another feature sometimes required when structural changes are contemplated.
5. Seat belts, together with some of the above modifications, must be altered as required. A determination has to be made as to whether a shoulder, chest, or waist harness is what is needed for the disability.
6. Steering wheel alterations, such as one of a smaller than usual diameter, should be considered if the thighs interfere with or hit the steering wheel itself.
7. Air conditioning is generally considered essential in hot climates, particularly for those with spinal cord injuries.
8. Two-way radio for communication is sometimes vital in rural areas, on freeways, or where vocational endeavors require it.
9. Distress signal flags are laudable safety features for the wheelchair bound.

Equipment charts have been devised to make selections easier to recommend. Table 17.2 shows modifications of vehicles to be considered depending on the nature of the primary diagnosis. Of course, the modification will then be determined by the functional disability.

TABLE 17.3. *Mobility Equipment*

Equipment	Supplier and address
Commercially available modified vans	
Braun	Braun Corporation 1014 South Monticello Winamic, Indiana 46996
Compass	Compass Industries, Inc. 715 Fifteenth Street Hermosa Beach, California 90254
Drive-Master	Drive-Master Corporation 61-A N. Mountain Avenue Montclair, New Jersey 07042
Helper	Helper Industries, Inc. 832 N.W. First Street Fort Lauderdale, Florida 33311
Motorette	Motorette Corporation 6014 Reseda Boulevard Tarzana, California 91356

Table 17.3 *continues*

Table 17.3—*continued*

Equipment	Supplier and address
Roycemobile	Royce International, Ltd. Department AL 4345 South Sante Fe Drive Englewood, Colorado 80110
Scott	Mobility Engineering and Development, Inc. 15936 Blythe Street Van Nuys, California 91406
Sevier	General Teleoperators,.Inc. P.O. Box 3584 Los Amigos Station Downey, California 90242
Speedy Wagon	Speedy Wagon Sales Corporation 2237 Harvester Road St. Charles, Missouri 63301
Servo systems *2-degree-of-freedom servo* *systems* CCI-Harden	Creative Controls, Inc. P.O. Box 412 Birmingham, Michigan 48012
3-degree-of-freedom servo *systems* Scott	Mobility Engineering and Development, Inc. 15936 Blythe Street Van Nuys, California 91406
Sevier	General Teleoperators, Inc. P.O. Box 3584 Los Amigos Station Downey, California 90242
Lunar Rover	Southwest Research Institute 8500 Culebra Road P.O. Box 28510 San Antonio, Texas 78284
Special Mobility Systems Advanced Wheelchair	National Welded Products 2900 Spring Street #6 Redwood City, California 94063
Chair-E-Yacht	Chair-E-Yacht P.O. Box 231 Shoshoni, Wyoming 82649

Table 17.3 *continues*

Table 17.3—*continued*

Equipment	Supplier and address
Everest & Jennings Mark 20 Power Cart	Everest & Jennings 1803 Pontius Avenue Los Angeles, California 90025
Indoor/Outdoor Wheelchair	General Teleoperators, Inc. P.O. Box 3584 Los Amigos Station Downey, California 90242
Para-cycle	The Benz Corporation P.O. Box 5703 San Jose, California 95129
Permobil	Permobil Box 90 86100 Timra Sweden
Steven Motorized Wheelchair	Steven Motor Chair Co. 120 North Gunter Siloam Springs, Arkansas 72761
Voyager	Voyager, Ltd. P.O. Box 1577 South Bend, Indiana 46634

TABLE 17.4. *Elevator (Lift) Manufacturers*

1. Braun Corp., 1014 S. Monticello, Winamac, Indiana 46996
2. Casady Safety Van Lift, 1627 Linnea Ave., Eugene, Oregon 97401
3. Collins Industries, P.O. Box 58, Hutchinson, Kansas 67501
4. Helper Industries, Inc., 832 N. W. 1st St., Fort Lauderdale, Florida 33311
5. Para Industries, Ltd., #6-4826, 11th St., N.E., Calgary, Alberta, Canada
6. Ricon Corp., 15806 Arminta St., Van Nuys, California 91406
7. Speedy Wagon Sales Corp., 2237 Harvester Road, St. Charles, Missouri 63301

TABLE 17.5. *Adaptive Automotive Equipment Manufacturers*

1. Blatnik Precision Controls, Inc.
   1523 Cota Avenue
   Long Beach, California 90813
   (213) 436-3275
2. Drive-Master Corp.
   61 North Mountain Avenue
   Montclair, New Jersey
   (201) 744-1998

3. Ferguson Auto Service
   1112 North Sheppard Street
   Richmond, Virginia
   (804) 358-0800
4. Gresham Driving Aids
   P.O. Box 405
   Wixom, Michigan 48096
   (313) 624-1533

Table 17.5 *continues*

Table 17.5—*continued*

5. Handicaps, Inc.
   4345 South Santa Fe Drive
   Englewood, Colorado 80110
   (303) 781-2062
6. Hughes Hand Driving Controls, Inc.
   Tevis Bridge Road
   Lexington, Missouri 64067
   (816) 259-3681
7. Kroepke Kontrols, Inc.
   104 Hawkins Street
   Bronx, New York 10464
   (212) 885-1547
8. Manufacturing & Production Services
   2932 National Avenue
   San Diego, California 92113
   (714) 292-1423
9. Mross Inc.
   Star Route Box 42
   Elizabeth, Colorado 80107
   (303) 646-4096
10. Nelson Products
    5690-A Sarah Avenue
    Sarasota, Florida 33577
    (813) 924-2058

11. Smith's Hand Control
    1472 Brookhaven Drive
    Southhaven, Mississippi 38671
    (901) 743-5959
12. Thompson Hand Control
    4333 NW 30th Street
    Oklahoma City, Oklahoma
      73112
    (405) 946-9517
13. Trujillo Industries
    5726 W. Washington Blvd.
    Los Angeles, California 90016
    (213) 933-7469
14. Wells-Engberg Co.
    P.O. Box 6388
    Rockford, Illinois 61125
    (815) 874-6400
15. Wright-Way Inc.
    P.O. Box 907
    Garland, Texas 75040
    (214) 278-2676

AUTOMOBILE VERSUS VAN

Whereas the automobile as a common type of vehicle for use by the disabled has been popular, it does present physically limiting problems. For example, ingress and egress pose serious obstacles. Paraplegic patients with good upper limbs often negotiate entry into the driver's side by sliding from left to right. A slide board is often used (Fig. 17.7). Alternatively, they may enter the passenger side of the vehicle and slide from right to left. Upper extremity amputees lower or raise the seat in order to slip behind the steering wheel either from the left or right. Spastic conditions like multiple sclerosis require door or seat modifications. Diseases where muscle strength or lack of coordination are predominant necessitate many special adjustments to the controls and addition of other adaptive devices. Hand control mounts must correspond to the opposite side of the disability. Consequently, interference by these mounts must be considered also. In addition, when using an automobile, storage for the wheelchair has to be arranged as shown in Fig. 17.8. If the chair is placed behind the driver's seat, additional leg room to accomodate the medical condition must be anticipated. All of the alterations in driver positioning, controls, or adjustments harass a person making adaptation changes in his vehicle.

With the advent of the truck or van type of vehicle, many of the frustrating physical problems associated with automobiles have been resolved to a major extent. The severe handicaps associated with paraplegia, quadriplegia,

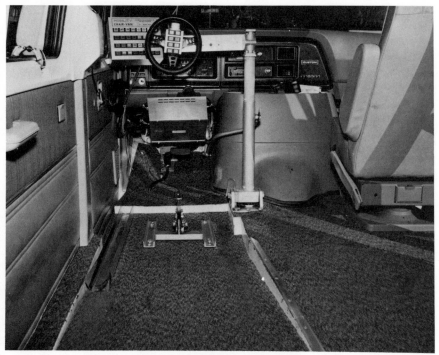

Fig. 17.6. Van floor channeling.

bilateral amputations, etc. almost necessitate the van vehicle. In particular, the van has made possible transportation mobility for such musculoskeletal disabilities as muscular dystrophy, multiple sclerosis, severe arthritis of the spine, etc. This category of the handicapped has become emancipated in transportation because of van "modifiers," as mentioned earlier. In the van, not only can the disabled person function as a driver but also he has the option of being a wheelchair passenger. Most high-level quadriplegic persons prefer a nondriving role.

The greatest advantage of the van is the convenience of entry and exit without leaving the wheelchair. All that is required is an elevation system for either rear or side entry.

We may now summarize the above comments as follow:

Advantages of Vans

    a. Entry and exit are easy and, generally, little or no other assistance is required, ensuring complete independence.

    b. Travel limits relatively unrestricted.

    c. Mobility within van is great.

    d. More roominess for self and passengers, etc.

    e. The disabled person does not have to leave the wheelchair.

    f. Storage room for adaptive equipment.

    g. Safety is greater.

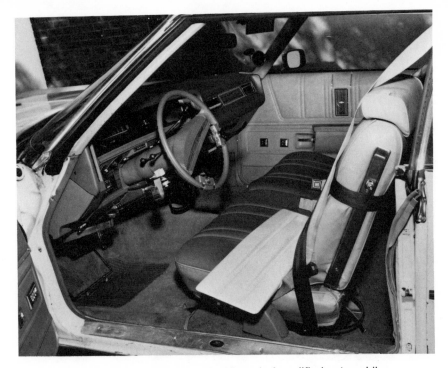

Fig. 17.7. Slide board and dashboard of modified automobile.

h. Floor can be leveled.

i. Roof can be raised.

j. Good recreational vehicle.

Disadvantages of Vans

a. High costs.

b. Adaptive equipment more complicated.

c. Body must be altered for doors, lifts, etc.

d. Floor must be modified.

e. Resale value poor except for another disabled person.

f. Security of driver and tie-down of wheelchair are essential, and wheelchairs do not stand up well in accidents.

g. Parking may be a problem—pavement, curbs, dirt road, etc.

h. Roof may be required to be raised—causing additional expense and inconvenience to travel in ferries, tunnels, etc.

Advantages of Automobiles

a. A standard automobile is usually available and costs less to buy and operate.

b. Modification costs are reasonable.

c. It is usable, generally, by unimpaired drivers.

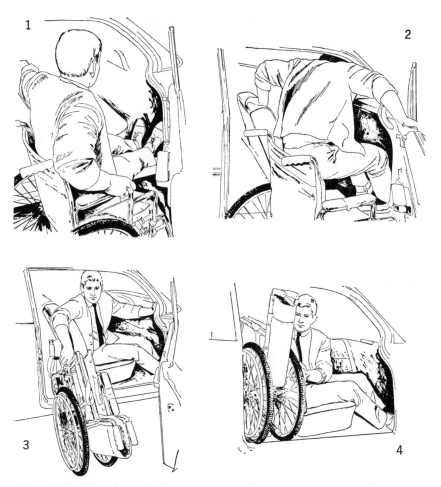

Fig. 17.8. Automobile wheelchair transfer—illustrating four sequential steps.

d. There is a resale value.
e. Dependability.

Disadvantages of Automobiles

a. Structural changes are expensive and permanent.
b. Only large cars can be used.
c. Ingress and egress can be slow and tedious.
d. Leg room is restricted by the hand control and other equipment.
e. Transfer activities are rather limited where there is no pavement or sidewalk.
f. Wheelchair transfer activities in parking lots can be difficult where parking spaces are slanted.

Disability Indications for Automobile Modifications

Requirements for particular modifications in or on the vehicle are dictated by a thorough knowledge of the level of injury (if spinal cord damage has occurred), the extent of the disability (bone, joints, muscles, nerves, etc.), and whatever function remains. Consequently, three fundamental data bases must be derived: manual muscle tests, joint ranges, and activities-of-daily-living (ADL) evaluations. Other considerations are related to the degree of brain damage and emotional stability, vocational requirements, and ability to satisfy the licensing laws of respective states. Social consequences to be considered relate to employment mobility, demands on family members, widening of recreational pursuits, and encouragement of independence generally.

UPPER EXTREMITY DISABILITIES

When single upper limb amputees require to drive a vehicle, few or no adaptations are necessary. This is especially true when an automatic transmission is provided and a prosthesis is utilized. Those desiring mechanical aids, on the other hand, can obtain these inexpensively, e.g., rings, or may purchase commercially available modifiers.

Bilateral upper limb amputees with prostheses are readily able to drive an automobile with few aids other than driving rings. Whether the disability is above or below elbow is of very little practical significance. By appropriate locations of hand controls, most variations of amputees can successfully drive safely.

When there is a combined upper and lower amputation on the same side, the patient is treated as a hemiplegic (see Table 17.2). More severely disabled cases involving three or even four limbs and who desire to drive may be considered more difficult, but not unsolvable problems.

In loss of function to the upper extremities an essential element in vehicular equipment prescription is ingress or egress ability. Many variations are available and must be tailored to the functional loss. A sliding board is often used in the automobile transfer from the wheelchair. It serves as a bridge from the car seat to the wheelchair and is utilized when muscle strength is impaired. There is an alternative to extension-pushdown type transfer: if normal flexor muscles are present in the elbow and shoulders, swinging into the car seat can be done by a gutter hand grasp on the roof edge of the car or an overhead grab bar. Other variations with automobiles are car seats that swivel outward, hydraulic lifts, and tilting steering wheels.

Total inability to transfer independently to an automobile makes the van a more acceptable alternative. With the van, door dimensions to adequately accomodate a full-size adult wheelchair (electric) require a minimum width of 57 inches. As mentioned, entry may be by side or rear loading, depending on patient requirements.

Lifts are usually electrically controlled and should be equipped with safety stops in front and rear so the user will not roll off. Swing down, swing out, unfolding, etc. are common varieties employed. Bleeder valve switches can be placed outside the van, on the lift, or on the door as required. Occasionally, sliding side doors may be desired.

Power steering, power brakes, etc. are often needed by those with weak muscles in the upper extremities.

LOWER EXTREMITY DISABILITIES

The ability to operate the brakes or accelerator may depend upon muscle strength in the leg or thigh muscles. Power brakes are the usual answer. With weak plantar flexion, it is possible to lessen the return spring of the accelerator pedal. A footholder on the accelerator or brake pedal itself may also be helpful.

Lower extremity amputees should use automatic transmission with the dimmer switch controlled by a hand switch. If both upper and lower limbs are absent, automatic transmission, hand control, gear shift, brake, accelerator, and switch modifications are required. Obviously, modifications will depend on whether the right or left limbs are absent.

In a below-knee amputation, if the patient wears adequate prosthesis and there is no other problem, such as limitation of strength or range of motion, no special alteration or restriction is imposed in driving. However, since the above-knee amputee, even with prosthesis, cannot tell the location of his foot, he usually must be considered limbless in respect to driving a vehicle. An unilateral above-knee amputee may only require moving the accelerator pedal but a bilateral above-knee amputee has essentially the same disability as a paraplegic.

SPINAL DISABILITIES

The patient with arthrodesis of the spine poses a driving problem. The most common cause of total spine arthrodesis is rheumatoid spondylitis, and although patients with this disability can usually drive a car safely, they have difficulty checking well on vehicles to the right or left of them. By providing enough mirrors to give a 360° field of vision, this problem can be partly solved.

Patients with back pain may not require any special driving aids, but alteration of seating may be important. The average automobile seat is not well designed for the patient with low back pain, as the angle between the lower extremities and the spine is often such that it may well aggravate the back problem. Furthermore, automobile seats are often too soft for many patients. It may be necessary to install a firmer seat in the vehicle or, more simply, to use a spinal supporting device that can be placed on the seat. These devices are usually readily available and can be contoured to accommodate the lumbar spine in an optimal position.

DISABILITIES ASSOCIATED WITH INCOORDINATION

Persons with incoordination, rigidity, and other involuntary movements are generally unable to drive a vehicle as, at present, we do not have any technological answer to their problems. However, if involuntary motions are very mild, it may be possible for some patients to drive a vehicle. A test of disability should not be made in the examining room but in a closely supervised situation behind the steering wheel. Ideally, the test should be made in a mock-up car in a rehabilitation department and, when practical, all such severely handicapped persons should be so tested before undertaking driver training programs with their equipment.

DISABILITIES WITH IMPAIRMENT OF CONSCIOUSNESS

Conditions in which there may be temporary loss of consciousness such as diabetes and epilepsy present a serious dilemma for licensing authorities and physicians who are asked to evaluate them. In giving permission to drive, the better the control of the condition that causes the disability and the more compliant the patient is with medical advice, the more liberal the advice should be. However, in many of these conditions, some patients exhibit genuine difficulty in remembering the hazards of failure to follow advice regarding their condition. Epileptics present a particularly complicated problem. There are many authorities that insist that no epileptic patient should be allowed to drive. This attitude has made it difficult to have an objective survey of the conditions of epileptics who drive automobiles, as not only patients but also physicians, when asked for information, refuse to list the epileptic patients that drive a car. The general opinion seems to be that an epileptic person can be allowed to drive if he is under strict medical supervision, if it is proven that he takes medication regularly, and if he has not had an attack of unconsciousness for at least 24 months.

The question that has been raised in regard to epileptics raises a broader problem concerning the ethical standards of the medical profession. The legal climate today demands that physicians report to the appropriate agencies uncooperative, unsafe, or newly handicapped drivers. Jacobs (4) has recently reviewed this problem. Although it may occur, he could find no instance of a physician being sued for breach of doctor-patient confidentiality for reports to authorities concerning patient's handicaps. We quote from a summary of his recommendations as follows:

> "A physician should counsel the handicapped patient and the patient's whole family knowledgeably. He should put his advice in writing and have the patient or a member of the patient's family sign the document. The physician should try to refrain from prescribing medications that impair driving ability. He should report the uncooperative patient to the state by notifying only the specific person of the specific department with jurisdiction over driver licensing. He should include

in his report his basic diagnosis, laboratory findings, and verifiable incidents supporting his opinion that the patient is an unsafe driver."

PRESCRIPTION OF ASSISTIVE AIDS

To facilitate prescribing of adaptive modifications, Table 17.2, which is by no means inclusive, may be consulted for common neuromusculoskeletal disabilities. Many of the recommended "modifiers" are based on the needs of those with spinal cord, brain, neuromuscular disease/injury, and amputations. Modification requires individual evaluation, including other related aspects such as, *e.g.*, terrain, climate, etc. Finally, reliability and design should be as fail-safe as possible.

Van Access Systems

Elevator and ramp methods for entry and exit depend upon the type of vehicle. Some of these rely upon the use of hoists, elevators, and ramps mounted on the side or rear. Cable winches, hydraulic components, or other devices employed work electrically, usually with a mechanical backup for emergencies. As these systems improve with advancing technological refinement, it is to be expected that the handicapped driver will still have to provide for his own individual requirements. The state-of-the-art is best served by intelligent assessment of a disability.

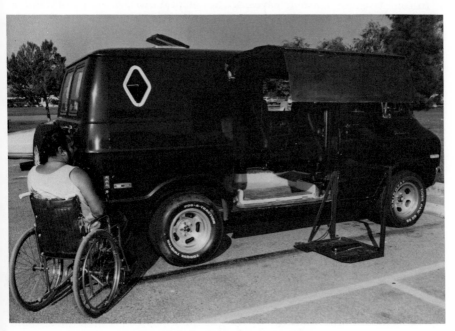

Fig. 17.9. Swing-out van elevator.

Two basic types of elevator modifiers are now available: swing-out and fold-down.

Swing-out Elevator

Fig. 17.9 shows a side loading method: the wheelchair is rolled on a platform which rotates 180° as it swings out and then is gently lowered to the ground level. Safety ledges, switches, and other mechanical controls for emergencies are handily mounted.

Fold-Down Ramp and Elevator

The fold-down platform is configured like an aircraft passenger step (Fig. 17.10). When a button is activated, a ramp is formed as it lays itself onto the road. Another type of fold-down elevator-type platform is shown in Fig. 17.11. Here the platform folds out parallel to the ground and lowers like an elevator. A safety guard is present to keep the wheelchair from rolling off. Switches and actuating devices are usually placed in accessible positions for the wheelchair user. The fold-down can also be employed for entry at the rear. In this instance, it is also invaluable for persons using a wheeled stretcher. One shortcoming here is that considerable road space is necessary to facilitate access.

Driver Training

Automotive aids, by themselves, are not helpful without adequate training in their use. The disabled person, in order to operate the vehicle, must

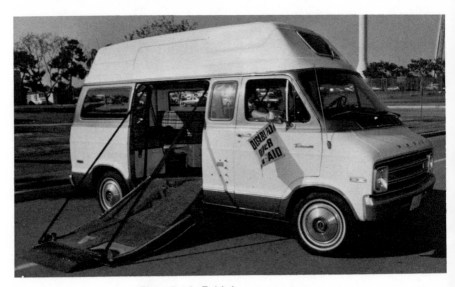

Fig. 17.10. Fold down van ramp.

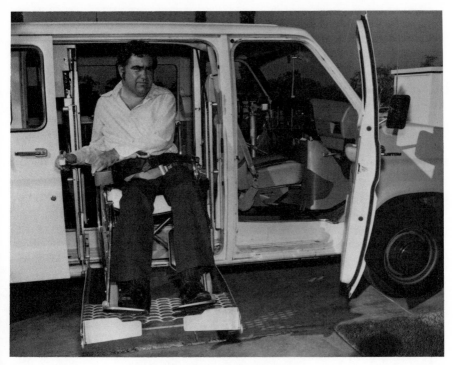

Fig. 17.11. Fold down van elevator.

satisfy current and local driving regulations. Therefore, often, special driving instruction is necessary, particularly when employment, social, and recreational goals are needed for independence. The ability to drive safely will determine whether the individual is an asset or burden to society.

The following conceptual outline (Diagram 17.1) of driver training for handicapped veterans was developed with much success at the Veterans Administration Medical Center at Long Beach, Calif. It illustrates what can be done to examine and validate driving performance.

Research in Automotive Modifications

Automotive modifications, practical and esthetic, are now used around the world. Sweden, Germany, Great Britain and, particularly, the United States are conducting a great deal of experimental as well as production effort. Push-button, "single-stick," and remote control servo systems are being developed. Fig. 17.12 illustrates one such experimental system. Its unique features are activated by use of a joystick. This system has three-degrees-of-freedom providing braking, acceleration, and steering. The ignition and operation of all accessories, including doors, lift, etc. are accomplished by activating push buttons on a panel facing the driver. When the joystick is pushed forward, acceleration occurs. Braking takes place by

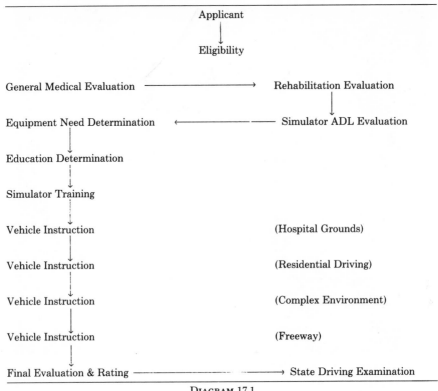

Applicant

Eligibility

General Medical Evaluation ————————————→ Rehabilitation Evaluation

Equipment Need Determination ←———————— Simulator ADL Evaluation

Education Determination

Simulator Training

Vehicle Instruction   (Hospital Grounds)

Vehicle Instruction   (Residential Driving)

Vehicle Instruction   (Complex Environment)

Vehicle Instruction   (Freeway)

Final Evaluation & Rating ——————— ————→ State Driving Examination

DIAGRAM 17.1

pulling backward. The small wheel, when rotated, steers the vehicle. A popular goal of most research is single-limb control for braking, acceleration, steering, signaling, switch lighting, etc. Special sizes of vehicle, access, powering methods, accommodations for wheelchair drivers, and unique transmissions and steering systems all have their advocates. The Germans, for example, have developed a driving modification that allows a vehicle to be completely driven by the lower extremities. One new development which should be mentioned is a specially designed two-driver vehicle which may be loaded either from the side or rear with dual controls (computer and standard).

In the future, power could be by solar, electric, or atomic energy. Entry and egress methods may see innovations such as jacking the vehicle to ground level or wheel retraction bringing the vehicle floor down. Finally, programmed or remote control of a vehicle is a future possibility.

Acknowledgments

Grateful acknowledgment is made to Marian B. Berman, Medical Illustrator, and the Medical Media Production Service, Veterans Administration Medical Center, Long Beach, Calif. for assistance with these illustrations.

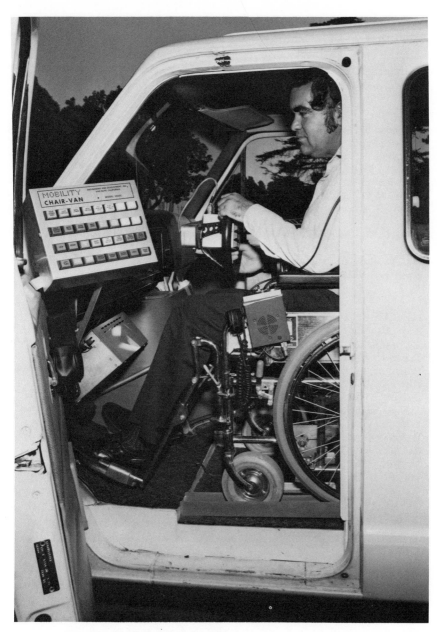

Fig. 17.12. Push button and servo controls in van (Scott).

Particular appreciation for use of Figs. 17.1, 17.2, 17.3, and 17.4*B* is directed to Frank D. Gentile, Vice President, and his staff at the Human Resources Center, Albertson, Long Island, N. Y. These figures were copied from illustrations 17.3, 17.5, 17.8, 17.23, and the accompanying text for *Hand Controls and Assistive Devices for the Physically Disabled Driver.*

REFERENCES

1. BLOHMKE, F. Proceedings. V. Traffic Medicine. D. The amputee in the road traffic. *Hefte Unfallheilkd, 114:* 238–242, 1973.
2. CRANCER, A., JR., AND McMURRAY, L. Accident and violation rates of Washington's medically restricted drivers. *J. A. M. A., 205:* 272–276, 1968.
3. HEIPERTZ, W. Proceedings. V. Traffic Medicine. C. The Severely Disabled in the Road Traffic. *Hefte Unfallheilkd, 114:* 232–238, 1973.
4. JACOBS, S. Reporting the handicapped driver. *Arch. Phys. Med. Rehabil., 59:* 8, 387–390, 1978.
5. LONG, C., II. The handicapped driver—a national symposium. *J. Rehabil., 40(2):* 34–39, 1974.
6. WALLER, J. A. Chronic medical conditions and traffic safety. Review of the California experience. *N. Engl. J. Med., 273:* 1413–1420, 1965.

SELECTED REFERENCES

1. FREEMAN, C. C. Evaluation of adaptive automotive driving aids for the disabled. *N. Y. Acad. Med. Bull., 50:* 536–544, 1974.
2. MENOHEM, L., *et al. Hand Controls and Assistive Devices for the Physically Disabled Driver.* Human Resources Center, Albertson, N. Y., 1977.
3. REICHENBERGER, A. J., AND NEWELL, P. H. Adaptive devices for automobiles. In *Atlas of Orthotics,* pp. 462–478. C. V. Mosby, St. Louis, 1974.
4. PERSONAL LICENSED VEHICLES FOR THE DISABLED. Report of a Workshop, June 14–17, 1976. Rehabilitation Engineering Center, Moss Rehabilitation Hospital, Philadelphia, Pa., 1976.
5. PROGRAM GUIDE—PROSTHETIC AND SENSORY AIDS SERVICE. *Add-on Automotive Adaptive Equipment for Passenger Automobiles.* M-2, Part IX, G-9, Washington, D. C. March 31, 1978.

18

Self-Help Clothing

MARY ELEANOR BROWN, M.A.

Clothing to match the needs of the disabled promotes motion and encourages the wearer to put it on. It has convenient openings where they are most time and effort saving and of proper size. Kinesiologically fashioned clothing makes the wearer feel good, because it is not too tight, too loose, too narrow, too wide, too short, too long. It does not restrict motion or hinder breathing.

Practical self-help clothing is adjustable and expandable according to desired functions. It protects its wearer without curtailing movement. The fabric is not too heavy, too light, too warm, too cool, too bulky, too flimsy. It is reinforced against wear occasioned by braces and crutches or other necessities associated with lost or impaired motion. Suitable clothing is safe to wear, easy to sew, maintain and repair, easy on the eye and pocketbook, easy off and on (Fig. 18.1), and nice to the touch.

Clothing can match physiologic needs. For warmth, patches or strips of insulating textiles may be inserted in the regions of ankles, wrists, neck, and ears. Some persons, particularly the elderly, may enjoy the thermal underwear for skiers and fishermen that retains the body heat (78). The same manufacturer supplies ankle, knee, and elbow warmers. Proper fit, flattering design, stretchable fabrics, and easy donning and doffing are desired by all of us but even more so by people of small stature (51) who need above-normal ranges of motion to perform daily activities in an average size world.

Before fabrics and scissors, people wore animal skins, fastening them with bone pins (66). Now clothes are the products of worldwide industries providing jobs and careers to millions (75). "The study of clothing is rooted in a number of natural and social sciences" (64). Clothes are symbols of cultures and have historical value (65, 66). "There is not a human institution which has not been importantly affected by the clothes we wear .... Modern civilization rests on clothing," said Lawrence Langner who wrote a play, "The Importance of Wearing Clothes," and later a book by the same title,

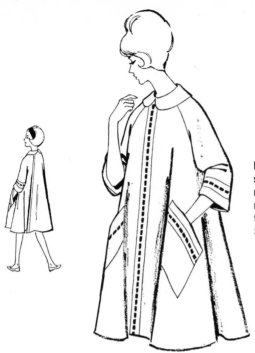

Fig. 18.1. Easy-on robe designed by Dorothy Behrens features pressure-tape back closure, accessible, roomy pockets, and three-quarter raglan sleeves. (Courtesy of Vocational Guidance and Rehabilitation Services of Cleveland, Ohio.)

now in paperback (65). Often writers begin with "clothes-make-the-man" quotations, alluding to the effect of clothing on self-confidence, healthy attitudes, and success in daily life and work. One writer stresses clothing as "a positive part of the rehabilitation process" (73). She says, "Clothes can help us to get and hold jobs or miss or lose them."

Self-help clothing for the disabled is a concern of the fields of health, medicine, social service, home economics, and psychology (53, 59, 63, references under IC). This chapter reports the work of physical and occupational therapists, nurses, home economists, social workers, physicians, psychologists and the projects and theses of university students (Fig. 18.2; 6, 33, 63). A historical account is in "Clothing for the Physically Handicapped 1937–1962" (67) and updated in two review-type references (69, 70). A handy chart identifies seven research approaches to the study of clothing for the disabled and supplies the chronology from 1927–1963 (68).

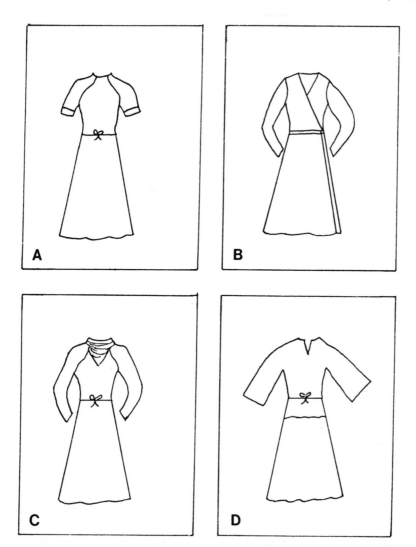

Fig. 18.2. Four basic garments for women with rheumatoid arthritis, designed by Barbara Kohlbeck (33). Comfortable, easy-on, easy-off, easy-care, they may suit many girls and women, regardless of age or degree of ability. *A*, A-line, tube dress with short raglan sleeves. Velcro strips on raglan seams provide bib-like, front opening extending from neckline downward to level of armpits on both sides. Tie-belt can be pre-tied and fastened with Velcro; *B*, Coat-type style, with enlarged armholes, long sleeves, and no fastening cuffs, wraps with Velcro inside front waistband; *C*, Same as *A* but with long sleeves, slightly gathered cuffs with elastic casing, and cowl neckline in front only. With no seam openings, this design may require knit fabric to permit dressing; *D*, Two-piece: top has kimono sleeves, front slit neck opening, and elasticized waist with decorative bow. Skirt is gored and has elastic waistband. (Courtesy of Barbara Kohlbeck.)

As with the hoopskirt, bustle, and leg-of-mutton sleeves, the development of self-help clothing has experienced periods of exaggeration. Preoccupation with buttons and shoelaces was followed by comprehensive collections of dressing aids (36, see also Chapter 19). To some, an apparatus for donning pantyhose (48) multiplies the complexities of putting on that fragile, unwieldy garment. Other ill-fitting, poorly made clothes may result in disabilities (44, 58).

However, inquiry has narrowed to basic elements of clothing and some garments adaptable to many disabled persons (Fig. 18.2). A British occupational therapist (37) offers a comprehensive work of 157 pages on clothing for adults. Clear and practical suggestions addressed to the disabled appear in an illustrated 12-page pamphlet from a State university extension service (62). The theme of simplicity is emerging in the variety of comfortable, casual, leisure-time clothing of nowadays. Flexible garments facilitate breathing, moving, walking, running, dancing and other physical fitness pursuits of persons of all ages and abilities. If abilities are lessened by accident or disease, clothing becomes a major problem.

Hospital garments soon become inadequate. It is natural to look forward to one's own clothes again. It is disastrous if no one goes over these clothing articles to make sure they can be put on and taken off. A physical therapist, an occupational therapist, or a nurse takes inventory of an individual's clothing and clothing skills. A stopwatch is used to learn how long it takes a person to dress and undress.

A manageable and attractive wardrobe is assembled by remodeling, shopping for self-help features, adapting patterns and designing one's own styles. Independent dressing and undressing need no longer go begging because no one pays attention to this aspect of well-being.

This chapter contains not only the story of self-help clothing. It also emphasizes the manner in which its wearer is assured, through evaluation by taking inventory, that clothing skills and clothing articles match each other. The case summaries which follow in Fig. 18.3 are self-help clothing stories of subjects, lettered *A* through *I*, and illustrate studies made by this writer at Sunnyview Hospital and Rehabilitation Center, Schenectady, N.Y. (19, 54). The procedure of matching the patient and his clothing through evaluation is responsible for the successes reported.

Case Summaries

SELF-HELP CLOTHING STORIES

(Sketches, Courtesy of Sunnyview Hospital, Schenectady, N.Y.)

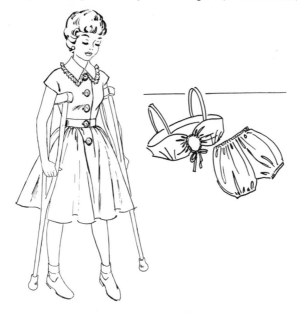

DAILY ACTIVITY RECORD OF **A**

INVENTORY		PROGRESS			
WITHIN TIME	BLACK	WITHIN TIME	R E D		DATE
		WITHIN TWICE TIME; LATER WITHIN TIME	RED	RED	DATE / DATE

INVENTORY DATE 3/3/50
EXAMINER'S SIGNATURE (R.)

CLASSIFICATION	INVENTORY LIST	TIME ALLOWANCE	NO.	GRAPH	SYMBOL	TIME	DATE
IV. DRESSING & UNDRESSING	Undressing.	10'	26	Black	UNDRESS	8'16"	
	Fastening shoes or tying shoestrings.	1'	24	Red Red	⌒	1'17" / 45"	6/16/50 / 11/26/50
	Dressing except for fastening shoes or tying shoestrings	15'	23	Red	DRESS	5'8"	5/23/5?

Fig. 18.3. *A*'s self-help clothing comprised bloomer underpants, brassiere with drawstring in front, dress with big buttons and front opening extending below waist, side zipper, and deep hem; no underskirt. Born August 19, 1939, with cerebral palsy (spastic quadriplegia and arrested hydrocephalus), *A* was dependent in clothing management in 1950. On June 1, 1951, she undressed, got into the tub, drew water, bathed, dried herself, got out of tub, and dressed without assistance. The time required was ½ hour. In 1 year 3 months and at the age of 11 years 9 months, this slow but amiable young girl became completely independent in all phases of clothing and toilet management.

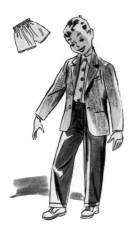

B's self-help garments included elastic-topped under-shorts, a roomy shirt with half-inch buttons, elastic-topped trousers, and a loose-fitting coat; no undershirt or tie. Born November 22, 1942, with cerebral palsy (rigidity quadriplegia), he had no clothing skills in early 1950. He learned to undress in 3 months, but buttoning and managing tight clothing, especially after toileting activities, were not possible. After 14 months his difficulties were solved by a better selection of purchased clothing. At 8½ years of age he was completely independent in handling his clothing.

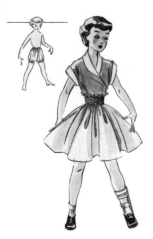

C's self-help costume included elastic-edged underpants suitable also for exercise, a blouse with deep-cut arm-holes and ample neckline without fasteners, a skirt with elastic-shirred waistband and deep hem making a slip unnecessary; no undershirt. Born July 1, 1942, with cerebral palsy (spastic quadriplegia), she was completely dependent in all clothing management in 1950. Two years 10 months later, at 10½ years of age, she became independent in undressing and dressing except for putting on and taking off her brace and fastening her shoes.

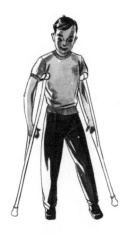

D's self-help clothing included elastic-topped under-shorts and trousers with no fasteners and a loosely woven knitted shirt; no undershirt. Born March 10, 1941, with cerebral palsy (spastic quadriplegia), he undressed in 2 minutes 3 seconds on March 3, 1950. In 14 months he learned to dress himself with selected bought clothing of suitable size. He gained complete clothing independence at the age of 10 years 2 months.

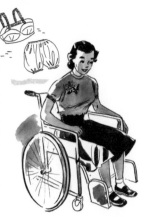

E's self-help clothing featured bloomer-type undershorts, brassiere with elastic back and shoulder straps, deep hem in skirt to eliminate slip, loosely woven pastel T-shirt, and elastic-topped skirt, to complete two-piece, overhead, easily donned costume; no undershirt. Born August 26, 1938, with cerebral palsy (rigidity quadriplegia), she was completely dependent in all clothing management until 1950. Two years later at the age of 13 years 9 months, she became independent in undressing and dressing except for putting on brassiere and fastening shoes. It took 3 months of daily practice for her to learn to adjust her clothing before and after toilet activities.

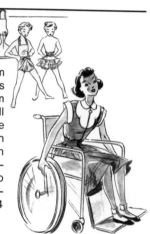

F's self-help wardrobe included two underwear-gym suits. The ruffled, bloomer-type swimsuit on right was purchased to serve as underpants, underslip, and gym suit. Her dress had a zipper with large ball-on-tab-pull and extended below elasticized waistband to eliminate need for belt and buckle. Born February 13, 1942, with cerebral palsy (athetoid quadriplegia), this little girl, in constant motion, was completely dependent in undressing and dressing in 1950. In 15 months she learned to undress in 9 minutes 27 seconds. Dressing independence except for fastening shoes was achieved in 4 years, when her age was 11 years 11 months.

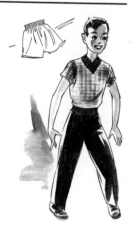

G's ready-made, self-help wardrobe consisted of elastic-topped shorts, blue jeans, and loose stretchable shirt with ribbing at neck and waist. Born March 3, 1941, with cerebral palsy (ataxic quadriplegia), he was completely dependent in clothing management in early 1950. Fourteen months later, aged 10 years 2 months, he was independent in undressing and dressing except for fastening his shoes.

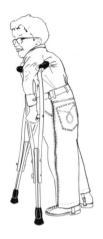

H's self-help clothing and equipment for dressing and undressing independence included a toilet seat specially designed for him (55). Main clothing items were charcoal jeans with wide pantlegs, completely zippered down both sides with easy-to-see pink zippers and easy-to-find loops for fingers for pulling up over braces; shoes opening to toes; diapers in organdy pocket inside incontinence pants (Figure 18.6d) to avoid bunching. Born June 21, 1945, with spina bifida, club feet, hydrocephalus, sensation losses, impaired bowel and bladder control, and eye defects, he was entirely dependent in 1950. At age 10 years 3 months, with an I.Q. of 65, he mastered getting on and off his toilet seat, managed his protective pants, and dressed and undressed, including putting on and taking off his braces. The 10 months with over 600 hours of instruction seem little compared with the years of complete dependence his parents would otherwise face.

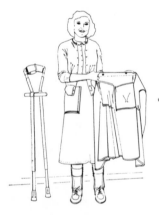

I's self-help clothing included a front-tying brassiere, short-sleeved blouses with front buttoning, side-zippered shorts for exercise and for easy donning over braces, wrap-around denim skirts with large pockets, and regular socks, shoes, and underpants (after practice with special styles). A right-handed girl, her involvement was mainly of the left upper limb and both lower limbs, requiring double long leg braces, pelvic band, and the use of below-elbow crutches. Born July 30, 1938, she contracted poliomyelitis October 12, 1954. On March 9, 1955, dressing and undressing were not satisfactory. On March 15, 1955, after 6 days of concentrated instruction and clothing study she became completely independent in dressing and undressing. She returned home and was married later that year.

Others report case studies. Two authors (59) give a case summary of a seven-year old girl with multiple amputations. Three writers (27) summarize their work with a 9-year-old girl with cerebral palsy and a teenage girl with spina bifida. A home economist (1) designed a basic pattern for a woman with quadriplegia which "could be used again and again, with variety derived from the fabric and trims selected, rather than from the garment design."

Clothing Entities According to Dressing Direction

The human body has a trunk as its largest mass, a somewhat spherical head on top with a cylindrical neck between the two, and two upper and two lower limbs. Clothes may be considered according to the way in which they are placed on the body: they may be wrapped around the body, placed over the head, or drawn over the feet. The elemental aspects of wearing apparel are used as a first guide to ferreting out ways to meet the special clothing needs of exceptional persons. Table 18.1 lists common clothing items showing the direction of motion required by the construction.

A coat-type garment goes around the body, has a complete vertical opening in the front or back, and two armholes or sleeves or shoulder straps. The coats may or may not have fastenings.

The coat-like garment usually opens down the front and has as its advantage the ease with which it may be worn over the clothing. If the full-length opening is in the back, as with smocks and operating-room gowns, the coat is harder to put on, adjust to the figure, and fasten. Women are familiar with the difficulty of fastening a bra in the back. Another advantage of the coat is that it avoids disarranging hair and headwear since it is not pulled over the head. A garment which is stepped into may become soiled. A coat-type garment may be put on in a lying, sitting, or standing position. Over-the-head and over-the-feet clothing may require combinations of lying, sitting, and standing positions.

Many of the same garments come in tube form, that is, without full-length openings. They have one opening for the head and sometimes additional openings at different locations. They require placing over the head or over the feet. In this group are many articles of underwear: garter belts, girdles, slips, and undershirts.

Wrap-arounds require no overhead or overfoot placement. They differ from coat-types in that they have no sleeves. They are wrapped around the trunk and fastened.

Pants are drawn over the feet. Limb, and head and neck articles are placed on the extremities and head, and around the neck. Many have fastenings.

TABLE 18.1. Clothing Entities According to Dressing Direction

Type	Coat	Tube	Wrap-Around	Pants	Limb	Head and Neck	Combined
Direction	Around	Overhead or overfeet if openings are large enough	Around	Overfeet	Toward center	Toward center	
Opening(s)	One complete vertical; Two armholes or sleeves or shoulder straps	One head with or without additional slits, armholes, sleeves, shoulder straps	One complete vertical	One trunk; Two pantlegs or holes for limbs			
Garments	Coats, Vests, Jackets; Dresses, Blouses; Sweaters, Shirts, Bras; Undershirts; Pajama tops, Bathrobes	Ponchos; Dresses, Blouses; Skirts; Sweaters, Shirts, Garter belts, Girdles; Slips, Undershirts; Pajama tops, Nightgowns, Nightshirts	Capes; Skirts; Garter belts, Girdles, Corsets, Slips	Pants, Slacks; Pedal pushers, Culottes; Shorts; Underpants, Briefs; Pajama bottoms	Gloves, Mittens; Socks, Stockings; Shoes, Overshoes, Boots; Slippers	Hats, Caps, Wigs; Scarves	Overalls, Jumpsuits, Ski-type coveralls in one piece, Wrap-around pants, Blouse-slips; Pant-skirts, Shorts plus wrap-around legs, Sweater-slips, Pant-shirts, Bra-slips, Panty girdles; Pant-slips, Wrap-around underpants, Crotch-fastening blouse-underpants; Tights, Pantyhose, Swimwear

Clothing Entities Related to Disabilities

Clothing articles may be changed from one entity to another, and also combined, to suit the needs of individuals.

COAT AND TUBE OPENINGS

The main openings of the garments may be critical. Open-down-the-front garments are easier to manage. Changing the back openings of dresses to front openings is a simple remedy. Coat-type clothing may be converted to tube-type by partially or fully fastening it after which it can be put on overhead, even in a lying position. This method has helped women with back-fastening and front-fastening brassieres.

Some tube-type clothing can be converted to full-opening, coat-like clothing. Pajama tops, undershirts, slips, nightgowns, and nightshirts are often opened fully down the front to facilitate their management.

Front-opening tube garments are made easier to get into by extending the opening below the waist. Side front openings are more easily seen and located by the dresser than outright side ones. Placket openings may be changed to the other side if they are more easily closed by the other hand. This may be the case with a patient paralyzed on the left side, since dresses usually have openings on the left. Head and neck openings on tube clothing, such as knit sweaters, shirts, undershirts, and pajama tops, are more stretchable if they have overlapping, expandable necklines. A bib-like panel opening to below the waist facilitates putting on a dress. It is easily fastened and decorative. A down-the-back split skirt on a dress may help a woman when in the bathroom especially if she can snap the bottom corners up in front and out of the way.

FASTENERS

"Do wear simple clothing with few or no fastenings," says the therapist when introducing the patient to the many action-requiring procedures of physical therapy and daily activities to relearn. Total-body activity demands maximal free range, and the patient must be free of encumbering clothing or apparatus which might interfere. Precious therapy minutes adding up to hours and days, have gone into unpinning, unbuttoning, unhooking, unsnapping, untying, unbuckling, and unzipping clothing in preparation for exercise. Even more time has been absorbed in replacing these clothes after exercise.

The Overhead No-Fastener Two-Piecer

The overhead, no-fastener, two-piecer has been a popular clothing style for girls and women, young and old. As seen on Subject E (Fig. 18.3), it is composed of a loosely fitting T-shirt top and an overhead, elastic-topped skirt with a deep hem making a slip unnecessary. Both items can be purchased ready-made. Attractive costumes are assembled by choosing a pastel T-shirt of good quality with contrasting or matching plain material or harmonizing print for the skirt. There are other no-fasten garments with stretchable and elasticized openings, gracefully overlapping (surplice) necks and sleeves and other draped arrangements over shoulders with folds and sashes for anchorage.

Velcro

Velcro (32) ("vel" for velvet; "cro" for French *crochet,* small hook) makes use of two dissimilar strips which adhere on slight pressure because one is composed of tiny loops and the other of tiny hooks, as shown in Fig. 18.4*b*. These strips survive hard usage. They are closed during laundering and should not be exposed to a hot iron.

With Velcro, we can convert a garment unhandy for a specific patient into another kind by introducing a slit at a crucial place, or by replacing a hard-to-fasten button-opening by two strips of Velcro. Details and instructions are easily found (5). An example is to slit undershirts down the front and install Velcro the full length whenever such an adjustment simplifies dressing and undressing. Dabs of Velcro available in fabric stores in various shapes and strengths may be sufficient. They are useful under buttons obviating button holes and for anchoring collars, belts, and scarves. Velcro and zippers should not touch the skin.

Zippers

The zipper (Fig. 18.4*c*) was on the market in 1927 and many a cerebral palsied child has benefited by long sturdy zippers extending under the arm from sleeve cuff to bottom of garment. Snowsuits can be zippered to open out into two flat pieces by having both sides thus treated. Blanket zippers and those used for furcoat linings are recommended. Zippers in contrasting

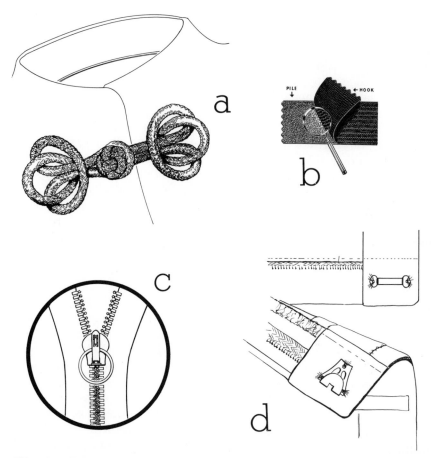

Fig. 18.4. Fasteners. *a*, Fur coat frog, easy to open and close with its large, soft, firm, flexible, and holding parts; can also be homemade; *b*, Velcro comes in many sizes and colors. Hooks of upper press-tape lock with loops of lower tape. (Courtesy of Smalley and Bates, Inc., Nutley, N.J.); *c*, Large-size zipper comes in different lengths, is solid, easy to lock, and decorative; *d*, Large-size bar and hook for pants and skirts are simple to handle.

colors aid visibility. Decorative tabs of shapes to suit the hands which pull them are also helpful. Metal rings and key chains are used. The zipper needs an underlay so as not to pinch or catch in other parts of the garment or the slip underneath it.

A reference (50) contains guides to the varieties of zippers, their insertion (in a pleat sometimes), ways of shortening, their pitfalls, their use with other fastenings for anchorage, and elements in their operation and care. A popular design (23) for pants makes use of double cam lock, two-way automatic slider zippers concealed stylishly within outside seams. They allow partial or full opening in either direction while pants are anchored around the waist.

One may install Velcro and zippers on a garment with sleeves, such as a jacket, the full length of the underarm sleeve to the bottom of the jacket on one or the other side, or on the outsides from the bottom upward (9). Crotch-opening underpants can be made by installing Velcro or zippers (or gripper snappers) along the bottom (crotch) edge. Similar openings may be inserted on one or both sides. Slits with zippers can provide for ventilation, as well as for reaching urinal bags or other appliances. There are also the overlapping slits so stitched that no fastening is necessary, as are found in the front of men's shorts and pajamas. Garments may be made to open out flat into one piece or form two separate pieces. Such flat clothing is easy to wash and iron and is particularly adaptable to the custodial care of severely disabled children and debilitated older persons.

Montessori (15, 40) dressing frames, sketched in Fig. 18.5, c and d and adaptations thereof are part of every occupational therapy program. In 1942 at New York's Institute for the Crippled and Disabled Rehabilitation and Research Center, eight authentic Montessori dressing frames equipped with snap-fasteners, three varieties of buttons, hooks and eyes, two kinds of laces, and one set of ribbons for tying and untying bows were used. It was soon obvious that undoing was easier than doing, and that the snaps were usually the easiest. The large buttons were next in difficulty, the laces and ribbons usually being even harder. Tying a bow is the hardest of all for many. For the one-handed, all fastenings present a challenge, and ingenious methods have evolved. There are step-by-step instructions describing in words and pictures the ways of manipulating the various fastenings. With their modern counterparts containing the latest in fasteners, such frames are excellent for evaluation. However, it is easy to be caught up in the zeal of teaching, only to realize after time has been spent that the particular situation would have been better solved by omitting the fastenings.

Besides Velcro and zippers there are a variety of fasteners on the notion counters of department stores (Figs. 18.4 and 18.5). In addition to the many sizes of ordinary snap fasteners, there are gripper snappers which snap with greater pressure. There is also a selection of hooks with bars for trouser and skirt tops, larger and more effective than the usual hooks and eyes.

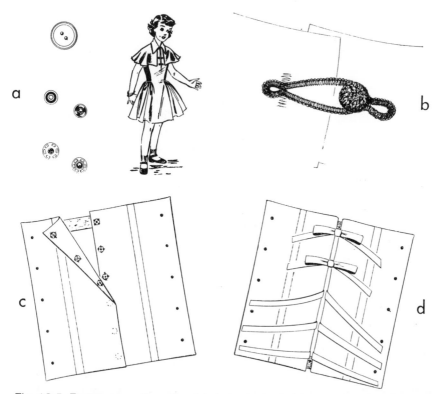

Fig. 18.5. Fasteners. *a*, Smooth, nickel-size button with rim and two holes allows use of electric sewing machine button attachment for sewing onto one-piece, self-help dress shown to right of it. Other features are stationary buttons with elastic between them permitting wide opening for head, cape-like sleeves, non-fastening collar, and elastically shirred panels, underarm to waist (Courtesy of *The Cerebral Palsy Review*). Also at *a*: gripper-snapper (⁷⁄₁₆ inch) and snap fastener (⁹⁄₁₆ inch); *b*, Homemade, elastic loop closure. Coarse nylon thread is crocheted around cylindrical elastic and looped over spherical button covered with the same crocheted nylon thread. Overall loop length, 4¼ inch, loop slit, 2½ inch; *c* and *d*, Authentic snap and ribbon-tying Montessori teaching frames made in Italy.

Buttons should be strong and durable (plastic may melt); of a size no smaller than a nickel; flat, round, smooth with a slight rim for easier handling (Fig. 18.5*a*); put on with long thread shank; in sight of buttoner; and in a color contrasting with the buttonhole for easier visibility. Buttonholes can be horizontal (25). They must permit pull in the line of stress. They need to be large enough to hold yet not allow the button to open. Fur coat frogs and other looping closures can be purchased or homemade (Fig. 18.4 and 18.5).

Shoelaces are a problem. Should we omit them for less effective substitutes? Loafers may not stay on. Elastic inserts may be tried. Elastic shoelaces and zippers, sports-shoe hooks instead of eyelets, with larger laces, and more manageable shoelace tips for holding are suggested. Various shoe-fastening devices are available (83, 85). Buckles have long been viewed by some therapists as superior to laces, especially on braces.

One of the most tantalizing of all fasteners is the garter. Sometimes it falls off. To reach it, to muster enough strength to secure it without tearing, to remain comfortable without losing one's stockings, weary the patience of many women. Pantyhose of fabric permitting ventilation may suit those who fit comfortably into available sizes and can put them on. Tights made by sewing ample stockings onto underpants may be stronger, less confining, and easier off and on. Stretch socks may be suitable if they do not reduce circulation. Tubular socks and stockings can be purchased that conform to the foot without having heel and toe shapes. A useful discussion of fasteners is given elsewhere (5).

SLEEVES

Sleeve variations are numerous and can be altered further to meet needs. The basic points are to avoid tight armholes and binding sleeves. Even the sleeveless garment needs a roomy, action-allowing but contour-fitting armhole. They may be altered to fit and to cover underwear if they are purchased too large. Wide sleeves cut from the same piece of material (kimono) are roomy. So are the kind that extend up to the neckline of a garment, giving a slanting seam line from the underarm to the neck in both front and back (raglan), as in Fig. 18.1. These allow action and tend less to split than the kimono. An underarm extension of blouse into sleeves allows extra "give" (46). Incomplete cap sleeves are favorites if underarms are well fitted so that underwear does not show. Butterfly sleeves are cool and becoming. No sleeves when possible is a good recommendation. In her back pack, a camper includes a pair of "sleeves" made from long underwear legs, each with an elastic loop for over the head. They take less room than a sweater. This design idea could suit a disabled person. Velcro patches might anchor better than loops.

Of the inset sleeves, short sleeves are preferred to long, except in special cases. Armhole tucks often given in patterns may be omitted so that sleeves can be roomier. Below-elbow sleeves may have a surplice cuff (46). Inverted, underarm seam pleats, gussets of pleasing design (23), and underarm, open-and-shut features (46) provide freedom of motion.

SKIRTS

Skirts, whether parts of dresses, separate tube-type or wrap-around, need adjustable waistlines. These may be elasticized all the way around or half way or with intermittent inserts of elastic. Adjustability may be afforded by the wrap-around if it ties.

If skirts are made with deep hems, slips may be left off. Some skirts are lined to eliminate slips. Skirts may be flared for action but should not be over-wide. Two to 2½ yards is recommended (46). Hip darts may be released. Inverted pleats and kick pleats may give extra roominess. Available on the market is a sheath style with action-full hidden pleats (53). Wrap-arounds may wrap toward the front or rear.

Capes have the easy feature of no sleeves. One design has two inside straps to keep it from falling off the shoulders (23). Ponchos are appealing garments that cannot fall off.

The dresses of very young girls may serve best without waistlines. They may be tent-style, that is, hung from the shoulders, or from a yoke. They may be jumpers with crisscross straps anchored one within the other in the back to stay over the shoulders, or some equivalent (8).

PANTS

Pants are overfoot trouser clothing to cover the lower trunk. They have two pantlegs for lower limbs or two thigh holes. Table 18.1 lists the usual kinds. This garment presents problems for the disabled, especially if it is of the form-fitting style. It has three major troublesome features: narrow pantlegs, the fly, and the perilous position when both hands are weak or paralyzed and cannot hold up the pants.

Designers and workers have faced all three. Pantlegs are wide regardless of style, unless tapering favors the individual's activities, such as might be the case in those who easily lose their balance when on crutches. Velcro is satisfactory for flies. A male nurse (30) describes straps attached to the trouser fly for the severely subnormal boy which allow for urination without need for unfastening the garment. Elastic webbing is used at the back of the waist, which is a half-style allowing the seat to drop while the pants do not.

For some, pockets are better in a blouse than in pants. Darts are omitted in front to reduce puffing up of material on the lap while sitting. Suspenders may be worn for convenience and safety in some cases. Belts can be omitted, simplifying the waist. A snap fastener is used at the top. For toilet purposes, an opening of 9 inches is best. The waist needs to adjust to weight changes. If the wearer is sedentary, the back is cut long and the front short to lessen puffiness on the lap. Custom-made, wheelchair suits are provided by a tailor (82).

Stretch fabrics are used for slacks. Darts are released if desired. Knee width is controlled in a number of ways. Hidden action pleats can be effective and decorative. A particularly attractive method is the shirring of side seams with replaceable elastic shown in a pair of self-help pedal pushers for non-brace users (46). The shirring provides extra length for knee action that contributes to comfort, yet permits safe, close fit.

Pantskirts are wide-legged pants simulating skirts. The wrap-around feature is applied to long pants and underpants. By separating pants into two garments each pantleg can be put on separately and tied like an apron or anchored with Velcro (73).

UNDERWEAR

For children, we can say, "Leave off the undershirt, and add a sweater for warmth." However, there is the problem of perspiration to say nothing of the nice feeling next to the skin of a light, soft, flexible, and comfortable piece of material with holes for ventilation. Some of the too closely woven and otherwise treated modern fabrics are cold, clammy, and airtight in winter. They are insufferably hot in summer; they are never comfortable. A soft piece of cotton underwear under a brace or prosthesis may feel good; it acts as padding and absorbs perspiration.

Slips may be opened down the front and split in the back. They may contain a terry-cloth panel for absorption in case of slight bowel and bladder or other discharge difficulties. Shoulder straps on slips and bras may be elasticized or otherwise adjustable.

Front-opening bras with drawstrings or Velcro are desirable. To make a back-opening bra into a front-opening bra (5), rip off the hook-and-eye piece in the back, seam the back together, cut the front and insert the hook-and-eye piece in the front. Some women like a short zipper in the front instead of the hooks and eyes. A third method is to use front drawstrings as shown in Fig. 18.3A. Shoulder-strap position is ensured by building up the straps or by horizontally strapping the straps in the back. Strapless bras may be tried for the more buxom.

Step-into bras, shoulder protectors, girdles, and slips are specialties of a mail order house (79). They feature front openings, Velcro fastenings, and four zippers on the girdle to allow staggered sequential closing; two extend from the middle downward and two from the middle upward. These items accommodate the one-handed dresser among others. Bra styles and sizes abound in the stores (86), so that it is worth shopping thoroughly for the style desired before resorting to items that need major changes.

LIMB CLOTHING

Mittens are easier to take off and put on, although gloves allow greater convenience and more exercise. The tethered gloves offered by one designer (23) have elastic bracelets which save the wearer from losing them.

Stockings are perishable and not easy-on or off for anyone. Seamless, stretch, no-run, mesh stockings, are relatively practical. Thigh-top stockings, some tubular, fit high in the groin with elastic tops and need no garters (86). Some of the elastic strands at the top may be cut at various spots to desired looseness.

Socks may have tabs sewed on their toes or to their sides to make flail toes possible to direct into shoes (29). Pantyhose have no garters but require a good fit.

Shoe soles may be patched with a round piece of non-slip material such as "Scotch-tred" for safety (29). Shoes may be open down to the toes, baseball fashion, for easier entry of the foot. In the opinion of this writer, shoes are among the most binding and crippling of all wearing apparel. To make shoes in pairs and nonadjustable seems contrary to nature, since no one has two feet identical in size or shape. Custom-made shoes from plaster casts conforming to the structure of each foot are a solution to many foot problems. Other approaches to footwear are included in the chapter on shoes.

HEAD AND NECKWEAR

The trend is away from hats and time-consuming hairdos toward scarves and hair-containing caps. If tying is difficult, the motion-handicapped person can use Velcro. Pull-on caps and stretchable, crocheted, and knitted winter hats protecting the ears are relatively easily put on. If firmer anchorage is necessary, a chin-strap can have a Velcro attachment. Wigs may simplify hair and headwear problems.

Special Clothing for Disabled

Some disabled have such complex clothing needs that special clothing must be obtained to meet them.

PANTS AND PROTECTIVE PANTS

An activity to be coped with about 10 or more times a day is emptying the bladder and bowels. For the person with motion difficulties, this may require more than usual attention to the selection of manageable underpants and the necessity for convenient openings and anchorage of other clothes. Such problems are multiplied when there is bladder or bowel dysfunction. Add to motor and voiding impairment, long double leg braces with or without a pelvic band and back brace, and personal hygiene and the use of the toilet may present sizable though not insurmountable hurdles. Underpants feel better under a brace than over it. Side-zippering one or both sides and providing snaps the full length of the crotch may be helpful. Velcro may be used in all three places if the strips do not touch the skin. Crotch pants with snaps are handy for those using bedpans. Under-brace pants protect the appliance from the soiling which causes undesirable odors, metal rust, and leather disintegration.

Special pants are available in many styles for protecting the disabled from the embarrassment of loss of control of bowels and bladder. The disabled person may not always be in a situation to make his elimination control work for him in time. He should be protected by padding.

The required features of incontinence protective garments are that they be waterproof, absorbent and washable or disposable; tight-fitting yet comfortable; functionally designed to permit easy and quick management, and as close to normal appearing as possible, even attractive. It is recommended that the site and type of openings and fastenings be chosen so that there is minimal movement of the person and minimal time spent. The requirements of those who need to undo protective clothing to attend to evacuation in a hurry must be considered.

Slip-on panties are hard to manage when long double leg braces on a pelvic band are worn. Panties with side or crotch openings are more convenient. It is wise to inform the orthotist ahead of time of protective padding needs so that details of the brace do not later complicate matters. There are plastic sprays available which may protect the leather and metal from the effects of incontinence.

A pair of ordinary bloomer-type panties was given a crotch opening with light snaps. These were used by an adult patient with residual poliomyelitis affecting the right upper extremity and causing flail lower extremities. They suited her because she did not have to raise herself but could unsnap the four snaps at the crotch when on the toilet. Without this crotch opening she was dependent on others for toilet needs in order to get her slip-on panties down.

The panties are usually worn under the braces. Because of the side or front openings, it is possible to open them, remove soiled filler, allow for bladder or bowel function, insert fresh filler, and close the openings. In this way the leather and metal of the braces are protected, and this means better hygiene and longer life for the braces.

A pair of practical protective pants is shown in Fig. 18.6. It can be put on in a sitting or lying position without pulling over the feet. It has a flap in the front which may be opened and closed without disturbing the waistband. For subject *H* (Fig. 18.3) this tricot pant treated for complete protection was purchased ready-made and an organdy pocket was sewed in to hold folded diapers as shown in the figure. Such strategic diaper placement prevents bunching yet concentrates layers according to need. Thus, the use of more than one diaper lengthwise is avoided. Organdy has body because it is finely woven, yet is soft after being washed. It may require such ingenuity on the part of a worker to make the difference between complete dependence and independence in daily activities. Disposable diapers having the stay-dry feature could be used or the pants could be made with a plastic covering.

For those wearing long double lower extremity braces, another design is the custom-made, plastic-lined, self-help panties used successfully in studying the toilet problems of seven children with spina bifida (20). They are cut short enough in the crotch to fit snugly, holding the padding close to the body and keeping it in place. The advantage in having the plastic inside is that these do not look like special panties. Furthermore, they do not need

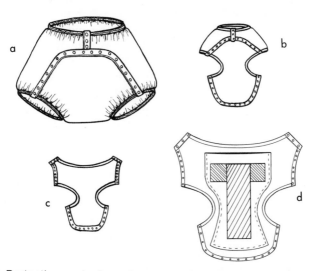

Fig. 18.6. Protective pants shown in consecutive stages of opening. *a*, Front view closed; *b*, Front flap dropped; *c*, Waistband opened; *d*, Pocket containing folded diapers. (Courtesy of Hilltop Supplies, Emerson, N.J.)

to be washed every time, since the padding inside can be changed. This model may be worn with the exact amount of padding needed. This is an additional advantage, inasmuch as one person's needs may vary at night and at different times of day. This also allows for improvement with training. To this model may be added the crotch opening with front panel or a pocket for holding a diaper or filler.

The filler or padding may be one or more regular diapers folded as desired, or cellucotton enclosed in gauze, such as that found in sanitary napkins, or disposable diapers ("Chux"). The dimensions of the pads depend upon the size of the individual wearing them and the amount of urine voided or feces eliminated. The raw cellucotton and other forms of layered absorbent paper may be purchased separately. By buying separately and in bulk, the exact amounts, sizes, and shapes can be cut as desired.

For non-brace wearers requiring incontinence protection, the side-opening designs are not usually necessary, unless such persons cannot reach their feet to put them on or encounter difficulty in lowering and raising panties. One 12-year old boy wore a rubber bloomer which anchored diapers.

Flip-on shorts are a novel idea for facilitating opening and closing of vents in front or back for bathroom purposes, especially in the care of the severely disabled. An overlapping pliable plastic hoop around the waist, upon which the garment is gathered, allows for easy separation of slitted garment and reclosing of it. If zippers are added, the hoop anchors the top as the one-handed person zips up the opening. The hoop procured was sold for making aprons.

Still more designs are to be found in the literature (5) and in the catalogues of supply houses (83, 86). Elasticized waist and thigh openings are desirable for adjustability and full protection of both person and appliance. Additional cotton-flannel panels may be inserted. Snap-in flannel liners may be purchased (83, 86).

The physical therapist's desire to study the limbs of the moving patient to correct his gait may be satisfied by the plastic pouch on a belt for men which fits comfortably around the buttocks and through the crotch and has ample space for disposable material or other filler (86). It provides safety day or night. Because it does not enclose the entire thigh, it is cooler than other protective garments.

A British fabric researcher (22) describes protective pants made of polypropylene, a fiber which permits liquid to pass through it without becoming wet itself while the skin remains dry. A disposable pad is held in a plastic kangaroo pouch on the outside of the garment (60, 96). As this design is for urinary incontinence only, one is needed for double incontinence. Colostomy pouches can be bought (86). A nurse (49) devised seatless clothing, saying, "We don't have to sit on our clothes." A Singapore physician (52) describes a sarong for hospital patients who wear indwelling catheter drainage of the bladder and need frequent nursing care. A bed jacket for the acutely ill patient in intensive care accommodates medical examinations and nursing procedures (31).

URINAL BAGS

Urinal bags are intimate and precarious appliances. They can be the source of great embarrassment and even injury if not kept immaculate, if the fit is incorrect, and if valves are faulty or not present to prevent backflow. Urinal bags can be purchased from supply houses (83, 86). They must fit perfectly and must be worn only according to the bladder and bowel training program meeting the individual's medical status and needs. One needs two urinal bags, as the airing of a cleansed urinal bag is imperative to control odor. Urinal bags need to be worn on a schedule which prevents skin irritation. If worn occasionally they may prove a boon in some situations. A man attending a theater, who cannot count on bladder continence over a period long enough to get him there and back without mishap, can enjoy himself more with a well fitting urinal bag which he does not use except in emergency. The clothing of the person wearing a urinal bag or other appliance must have suitable openings.

MENSTRUATION PROTECTION

Just as intimate and precarious as managing incontinence is the problem of menstruation in the case of motor impairment. Severely disabled women need the protection of plasticized and elasticized bloomers, over and above the necessary padding. An incontinent girl with spina bifida wore sanitary napkins against her body, topped by a cellucotton filling covered with gauze, held in place by incontinence pants (20) of the design shown in Fig. 18.6a and described earlier. The outermost layer was her snugly fitting, custom-made underwear doubling for gym suit (Figure 18.9). She was overweight and desperately needed her scheduled exercise periods. These were curtailed if her clothing ceased to protect her. One continent girl merely anchored her sanitary napkins to her gym-suit underwear by means of adhesive tape. Adhesive-backed napkins and sanitary pants made of stretch fabrics to anchor them are found in drug stores. Tampons should be tried when there is possibility of successful management.

BREAST FORMS

Breast forms for mastectomy patients were the invention of a compassionate corsetiere, Ella H. Bernhardt (7, 47). She struggled to simulate the normal breast with padding and other solids and later with liquids that at first gurgled and leaked. Her lifelike breast forms come in 26 sizes and are sold worldwide (81).

A nurse (61) describes other prostheses and gives addresses of mastectomy specialty shops selling forms and clothing (80, 88), and of companies which provide lists of stores selling their products. Some department stores carry mastectomy bras and fillers (86).

The American Cancer Society (34) has a "Reach to Recovery Program" for women who have had a mastectomy. At the request of the attending surgeon, a trained volunteer, who herself has had a mastectomy and returned to normal life successfully, visits the patient in the hospital. "Living proof" of the ability to resume normal life, the volunteer offers information on breast forms and clothing, answers the patient's nonmedical questions, and assists in the performance of exercises approved by the surgeon.

In a booklet, written by the Program's Founder (34), a good fit by a qualified corsetiere is recommended, and instructions are given for making your own breast forms and swimsuits, and adjusting your own bras and other clothing articles.

GYM SUIT DOUBLING FOR UNDERWEAR

An intriguing idea emanating from the exercise tables, platforms, and floor mats in schools and clinics, is that of the exercise costume doubling for underwear. Most persons who have suffered loss or impairment of motion are likely to need exercise. The chore of removing school or street clothes, putting on gym suits, then the reverse process, is time-consuming, and underwear doubling for the gym suit has been found practicable. The top clothing if cleverly designed may be removed and replaced quickly, often by the disabled person himself.

The play suit with halter strap in Figure 18.9 is also shown in the upper left sketch above subject F (Fig. 18.3). Many attractive, ready-made play-suits are suitable for mat exercises and may serve as underwear, too. Colored cotton panties with closed thigh bands can be purchased inexpensively. The child's self-help development should be the guide to the selection of the gym suit doubling for underwear. A bra top was added to this pattern for a developing girl with a spina bifida mentioned above (20). An elasticized halter strap was attached to the bra which was in turn anchored to the bottom of the playsuit by two elasticized bands. The entire garment was made of strong material to allow minimal yet adequate coverage for exercise freedom, at the same time encouraging self-help.

CLOTHING ADAPTATIONS FOR WHEELCHAIRS, CRUTCHES, AND CANES

Equipment and appliances are hard on clothing. Ready-made clothes are best purchased with attention to fabric, quality, and workmanship. Reinforcements are recommended, especially under arms, in crotch, over elbows, around knees, and where braces or other appliances touch. The management of clothing worn by wheelchair users can be eased by noting the following points:

For wheelchair wear a) a two-piece dress does away with the pull on the neck occasioned by sitting on a dress which does not give; b) a blouse may get dirtier sooner and can be easily changed; c) long sleeves are cumbersome and are easily soiled; d) a wrap-around skirt makes raising the body unnecessary and facilitates preparation of clothing for use of toilet; e) a slip can be omitted and a camisole-type garment worn over the bra if the blouse is thin; f) a stadium rug with full-length zipper may tuck in both lower limbs for warmth and glamor (23); g) short jackets to the seat of the chair prevent sitting on them which restricts movement; h) pant seats, longer and more ample than usual, prevent binding; i) fewer front tucks and fullness at the waist of pants, dresses, and skirts prevent bulkiness in lap; j) zipper and other openings are less puckering if not centered; and k) capes, seat-length in back and with side slits, are easy to manage and have an air of distinction (23).

Dressing the severely incapacitated has been studied by a nurse (49), resulting in apron-style, seatless pants, and backless dresses that can be tucked around the body for normal appearance.

For crutch-users, clothes can be hazardous, and the following points are given: a) because of the wide range of shoulder joint and shoulder girdle movement, extra fullness of men's sleeves is recommended; b) women crutch-users do better with inset rather than kimono or raglan sleeves; and c) excessive fullness of skirts, jackets, and pantlegs may entangle person and crutches, especially if balance is uncertain.

Brace-users soon find clothing details of concern. The following hints are offered: a) pantlegs must be wide enough to encompass the braces and allow easy donning, whatever openings are devised; b) all lower trunk garments must be larger if pelvic bands and incontinence protection are worn; c) loosely knit underwear catches in brace locks; d) two-piece dresses allow for the greater amount of wear and tear on skirts; e) culottes may serve to conceal braces better than skirts and be more easily donned than slacks; f) inside seams of trousers need finishing off so as not to get caught on brace latches; g) hard-finished, oil-resistant, and anti-static treated fabrics are desirable; and h) in cold climates, pajama bottoms under braces can give warmth and circulation in spinal-cord injuries when sensation is defective. They can also ensure comfort, warmth, and circulation in post-poliomyelitic patients as well as in other conditions in which circulation is under par. Colored ski underwear or tights with necessary zipper adaptations added might serve some disabled as long underwear under braces. This would keep extremities warm, protect them from the coldness of the metal, yet allow opening for toilet activities.

Our woman hiker of the light pack wears short pants. When she gets cool, she elongates them by applying wrap-around legs with Velcro fasteners. Layered clothing is handy in that one can peel off according to need. A three-piece pantsuit can be worn all at once, with a sleeveless blouse underneath and an added cape.

In Accent on Living, Fall 1977, a woman writes, "My brace made shambles of my underwear till I began making pants of nylon tricot. The fabric stands up like iron"(90, 42). Two authors (56) describe adapting Simplicity patterns to subjects wearing Milwaukee body braces.

APRONS AND BIBS

Apron patterns with purposes and special features are analyzed and detailed by Scott (46). Among the many designs are a plastic hoop at the waist to eliminate tying, a corded rim to secure contents, and a crumb-catcher. Easy-to-don, utility aprons, bibs, and "stay neat" dresses with decorative, detachable bibs, and full-length panels can be purchased (53). Laryngectomy bibs and scarves for protection and camouflage are crocheted or made from knitted dishcloths (34).

COMBINATION GARMENTS

The disabled wardrobe shopper may consider the possible advantages of combined pieces of clothing in order to reduce the number of garments needed (5). Table 18.1 lists them and some are given below: a) If a knee-length pant-slip is worn, a slip can be omitted; b) the bra-slip, sweater-slip, and blouse-slip may facilitate undressing and dressing and can be easily adjusted to accommodate front-center openings; c) ski-type pajamas and coveralls in one piece with stretchable head and limb openings may be swiftly donned and zipped up.

NECKTIES

Although men's neckties can be omitted, pictorial, step-by-step instructions are available from clothing manufacturers. Some like to pre-tie, slip over head, and adjust. Bow-tie and four-in-hand styles can be purchased with clips or snaps. Bolo ties from the West have colored cords with sliding holders which do not require tying; they are put over the head and the ends pulled to the desired length. They are worn on informal occasions and may match or harmonize with the shirt or suit. A necktie of the same fabric as the shirt makes a pleasing outfit (23).

BELTS, BUCKLES, COLLARS

Other better-left-off items are belts, buckles, and collars. If belts are worn, they should be attached and longer than normal for adjustability. An idea is to pre-tie a sash and use Velcro to attach. If a belt is used for lifting a patient to a standing position, it must be of good leather and be anchored by sufficient sturdy loops to ensure safety (29). A collar can ride up while its wearer propels a wheelchair. If collars are desired, they can be sewed down. High necklines and collars may be used to hide irregularities.

POCKETS

No pockets are better than those out of reach and too small, such as tiny, high-up, blouse pockets and most pants pockets. Ample front pockets on shirts are preferable (9). A well designed pocket can be especially helpful to the disabled housewife (46). Useful pockets are easy to reach, large enough to hold many articles, and slanted so that objects do not fall out. Velcro or a zipper may be used to lock them. A bellows-designed, pouch pocket has further expandability and can be conveniently and modishly worn on a dress or on a belt (23).

Bags, purses, and carry-alls for the wheelchair, crutch, and cane-user are suggested, and some are available commercially (53, 87). These include a purse-cane or crutch combination, a carry-all to fit onto a crutch, and bags of various designs for wheelchair arms.

Suggested also are roomy, dress or skirt pockets placed low enough for easy access and away from the lap. The pocket may be worn on a belt which can ride forward or backward as desired. Detaching snapped-on pockets from aprons converts them to handbags. A small coin pocket on a sleeve is suggested by a bus rider.

Self-Help Clothing Studies

Three self-help clothing studies conducted by this author culminated in results illustrated in the nine case summaries at the beginning of the chapter. Daily activity inventories were taken of 47 children with cerebral palsy in four classes in three public schools as part of the Cerebral Palsy Program of the New York State Department of Health (11). This study revealed that:

"Thirty performed no dressing and undressing; fourteen, undressing, but not dressing; none accomplished all dressing and undressing ... ; nineteen in the upright position did not readjust clothing after toilet activities. Dressing and undressing have been outstandingly difficult. These activities require considerable coordination. A very great difficulty, however, is the unsatisfactory clothing—fastenings which do not fasten; shoe-strings that are too short and often untipped, tearing at the least force; overalls and suspenders that are too tight and do not hook or stay hooked; buttons on trousers which are so small as to defy buttoning, or which have buttonholes which do not permit the entrance of the buttons; long underwear, buttoning in the back with tiny ineffectual buttons; dresses with minute buttons at the top of a tight neckband; slip-over sweaters often too small, in layers .... Inability to adjust and readjust clothing before and after toilet activities reinforces further the need for more care with children's clothes, as well as a better selection. The minutes per day spent on such activities by parents and therapists add up to hours that might be turned to better account for all concerned.

"Why not capes, instead of layers of tight turtleneck sweaters? Why not sturdy diaper-like pants with snaps, instead of flimsy ones which get torn being pulled off and on over braces? Why not wrap-around skirts, or culottes, instead of tight overalls or slacks? Why not ski pants that zip up the side? Why not dresses and blouses with zippers or large buttons and buttonholes in front, rather than unreachable ties and microscopic buttons in the back? Why not narrow bands with buckles on braces instead of wide bands with laces? And why not shorter hair on those who cannot manage their own, instead of long curls which get tangled up in the sweaters, bibs, slings and back braces?"

A second study (14) used a daily time schedule. An analysis of 26 categories of activities performed by a school staff included undressing and dressing children and taking them to and from the bathroom. An excerpt follows:

" ... One of the major time-consuming, annoying and frustrating features was the clothing worn by the children. There are two reasons why this subject needs study: a) Independence in dressing and undressing is a foremost aim (and this includes toilet mechanics and hygiene: adjusting clothes before and after bladder and bowel evacuation, and also attention to menstruation needs). Clothes must be such that it is mechanically and humanly possible for the children to handle them. b) Manageability of severely disabled who cannot be taught, needs to be facilitated, and one very important method is workable, manageable clothes."

An undressing and dressing study based on total-person inventory-evaluation was done at Sunnyview Hospital and Rehabilitation Center, Schenectady, N.Y. (19, 54). The undressing and dressing achievements of subjects A through I (Fig. 18.3) are taken from their daily activity inventories. Inventory-evaluation details on seven of the nine subjects are charted in a prevocational evaluation study (18).

Inventory-evaluation means taking inventory of what the disabled person does in the motions and activities required for daily life and work, including undressing and dressing. It also means taking inventory of the clothing itself, in order to isolate features causing difficulties and hampering independence.

The first edition of this book (68) carries a fuller discussion of our inventory-evaluation method and describes 18 checklists, examinations, and evaluations which we assembled to obtain our best estimate of the motor status and potential of one with motor handicaps. Samples may be available (13).

The two most critical inventories concerning clothing are the daily activity inventory (12) and the clothing skill inventory reproduced in Table 18.2. This chapter advocates the evaluative process (12, 16–20) as the foundation for an effective teaching program.

Teaching Undressing and Dressing

"The two-year-old can take off his shoes as well as his stockings and pants .... When being dressed he is not only cooperative but definitely helpful .... Some children ... like to undress over and over again as a game ... " (28). The young child's natural interest is stirred by giving him

TABLE 18.2. *Clothing Skill Inventory*

The page is lined horizontally to form blocks. Items performed within times set by the therapist as adequate are filled in. Date and time columns allow a variety of uses. Reverse order of items provides a mounting direction for achievement, especially effective if date column is filled in at first inventory. Other color coding can indicate later achievements.

Name			Blue, with help Red, independent						
No.	Inventory List	Date	Time	Date	Time	Date	Time	Date	Time
50.	Manage fastenings in back of dress								
49.	Overcoat on								
48.	Overcoat off								
47.	Turn clothes right side out								
46.	Small buttons, button								
45.	Small buttons, unbutton								
44.	Snap, fasten								
43.	Bowknot, tie								
42.	Bowknot, untie								
41.	Zipper, up								
40.	Zipper, down								
39.	Simple knot, tie								
38.	Lace shoes								
37.	Belt through loop on trousers/dress								
36.	Trousers on								
35.	Trousers off								
34.	Skirt on								
33.	Skirt off								
32.	Dress on								
31.	Dress off								
30.	Shirt on								
29.	Shirt off								
28.	Shirt on over undershirt								
27.	Shirt off over undershirt								
26.	Undershirt, no sleeves on								
25.	Undershirt, no sleeves off								
24.	Large buttons, button								
23.	Large buttons, unbutton								
22.	Shoes on								
21.	Shoes off								
20.	Socks with elastic tops on								
19.	Socks with elastic tops off								
18.	Socks with ribbed tops on								
17.	Socks with ribbed tops off								
16.	Sweater on								
15.	Sweater off								
14.	Buckle, fasten								
13.	Buckle, unfasten								
12.	Jersey loop around waist, on								
11.	Jersey loop around waist, off								
10.	Jersey loop on head								
9.	Jersey loop off head								
8.	Jersey loop on right leg								
7.	Jersey loop off right leg								
6.	Jersey loop on left leg								
5.	Jersey loop off left leg								
4.	Jersey loop on right arm								
3.	Jersey loop off right arm								
2.	Jersey loop on left arm								
1.	Jersey loop off left arm								

clothes he can manage. By the time he is 4 "the child . . . usually dresses and undresses himself with very little assistance, though he may need his clothes laid down on the floor, each garment separately oriented so that he can slip into it . . . . Almost all children, even though they dress themselves poorly, enjoy dressing up in adult clothes, especially in hats, gloves, shoes, belts and with pocketbooks" (28).

This natural interest is used by a school teacher who provides her therapist teamworkers with a "fireman's vest" of scarlet hue to add zest to teaching dressing and undressing. Concentration and effort are obvious as the child furiously struggles to get into the glorified coat-type garment. Undressing and dressing are willingly undertaken by many of his playmates just to wear the "fireman's vest." A play approach interests children in learning to put on and take off hats, scarves, gloves, and many other clothes.

No matter how simple clothing skills may seem to adults, childhood is the time to learn them. Self-care learning is as dependent upon intelligence and application as learning to read and write. Daily scheduled practice at home and at school keeps the child's clothing management skills apace with his academic learning. In fact, the child's development is advanced if physical and academic programs are carried on at the same time rather than one lagging behind the other or being neglected altogether. Concentration and work habits become more solidly established by consistently encouraging and expecting them at an early age, whether for dressing, study or playing a game.

The skills of undressing and dressing require learning ability and readiness. Some children master them quickly and easily. Some need repetition and practice for long periods of time. Others need simple changes made to their present wardrobes. And still others need specially designed articles of clothing cut to individual measurement. The child first needs an evaluation of his abilities in undressing and dressing. Then he needs to master the skills of undressing and dressing at an age comparable to that at which such skills are usually learned (24, 28, 38, 39). He needs graduated methods and a program geared to his own growth pattern.

For the adult, the same principles of evaluation and graduated teaching methods pertain. The challenge lies in the mutual conviction of patient and therapist that the roads to independence are worth the traveling.

Once the evaluation details are known, the teaching program begins. The clothing entity chart (Table 18.1) and the clothing skill inventory (Table 18.2) can be guides for assembling the most common garments. When the evaluation shows little or no accomplishment, the therapist is obliged to think analytically. For instance, the therapist seeks a method for teaching the overhead placement of a circular piece of clothing with hole for head such as T-shirt, skirt with elastic waistband, or tube dress. The following materials are prepared, as shown in Figure 18.7:

a. Three rings of cotton roving, the rings being thick enough to grasp, and graduated in size from a diameter of 12 inches to the size of the opening wanted, for instance, 12 inches, 10 inches, 8 inches.

b. Three pieces of soft, stretchable, loosely-knit jersey tubing of varying degrees of width and stretchability, about 12 inches in depth, narrowing to size wanted.

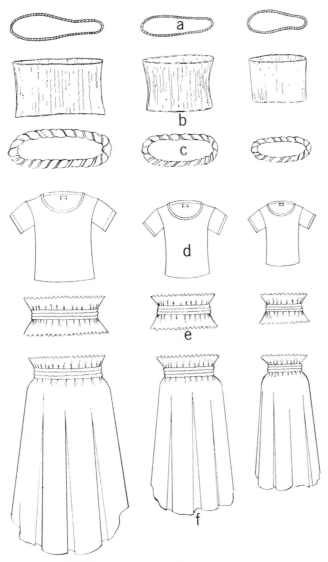

Fig. 18.7. Graduated teaching materials in three sizes for step-by-step instruction in removing and putting on tube-type and T-shirt garments. a, Rings of cotton roving; b, Jersey tubing before rolling; c, Jersey tubing softly rolled to form rings; d, T-shirts; e, Elasticized skirt bands; f, Complete skirts with elasticized waistbands.

c. Three sizes of jersey tubing like those in *b* but softly rolled to form rings.

d. Three sizes of actual T-shirts graduated in size and from loosely-knit to tighter mesh, all stretchable.

e. Three elasticized bands similar to waistbands.

f. Three entire skirts with three-rowed elastic waistbands from large to approximately one desired.

Undressing is easier than dressing because the pieces are withdrawn with no necessity for the withdrawn article to be in any one position as is the case with putting on clothing. Therefore, the various items are tried out with the individual one by one. The steps in teaching the overhead removal and placement of the loops, tubing, elasticized bands, and skirts may be as follows:

To take off: a) insert hands under loop; b) raise loop to neck over shouldertips; c) pull loop over head.

To put on: a) place formed loop on head; b) pull down around neck; c) pull down over upper extremities to waist; d) release upper extremities.

For those attracted to such graded teaching procedures, the Montessori Method (15, 40) has sensorial materials especially suitable to work with the disabled.

For T-shirts, the steps are:

To take off: a) pull assisting (not lead) arm out of sleeve into shirt, grasp underarm seam with lead hand and pull it over assisting elbow; b) pull back of shirt over head, head coming free of neck opening of shirt; c) shake shirt off lead arm.

To put on: a) spread garment in front of subject; b) run each arm into its respective sleeve; c) grasp entire back of garment in fingers with thumb through back of garment's neck hole; d) pull over head, stretch, then adjust shirt.

A coat dress may be donned in various ways, three of which are given here. The usual way is to insert one hand, then the other. The assisting hand goes first. Before inserting the better limb into the second sleeve, it is good to reach to the back of the neck and adjust the garment by pulling it over the shoulder so the sleeve is in place. Another way is to place the coat, neck toward subject, lining uppermost. He then runs both arms into the sleeves and takes the coat over head to fall in place on his back. A third way is to hang the coat, with lining facing out, on the back of a chair or hanger at a height corresponding to the wearer. He backs up to the coat and slips hands into dangling sleeves. Squatting down, he pushes his arms into the sleeves to the point where the coat can be drawn up over his shoulders.

Two self-help hints for teaching putting on brassieres are: a) put brassiere on backwards and fasten back-opening in front. Turn garment. Pull shoulder straps up. Adjust. b) fasten and adjust opening, whether in front or back, and put on overhead as tube garment. Adjust shoulder straps and body of garment.

It is always rewarding to this therapist to evoke from the individual his own maneuvers before giving him suggestions. Three persons with similar appearing hemiplegia may devise different methods. A woman with left hemiplegia learned to dress herself completely with wrap-around skirts and front-fastening dresses and brassieres. Another woman with left hemiplegia became independent in her dressing and undressing activities by having all her zippers moved to the right side from their usual places on the left as is the case with women's slacks, blouses, and other side-opening garments. A third patient with left hemiplegia fastens her favorite form-fitting, back-zipping slacks by bending forward from a standing position. She reaches behind her and with her right hand grasps the zipper. Because of her bent-over position, the seat of the garment is stretched taut over her buttocks, and there are no wrinkles. She moves the zipper upward smoothly as she resumes the upright position. Then she fastens the man-size hook and eye at back of waistband. Still another, Mrs. Odell, the founder of FashionABLE (79), allows the following quotation:

"As to your questions about side openings for hemiplegics—on the basis of my personal experience, plus considerable observation, I couldn't agree with you more that you should think of the individual rather than disability groups. I have hemiplegia of the left side, am left handed, with that hand so spastic it is useless in dressing, and I assure you it doesn't make a bit of difference which side the opening is on. The only exception I could possibly see to this would be in the case of obesity, in which the longer reach might be complicated by excess fat. I'm sure you are familiar with stroke cases who, with only limited return, manage better than others who are basically better off. Much, I'm afraid, depends upon the attitude."

Other teaching methods have been described (3, 10, 26, 77). A set of 27 slides from the Sister Kenny Institute shows dressing operations (97). A one-handed author uses body parts, such as catching long-sleeved garments between the knees (57). A Canadian nurse gives attention to the clothing of the elderly in nursing homes (41), and a home economist studies preferred style features in dresses for physically handicapped elderly women (45). Tips for the blind include coding with buttons, lace, and rickrack (70, 75). Braille color clothing tags are available (21). A method of teaching dressing to mentally retarded is described (4). Dressing aids are the special province of occupational therapists (see Chapter 19; 36, 37, references under IIA). Dressing and undressing, with and without aids, can be exercise if repeated as a drill, once a method has been established.

Assembling a Self-Help Wardrobe

Self-help styles are like any others. One design or feature appeals to some and fails to satisfy others. One person says vehemently, "I do not like Velcro ... give me a nylon zipper with a grabber any day." The individual benefits most if he can help to choose the styles and self-help features which please and work for him.

Styles for self-help may be grouped into those which can be remodeled from presently existing wardrobes, bought ready-made, homemade from patterns, and specially created or assembled according to the need, such as the popular Sunnyview Style.

REMODELING GARMENTS

It is not necessary to throw away the entire wardrobe. Remodeling ideas are plentiful (9, 37). With self-help clothing features in mind, remodeling can be rewarding. A common first step is making a button-down-the-back dress into a button-down-the-front dress by remodeling collar and belt. Many mothers substitute elastic around the waist for a tight waistband. Armholes can be enlarged. Openings can be extended to below the waist. Hems can be faced to make deeper, or skirts lined, so slips can be eliminated. Fastenings can be simplified by making them bigger and more manageable. Buttonholes can be changed to suit the need. All openings can be enlarged. Sometimes a one-piece dress requiring help for putting on can be made into a two-piece allowing complete independence. Inserting side zippers on shorts and trousers is another popular remodeling feature. Zippers may have tab pulls or loops added. Sewing circles can be formed, so that mothers of crippled children can exchange ideas with each other. Therapists and teachers can interest volunteers in the universal subject of clothes.

BUYING READY-MADE CLOTHING

With self-help features in mind, a mother can select appropriate items from ready-made clothing. Sometimes the clothing can be adjusted easily. The following ready-made clothing articles have self-help features and are worn by many crippled children and adults: undershorts for boys, enclosed boxer-top, front opening; shorts for girls, to which luggage side zippers may be added; jeans, in which full-length side zippers can be inserted; pants, boxer-top, complete waistband, no opening; shirts for boys and girls, stretchable T-shirt-type; loosely woven sweatshirts and sweater-like slipovers with and without collars in different colors, striped or plain; shirts for boys, short-sleeves, coat-type with half-inch buttons; coats for boys, loose-fitting with large buttons; skirts for girls and women, wrap-around in denim; playsuits for girls to double for underwear and gym suits; tubular jersey dresses with no fastenings; popular knitted two-piece dresses; loosely knit jersey blouses with bat wing sleeves and woolen skirts that have wide elastic at top; open-down-the-front, printed nylon jersey dresses, easily laundered and requiring no ironing.

CHOOSING AND ADAPTING PATTERNS

With self-help clothing features in mind, it is possible to find the desired pattern in pattern books, which contain pull-over garments, wrap-arounds, tunics, caftans, stretch slacks of varying lengths and with built-in growth features, in a wide choice of accommodating fabrics (2, 35, 43, 50, 75, 96). One McCall pattern was suitable without any changes (19). Others have been adapted from Simplicity and Butterick patterns. Occupational therapists modify patterns and suggest specific patterns (29). Other pattern companies are Vogue, Kwik-Sew, and Folkwear. Sister Kenny Institute has a booklet with over 30 fashion designs adapted from available patterns (9), and a team collaborates on a pattern study (59). The Texas Research Center (77) sells clothing patterns for physically and mentally handicapped persons.

"Middy" Blouse and Skirt

Here are the changes made on a Simplicity middy blouse and skirt. Omit neck fastenings. Enlarge armholes 1 to 1½ inches to fit ungathered sleeves. Insert side zipper in blouse on left or right according to needs of child, or leave both sides of blouse slit 3 inches in middy-blouse fashion. Use 2½ inch elastic on waist of skirt instead of band made of material. Side-zippered, having no neck fastenings, this ample middy blouse and pleated skirt in a cotton broadcloth are easy to put on, loose, comfortable. This is a style repeatedly recalled by fashion designers. A costume of such long-standing popularity and sketched in Figure 18.8 has appeal because it lends itself to many variations, including its traditional sailor's "middy" backdrop collar when desired.

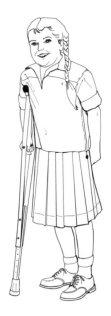

Fig. 18.8. Two-piece middy blouse and skirt with no neck fastenings, side zipper on blouse, and elastic in waistband, adapted from a Simplicity pattern. (Courtesy of Sunnyview Hospital, Schenectady, N.Y.)

Playsuit

A Simplicity playsuit pattern served for the underwear-gym suit shown in upper left sketch above subject *F* (Fig. 18.3), with the following changes. Make a newspaper pattern from the playsuit pattern extending the sides for ties to wrap around the waist instead of buttoning down the sides. Insert elastic in the halter strap and at the back of the waist (Fig. 18.9). This playsuit is put on in the morning as underwear. A self-help two-piece dress worn over it is removed for exercise. This same pattern may be further adapted to provide an elastic-backed brassiere moored to the wrap-around by elastic bands.

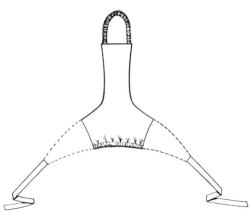

Fig. 18.9. Playsuit doubling as underwear and gym suit, adapted from a Simplicity pattern. Elastic in halter (at top) and at back of waist (at bottom). The garment is held in front as the halter is put on over the head, then taken between the legs and wrapped around the waist. (Courtesy of Sunnyview Hospital, Schenectady, N.Y.)

MAKING A SUNNYVIEW DRESS

The popular Sunnyview two-piece dress was first made in 1950. It is worn by subjects *C* and *E* (Fig. 18.3). It can be assembled from ready-made or homemade garments. It is a deep-hemmed elastic waist-banded tube skirt with no fastenings. It has a matching or contrasting ready-made T-Shirt or other ready-made blouse with trim to go with the skirt or homemade blouse. The skirt pattern (Fig. 18.10) and the instructions follow. Take 2 yards of cotton dress goods 36 inches wide, and seam A and B together. Turn hem at the top 3 inches in width. Measure 1 inch down from the top, and mark this 1 inch width all the way around. Stitch along the other three lines which are ⅝ inch apart. Measure three strips of ¼ inch elastic to fit the waist of the individual. Run it through the three lower parts of the top hem, leaving the top to frill. Turn up the bottom hem the desired length, making it 8 to 10 inches deep.

This style is popular because of its simple design, quick assembly, and

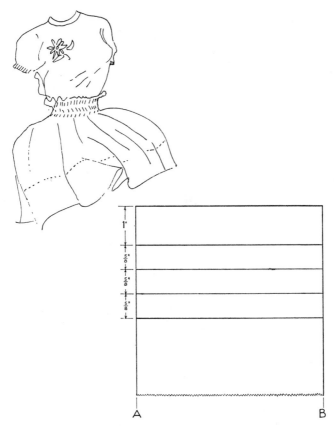

Fig. 18.10. Sunnyview two-piece dress combines trimmed T-shirt with homemade skirt. Deep hemmed, tubular skirt needs no fastenings because of its stretchable, three-rowed, elastic waistband. Simple design, quick assembly, wide size range, and combining possibilities make it practical and popular for girls and women of any age for day or evening wear with long skirt and fancy top. (Courtesy of Sunnyview Hospital, Schenectady, N.Y.)

matching possibilities for change of costume. It meets the needs of many girls and women of different ages, conditions, and disabilities. It has a wide size range, the same size pattern encompassing the usual sizes 6 to 10. Therefore, it is outgrown slowly, because of its adjustable waist and deep hem. The skirt has the additional advantage of being easy to remove for exercise periods and put on again.

Prepleated materials, with the option of tapered pleating, can be bought to individual measurement which need only one vertical seam to make a flattering skirt with a soft elastic at the waist. Shirred-top fabrics can be purchased for instant skirts (and also dresses) requiring one seam and no waistband.

Clothes Consciousness Through Teamwork

Four ways to enlist interest in self-help clothing are 1) to teach children and adults to make their own, 2) to form sewing circles for parents, patients, and other family members, 3) to foster volunteer services among hospital women's auxiliary groups, and 4) to have fashion shows for fun and education (13, 54).

Subjects *A* and *F* (Fig. 18.3) learned to make their own self-help clothes. The Schenectady parents met with the occupational therapist at lunchtime and after school once a week and were shown ways to remodel their children's clothing toward self-help.

An undergraduate senior (6) undertook to teach dressmaking to four children in a crippled children's school. They helped to choose and buy their materials and made simple ponchos and dresses.

Making your own clothes can be a hobby for men, women, and children. All can learn with the easy-to-sew patterns marked for different sizes, wide choice of fabrics (2), versatile sewing machines, and sewing aids (36, 50, 57). Fabric stores can suggest sewing books, classes, and patterns. One source provides sew-it-yourself kits (87). An article gives directions for making underwear with nylon tricot fabric (42). All about textiles and their maintenance is given in a booklet (2).

Children and adults with atypical motion benefit from comprehensive care offered by a wide variety of persons with specialized training. Because of its universal appeal, clothing lends itself to the interests and skills of many persons. Clothing for the disabled is naturally conducive to the delicate human activity of interprofessional teamwork (references under IC).

Another teamworker might be a computer researcher who would use the clothing information centers (references under IIB) to retrieve from the mass of reported details a basic wardrobe suitable for a large enough group of disabled persons to support manufacture. Some authors are pointing the way (27, 35, 43, 59, 63, 69, 70). One (35) cites the "cardigan" (a warm jacket of knit worsted, with or without sleeves) as the most likely ready-made garment to accommodate a large population.

We list some principal self-help clothing features as an aid to team workers: Loose fitting garments with openings easily seen and reached; generous armholes; nonstick linings for coats and blouses; action features such as hidden pleats and underarm inserts; roomy, two-piece dresses; skirts with elastic waistbands; stretchable T-shirt tops with large openings for head; well-fitting, attractive colored bathing and playsuit type underwear doubling for gym suits; front dropping underpants with snaps on sides for use when braces are worn; side-zippered shorts and pants for severely disabled, especially when braces are needed; simple fasteners, preferably none; if used, buttons to be large with buttonholes to fit, directed along line of stress and placed for manageability; zipper pulls large enough to grasp, placed on sides of shorts and pants when braces must be covered; elastic necks, waists, leg openings; front drawstrings and zippers when necessary for girdles and brassieres; ample openings for extremities with elasticized leg openings for protection; tube-type, or with opening extending below waist if dresses are one-piece; stretchable materials when possible, such as in T-shirts; deep hems to avoid slips; slide hooks rather than lacings or leather straps with holes and a pointed prong; loafer-type shoes rather than shoes with laces; rubber shoelaces, if laces seem desirable, or zippers hidden by flap or decoratively placed with permanently tied shoelaces.

The cardigan sweater (35), the Sunnyview Dress (Fig. 18.10), and the designs shown in Fig. 18.2 are principal examples of practical and versatile garments most adaptable to the needs and tastes of large numbers of people, regardless of age, size or degree of ability or disability.

Our team's aim is to find simple garments to clothe the person, so that our "second skin" (64), our "nearest environment" (75), fosters growth of the being within.

Acknowledgments

The author of this chapter owes special recognition and gratitude to five teamworkers for their invaluable roles, under many circumstances and over many years, in the development of the information on self-help clothing summarized in this chapter. They are Miss Moira M. Ward, R.N., Mrs. Mary Easton van der Bogert, O.T.R., Mrs. Evelyn Hall Johnson, O.T.R., Mrs. Elizabeth M. Wagner, O.T.R., and Miss Blanche Talmud, R.P.T.

I. SELECTED REFERENCES*

1. AHRBECK, E. H., AND FRIEND, S. E. Clothing—an asset or liability? Designing for specialized needs. *Rehabil. Lit.*, *37:* 295, 1976.
2. AMERICAN HOME ECONOMICS ASSOCIATION. *Textile Handbook*, ed. 5. The Association, Washington, D.C., 1974.
3. AMERICAN OCCUPATIONAL THERAPY ASSOCIATION. Dressing techniques for the cerebral palsied child. *Am. J. Occup. Ther.*, *8:* 8, 48, 1954.
4. AZRIN, N. H., SCHAEFFER, R. M., AND WESOLOWSKI, M. D. A rapid method of teaching profoundly retarded persons to dress by a reinforcement-guidance method. *Ment. Retard.*, *14:* 29, 1976.
5. BARE, C., BOETTKE, E., AND WAGGONER, N. *Self-Help Clothing for Handicapped Children.* National Society for Crippled Children and Adults, Chicago, 1962.
6. BATINALE, M. Adaptive dressmaking for handicapped children. Senior project submitted in partial fulfillment of the requirements for the degree of bachelor of science in home economics. California Polytechnic State University, San Luis Obispo, 1977.
7. BERNHARDT, E. H. The rehabilitation of mastectomy patients. *R.N.—A Journal for Nurses*, October, 1953.
8. BOETTKE, E. M. *Suggestions for Physically Handicapped Mothers on Clothing for Preschool Children.* Bulletin I. School of Home Economics, University of Connecticut, Storrs, 1957.
9. BOWAR, M. T. *Clothing for the Handicapped: Fashion Adaptations for Adults and Children.* Sister Kenny Institute, Chicago Avenue at 27th Street, Minneapolis, Minn. 55407, 1977 (Revised 1978).

10. BRETT, G. Dressing techniques for the severely involved hemiplegic patient. *Am. J. Occup. Ther.*, *14:* 262, 1960.
11. BROWN, M. E. Daily activity inventories of cerebral palsied children in experimental classes. *Phys. Ther. Rev.*, *30:* 415, 1950.
12. BROWN, M. E. Daily activity inventory and progress record for those with atypical movement. *Am. J. Occup. Ther.*, *4:* 195, 1950; *5:* 23, 1951.
13. BROWN, M. E. *Fashion Show and Folk Dances.* Prepared for Second Congress World Confederation for Physical Therapy, 1956. Available from M. E. Brown, 684 Bernardo Ave., Morro Bay, Calif. 93442.
14. BROWN, M. E. Fashions for C.P.'s. *Cerebral Palsy Rev.*, *12:* 3, 1951.
15. BROWN, M. E. MARY ELEANOR BROWN: Montessori Pupil/Physical Therapist. Communications, No. 1, 1978, p. 26 (Amsterdam, The Netherlands).
16. BROWN, M. E. The patient's motion ability: evaluation methods, trends and principles. *Rehabil. Lit.*, *21:* 46, 78, 1960.
17. BROWN, M. E. Physical and occupational therapy in stroke care. *J. Rehabil.*, *29:* 33, 1963.
18. BROWN, M. E. AND VAN DER BOGERT, M. E. Pre-vocational motor skill inventory: preliminary report. *Am. J. Occup. Ther.*, *7:* 153, 1953.
19. BROWN, M. E., VAN DER BOGERT, M. E., WARD, M. M., AND HALL, E. Why should children dress themselves? Self-help clothing stories of nine crippled children, with patterns. Unpublished report of studies done at Sunnyview Hospital and Rehabilitation Center, Schenectady, N.Y., 1957.
20. BROWN, M. E., AND WARD, M. M. Toilet problems of seven children with spina bifida. *Phys. Ther. Rev.*, *33:* 632, 1953.
21. BRUCK, L. *Access: The Guide to a Better Life for Disabled Americans.* Random House, New York, 1978.
22. CLULOW, E. E. Clothes for the handicapped. *J. R. Coll. Gen. Practitioners*, *24:* 362, 1974.
23. COOKMAN, H., AND ZIMMERMAN, M. E. *Functional Fashions for the Physically Handicapped.* Institute of Rehabilitation Medicine, New York, 1961.
24. DAVIS, V. Clothing for the pre-school child. Leaflet 191. Extension Service, University of Massachusetts, Amherst, 1954.
25. DAVIS, V. Self-help fasteners. Leaflet 281. Extension Service, University of Massachusetts, Amherst.
26. FOWLES, B. H. Dressing techniques for the hemiplegic patient. In *Syllabus of Rehabilitation Methods and Techniques*, 1963. Available from author, 7520 Curtiss Ave., Sarasota, Fla. 33581.
27. FRIEND, S. E., ZACCAGNINI, J., AND SULLIVAN, M. B. Meeting the clothing needs of handicapped children. *J. Home Econ.*, *65:* 25, 1973.
28. GESELL, A., AND ILG, F. L. Infant and Child in the Culture of Today. Harper, New York, 1943.
29. HALL, D. S., AND VIGNOS, P. J., JR. Clothing adaptations for the child with progressive muscular dystrophy. *Am. J. Occup. Ther.*, *18:* 108, 1964.
30. HILL, N. J. W. Special trousers for the subnormal child. *Nurs. Times*, *58:* 818, 1962.
31. JONES, E. S., AND CARTER, R. J. A bed jacket for the acutely ill patient. *Nurs. Times*, *60:* 894, 1964.
32. KENT, G. Velcro: Newest magic fastener. *Reader's Dig.*, March, 1959.
33. KOHLBECK, B. Clothing for the arthritic: practical yet fashionable. Senior project submitted in partial fulfillment of the requirements for the degree of bachelor of science in home economics. California Polytechnic State University, San Luis Obispo, 1977.
34. LASSER, T. *Reach to recovery.* American Cancer Society, 777 Third Ave., New York, N.Y. 10017, 1974.
35. LORD, J. Clothing for long-stay patients. Parts I and II. *Nurs. Mirror*, *132:* 14, 40, 1971.
36. LOWMAN, E. W., AND KLINGER, J. L. *Aids to Independent Living: Self-Help for the Handicapped.* McGraw Hill, New York, 1969.

37. MACARTNEY, P. *Clothes Sense for Handicapped Adults of All Ages.* Disabled Living Foundation, London, England, 1973.
38. MOELLER, F., AND TINGLEY, K. A. *Children and Their Clothing.* Cooperative Extension Service, University of Connecticut, Storrs, 1962.
39. MOELLER, F., AND TINGLEY, K. A. *Girls from Nine to Thirteen—Their Clothing Abilities.* Cooperative Extension Service, University of Connecticut, Storrs, 1952.
40. MONTESSORI, M. *The Montessori Method.* Frederick A. Stokes, New York, 1912.
41. MORGAN, D. M. Sensitivity programs and special clothing for the elderly. *Dimen. Health Serv., 54:* 44, 1977.
42. NEMETH, K. Undergarments for the woman with special needs. *On Your Own, 5:* 1, 1975 (Division of Continuing Education, Box 2967, University, Ala. 35486).
43. REICH, N. Clothing for the handicapped and disabled. *Rehabil. Lit., 37:* 290, 1976.
44. SAVASTANO, A. A. Shoulder straps, girdles and garters. *Rhode Island Med. J., 49:* 664, 1966.
45. SCHUSTER, J. D., AND KELLY, D. Preferred style features in dresses for physically handicapped elderly women. *Gerontologist, 14:* 106, 1974.
46. SCOTT, C. L. *Clothes for the Physically Handicapped Homemaker, with Features for All Women.* Home Economics Research Report No. 12, Government Printing Office, Washington, D.C., 1961.
47. SELIGMANN, W. New breast form for mastectomy patients. *Am. J. Surg., 86:* 466, 1953.
48. SEPLOWITZ, C. Panty hose aid. *Am. J. Occup. Ther., 29:* 424, 1975.
49. SMITH, R. They were dressed! *J. Psychiatr. Nurs.,* May–June, 1966.
50. Talon/Velcro Consumer Education, 41 E. 51st St., New York, New York 10022. Convenience clothing and closures booklet.
51. THIEL, L., AND SHAW, L. Little people have big problems. *On Your Own, 8:* 1, 1978 (Newsletter, Division of Continuing Education, Box 2967, University Ala. 35486).
52. TINCKLER, L. Urological sarong. *Br. J. Urol., 42:* 496, 1970.
53. VOCATIONAL GUIDANCE AND REHABILITATION SERVICES, Cleveland, Ohio. Functionally Designed Clothing and Aids for Chronically Ill and Disabled. Report on National Seminar, November 9-10, 1966.
54. WARD, M. M. Self-help fashions for the physically disabled child. *Am. J. Nurs., 58:* 14, 1958.
55. WARD, M. M. Toilet seats for disabled children. *Am. J. Nurs., 57:* 127, 1957.
56. WARDEN, J., AND DEDMON, K. Clothing design uses style and utility. *J. Rehabil., 41:* 17, 1975.
57. WASHAM, V. *The One Hander's Book.* John Day, New York, 1973.
58. WATSON, C. C. M. Zipper injuries. *Clin. Pediatr., 10:* 188, 1971.
59. WHITE, L. W., AND DALLAS, M. J. Clothing adaptations. The O.T. and the clothing designer collaborate. *Am. J. Occup. Ther., 31:* 90, 1977.
60. WILLINGTON, F. L. Marsupial principle in maintenance of personal hygiene in urinary incontinence. *Br. Med. J., 3:* 626, 1973.
61. WINKLER, W. A. Breast cancer: Confronting one's changed image. *Am. J. Nurs., 77:* 1433, 1977.
62. YEP, J. O. *Clothes to Fit Your Needs.* Leaflet Pm-570. Cooperative Extension Service, Iowa State University, Ames, June, 1973.
63. YEP, J. O. Tools for aiding physically disabled individuals increase independence in dressing. *J. Rehabil., 43:* 39, 1977.

A. Clothing

General encyclopedias have historical accounts.

64. HORN, M. J. *The Second Skin,* ed. 2. Houghton Mifflin, Boston, 1975.
65. LANGNER, L. *The Importance of Wearing Clothes.* Hastings House, New York, 1959 (Paperback, 1977).

66. MANCHESTER, H. H. *The Evolution of Dress Fastening Devices from the Bone Pin to the Koh-i-noor*. Written for Waldes and Company, Inc. Long Island City, New York, 1922.

B. Chronology of Clothing for Disabled

67. WAGNER, E. M. Clothing for the physically handicapped 1937–1962. In *Rehabilitation of the Physically Handicapped in Homemaking Activities*, American Home Economics Association Workshop Proceedings. Government Printing Office, Washington, D.C., 1963.
68. BROWN, M. E. Self-help clothing. In *Orthotics Etcetera*, edited by S. Licht, ed. 1, Elizabeth Licht, Publisher, New Haven, 1966.
69. HALLENBECK, P. M. Special clothing for the handicapped: Review of research and resources. *Rehabil. Lit.*, 27: 34, 1966.
70. LAMB, J. M. Clothing for handicapped children: Recent developments. *Rehabil. Lit.*, *38:* 278, 1977.

C. Interprofessional Teamwork

71. WHITEHOUSE, F. A. Some characteristics of comprehensive rehabilitation teamwork. In *Contemporary Vocational Rehabilitation*, edited by H. Rusalem and D. Malikin. New York University Press, New York, 1976.
72. JUDSON, J. S. The team approach. *J. Home Econ.*, *50:* 702, 1958.
73. NEWTON, A. Clothing: a positive part of the rehabilitation process. *J. Rehabil.*, *42:* 18, 1976.
74. SCHWAB, L. O., AND SINDELAR, M. B. Clothing for the physically disabled homemakers. *Rehabil. Rec.*, *14:* 30, 1973.
75. WATKINS, S. M. New careers for home economists: Designing functional clothing. *J. Home Econ.*, *66:* 33, 1974.

II. SOURCES

Classified telephone directories; public health nurses; local libraries; local department, fabric, and speciality stores; local units of groups serving specific conditions, such as The American Cancer Society (34); local schools and adult education programs; State university extension services; State and Federal government services through Department of Health, Education and Welfare, Washington, D.C. 20201 or call Federal Information Center.

A. Clothing and Aids

76. American Foundation for the Blind, 15 W. 16th St., New York, 10011.
77. Caddell, K., Textile Research Center, Box 4150, Lubbock, Texas 79409. Clothing for physically and mentally handicapped persons.
78. Damart, Inc., 1811 Woodbury Avenue, Portsmouth, N.H. 03801. Thermal underwear.
79. FashionABLE, Rocky Hill, N.J. 08553. Special clothing for women and aids.
80. Joyce Hart Salon, 709 Madison Ave., New York, N.Y. 10021. Complete mastectomy fashion service.
81. Identical Form, Inc., 17 W. 60th St., New York, N.Y. 10023. Breast forms.
82. Leinenweber, Inc., 69 W. Washington St., Chicago, Ill. 60602. Men's clothing for wheelchair-bound.
83. J. A. Preston Corporation, 71 Fifth Ave., New York, N.Y. 10002. Incontinence pants and aids.
84. PTL Designs, Inc., Box 364, Stillwater, Okla. 74074. Apparel manufacturing for the elderly and physically handicapped.
85. Fred Sammons, Inc., Box 32, Brookfield, Ill. 60513. Shoe fasteners and aids.
86. Sears, Roebuck and Company. Sanitary and incontinence pants, mastectomy bras, breast forms, and thermal underwear.
87. Smith, C. O., 7674 Park Ave., Lowville, N.Y. 13367. Custom-made garments and sew-it-yourself kits.

88. "Miss Stevens," 321-A South Robertson Blvd., Beverly Hills, Calif. 90211. Mastectomy clothing.
89. Vocational Guidance and Rehabilitation Services, 2239 E. 55th St., Cleveland, Ohio 44103. Manufacturer of special clothing and aids.

B. Clothing Information Centers

90. Accent on Living, Inc., Box 700, Bloomington, Ill. 60701. Publishers of Accent on Living Magazine and Buyer's Guide for Disabled.
91. American Home Economics Association, 2010 Massachusetts Ave., N.W., Washington, D.C. 20036.
92. Clothing Information and Research, School of Home Economics, University of Arizona, Tucson, Ariz. 85721.
93. Disabled Living Foundation, 346 Kensington High St., London, W 14 8 NS, England.
94. Institute of Rehabilitation Medicine, 400 E. 34th St., New York, N.Y. 10016.
95. National Easter Seal Society for Crippled Children and Adults, 2023 W. Ogden Avenue, Chicago, Ill. 60612.
96. Shirley Institute, Didsbury, Manchester M 20 8 RX, England.
97. Sister Kenny Institute, Chicago Ave. at 27th St., Minneapolis, Minn. 55407.

*RECENT REFERENCES

HOFFMAN, A. M. *Clothing for the Handicapped.* Charles C Thomas, Springfield, Ill., 1979.

KERNALEGUEN, A. *Clothing Designs for the Handicapped.* University of Alberta Press, 1978.

19

Self-Help Aids

BECKY MONNARD LOOSEN, M.A., O.T.R.

Self-help aids can be defined as devices which enable a person with a physical disability to function more independently. More specifically, they are frequently standard objects of daily use, *e.g.*, comb, spoon, shoe laces, modified in their design or construction to enable the user to become more self-sufficient. Orthoses and therapeutic equipment are generally not considered to be self-help aids in the true sense of the definition and will not be considered in this chapter.

A self-help aid should be designed and selected primarily to increase a person's independence, allowing the user to perform some task or activity that he could not perform without it. Furthermore, the self-help aid could allow a person to perform a selected activity in a shorter time or with less expended energy. If self-help aids are to fulfill this major purpose, the user must regard the task or activity to be of personal importance. He must recognize the need for the device, be committed to learning to use it, and be willing to incorporate its use into his daily activities.

Self-help aids are but one means to accomplish specific rehabilitation goals. The selection and use of these devices should be an integral part of the entire rehabilitation process and should be considered in conjunction with other treatment goals and alternative methods of meeting those goals. While self-help aids can be used either temporarily or permanently, it is important to establish long-term goals and to avoid sacrificing these goals for short-term functional gains which preclude the attainment of the long-term goals. When considering a person for a self-help aid, it is important to assess the whole person, determining his abilities, needs, and those factors which will potentially influence acceptance of the proposed aid. Of equal importance is the assessment of the device's intended purpose, limitations, construction, and prerequisite functions required for utilization. Only after considering all of these factors should one decide whether the person should receive a self-help aid.

Personal factors potentially influencing the selection and acceptance of the self-help aid include: (a) physical function; (b) cognitive abilities; (c) psychological acceptance of the disability; (d) social and cultural pressures; and (e) economic and vocational factors.

Personal Factors

PHYSICAL FUNCTION

Some areas of function are routinely evaluated in persons having a physical disability. These include: range of motion, muscle strength, prehension, hand placement, sensation, coordination, muscle tone, balance, and ability to perform activities of daily living (ADL). To evaluate selection of self-help devices, it is imperative to determine exactly what the individual can do. If he is unable to complete an activity independently or uses an unreasonable amount of time or effort, what specific factors contribute to his inability to perform adequately? Given this information, one can determine what specific areas of daily function may be improved with the use of a self-help aid. One can also decide the availability of physical resources and their adequacy to meet the physical requirements to utilize certain devices.

Self-help devices are not intended to replace general areas of physical function but to compensate for physical limitations for a specific activity. Indications for the use of these devices include: (a) position or support of the body, as with the elevated toilet seat with safety bars; (b) stabilization of objects, as with the use of a suction holder or Dycem matting; (c) compensation for loss of function of a body part due to paralysis, as with a utensil cuff, rocker knife, or adjustable head pointer; (d) compensation for loss of range of motion due to muscle weakness or structural limitations, as with a curved bath brush, long-handled shoehorn, or extension eating utensils; (e) compensation for increased involuntary motions, as with the use of weighted utensils, a typewriter keyboard shield, or weighted wrist cuffs; (f) compensation for sensory deficits, as with the vibrating alarm clock or Braille wrist watch.

PSYCHOLOGICAL FUNCTIONING

Self-help aids vary in design and operation, ranging from simple to complex. If a device is to become a part of an individual's daily routine, he must understand how the device works and must have the necessary cognitive abilities to utilize the device. Consideration should be given the cognitive abilities of the individual, the skills required to manage the device, and the complexity of the training program required for its use. Simplifying existing devices by modifying, combining, or deleting certain portions of the device may make operation easier.

It may be argued that most handicapped people never completely accept their disability, continuing to question why it happened to them and to believe that they will one day return to functioning "normally." This lack of disability acceptance should not be confused with an individual's inability to acknowledge specific functional deficits. However, only after a person has admitted his limitations and wishes to improve his functioning capabilities can he be expected to see the merit of accepting and utilizing a self-help aid. An individual who has not recognized and accepted the functional limitations of his disability is an unlikely candidate for self-help devices. Several factors directly related to the disability will influence the speed and degree to which an individual is likely to accept self-help aids. These include the age at which the disability developed, the individual's perception of its functional effects, and the duration and prognosis.

In general, very young and middle-aged persons are more likely to accept an aid than are teenagers or the elderly. Presumed unfavorable reactions from peers frequently discourage a teenager from accepting and using a self-help device. Reluctance to incorporate new patterns into long-established habits and belief that little time remains often contribute to rejection by an elderly person.

Frequently, how a person perceives his disability is as important, if not more important, than the actual pathological changes. Given the same physical status, some persons will perceive the impairment as altering their capabilities while still leaving them with many resources; others will perceive it as an inconvenience, but a few, at the other extreme, will perceive an impairment of a similar type as a devastating hopeless problem. Those who believe that they have certain functional problems but are capable of altering some of them are most likely to accept self-help aids. In contrast, persons who perceive their impairment as either an inconvenience or a hopeless problem are least likely to use aids.

How an individual accepts a needed self-help device usually correlates positively with the duration of the disability. Persons with long-standing disabilities who have passed through the stages of denial, anger, and depression concerning their disability are in a better position to work toward functional improvements. However, individuals with long-standing disabilities who have functioned for years without self-help devices are likely not to accept devices not providing significant functional gains.

The prognosis of a disability may influence the acceptance of a self-help device. Individuals with a stable prognosis and a permanent disability more than likely will accept a device. In contrast, those with the prognosis of ultimate deterioration or steady improvement may reject the device. If the individual believes that the pending functional deterioration will happen so rapidly and will be very severe, he may reject the device as a waste of energy and time. If the individual believes his prognosis is to return to normal, he may reject a device because he feels that engaging in other therapeutic activities is more profitable.

Accurate assessment of an individual's psychological readiness to accept a self-help aid is imperative. Introduction of the device too early in the rehabilitation process may create a rejection unfavorably influencing later attempts to incorporate its use into daily activities. On the other hand, the aid should not be introduced too late, as this may convey that it is a last resort. Because self-help devices are frequently foreign to the average person, one must judge the timing and manner of introduction correctly. Efforts should be made to introduce the device to the patient in a non-threatening manner, assuring him that he will not fail in its use. It is important that the device's capabilities be accurately portrayed. The user should not misconstrue a device's limitations as a result of his inadequacy.

Social and Cultural Factors

Beauty, strength, and self-sufficiency are three characteristics highly valued and sought by many because of social and cultural pressures. A person with strong internalization of these values may believe that a self-help device is, or is perceived by others, to be a violation of these values, and so may reject or rarely use a device. Such a person may make certain assumptions that outweigh its functional merits or restrict its use to "protected environments" such as the clinic, institution, or home. The following assumptions influence decisions as to use. Self-help devices are objects generally thought to be unesthetic or obtrusive, which may draw attention to the user and his problem. Using a self-help aid may be interpreted as a sign of physical and mental weakness, suggesting that a person lacks the strength or mental fortitude to overcome his problems. Lastly, although devices increase function in many individuals, their use may connote dependency. If an individual characterizes the device as being cosmetically unacceptable or a sign of weakness or dependency, rather than as a functional tool, he is unlikely to accept it.

Social and cultural factors also determine roles as well as behaviors and expectations for those roles. Devices which assist a person in accomplishing tasks perceived by that individual and those around him as appropriate are most readily accepted. However, aids which require the individual to assume different responsibilities or an unacceptable role are frequently considered as unnecessary or frivolous. For example, an individual whose entire family has been involved in ranching and farming for generations may be reluctant to accept communication aids that will enable him to assume a desk job. One should be aware of social and cultural factors influencing the client which may determine his acceptance of a self-help device. The initial impulse of a therapist or other health personnel may be to establish different values for the client, but this is usually unrewarding. A more productive approach is to select, present, and construct a device that meets the client's values and expectations.

Economic and Vocational Factors

Cost factors may influence willingness to purchase and use self-help aids. Economic gains derived from using devices may also be influential. If the functional aid will enable a person to earn a living, the cost is of secondary importance. This is particularly true if the individual perceives that his employer's and associates' reactions are favorable. Devices which make attendants unnecessary or simplify care may also be willingly purchased. Whether a person chooses to purchase self-help aids is to some extent influenced by the economic needs and resources of the family. Although the cost cannot be ignored, it should be of secondary importance to function, as often a variety of financial resources are available to secure needed devices.

The Device

The features of a self-help aid which determine selection and use include: (a) design; (b) construction; and (c) availability.

DESIGN

Self-help devices should be selected on the basis of their ability to provide a specific function. Their design should accomplish the desired purpose as simply and efficiently as possible. A versatile device is frequently more readily accepted than several different devices. For example, an individual may prefer a utensil cuff for feeding, facial hygiene, and typing over utensils and objects, each of which has been adapted with a palmar cuff. Complicating a device with "gadgetry" that provides no additional or needed function should be avoided. The user must have the skills needed to manage the device, and one should use an individual's physical abilities, instead of overriding them. Design should be consistent with good body mechanics and should allow the user to conserve energy. Motions required to use the device should duplicate, where possible, those normally utilized for that specific activity. One should avoid devices which pose potential safety hazards due to the patient's medical complications. Although a self-help aid may be operationally safe, it may be contraindicated due to the physical or psychological status of the user.

The self-help aid should have clean simple lines which are cosmetically pleasing but still achieve the desired mechanical goal. It should be as compact and lightweight as possible to allow for easy use, storage, and transportation. To decrease the amount of adjustments and maintenance required for operation, avoid unnecessary appendages and articulations. When a device includes mechanical parts subject to large amounts of stress and use, care should be taken to ensure that the parts can be easily obtained and replaced.

CONSTRUCTION

Careful consideration should be given the construction of a self-help aid relative to its design and use. Quality of construction depends upon materials and workmanship inherent in fabrication. As no device can function beyond its physical capabilities, proper selection of materials and quality workmanship enhance these capabilities. Materials may differ as to their durability, elasticity, flexibility, mechanical strength, corrosion resistance and heat tolerance. They also differ in ductility, elastic memory, compressibility, weight, choice of color, texture, shrinkage, hardness, and life expectancy. No one material should be universally used for all devices. The material selected should meet both the mechanical needs of the device and the needs of its user. For example, if an individual needed an assistive device for washing dishes, it should be constructed from corrosion-resistant material with high heat tolerance. Also consider the anticipated duration of use. Since the material in the device must maintain its appearance and form after continual use, it should be durable and easily cleaned and should require minimal maintenance. Materials cosmetically pleasing to the user may increase the device's acceptance and use.

Color is probably the factor that most determines a material's cosmetic appeal. The quality of construction of a self-help aid is as important as the quality and type of materials selected in determining patient acceptance. Fastenings should be secure and placed to avoid bony prominences or hypersensitive areas. Edges should be smooth and, if possible, rounded to prevent any potential injury. In devices needing assembly or interlocking parts, components should fit snugly and provide mobility only where needed. Surface finish should be smooth and clean, absent of tool marks, excess materials, gouges, or other demarcations. Seams and joints should be appropriately finished to prevent separation, fraying, and excessive bulk. Most importantly, the device must fit its user. Although a device may be purchased ready-made, it is still necessary to evaluate its fit and make any modifications required for use.

AVAILABILITY

Self-help devices may be obtained through commercial sources or fabricated by appropriately skilled personnel. Each method has both its advantages and disadvantages. It is generally to the user's benefit to purchase devices commercially, as they are relatively low in cost and of high-quality design and construction. However, as the number of devices commercially available is limited, it may be necessary to fabricate the desired aid. The availability of these devices is influenced primarily by the skills and creativity of the personnel constructing the device and their access to the needed materials and equipment. Those devices that can be quickly obtained and require a minimal number of modifications will tend to be the most readily accepted.

TRAINING

Once the device has been appropriately selected and constructed, the individual needs instruction in its use and care. A training program should teach the application, use, and maintenance of the device and allow the individual sufficient time to master each of these. Factors which are believed to influence learning should be considered, such as the user's attention span, motivation, need for reinforcement, level of verbal and written comprehension, and ability to retain and generalize information. The method of instruction and the environment in which it will occur should be structured to maximize the user's ability to learn the needed skills. The user should first learn to apply and remove the device properly and as independently as possible. Incorrectly applied devices will not work to their mechanical advantage or feel comfortable. Next, the individual must be able to position and grasp the device, accurately place the extremity, and release the device. If grasp is not required, placement and control of the extremity become the most crucial preactivity skill. The user should then be ready to learn use of the device with specific activities. Each activity should be analyed for prerequisite functioning and logical sequencing and then presented in small graded units so that the user is not overwhelmed by detail. As the user's abilities, confidence, and tolerance increase, higher expectations can be set for the devices use until long-term goals have been met. Throughout this training program, the device should be periodically rechecked and modified for proper fit and mechanical functioning. Although the user may make mistakes and become frustrated, he may have valuable suggestions to offer the trainer about his specific problems. The user should learn care of the device, such as storage and cleaning, minor adjustments needed, and remedies for frequently encountered problems, as well as the guarantee or warranty and where service and parts are available. This information should be provided in writing. Since it is a long-term goal for the user to regard the aid as an essential tool and incorporate it into daily activities, one should maintain contact with the user and family to help with unanticipated problems. One should also periodically re-evaluate the device to ensure that it continues to operate effectively, and to introduce new or improved aids when feasible.

Self-Help Devices

On the following pages are a few examples of self-help aids that have been described in books, journals, or catalogs. Some of these are commercially available, and others have been constructed for a specific individual but offer alternatives to related problems. They are only a small representation of those available and are grouped by specific ADL with reference to their compensating abilities.

EATING

Compensation for Loss of Function of a Body Part due to Paralysis

Loss of grasp is a frequently encountered problem. Devices that compensate for grasp replace the holding component of the hand, for example, a cuff which surrounds the hand or several digits. It may be attached individually to each utensil and object or it may consist of one cuff which has a pocket for fitting many utensils and objects. Some examples of these are as follows.

(a) A utensil holder is an encircling cuff made of plastic, Velcro, or leather, with a pocket on the palmar aspect to hold the utensil. It is available in various sizes and may be further adjusted with elastic or Velcro closures (Fig. 19.1). Adaptions of this cuff include the Quad Utensil Holder and Right Angle Pocket. The Quad Quip Utensil Holder has a tapered semi-rounded wooden base that supports the palmar arch of the hand and positions the utensil at a distance from the palm. For fastening, it has a continuous loop of Velcro passing through a rectangular ring and securing on itself with a "D" ring pull (Fig. 19.1). The Right Angle Pocket slides into the pocket of a cuff and holds utensils, such as a knife used for cutting meat, that need to be positioned somewhat perpendicular, rather than parallel, to the palm (Fig. 19.1).

(b) A U-shaped cuff fits partially around the hand, with a pocket on the palmar aspect for the insertion of utensils. The pocket adjusts to various angles to position the utensil for effective use. Constructing the device of a

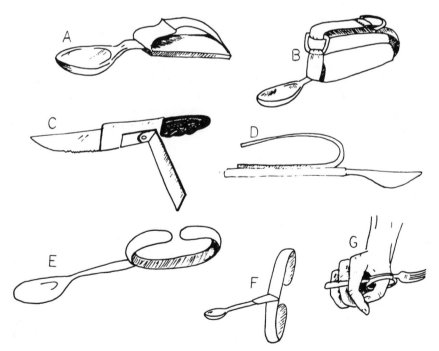

Fig. 19.1. Eating utensils. *A*, utensil holder; *B*, Quad Quip utensil holder; *C*, right angle pocket; *D*, U-shaped cuff; *E*, horizontal utensil; *F*, vertical utensil; *G*, thumb loop utensil (C. E. Nelson).

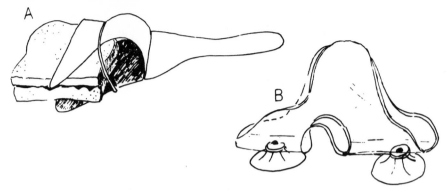

Fig. 19.2. Sandwich holders. *A*, designed for utensil holder; *B*, table-suction sandwich holder (Weiss).

plastic that retains its shape will allow its user to slide his hand securely into the cuff without using closures (Fig. 19.1).

(c) Utensils may be individually attached to a cuff that partially surrounds the hand, having a dorsal opening and no fastenings. Spoons and forks attached parallel to the palmar bar require a fully pronated position. Those attached at a right angle allow for the forearm to be in midposition (Fig. 19.1). A knife may be attached to this type of cuff at a different position and angle to allow for lever action and clearance of the digits when cutting.

(d) A thumb loop of plastic or metal attached to a fork or spoon allows the utensil to rest on the dorsal aspect of the thumb. A handle laced between the first and second fingers gives added support (Fig. 19.1). Cuffs which are permanently attached to utensils should be of durable plastic or plastic-coated metal to withstand corrosion, dishwashing detergents, and high temperatures.

(e) A sandwich holder may be inserted into a cuff or stabilized on a table (Fig. 19.2).

(f) A glass or cup may be supported in a holder with one or two cuffs mounted on the side for use with the forearm in midposition. The user slides his hand through the cuff, allowing the top of the cuff to rest on the radial side of the index finger (Fig. 19.3).

(g) By using a hose clamp and thumbscrew, a glass or cupholder may be adapted to various circumferences (Fig. 19.3).

(h) A long straw with a holder allows the user to consume liquids without picking up a glass or cup. The diameters of the straws may vary from 1/8 inch to 1/4 inch to accommodate different consistencies of liquids. Plastic couplers may be used to gain additional length by attaching two straws together (Fig. 19.3).

(i) The glass or cup can be positioned in an adjustable base to prevent tipping or can be held at a designated angle (Fig. 19.3).

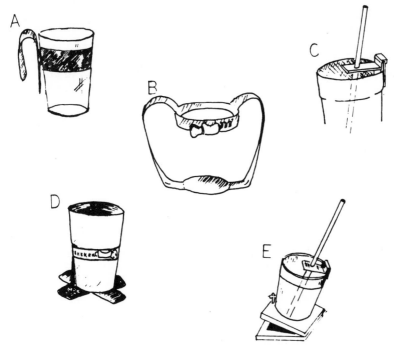

Fig. 19.3. Glass-and-Straw adaptions. *A*, glass holder; *B*, bilateral glass holder; *C*, straw holder; *D* and *E*, glass stabilizer.

As feeding is primarily a unilateral activity, persons with complete functional loss of one upper extremity can usually feed themselves after instruction in adapted techniques. One problem frequently encountered is cutting meat. A knife with a curved blade used in one hand with a rocking action, rather than the sawing motion of a table knife, allows stabilization and cutting of the food (Fig. 19.4). A pizza cutter also may solve this problem. An adaptive fork with curved side blade or rocker knife with tines will accomplish the combined purposes of a fork and a rocker knife (Fig. 19.4).

Compensation for Loss of Range of Motion due to Muscle Weakness or Structural Limitations

(a) Objects and utensil handles may be enlarged with foam padding, Plastisol-coated aluminum cylinders, bicycle grip handles, wood, plastic, or other materials. However, one should avoid adding too much weight for upper extremity strength. Using built-up utensils with hollow handles and selecting materials by their cubic weight are two means of eliminating significant weight gains (Fig. 19.4).

(b) Utensils with expandable stainless steel handles are easily bent to the size required.

(c) Swivel and bent-angle utensils are two types of devices used effectively with a pronated forearm. Selection of the size and type of handle grip should be made according to the user's hand function (Fig. 19.4).

(d) Extended handles compensate for loss of range of motion of the elbow or shoulder. Utensils of standard size may be interchanged in an extension handle with a pocket or they may be individually lengthened, with extended handles permanently attached. A wing nut on the extension handle or an adjustable pocket will allow the angle of the utensil to vary (Fig. 19.5).

Compensation for Increased Involuntary Motion

(a) Weighted utensils or weighted wrist cuffs may temporarily decrease involuntary motions to the point where self-feeding is possible. Too much weight should be avoided, as long-term use may increase involuntary motions.

(b) Several types of automatic feeders are available for persons with severely impaired function due to involuntary motions. These feeders are generally activated and controlled by gross upper extremity movements or by a head stick (Fig. 19.5).

(c) A weighted cup or a covered cup with a spout may be used to drink liquids and decrease spilling (Fig. 19.5).

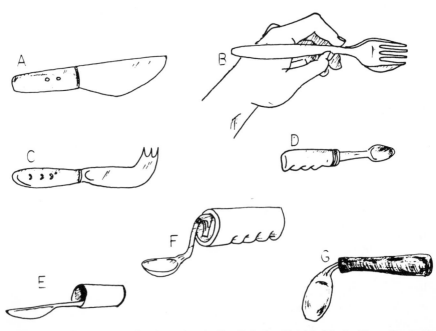

Fig. 19.4. Eating utensils. *A*, rocker knife; *B*, fork with side blade; *C*, rocker knife with tines; *D*, built-up-handled spoon; *E*, built-up-handled knife; *F*, swivel spoon; *G*, bent-angle spoon.

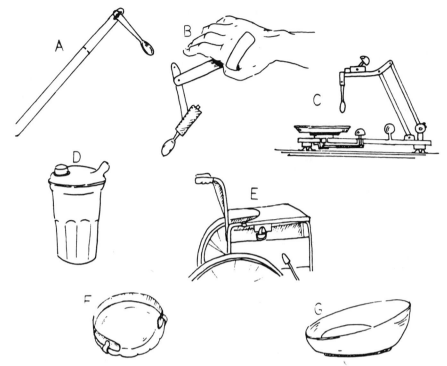

Fig. 19.5. Eating utensils and aids. *A*, adjustable-extension spoon; *B*, extension handle with adjustable pocket; *C*, automatic feeder (Orthopop); *D*, covered cup with spout; *E*, lapboard; *F*, plate guard; *G*, scoop dish.

Position and Support

Lapboards and trays help position the wheelchair bound individual for eating and accomplishing other activities. Rubber "O" rings and T-bar supports may be used to attach the lapboard to the chair arms. A self-locking bracket on one side of the chair will suspend the lapboard from the desk arm when not in use and keep it within easy reach when needed (Fig. 19.5).

Stabilization of an Object

(a) A plate guard or a scoop dish helps the patient to get food onto the utensil and prevents it from being pushed off of the plate. A Lazy Susan Plate Guard allows the plate to rotate until the desired food is within reach and aligned with the stationary guard. Hooks, clips, clamps, rubber bands, or a grooved surface will hold the guard onto the plate (Fig. 19.5).

(b) Rubber matting, Dycem, and suction cups under plates, bowls, and other objects can be used to increase stability.

WRITING AIDS

Compensation for Loss of Function of a Body Part due to Paralysis

Where functional grasp is absent, self-help devices either securely position the digits around the pen/pencil or hold it diagonally across the web space with a clip, loop, or casing attached to a metacarpal cuff. With the first design, the radial three digits are partially encased and held in a modified palmar prehension. With the second design, hyperextension of the wrist will usually produce enough modified lateral prehension to assist in supporting the lower end of the writing utensil. Following are some examples.

(a) A pencil or pen is inserted into a rectangular Velcro or leather pouch which is placed between the thumb and index finger, with the long finger stabilizing the lower end of the writing utensil. Digits are secured with an encircling elastic strap attached to the pouch (Fig. 19.6).

(b) A leather index finger cuff can support the lower portion of the pencil or pen along the side of the second digit. The upper portion of the writing utensil is supported by the strap, which secures on itself. Proper adjustment of this strap will draw the thumb against the pen for additional stability and control (Fig. 19.6).

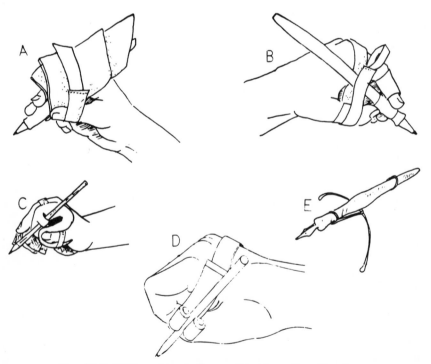

Fig. 19.6. Writing aids. *A–D*, pencil holders; *E*, writing frame.

(c) A low-temperature plastic writing device, similar to a lengthened C-bar, holds the thumb in abduction and opposition under the first two fingers, which it partially supports. One strap proximal to the proximal interphalangeal joints of the two fingers and one strap proximal to the interphalangeal joint of the thumb secures the device to the hand. The pen is held for writing and secured to the device along the lateral aspect of the index finger (Fig. 19.6).

(d) One can insert an attachment having a dual roller pincher clip, metal sleeve with a self-locking mechanism, or a similar holder into the pocket of a utensil cuff to hold a pen. (Fig. 19.6).

Compensation for Loss of Range of Motion due to Muscle Weakness or Structural Limitations

(a) The circumference of pens and pencils can be increased with foam padding, foam tubing, wood, tape, plastic tubing, or similar materials.

(b) Pens or pencils can be inserted into a triangular-shaped rubber sleeve which is commercially available.

(c) By purchasing writing utensils of larger diameters, there may be no need to adapt those of a smaller diameter.

(d) A tripod-shaped semicircular writing frame which holds the pencil in position and supports the hand is commercially available. Some gross grasp is required for best control (Fig. 19.6).

Compensation for Increased Involuntary Motion

(a) A writing utensil can be weighted with lead pieces or inserted into a wooden or plastic casing filled at the bottom with lead shot.

(b) A magnet attached to a wrist strap can be used on a flat metal surface to position the wrist and lower forearm for writing.

(c) For information on weighted cuffs see "Eating."

Compensation for Sensory Deficits

Elastic string can be attached to a clipboard or similar surface for a writing guide for those having visual deficits.

Stabilization of an Object

A clipboard, writing board with a clamp at the top and on one side, magnetic board, or paper weights will keep the paper in place. Applying small rubber pads, Dycem, or other nonskid materials to the back of writing boards will stabilize the paper holder.

TYPEWRITING AIDS

Compensation for Loss of Function of a Body Part due to Paralysis

(a) A pencil or rubber tip dowel can be inserted into the pocket of a universal cuff for typing. With the forearm in midposition, the eraser or rubber-tip surface should project from the ulnar side of the cuff.

(b) Plastic-coated typing sticks with adjustable plastic metacarpal cuffs are commercially available for use with the forearm in midposition (Fig. 19.7).

(c) For use with the forearm pronated, a T-shaped typing stick may be made from two dowels and held in the hand with a Velcro or elastic strap attached to both ends of the dowel that spans the hand (Fig. 19.7).

(d) Index fingers may be individually kept in position for striking the keys with plastic finger shells having extended rubber-covered tips. Lengthening the shell beyond the fingertip prevents the other digits from dragging the keyboard (Fig. 19.7).

(e) Headsticks or mouthsticks may be used by those having no functional use of either upper extremity.

(f) Electromechanical typing systems activated with gross lower or upper extremity movements, a mouthstick, or breath controls may be useful to those having severely impaired upper extremity function.

(g) A continuous roll of paper suspended from a wooden frame above the typewriter eliminates the need to insert paper more than once (Fig. 19.7).

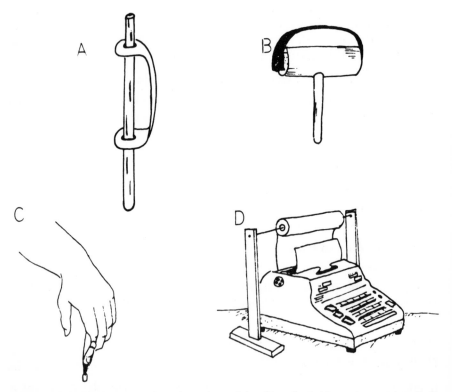

Fig. 19.7. Typewriting aids. *A*, typing stick with adjustable metacarpal cuff; *B*, typing stick; *C*, finger shell (P. N. Craver); *D*, paper roll holder.

(h) The Bird Beak Paper Inserter is held in the mouth, and the tongue is used to activate the gripper, which holds the paper while it is inserted.

Compensation for Loss of Range of Motion due to Muscle Weakness or Structural Limitations

(a) The circumference of a typing stick may be increased with foam padding or tubing, wood, tape, or a rubber ball.

(b) Enlarging or attaching spokes to the paper roller wheel on a manual typewriter simplifies the positioning of typing paper.

(c) If the vertical line spacer lever is lengthened, less strength is required to activate it.

(d) Constructing an inclined plane to support the forearms may benefit patients unable to maintain this position without early fatigue.

Compensation for Increased Involuntary Motion

(a) A keyboard shield made of plastic or wood with a hole over each key prevents unintentional striking of the keys. The raised guard should be designed for specific keyboards, as typewriters differ.

(b) Typing sticks, mouthsticks, headsticks are used as discussed previously.

(c) Electromechanical typing systems are used as discussed previously. Electric typewriters are frequently more manageable than the manual style because of the amount of pressure required to depress the keys. They can be self-correcting and thus eliminate the need for erasing, correction fluid, or strikeovers. A lapboard may be necessary to position the typewriter for those who cannot use one on a table due to standard wheelchair arms or limited range of motion.

TELEPHONING AIDS

Compensation for Loss of Function of a Body Part due to Paralysis

(a) Many of the same writing and typing devices previously described may be used on dial or pushbutton telephones.

(b) A metal or plastic cuff attached to the back of the telephone headset (receiver) with a wide Velcro strap helps bring the receiver to the ear.

Compensation for Loss of Range of Motion due to Muscle Weakness or Structural Limitations

(a) A gooseneck arm clamped to the edge of a table will hold a telephone at ear level. A narrow plate across the cradle of the telephone or one with an on-off switch will open and close the circuit (Fig. 19.8).

(b) The Drop-In Telephone Amplifier, positioned on a table to hold the handset and amplify the sound, is helpful to those who have sufficient hand function to place and remove the receiver from the amplifier.

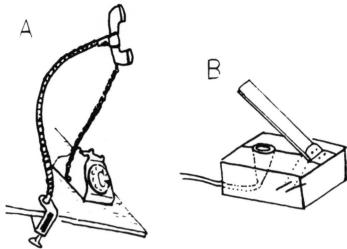

Fig. 19.8. Communication aids. *A*, gooseneck handset holder; *B*, call signal.

(c) Telephones especially adapted and commercially available include the Speakerphone, the Card Dialer, and the One-Number Dialer.

Compensation for Sensory Deficits

(a) For those with hearing impairments, telephones with handset amplifiers, receivers that transmit sound vibrations to the inner ear, or other adaptations may prove helpful.

(b) A loud gong, a specified frequency range, or a flashing light may replace the usual telephone ring.

(c) For those with some visual impairment, a shield with enlarged keys and numbers can be placed over the face of a pushbutton phone.

OTHER COMMUNICATION AIDS

(a) A call signal can be adapted by encasing the control unit in a wooden block and attaching a lever to depress the call button (Fig. 19.8).

(b) Puff 'N Buzzer is a call signal which is activated by a breath-controlled switch.

(c) Gross arm motion may be used to control the long lever of the Hand Touch Call System.

(d) Longer keys provide more leverage for operating a portable tape recorder and, thus, require less pressure.

PERSONAL HYGIENE

Compensation of Loss of Function of a Body Part due to Paralysis

(a) Toothbrush, rat-tail comb, nail file, rat-tail brush, and flat-handled makeup applicators may be inserted into the pocket of the utensil holder.

(b) A cuff or strap with a "D" ring closure may be attached to a hairbrush. Recommended materials for adaption include leather, plastic, Velcro, or elastic (Fig. 19.9).

(c) A mitt made of terry cloth or sponge with Velcro straps around the wrist and a "D" ring closure substitutes for a wash rag (Fig. 19.9).

(d) A back scrubber with two adjustable hand loops can be made from a continuous length of webbing covered with a sponge pad (Fig. 19.9).

(e) A commercially available rubber cap with slots replaces the screw-type caps of toothpaste, shaving cream, and hair cream tubes. Once the cap is installed, no prehension or grasp is required to dispense the contents of the tube.

(f) Razors can be adapted with a palmar cuff or a continuous piece of metal which wraps around the first and third fingers and spans the palmar aspect of the second finger (Fig. 19.9).

(g) For individuals with only one functional upper extremity, a commercially available denture brush is held to a flat surface with suction cups (Fig. 19.10). Cleaning the unaffected hand can be accomplished with a flat brush or sponge having a suction cup base. A T-strap Velcro strap attached to a plastic base holds eye glasses for cleaning (Fig. 19.10).

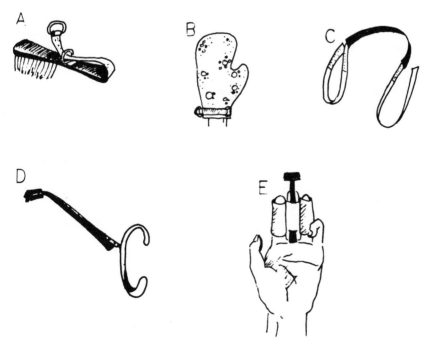

Fig. 19.9. Personal hygiene items. *A*, adapted hairbrush; *B*, wash mitt; *C*, back scrubber; *D–E*, safety razor holders.

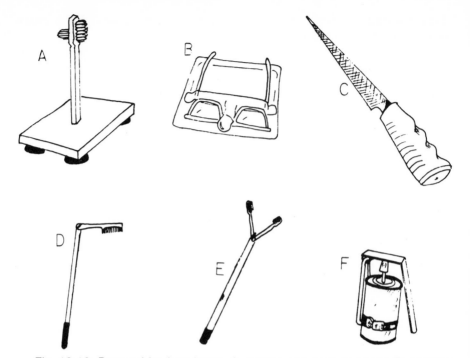

Fig. 19.10. Personal hygiene items. *A*, suction cup denture brush; *B*, eyeglass holder; *C*, built-up-handled nail file; *D*, adjustable extension comb; *E*, adjustable extension toothbrush; *F*, aerosol can dispenser.

Compensation for Loss of Range of Motion due to Muscle Weakness or Structural Limitations

(a) To compensate for limited finger flexion, the handles of a comb, brush, toothbrush, safety razor, and fingernail file can be enlarged with foam padding and other materials, as previously described (Fig. 19.10).

(b) Objects with extended handles compensate for loss of range of motion of the elbow and shoulder. Objects of standard size may be altered by using an extension handle with a pocket similar to that of the utensil holder or lengthened by extended handles permanently attached. One may vary the angle of the utensil with a wing nut on the extension handle or an adjustable pocket (Fig. 19.10).

(c) Individuals with limited grasp may dispense aerosol from cans having a lever that depresses the valve control. A hose clamp and thumbscrew makes the device adjustable to cans of various sizes (Fig. 19.10).

(d) A long-handled sponge, curved bathbrush, or hand-held shower head enable those with limited shoulder or elbow motion to bathe.

(e) Toilet activities for an individual with unilateral limitation of flexion may be accomplished with a raised commode seat having one sloping side.

If there is difficulty with reach or grasp of toilet tissue, long-handled tongs with curved plastic covered grippers may be used.

(f) Commercially available sanitary napkins with strips of adhering tape eliminate the need for a belt or manipulation of fasteners.

Position and Support—Stabilization of an Object

(a) A commercially available chair with removable cushion, commode bucket, removable arm rest, casters, and a toilet tissue holder which snaps onto the tubing on one side of the chair enables individuals to shower and use the toilet without leaving the chair.

(b) A raised commode seat with safety side bars assists with standing or sitting, as well as providing a safety factor where there is impaired balance.

(c) Tub rails, grab bars, and a tub seat may simplify tub transfers.

(d) Nonskid appliques on tubs, showers and other floor surfaces prevent slipping.

DRESSING

Compensation for Loss of Function of a Body Part due to Paralysis

(a) A Plastisol-covered metal cuff with a zipper pull extending from one end and a buttonhook extending from the other end may be used by individuals having no prehension and grasp (Fig. 19.11). A buttonhook with a flat handle inserted into the pocket of a utensil cuff and a loop of leather lacing through the eyes of zippers is an equally effective alternative.

(b) The cuff of a long-sleeve shirt on the unaffected side can be buttoned with a buttonhook having suction cup base secured to a flat surface.

(c) A flat plastic hook with a series of webbing loops attached may be inserted into the belt loops of trousers. The loops are placed over the forearms, and as the user rolls from side to side, he pulls up his pants by moving from one loop to the next until he is at the loop closest to the hook. Shoulder flexion and/or abduction and elbow flexion are required to use this device in dressing (Fig. 19.11).

(d) Commercially available mitts with a rubber-faced surface draw a wool sock across the foot and up the leg.

(e) When only one upper extremity is functional, various self-help devices are commercially available that help don shoes without tying laces. These include those that have a zipper that is laced into the shoe, elastic shoelaces, and laces that are wrapped around plastic buckles. Velcro closures are simple substitutes for shoe laces and can be used on any shoe.

(f) For individuals having no bilateral grasp, one may sew leather thumb loops to both sides of the shoe, and the same type of loop may be applied to socks.

(g) The shoehorn which holds a tie shoe open while the foot is inserted

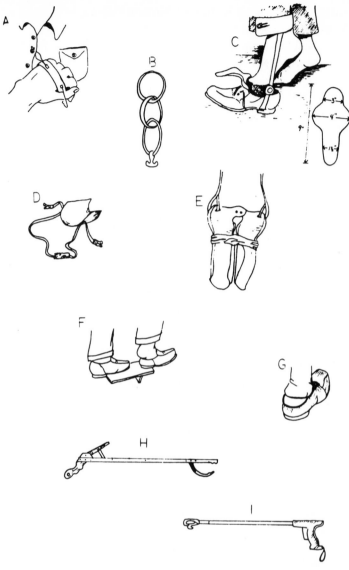

Fig. 19.11. Dressing aids. *A*, combination zipper pull and buttonhook; *B*, trouser pulls; *C*, dorsal arch shoehorn (Seplowitz); *D*, sock pull; *E*, panty hose aid (Seplowitz); *F*, bootjack; *G*, counter protector; *H*, lever-action reacher; *I*, pistol-grip reacher with adjustable terminal unit.

will help those who have one functional upper extremity and must wear a lower extremity orthosis attached to a shoe. For optimal fit, the shoehorn made of low-temperature plastic can be molded directly to the shoe (Fig. 19.11).

Compensation for Loss of Range of Motion due to Muscle Weakness or Structural Limitations

(a) Buttonhooks assist those who lack sufficient prehension to manipulate buttons. Handles of plastic or wood should be selected after assessment of the user's ability to grasp.

(b) A small metal cup hook inserted into the end of a dowel will help pull zipper tabs. Length and width of the dowel depend on location and severity of the limitations.

(c) Persons with shoulder limitation can use a long chain or cord zipper pull for back zippers if they can attach the pull to the zipper.

(d) For lower extremity dressing, long plastic-covered dowels with garter clips attached to one end may be used to pull on socks, but hand function is needed to attach garter slips to socks. The sock is pulled into place above the ankle and released from the device by pushing the garter slip downward. A second alternative is to place a sock over a plastic or aluminum trough and draw it over the foot with long cotton webbing straps or two rods attached to each side of the trough which keep the top of the sock open while the foot is inserted (Fig. 19.11). This may be modified to include one long handle attached to the center of the trough when bilateral use of the upper extremities is absent.

(e) For panty hose, two troughs attached to one another are made from cloth-covered polyethylene, cotton webbing, and garter clips. The panty hose is drawn over the troughs and attached in back to the garter clips. Feet are inserted into the top of the panty hose, held open by the troughs. Long webbing straps attached to the troughs pull the panty hose up the legs, and when the garter clips are within reach, they are released and the individual completes the process with his hands (Fig. 19.11). The same basic principle is applicable for constructing devices to assist in putting on trousers or underwear.

(f) A long-handled shoehorn, counter protector, and bootjack may be utilized to apply and remove slip-on shoes or tie shoes that have been modified to include elastic hose laces if the individual is unable to reach the feet due to limited range (Fig. 19.11). (g) Reachers provide a means of obtaining articles that would otherwise be out of reach. Styles of reachers commercially available are voluntary opening or voluntary closing, collapsible, magnetic holder, lever- or trigger-operated, swivel head, and pistol grip handle of scissors-like action (Fig. 19.11).

HOMEMAKING

The rehabilitation program frequently includes work simplification and energy conservation, which involve using appropriate equipment, technique, and work surfaces. Self-help devices for homemaking may be purchased through rehabilitation equipment suppliers or they can be fabricated. Many are also readily available at local stores in the houseware section. These utensils and objects that may be designed for homemaking convenience are excellent substitutes for self-help devices.

Compensation for Loss of Function of a Body Part due to Paralysis

With only one functional upper extremity, stabilizing objects is frequently the primary intent of self-help aids.

(a) Suction cups or rubber feet may be applied to the base of an upright grater, rectangular brush, bottle brush, cutting board with a corner guard and stainless steel spikes, and other similar objects to stabilize them (Fig. 19.12).

(b) Utensils such as a potato peeler or apple corer attached to a clamp may be mounted on the edge of a counter or table.

(c) A U-shaped frame with a suction cup base stabilizes the handles of pans and skillets to allow stirring on the stove (Fig. 19.12).

(d) A commercially available pan strainer, a jar opener that permanently attaches on the underside of a cabinet, and a bowl holder for mixing and pouring assist in food preparation (Fig. 19.12).

(e) A pizza roller or rolling pin with an upright frame simplify rolling pastry dough (Fig. 19.13). A length of material attached to a plastic hoop which slips around the waist eliminates tying apron strings.

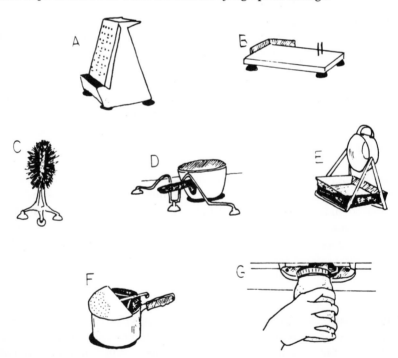

Fig. 19.12. Homemaking aids. *A*, food grater; *B*, cutting board; *C*, bottle brush; *D*, pan stabilizer; *E*, bowl holder; *F*, p   r;   ar opener.

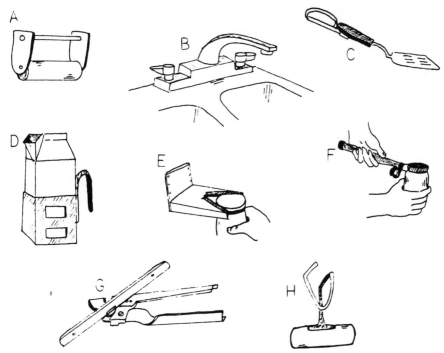

Fig. 19.13. Homemaking aids. *A*, rolling pin; *B*, faucet control extensions; *C*, loop-handled utensil (Burkhardt); *D*, milk carton holder; *E* and *F*, jar opener; *G*, extension handle can opener; *H*, stove control.

(f) A commercially available can opener that is held in one hand pierces the can and starts the opening process with a squeeze of the lever. Interchangeable attachments include a mixing unit and knife sharpener.

(g) Lever action may be used to turn round faucet controls having rubber, metal, or plastic extensions (Fig. 19.13).

(h) Individuals with no hand function bilaterally can benefit from many of the stabilizing devices described for the one-handed homemaker when these devices are used in conjunction with utensils adapted with a cuff or strap. An aluminum or high-temperature plastic sleeve is attached to the handles of a variety of kitchen utensils. A cuff-like handle of the same material constructed to fit the user's hands is inserted into the sleeve and easily removed for use with other similarly adapted utensils (Fig. 19.13). Table utensils inserted into the pocket of utensil cuffs are useful for food preparation.

(i) When grasp is absent, bottles with hand pumps can be activated with palmar pressure to dispense juices, sauces, or other liquids.

(j) Commercially available milk carton holders with a plastic frame and cuff-like handle assist in pouring liquids from any half-gallon carton (Fig. 19.13).

Compensation for Loss of Range of Motion due to Muscle Weakness or Structural Limitations

(a) Building up handles of cooking utensils will compensate for limited range of motion of the fingers.

(b) Jar openers with a long handle, a serrated V-shaped opening, or rubber grippers assist those with muscle weakness of the hands (Fig. 19.13).

(c) Extending the length of handles and cutter wheel crank of a manual can opener decreases the range of motion and strength required to operate it (Fig. 19.13).

(d) Those with limited range of motion or confined to a wheelchair can perform many activities using a long-handled dust pan, feather duster, and sponge.

(e) A platform placed in the sink enables individuals with limited range of motion or wheelchair occupants to reach the bottom of the sink.

(f) Reachers or long-handled tongs obtain objects otherwise unavailable.

(g) An angle rod attached to a cylindrical wooden handle is useful to turn stove controls (Fig. 19.13).

(h) A lapboard or small utility cart with casters transports items from one location to another.

VOCATIONAL ACTIVITIES

Many of the communication devices discussed previously will assist individuals in assuming vocational responsibilities. Applying the principles used in their construction will be useful in modifying equipment and instruments peculiar to a specific job. The following are a few examples.

(a) For office work involving the lifting and replacing of file folders, a device may be constructed from a piece of stainless steel and a scissor bill clamp. The plastic-covered thumb loop and the leverage action of the clamp eliminate the need for fine finger dexterity (Fig. 19.14). Comfortable and efficient work stations may require specifically designed chairs such as the Arthro Chair, a Catapult Chair, or one adapted with leg extensions. A table with a hydraulic lift or a specially designed desk with options such as a magnifying frame, tiltable desk top, removable arm supports, and adjustable height may also be necessary. Additions of electrically powered office equipment, such as a pencil sharpener, and adding machine may assist those with poor upper extremity function.

(b) For adaptations in industry, those with unilateral function or impaired grasp may benefit from pneumatic-powered tools with compressed air source and ratchet or pistol-grip handled tools.

TRANSFER AND TRAVEL

(a) For a patient who cannot readily arise from a bed, a webbing ladder may be attached to the end frame of the bed to assist in coming to a sitting from a supine or sidelying position (Fig. 19.14).

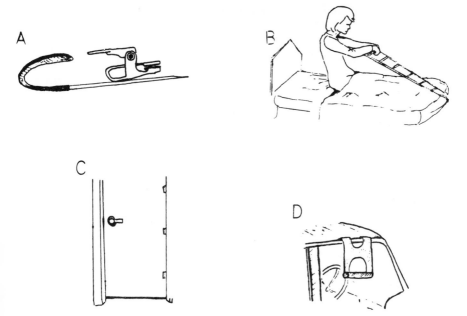

Fig. 19.14. Vocational, transfer, and travel aids. *A*, filing device; *B*, bed ladder; *C*, door knob extension; *D*, handgripper for car.

(b) For sitting transfers, a board approximately 24 to 30 inches long and 8 inches wide having tapered ends will provide a sliding surface. A commercially available, pear-shaped board has loops on each side which allow handling it without hand function. A spring-loaded rod fitting into the wheelchair tubing after removal of the armrest keep the board securely in place and level with the seat cushion of the wheelchair.

(c) Gloves or cuffs with a nonskid outer surface provide traction on the wheelchair rim and offer some protection for the palmar surface.

(d) Baskets or pouches may be attached to walkers or wheelchairs to transport and store items.

(e) A commercially available gripper attached to a cane or crutch slides under the edge of a flat horizontal surface to keep the walking aid upright and close to its user.

(f) For additional clearance for wheelchairs, a door hinge is commercially available that allows the door to open flush with the door jamb.

(g) To improve lever action on door knobs, rubber, metal, or plastic extensions are available which fit over the door knob (Fig. 19.14).

(h) Extended door pulls and a hand gripper suspended from the rain gutter of a car simplify transfers.

Avocational Interests

READING

Compensation for Loss of Function of a Body Part due to Paralysis

(a) Pages of a book or magazine may be turned using a mouthstick, headstick, or rubber-tipped dowel inserted into the pocket of a utensil cuff and drawn across the page. Another alternative is to form a continuous piece of plastic into a cuff, extending beyond either the ulnar or radial side of the hand, depending upon the need. Covering the end of the extension with a nonskid material provides traction to turn pages (Fig. 19.15).

(b) Electrically driven or battery-operated page turners may be activated with light touch, breath controls, or gross head, upper, or lower extremity movements.

Stabilization of Objects or Compensation for Positioning

(a) Bookstands position reading material at an angle suitable for reading. Page holders may be attached to a bookstand or clipped to the hard cover of the book (Fig. 19.15).

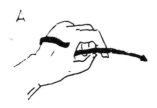

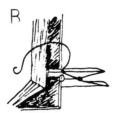

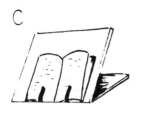

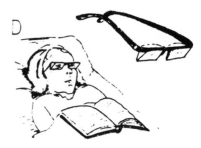

Fig. 19.15. Reading aids. *A*, page turner; *B*, page holder; *C*, book stand with page holder; *D*, prism glasses.

(b) Prism eyeglasses allow the supine individual to read while in bed (Fig. 19.15).

(c) A book holder suspended from a frame resting on the bed is useful when some elevation of the head is tolerated.

GAMES AND SPORTS

There are a large number of adaptations for special sports, and the following are only a few examples.

(a) Card holders and shufflers are commercially available for those with only one upper extremity or limited hand function (Fig. 19.16).

(b) Large-face playing cards can be used by those with visual deficits.

(c) Board and playing pieces of table games such as checkers, cribbage, tic tac toe, backgammon, and chess can be enlarged and made from wood or plastic. For patients with incoordination, playing pieces may be weighted.

(d) For racket games such as ping pong, the racket may be secured across the hand with a strap or cuff when grasp is absent.

(e) A retractable handle on a bowling ball, a long-handled ball pusher, and a bowling ramp may be useful to individuals confined to a wheelchair or to those with limited upper extremity function (Fig. 19.16).

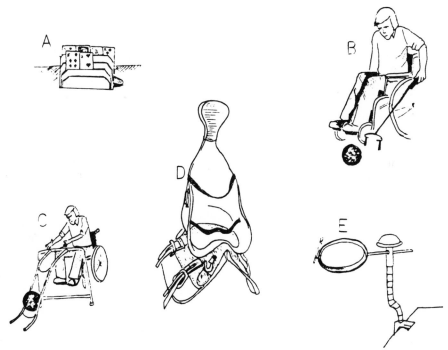

Fig. 19.16. Avocational aids. *A*, card holder; *B*, long-handled ball pusher; *C*, bowling ball ramp; *D*, Maddasaddle; *E*, gooseneck embroidery hoop.

(f) The Maddasaddle provides trunk support for horseback riding (Fig. 19.16).

SEWING AND NEEDLEWORK

(a) To perform needlework, attach an embroidery hoop to a vertical rod or a gooseneck arm. An expandable leg band or clamp attached to a table holds the device in place (Fig. 19.16).

(b) Needle threaders and electric scissors are commercially available for those with poor grasp.

(c) By placing the foot pedal of a sewing machine under the forearm on the cabinet top, a paraplegic can use both hands to control the machine.

RADIO AND TELEVISION SET CONTROLS

(a) Control units will remotely turn on and off a television, radio, light or other electric appliances and can be activated by using breath controls, auditory sounds such as whistling, sensitivity to beams of direct light, or gross movement of the head, upper, or lower extremities.

(b) For those with limited range of motion or weakness, control knobs may be enlarged in size or typing sticks may be used to depress the control buttons or levers.

SMOKING

(a) The Smoker's Robot, similar in principle to the oriental water pipe, increases the safety of smoking in bed where prehension is absent. The cigarette is securely held in a metal ashtray which can be placed on a tray or table. Tubing connects the cigarette holder to the mouthpiece.

(b) A filter holder may be attached to a metal cuff which fits around the hand or fingers, and a metal ashtray with a spring clip may be secured to the arm tubing of a wheelchair.

(c) Chemically, electrically, or lever-operated cigarette lighters are available and can be ignited with pressure from the palm of the hand.

Other Functional Aids

Individuals needing self-help aids for daily activities may also have medical complications or secondary conditions that require some kind of attention. The following are some examples of helpful devices.

(a) Inspection of the skin, including the buttock area, may be accomplished without grasp, using a gooseneck mirror with two adjustable plastic cuffs along its shaft.

(b) The Digi-Sert Stimulator, replacing manual stimulation, and the Supp-a-Sert Suppository Inserter, inserting a rectal suppository, may be used without grasp (Fig. 19.17).

(c) Urinary collecting bags may be emptied using a cylindrical valve with

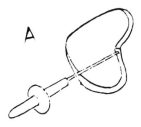

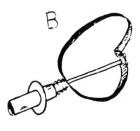

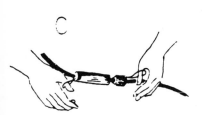

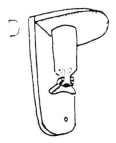

Fig. 19.17. Other functional aids. *A*, Digi-Sert stimulator; *B*, Supp-a-Sert suppository inserter; *C*, urinary collection bag drainage valve; *D*, insulin bottle stabilizer.

one or two loops for insertion of a digit, usually the thumb. These commercially available devices empty when pressure is applied against the loop; the valve closes when the pressure is discontinued (Fig. 19.17).

(d) Catheter clamps may be fitted with loops to open and close them.

(e) Fastening a broom clip to a board will stabilize an insulin bottle and allow a diabetic with functional use of one extremity to fill a syringe (Fig. 19.17).

(f) Visually impaired diabetics may use a syringe gauge constructed of a ½-inch dowel rod for measuring the desired number of insulin units. The rod is sized according to the length of the needle plunger when it is pulled out to the desired number of units. Cutting a lengthwise groove in the dowel allows the gauge to fit securely over the plunger. The syringe is filled, the gauge is placed over the plunger while the needle remains in the bottle, and the excess insulin is returned to the bottle until the desired amount remains in the syringe, as determined by the gauge. The needle is withdrawn from the bottle, the gauge is removed, and the insulin is injected. One may need to construct gauges for each style or brand name of syringe utilized, as the diameter of syringes varies causing the length of the plungers to differ.

Advances in technology and the ingenuity and innovation by those with physical disabilities have produced a significant increase in the number of self-help aids commercially available or individually designed. Many devices currently available cannot be covered in this short summary. For example, self-help aids to the visually impaired were barely mentioned, as there are an abundance of resources available from organizations helping those with impaired sight. We have also not reviewed the many types of orthoses and adapted techniques which play an important role in increasing function, as they are covered elsewhere in the book. When combined with self-help aids, they offer many individuals a new sense of independence.

Resources

Many of the self-help devices mentioned in this chapter are available from one or several of the companies listed below. Catalogs, locations of area representatives or distributors, and additional information about specific devices may be requested from each. In addition to these and the publications listed at the end of this chapter, other resources include companies and organizations such as Bell Telephone, The Division of the Blind and Physically Handicapped of The Library of Congress, and the Arthritis Foundation, to mention a few.

Abbey Medical
Division of Abbey Rents
600 S. Normandie Avenue
Los Angeles, California 90005

Medical Equipment Distributors,
Inc.
1215 S. Harlem Avenue
Forest Park, Illinois 60130

Carters Rehabilitation Equipment
Alfred Street
Westbury, Wilts BA13 3D2
Great Britain

G. E. Miller, Inc.
484 S. Broadway
Yonkers, New York 10705

Cleo Living Aids
3957 Mayfield Road
Cleveland, Ohio 44121

J. A. Preston Corporation
71 Fifth Avenue
New York, New York 10003

Maddak, Inc.
Industrial Road
Pequannock, New Jersey 07530

Fred Sammons, Inc.
Box 32
Brookfield, Illinois 60513

Illustrator—Lou Anne Cooke, OTR. The Capper Foundation for Crippled Children, Topeka, Kansas.

REFERENCES

1. ALEXANDER, B., AND REID, E. A drainage valve for urinary leg bags. *Am. J. Occup. Ther.*, 28: 10, 1974.

2. AMERICAN FOUNDATION FOR THE BLIND, INC. *Internal Guide to Aids and Appliances for Blind and Visually Impaired Persons,* ed. 2. Port City Press, Baltimore, 1977.
3. Bell Telephone. Services for Special Needs. USA, 1975.
4. BOYER, J. Syringe gauge. *Am. J. Occup. Ther. 30:* 8, 1976.
5. BURKHARDT, B. Loop-handled utensils. *Am. J. Occup. Ther.,* 29: 7, 1975.
6. CARVER, P. Typing splints for the quadriplegic patient. *Am. J. Occup. Ther., 29:* 9, 1975.
7. FEINBERG, J. Writing device for the quadriplegic patient. *Am. J. Occup. Ther., 29:* 2, 1975.
8. HENNEQUIN, C. Aid technique for writing for a quadriplegic. Can. J. *Can. J. Occup. Ther., 44:* 33, 1977.
9. HOPKINS, H. L. Self-help Aids. In *Orthotics Etcetera,* edited by S. Licht. Elizabeth Licht, New Haven, 1966.
10. MEYER R. The sock aid. *Am. J. Occup. Ther. 29:* 4, 1975.
11. NELSON, C. E., AND RANKA, J. L. CHRC eating aid. *Am. J. Occup. Ther., 29:* 6, 1975.
12. Orthopop. Independently Controlled Feeding Apparatus. Aptos, California, 1976.
13. RUSK, H. A. Principles of Self-Help Devices. *Rehabil. Medicine,* ed. 4. C. V. Mosby Co., St. Louis, 1977.
14. SEPLOWITZ, C. Dorsal arch shoehorn. *Am. J. Occup. Ther., 27:* 6, 1973.
15. SEPLOWITZ, C. Panty hose aid. *Am. J. Occup. Ther., 29:* 7, 1975.
16. WEISS, D., AND WEISS, L. The sandwich holder. *Am. J. Occup. Ther., 30:* 6, 1976.
17. ZIMMERMAN, M. E. Occupational Therapy in the A. D. L. Program. In *Occupational Therapy,* edited by H. S. Willard and C. S. Spackman, ed. 4. J. B. Lippincott Co., Philadelphia, 1971.

20

Introduction to Systems and Devices for the Disabled

C. GERALD WARREN, M.P.A.

Disabled people have the right to be provided access to education, vocations, and an improved quality of life. For this reason, they are rapidly bcoming consumers of technology. To date, however, technology has not been applied to problems of the disabled as vigorously as it has been used to enhance the quality of life of the able-bodied. This is usually attributed to the demand on the market being too small to motivate industry to provide goods and services for the handicapped. Nevertheless, the situation is currently changing with the advent of legislation to improve accessibility to all types of environments and to support independent living for disabled persons. This, in turn, is causing a significant increase in the demand for sophisticated equipment by the disabled population. We may soon see a great expansion in manufacturing and marketing in this area.

Systems and devices for the disabled include a large variety of equipment to provide communication, mobility, and environmental control. These systems usually involve sophisticated technology and go beyond equipment usually provided by physical therapy, occupational therapy, and prosthetics and orthotics. Consequently, comprehensive rehabilitation services now include an engineering component to apply current and developing technology.

This chapter discusses the basic equipment available to improve the quality of life for the severely disabled, with emphasis on actuators and their operation. It is important that clinicians and counselors in rehabilitation develop an understanding of the concepts and categories of this equipment so that they will recognize its potential value for their patients and clients. Determining the optimum operating method or actuator is crucial to success of an application; therefore, basic principles are presented for a wide variety of actuators. Appendix 1 provides references to manufacturers of systems and devices for the disabled and to major information sources in the field.

Types of Disability

Systems and devices are prescribed for two general categories of disability, the physically disabled and the sensory disabled. Those who are physically disabled are mechanically limited in their activities through loss of motor function from paralysis, loss of range of motion from structural deformity, or lack of motor control. There are also many varying combinations of these limitations. Severely disabled people, such as those with high-level quadriplegia, are candidates for powered wheelchairs, environmental control systems, and communication systems which augment or substitute for lost motor or control functions.

The sensory disabled, on the other hand, most commonly have lost the ability to see or hear. Other sensory losses, such as loss of perception, proprioception, pain, or touch, commonly accompany physical disability. Sensory losses also occur in multiple combinations such as blindness-deafness, blindness and peripheral neuropathy due to diabetes, etc. People with sensory loss are often candidates for comunication systems, environmental control systems, and systems which assist in mobility or safety by augmenting the lost sensory function with feedback about the immediate environment.

Communication Aids

Providing the ability to communicate may release unrecognized ability and provide new satisfactions for a severely disabled person. Systems which aid or provide communication have input or output functions, while some incorporate both. Speaking and writing are typical output functions; hearing and reading are typical input functions.

People who require assistance with output functions are usually physically disabled due to lack of motor control. Some deaf persons, however, may require equipment to comunicate because of the inability to speak resulting from their lack of auditory feedback. The topic of communication systems has been studied extensively by the Trace Center, and more details are available from this source (10).

The equipment used to provide output communication functions can be classified by one of these methods of operation: direct selection, scanning, or encoding. The most common direct selection method uses a pointer board on which the person points to a sequence of letters or symbols to convey a message, leaving the message to be compiled by the recipient. Although inexpensive in terms of equipment and cost, this method is very slow, requiring considerable concentration and time on the part of the recipient. The same principle has been used with much greater effectiveness in systems in which each letter or symbol on the board is electrically selected through pressure or magnetic switches in the board. The user is able to compile a message directly on an electronic display or small printer, and the entire message or segment can be communicated at one time (Figure 20.1) (2) This method has been expanded to incorporate the direct selection of words, message segments, or complete messages, which may be stored in a small memory within the machine. The equipment may be connected to an electronic display so that the text can be edited before it is transferred to a printer.

The second category of output communication systems includes those which use scanning. Typically, the user operates a switch which causes an electronic pointer to scan down the row of a matrix, stopping at the row which holds the letter or symbol desired. The operator then scans along the row, stops at the letter or symbol, and actuates a second switch to direct this information to the printer or display where the message is being compiled. Some systems then return the pointer to a fixed location on the display, while others alow scanning to continue from the last location. Because scanning systems are inherently slow to operate, they are most appropriate for persons who have limited mobility or response times and who are unable to use direct selection or encoding methods.

In the third category, encoding systems, the individual converts the message into a code which a machine can accept, process, and display, or convert into electronically generated speech. The code can be combinations

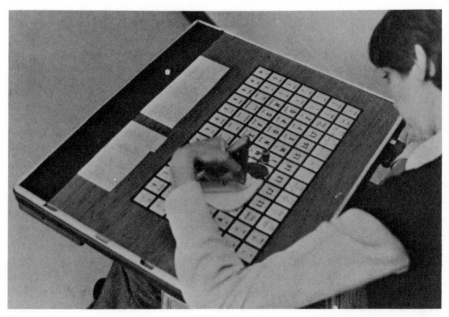

Fig. 20.1. The autocom-E portable communication aid with ¼-inch "ticker tape" printer.

of switch operations comparable to Morse code, or sequences of numbers that the operator can use to formulate word segments, words, or phrases.

Electronically generated or prosthetic speech can be used as the output of direct selection and encoding communication systems. Although these systems are capable of producing very intelligible speech at present, the quality of this speech is currently "machine-like." This may soon be overcome by producing prosthetic speech with improved control of inflection and tone modulation.

When communication is limited by the inability to receive sight or sound, a different class of communication aid is required. Deaf people can communicate with each other over telephone lines by using encoding systems. The message is typed on a keyboard, converted into electronic pulses or tones, and then transmitted over telephone lines to a similar device that decodes and displays it. An example of this type of system is the Portatel (11), shown in Fig. 20.2. Deaf persons may also use encoded or direct access devices which display or print messages when they are communicating with persons who do not understand sign language.

Blind persons are also benefiting from new engineering developments. For example, devices using pattern recognition techniques are capable of "reading" the printed word and converting it into prosthetic speech or into Braille via an embossing system. These systems are currently very expensive but allow blind persons to read virtually any printed material available to them (8, 15).

People with low vision who have difficulty reading regular print are often able to read using video systems. These systems use a small television

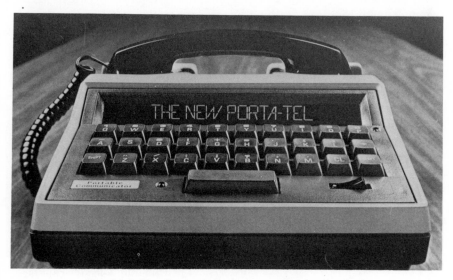

Fig. 20.2. The Portatel telephone system for the deaf.

camera to scan the printed material and display the words on a television screen at whatever size is legible to the individual (1, 17).

Mobility Control Systems

People are generally limited in mobility in two ways: they may be unable to find their way safely because of impaired vision, or they may be limited by lack of muscular power or control.

Devices referred to as electronic travel aids (ETAs) have been developed to aid persons with impaired sight to travel more safely or conveniently in their environment. These systems currently use beams of infrared light or ultrasound to sense objects or discontinuities in the immediate surroundings. Energy leaving these devices bounces off objects or changes its reflection pattern due to discontinuities in the environment. Sensing circuits in the devices provide either a tactile or an auditory output. The Laser Cane projects a light beam from a small laser to sense discontinuities in the direction in which the cane is pointed (3). Either auditory or tactile feedback provides information from the handle of the cane. A second system, the Sonicguide, worn like a pair of eyeglasses, emits ultrasound beams which similarly detect discontinuites and provide an auditory output (15). This manufacturer also produces a hand-held unit used like a flashlight to probe the immediate surroundings. It also provides an auditory output. The value of current ETAs, however, has been contested by many users of conventional cane and canine assistance.

A variety of powered equipment can now provide mobility for people with severe physical disabilities. Features of powered wheelchairs and powered platforms can vary widely according to each individual's specific needs. For example, with the right combination of chair features and on-board equipment, persons with very high-level quadriplegia can achieve independent mobility. The wheelchair can incorporate powered recline to allow the user to change his position periodically, thus resting the residual respiratory musculature and relieving pressure on the seating surface. It can also carry a respirator and communication equipment with remote actuators to operate environmental control systems. Joysticks are commonly used to control the direction and speed of powered wheelchairs. The stick is moved in the direction of desired travel, with the displacement of the stick controlling the speed and/or power. A joystick can be located in any area in which the person can produce motion in one plane; for example, people with high level spinal cord injuries can use chin controls. Many forms of switching, including sip-and-puff actuation, can be used to operate features of the wheelchair and the equipment it carries. This is more fully explained in the actuator section later in the chapter.

Severely disabled persons can achieve long-range mobility by using vans equipped with ramps or powered lifts to load wheelchairs. Specially designed controls allow a person to drive a vechicle from his wheelchair. These controls range from relatively simple lever and linkage systems using hand power to steer and control the pedals to servo-controlled systems. Hydraulic and electronic equipment permit driving with low force and displacement applied to the steering, braking, and acceleration controls (9, 14). Accessory controls can be clustered in a convenient location and operated with suitable low force and displacement switches. Standards for transportation equipment have been published by the Veterans Administration (16), and more details are given in the chapter on automotive aids.

Environmental Control

Environmental control systems allow severely disabled people to perform tasks in their homes or places of employment by controlling a wide variety of appliances or devices through any residual voluntary motion. A single actuator may operate many electrically operated or controlled devices or appliances. A survey and evaluation of different environmental control systems can be obtained from the Institute of Rehabilitation Medicine at New York University (7).

Four basic elements make up environmental control systems: the actuator, the display, the control unit or controller, and the controlled appliances. This is shown schematically in Fig. 20.3. The actuator is the interface between the person and the equipment. It can be any variety of switching input, as described in the actuator section. It may be connected by running wires directly to the control unit, or it may be operated by remote control.

There are two types of remote controls currently in use. In one, an FM transmitter is carried with the person (usually on the wheelchair), with a receiver located near the control unit. The operating range of this unit is primarily limited by the power of the transmitter and is usually not affected greatly by opaque objects such as walls between the transmitter and the receiver. A second type of transmitter currently in use generates a beam of

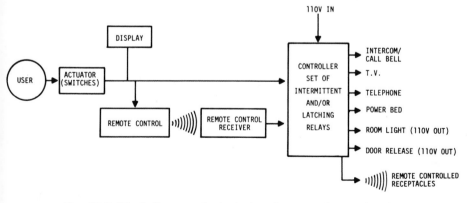

Fig. 20.3. Block diagram of a typical environmental control system.

infrared light which is directed to a receiver. Consequently, the transmitter must be in line of sight of the receiver or in a position in which the infrared beam can be reflected to it. These systems are especially valuable in areas where radio interference would cause inadvertent actuation of FM systems. Specific methods used for actuation are described in the actuator section.

Because most environmental control systems operate a number of different appliances, a scanning device usually selects and operates all appliances to be controlled. This requires a display panel to show the state of the scanner of all appliances. The user presses the switch to cause the system to scan through the functions to be controlled. Release or reactuation of the switch at the time the function desired is reached stops the scan. By operating a second switch, the selected function is activated.

The control unit is the part of the system where switching of selected functions or appliances takes place. The desired appliances or devices are usually connected electrically to the control unit. Fans, television sets, television channel selectors, radios, tape recorders, electric beds, remote receptacles, intercoms, telephone dialers, stereo systems, and lamps are all types of appliances which can be electrically controlled. The user can switch these appliances on or off, controlling them in response to inputs from the actuators.

Safety is a primary consideration in the design of the control unit. The user must be isolated from high voltages or currents. Relays are typical of switching devices used to perform this function because they use low voltages in the actuator circuit to control the higher voltages and currents necessary to power and/or control most appliances.

Switching devices provide either momentary functions or latching functions. Momentary functions remain on only during the time during which the individual is operating the actuator. Latching functions, on the other hand, are turned on by one operation of the actuator and remain on until the actuator is operated again to turn them off. Momentary functions are used for appliances such as intercoms, door latches, and electric bed controls, for all of which intermittent control is desirable. Latching functions are used for appliances such as lights, television sets, and radios, for all of which an on-off control is desired.

Appliances can also be operated remotely from the control unit, using a transmitter plugged into one of the receptacles. The relay normally used to control the appliance actuates the trasmitter. This radiates energy to a remote receiver which controls the desired appliance.

Environmental control units can also provide access to specially designed equipment such as automatic dialing telephones. These systems allow persons with limited manual control to answer incoming calls and to dial any number by using a dual function control switch. Specially designed intercom systems are available which can be operated through environmental control systems, as well as specially designed tape recorders which allow a disabled person to record continuously for 4 hours and which include such functions as underlining and scanning of tapes (12).

In the future, environmental control systems will be greatly improved, microcomputers will be used in the control units, and actuators will take on more remote functions. Experimental units are currently being used which require no direct wiring from the control unit to the appliance. They transmit encoded signals over the 110-volt house wiring system to specific sites within the home where receivers decode the signals and operate the desired appliances (4, 13).

Actuators

In all of the systems described, it is crucial that the user be able to control the unit easily, adequately, and in a manner which he feels is appropriate. To provide adequate control, motions or actions the person can reproduce consistently must be determined and evaluated for reliability, fatigue, and appearance. This motion or action is harnessed to some form of actuator to provide the person-machine interface. For a particular application, the four following criteria should be considered in selecting the actuator:

1. It must effectively and reliably control the desired equipment, and it must be safe from both electrical and mechanical hazards.
2. It must be easy to use: the required function must not exceed the physical capabilities or skill level of the user.
3. It must meet the expectations of the user in terms of appearance. Its level of intrusion into the person's domain must be acceptable, both visually and acoustically. Its operation should not require motions or efforts which the user does not feel are appropriate.
4. Its physical size and placement should not interfere with other desirable or necessary functions that the person may wish to perform.

For any system to function effectively, it must aid the individual to accomplish a specific task, whether it be mobility, communication, or control of appliances. These tasks require either discrete control or proportional control. Discrete control is provided by actuators which use on-off functions to control a system. The most common discrete actuators range from simple switching techniques to systems which require extensive electronic support. Mechanical switches, which are often the easiest to implement, usually provide the simplest and most direct approach. These actuators, which require some force and displacement, exist in various forms, the most common being sip-and-puff actuators and microswitches.

The sip-and-puff actuator is commonly used when there is little power or range of motion in the extremities. It allows the user to control a complex system by sipping or puffing on a straw. The function of this pressure-operated actuator is shown schematically in Fig. 20.4. The two switching functions are provided by using two switches connected to the same air tube. One of the switches is oriented so that a positive pressure in the tube will cause the diaphragm contact to touch a fixed contact, while the other is oriented to respond to a negative pressure. These switches can also be used as puff switches only by connecting the air tube to a bladder of bellows which is mechanically operated. Sip-and-puff switches are manufactured with various levels of pressure required to actuate them; therefore they can be stacked (connected to the same air tube) to allow operation of four functions (two sip and two puff).

Microswitches are available in a wide variety of sizes, shapes, and configuration. These switches are so named because of the low forces and displacements required to operate them. They can be incorporated into a multitude of switching designs to convert any small reliable motion into a switching function. Microswitches can also be incorporated into mechanically amplifying systems. Most equipment manufacturers sell various types of switches for their equipment, providing some latitude in actuator selection. The potential for custom fitting of microswitches to specific disabilities, however, is limited only by the imagination of the technician, clinician, or engineer assigned the task of providing a control method.

Industry has produced a wide variety of switching methods. Switches in general, or any method of closing a contact, can be as simple as the common wall light switch, or as complex as a switch in which the user bridges two contacts with his tongue and causes the dissolved electrolytes in the saliva to conduct a very low current. This current can then be amplified to control a relay or other switching device.

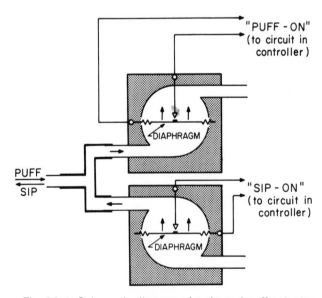

Fig. 20.4. Schematic diagram of a sip-and-puff actuator.

Fig. 20.5 shows many of the options that are available when choosing actuator sites for specific disabilities. It demonstrates a variety of locations where any movement of a body part can be used to control a system or device (16).

In cases in which the person is capable of only one motion, a circuit can often allow one switch to perform a double function by using a timer which distinguishes between long and short actuations of the switch. Typically, release of the switch less than ½ second after the actuation will select one function, while release more than ½ second after actuation will select another function. The time threshold is usually variable, which allows adjustment so that the person can activate two functions by any long and short motions that he can perform.

Light-operated actuators represent another category, which can be divided into three groups: beam-breaking, beam selection, and beam reflection. Beam-breaking actuators use a light source and photosensor for each required function, as shown in Fig. 20.6. To operate these actuators, the person moves his body, body part, or any opaque object to break the beam of light.

In a beam selection system, light is directed from a light source to a photosensitive surface or an array of photosensitive surfaces. The light source can be placed on any part of the body capable of accurately directing the light beam. For a large number of functions, as in a light-operated typewriter, a large array of photosensitive surfaces can be controlled by a single light source.

A recent and promising development uses a reflected beam of infrared light to control a number of functions (6). In this system, an infrared light-emitting diode (LED) is mounted on the temple of a pair of glasses. It

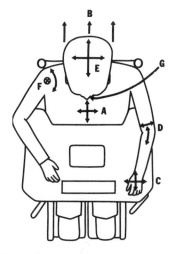

A.	Chin Control
B.	Head Rest Control
C.	Joystick
D.	Arm/BFO
E.	Head Control
F.	Shoulder Position
G.	Pneumatic Control (Puff/Sip)

Fig. 20.5. Control options available to the high-level spinal cord injured.

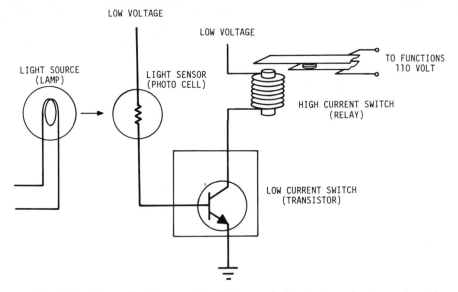

Fig. 20.6. Schematic diagram of a light-operated actuator using beam breaking or beam selection.

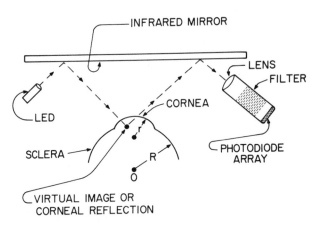

Fig. 20.7. The eye position monitor actuator, using infrared light.

bounces a light beam obliquely off the inside of the glasses and the cornea of the eye, as shown in Fig. 20.7. Motion of the eye then directs the reflected light through a lens and infrared filter to a photodiode array which can activate a large number of functions. Since the energy levels required are very low, and the light beam is directed obliquely toward the cornea, no adverse effects are anticipated. Although still in the development phase, this form of control appears to offer multiple control capability to high-level quadriplegic persons and other equally severely disabled.

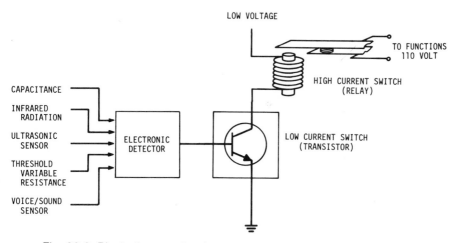

Fig. 20.8. Block diagram showing various types of electronic actuation.

A variety of other actuators may be used to control a system, as shown in Fig. 20.8. Of these, proximity detectors sense when the person places a body segment close to the detecting surface. These detectors can be grouped into those which sense capacitance, those which detect infrared energy radiated by the body, and those which respond to the absorption of ultrasound energy.

In capacitance-sensing detectors, placing a body segment close to the detector changes the capacitance in the circuit and activates the selected appliance. To operate this type of actuator, a person must have some muscular control, but little motion and no force are necessary.

Another type of proximity detector senses infrared or heat energy radiated by the person's body. An extremity placed close to or barely touching the surface emits heat which is sensed and actuates the switching function.

In a third type of proximity detector, the sensing element is an ultrasound transducer which emits a low-power ultrasonic beam. A body segment placed in or moved in the beam changes the absorption pattern of the ultrasound, affecting the circuit generating the beam. This change is sensed electronically, actuating a switching function.

Variable resistance elements include a variety of transducers in which the electrical resistance of a sensing element responds to displacement or force. These may be potentiometers which respond to rotary or linear motion, or they may be strain gauges which sense force on the transducer. Variable resistance devices are inherently analog devices producing an output proportional to the input. Analog controls are commonly seen in joysticks used to control powered wheelchairs, but they may also govern other equipment for which proportional control may be desirable. Variable resistance elements may be used for discrete on-off functions by using a circuit which detects a threshold to separate what are defined to be the on and off states of the actuator.

Sound actuation can provide a switching function by using a microphone and electronic circuit to sense sound levels or tone. Erroneous actuation by ambient noises often creates problems for such systems. Therefore, they can only be used in areas where noise is well-controlled, or where the microphone is positioned to receive selective input.

Electromyographic (EMG) signals may also be used to provide actuation. Surface electrodes detect electrical potentials from contracting muscle fibers. These signals are amplified and processed to control a system or device. These detection methods can use threshold detectors or can rely on pattern recognition techniques to determine when specific muscles or muscle groups are tensed. Thus, several control functions may be provided by a system which detects the EMG signals in a single area of muscle activity.

Systems which perform voice and word recognition hold much promise for the future. They use systems programmed to perform pattern recognition. The machine detects specific frequencies and tonal patterns in an individual's voice as he speaks certain command words, allowing the system to recognize and respond to those words only when spoken by that individual. These systems can detect a considerable vocabulary and can be used to operate a large variety of functions with random access. Cumulative or serial instruction may be used in which a series of words implements a specific function, such as "TV, CHANNEL, UP." This instruction would cause the system sequentially to select the television set, recognize the channel selector and, finally, to change to the next higher channel. At present, these systems seem exotic and are very expensive. However, if computer technology advances as rapidly in the next few years as it has in the recent past, very soon these systems may become available on a large scale.

Acknowledgments

The author wishes to thank John Imre for his editorial assistance in preparing this chapter.

REFERENCES

1. APOLLO LASERS, INC., 6357 Arizona Circle, P.O. Box 45002, Los Angeles, Calif. 90045
2. Autocom-E-Portable Communication Aid with Built-in Printer, TRACE CENTER, 1500 Highland Ave., University of Wisconsin-Madison, Madison, Wisc. 53706
3. BIONIC INSTRUMENTS, 167 Old Belmont Ave., Bala-Cynwyd, Pa. 19004
4. CLINICAL CONVENIENCE PRODUCTS, INC., 2066 Helena St., Madison, Wisc. 53704
5. COURTESY OF PRENTKE ROMICH COMPANY, R.D. Box 191, Shreve, Ohio 44676
6. DENVER RESEARCH INSTITUTE, P.O. Box 10127, Denver, Colo. 80208
7. INSTITUTE OF REHABILITATION MEDICINE, New York University, 400 East 34th St., New York, N. Y. 10016
8. KURZWEIL COMPUTER PRODUCTS, INC., 68 Rogers, Cambridge, Mass. 02142
9. MOBILITY ENG. AND DEV., INC., 6905 Shoup Ave., Canoga Park, Calif. 91306

10. NON-VOCAL COMMUNICATION RESOURCE BOOK, Trace Center (see Appendix)
11. Portatel portable telephone communicator for the deaf, SPECIALIZED SYSTEMS, INC., 215 South Highway 101, Suite 203, Solana Beach, Calif. 92075
12. PRENTKE ROMICH COMPANY, R.D. Box 191, Shreve, Ohio 44676
13. REHABILITATION ENGINEERING CENTER, Northwestern University, 345 East Superior St., Room 1441, Chicago, Ill. 60611
14. TARGET INDUSTRIES INC., 1264 Union St., W. Springfield, Mass. 01089
15. TELESENSORY SYSTEMS, INC., 1889 Page Mill Rd., Palo Alto, Calif. 94304
16. VA STANDARD DESIGN FOR SAFETY AND QUALITY OF AUTOMOTIVE ADAPTIVE EQUIPMENT
17. VISUALTEK, 1610 26th St., Santa Monica, Calif. 90404

Sources and Systems for the Disabled

This section lists primary sources of systems and devices for the disabled, along with basic references in the field.

Communication Aids

An excellent reference exists in this area, prepared by the Trace Research and Development Center. This is a continuously updating comprehensive listing of all communication devices, obviating the need for individual manufacturer listings. This reference can be purchased directly from Trace Center:

> *Non-Vocal Communication Resource Book,* edited by Gregg C. Vanderheiden, Trace Center, 1500 March Lane, University of Wisconsin, Madison, Wisc. 53706. Published by University Park Press, 233 East Redwood St., Baltimore, Md. 21202.

Mobility Aids

Manufacturers and distributors of powered wheelchairs and accessories:

American Stair Glide Corp., 4001 E. 138th St., Grandview, Mo. 64030

American Battery Car, Inc., R.R. 2, Box 126, Bristol, Ind. 46507

Amigo Inc., 6693 Dixie Highway, Bridgeport, Mich. 48722

ASKOM, Executive Building, 521 S. 14th St., Lincoln, Nebr. 68508

The Braun Corp., 1014 S. Monticello, Winamac, Ind. 46996

Braune Batricar Ltd., Griffin Mill, Trupp, Stroud, Gloucestershire, England, GL5 2AZ

E. F. Brewer Co., Box 159, 13901 W. Main St., Menomonee Falls, Wisc. 53051

Center for Orthotic Design, 325 Princeton Road, Menlo Park, Calif. 94025

The Chair Concern, 11825 Alondra Boulevard, Norwalk, Calif. 90650

Double DD, 341 North Dr., St. Charles, Mo. 63301

Everest & Jennings, Inc., 1803 Pontius, Los Angeles, Calif. 90025

Gendron Inc., Lugbill Rd., Archbold, Ohio 43502

General Teleoperators Inc., P.O. Box 3584, Los Amigos Station, Downey, Calif. 90242

Howard Mobility-Plus Inc., 124 W. S. Boundary, Perrysburg, Ohio 43551

Lic-Sweden, Stetsav vagen 4, 17183 Solna, Sweden

Lakeside Manufacturing Inc., 1983 S. Allis St., Milwaukee, Wisc. 53207

Lift Aids of Texas Inc., Custom Home Elevator Co., Inc., P.O. Box 18627, Fort Worth, Texas 76118

Medical Equipment Distributors, Inc., 1701 S. First Ave., Maywood, Ill. 60153

Mobility Dynamics, Inc., 21029 Itasca Ave., Unit D, Chatsworth, Calif. 91311

Nelson Medical Products, 5690 Sarah Ave., Sarasota, Fla. 33581

SAAB-SCANIA, Fack S-551 01, Jönkoping, Sweden

Sherry Products Inc., 1501 Pacific Coast Highway, Hermosa Beach, Calif. 90254

Voyager Inc., Box 1577, South Bend, Ind. 46634

Manufacturers of Electronic Travel Aids (ETAs):

Laser Cane: Bionic Instruments, 167 Old Belmont Ave., Bala-Cynwyd, Pa. 19004

Sonicguide: Telesensory Systems Inc., 1889 Page Mill Rd., Palo Alto, Calif. 94304

The standards for adaptive automobile equipment, including lifts, are listed in the VAPC Standards. They also list the manufacturers who are in compliance with these regulations for controls and wheelchair lifts:

Va Standard Design for Safety and Quality of Automotive Adaptive Equipment VAPC-A-7508-8

Included in *Bulletin of Prosthetics Research*, Veterans Administration, Washington, D. C., Spring 1976, BPR 10-25, pp. 162–170.

Environmental Control Systems

Manufacturers:

C. R. Bard, Inc., 731 Central Ave., Murray Hill, N. J. 07974

Cascade Medical Equipment, 6500 6th N. W., Seattle, Wash. 98117

Down East Electronics Mfg. Co., 44 Bucknam Rd., Falmouth, Maine 04105

Fidelity Electronics Inc., 5445 Diversey Ave., Chicago, Ill. 60639

General Telco Operators Inc., P.O. Box 3584, Los Amigo Station, Downey, Calif. 92042

Possum Inc., 6447 Forbes Ave., Van Nuys, Calif. 91409

Prentke Romich Co., R.D. 2, Box 191, Shreve, Ohio 44676

Scientific Systems International Inc., 506 B Oakwood Ave., N. E., Huntsville, Ala. 35811

Western Technical Products, 923 23rd Ave., E., Seattle, Wash. 98112

Information Sources

Accent on Living, P.O. Box 700, Gillum Road & High Drive, Bloomington, Ill. 61701

Produce a consumer magazine quarterly. Originate special publications dealing with specific problems on the disabled population. Maintain a computer information retrieval system on systems, devices, and how-to information on activities of daily living. The system is lay-oriented in terms of using a terminal to access information. Also developing a buyer's guide to equipment for the disabled.

Green Pages, P.O. Box 1586, Winter Park, Fla. 32289

This directory is published twice yearly with quarterly supplements, functioning as a "Yellow Pages" of products and services for the physically disabled.

International Commission on Technical Aids, Housing and Transportation, ICTA Information Center, FACK, S-161 25, Bromma 1 Sweden. This organization, which is housed in the Swedish Institute for the Handicapped, maintains a data base for international exchange. It is sponsored by the International Society for Rehabilitation of the Disabled. Write for a list of publications.

Prosthetics/Orthotics Research Reference Catalog

Available from the Printing and Publishing Office, National Academy of Sciences, 2101 Constitution Ave., N. W., Washington, D. C. 20418

This is an extensive cross referencing system of prosthetics and orthotics research, which includes some information on adaptive equipment and environmental control systems.

21

Eponymic Orthoses

HERMAN L. KAMENETZ, M.D.

During the 20th century, there has developed a tendency to turn away from eponyms. Medicine participated in this movement. In one of its branches, this resulted in the total abandonment of eponyms—at least theoretically. Indeed, only one exception has survived in *Nomina Anatomica*, the official internationally adopted list of anatomic terms: *tendo Achillis* has remained as an alternative to *tendo calcaneus*.[1] Likewise, diseases, procedures, instruments, signs, and symptoms have progressively become less associated with proper names, and the same effort has extended to the field of orthotics.

An eponym does not express anything about the use of a brace, not even about its anatomic area of application. In fact, certain proper names are associated with more than one device, *e.g.*, Hugh Owen Thomas devised splints for many body parts. Moreover, not every "Thomas" splint was conceived by the same person. Thus, eponymous terms are not always specific, and many need an additional description. Furthermore, two similar appliances, developed by two different individuals, may be called by different names of persons or places, instead of sharing a name revealing their common purpose. Later modifications might bring the devices even closer together, while parochialism keeps them separate.

If these facts apply within one and the same country, they become even more important as international communication and exchange increase. Therefore, the search for standardization, for the institution of an anatomic or physiologic (*i.e.*, functional) nomenclature or—even better—a combination of both, is very much justified, and great strides have been made in this respect in the 1970's.[2]

However, several points can be made in favor of orthotic eponyms (vanity, flattery, and chauvinism are not among them). The relative ease with which

---

[1] International Anatomical Nomenclature Committee. *Nomina Anatomica*, ed. 4, Amsterdam, 1977. As noted in the first three editions (London, 1955; Amsterdam, 1961 and 1966), Achilles tendon "is not regarded as a true anatomical eponym."

[2] Harris, E. E. A new orthotics terminology. A guide to its use for prescription and fee schedules. *Orthotics Prosthet.*, 27 (2): 6–19, 1973.

eponyms were eliminated from the anatomic terminology and will one day be eliminated from diagnoses cannot apply to objects. Diseases, and even more so, anatomic structures are limited in number; braces are not.

Furthermore, even functional names leave something to be desired since a complex orthosis may require too unwieldy a name. As opposed to this, an eponym is a convenient abbreviation.

Eponymous terms may also be justified for objects which can be considered historically. Just as we should relegate eponyms more and more into oblivion, there is no need to delete an old-fashioned name for an old-fashioned device. This attitude could be applied to other fields as well, notably to the one closest to orthotics, that is, prosthetics, and to medical technology and medicine in general. Thus, deserved credit (at least in some cases), historic data and, hence, intellectual delight inherent in eponyms can be conserved in terms such as Hessing brace, Thomas ring, and Taylor back support. Indeed, Hessing braces, notwithstanding their many types and variations, have been well established in their features, no material of modern invention will change them, and no further type will be added. Moreover, their importance in history is well established, and the implied honor is well deserved.

Under certain conditions, an eponym might also be applied to an object whose history is not as yet concluded. It may represent a significant advance, its development might continue, and its reputation might be so great that to replace the proper name with a descriptive name might not add to its clarity.

The mentioned principles apply to only a few of the names in this chapter, but they might serve as a guide for the future. The main reason for the following list is the fact that orthotic eponyms are still found in great numbers, and many a reader of this book might ask "What is it?" Here, he will find an immediate answer. Even if the latter does not include a full definition or description, it may give a reference (sometimes the one to the original publication) or some other information which will guide the searcher to his next step. References to this book are included here by chapters and in the Index by pages. Another reason for this chapter is historic curiosity.

In order to fulfill these two purposes I was forced to make the list discouragingly long, with many obsolete terms, although it represents only a selection. Yet, I hope that even more of the eponyms will become obsolete, that the given definitions will help in the use of a more appropriate nomenclature, and that this chapter will soon be only of historic interest.

A

Abbott, Edville Gerhardt. Portland, Maine, orthopedic surgeon, 1870–1938.
    Abbott jacket
        A plaster jacket with pressure pads used in the treatment of scoliosis.
        Abbott, E. G. Correction of lateral curvature of the spine. *N. Y. Med. J.*, *95:* 835, 1912.

Arnold-Abbott brace

Thoracolumbosacral orthosis with two paraspinal uprights, to which are attached three crossbars between the pelvis and the lower angles of the scapulae.

Abouna splint

Distal interphalangeal orthosis. Made of one piece of steel wire enclosed in a tube of latex rubber, it is shaped to fit over the two distal phalanges. Used in the treatment of mallet finger. Abouna, J. M., and Brown, H. The treatment of mallet finger. *Br. J. Surg., 55:* 653–667, 1968. Abstract in *Mod. Med., 38:* 124–125, July 27, 1970.

Adams metacarpal splint

Adams, J. E. A new metacarpal splint. *Lancet, 1:* 194, 1916.

Adams varus splint

Single upright attached to a shoe insert. In *Orthopaedic Apparatus,* edited by F. G. Ernst, p. 94. London, 1921.

Adams wrist splint

Adams, A. W. Cock-up wrist splint of duralumin wire. *Br. Med. J., 2:* 287, 1923.

Agnew, David Hayes. Philadelphia surgeon, 1818–1892.

Agnew thigh splint

Hip-knee-ankle-foot orthosis with pelvic band and ischial-weight-bearing thigh corset. Agnew, D. H. *Principles and Practice of Surgery.* Philadelphia, J. B. Lippincott Co., 1883.

Alexander-Kountz abdominal belt

Lower abdominal support with compression of the lower mid-portion by a pad. Alexander, H. L., and Kountz, W. B. Symptomatic relief of emphysema by an abdominal belt. *Am. J. Med. Sci., 187:* 687–692, 1934.

AMBRL or USAMBRL

Abbreviation for (United States) Army Medical Bioengineering Research and Development Laboratory, where several orthoses and prostheses were developed.

American hip splint

Judson, A. B. The American hip splint. *Lancet, 2:* 1225, 1888.

Anderson abduction splint

Shoulder abduction splint with adjustable shoulder and elbow. Described by Lawrence Noall. Upper extremity braces. *Instructional Course Lectures, 9:* 221–232 (p. 223), 1952.

Anderson, Roger. Seattle, Washington, orthopedic surgeon, 1891–1971.

Roger Anderson splint

Splint for external fixation of fractures of long bones. The fragments above and below the fracture are transfixed by pins which are then attached to rods. *British Medical Dictionary* (7).

Roger Anderson well-leg traction

Traction on the femur by incorporating both legs in plaster. The feet are then connected by an apparatus which forces the affected leg into full abduction and the well leg into full adduction, thus producing traction on the abducted leg. *British Medical Dictionary* (7). Anderson, R. New method for treating fractures utilizing the well leg for countertraction. *Surg. Gynecol. Obstet., 54:* 207, 1932.

Andrews ischiatic crutch

A half ring for ischial weightbearing attached to the pelvis and mounted on a rod attached to a shoe. Devised in 1860 by E. Andrews to avoid weightbearing on a lower limb. *Orthopaedic Appliances Atlas* (1), p. 350.

APL

Abbreviation for Applied Physics Laboratory of Johns Hopkins University, Baltimore, where electromechanical devices were developed to be used in conjunction with orthoses. Staros, A., and Rubin, G. The orthopedic surgeon and rehabilitation engineering. *Orthopedics, 1* (2): 118–124, 1978.

Arnold brace

Trunk support consisting of a large belt covering the entire pelvis, two paraspinal uprights, and a transverse band at a high dorsal level which drops to pass under the axillae, to rise again to the subclavicular regions, from where a pair of shoulder straps go to the back. Arnold, Hubert R. An efficient back brace. *Calif. West. Med., 46:* 323, 1937. *Orthopaedic Appliances Atlas* (1), pp. 219–220; see Fig. 6.18 of this book.

Arnold-Abbott brace

See under Abbott, Edville Gerhardt.

Ashhurst splint

A bracketed knee-ankle-foot wire splint used following excision of knee joint. Developed by John Ashhurst, Philadelphia surgeon, 1839–1900. *Dorland's Illustrated Medical Dictionary.* (9).

Ashley heel

A shoe heel with particularly large base of support built for greater stability in walking.

Augustine hyperextension brace

Similar to the Jewett brace. Augustine, Robert W. Brace for extension of the spine. *J. Bone Joint Surg., 30*(A): 784–785, 1948.

B

Baeyer, Hans von. German orthopedic surgeon (1875–1941) who developed various orthoses, some of which are described in this book, *Grundlagen der orthopädischen Mechanik.* Berlin, Julius Springer, 1935.

Baeyer dropfoot brace

A short ankle-foot orthosis with posterior upright and a pair of elastic or leather straps from the calfband to the lace stays of the shoe. *Orthopaedic Appliances Atlas* (1), p. 426; Jordan (11), p. 141.

Baeyer lock
> An automatic joint lock. Jordan (11), p. 91.

Baeyer tonus bandage
> Circular webbing straps around body to give tension to lower limbs while walking. Hohmann (10), p. 171.

Baker spinal brace
> A hinged brace with pads and "active" straps across back. Baker, L. D. Rhizomelic spondylosis. *J. Bone Joint Surg.*, 24: 827, 1942.

Bal, Balmoral (bal, balmoral) shoe
> Front-laced shoe of the Oxford type (*q.v.*), in which the lace stays meet in front, being stitched along their anterior borders to the vamp. Named after Balmoral Castle in Scotland, the then-center of fashion where the shoe was introduced in 1853 by Queen Victoria's consort Prince Albert.

Baldwin aeroplane splint
> A shoulder-abduction orthosis secured to the body by a half pelvic band and a posterior upright. Baldwin, C. H. A light aeroplane splint that permits mobility of the elbow. *J. A. M. A.*, 83: 687, 1924.

Balmoral (balmoral) shoe
> See Bal, Balmoral shoe.

Barlow splint
> X-shaped metal splint applied to the back of an infant with congenital dislocation of the hip. The four ends of the splint are molded over the shoulders and thighs to keep the latter abducted and flexed. Barlow, T. G. Early diagnosis and treatment of congenital dislocation of the hip. *J. Bone Joint Surg.*, 44(B): 292–301, 1962.

Barr-Buschenfeldt brace
> A scoliosis brace including turnbuckle and levers. Barr, Joseph S. and Buschenfeldt, Karl. A three-point-pressure brace for the corrective treatment of ambulatory cases of scoliosis. *J. Bone Joint Surg.*, 18: 760–765, 1936. Blount in Licht (13), p. 308.

Barton wedge
> A wedge inserted inside the shoe at its medial border.

Barwell bandage
> A device for the correction of scoliosis called "Oblique and Spiral Bandage", developed in 1868 by Richard Barwell, London surgeon, 1826–1916. Thomas in *Orthopaedic Appliances Atlas* (1), p. 182.

Bateman hand splint
> Dorsal wrist-hand orthosis with adjustable tension in flexion or extension, using spring steel bands. Bateman, J. E. A universal splint for deformities of the hand. *J. Bone Joint Surg.*, 28: 169, 1946.

Batts hallux valgus splint
> A traction device cut from a rubber glove. Batts, M., Jr. A simple corrective device for hallux valgus. *J. Bone Joint Surg.*, 23: 183, 1941.

Bavarian splint
>This term refers not to a specific part of the body but to the material used. Two pieces of flannel or cloth are folded once and sewn along the fold. A layer of fine plaster of Paris paste is introduced between each two layers of textile, and the splint is molded to the body. To remove it, it is cut along the seam. It was used similarly to plaster splints, probably as early as 1860. Peare, R. J. Bavarian splint modified. *Peninsula J. Med.*, 1: 8, 1876. Croft, J. Plaster of Paris splints for fractures of the leg. *Lancet, 1:* 819, 1878.

Baylor metatarsal splint
>An aluminum foot splint manufactured by the Zimmer Company.

Beattie splint
>A wrist cuff with an extension to immobilize the third digit. In *Orthopaedic Apparatus*, edited by F. G. Ernst, p. 14. London, 1921.

Becker brace or joint
>Both terms refer to an ankle-foot orthosis with a Becker joint, *i.e.,* a double adjustable ankle joint with two spring channels placed at the anterior and posterior borders of the uprights. Made by the Becker Company. Heizer, D. Short leg brace design for hemiplegia. *Phys. Ther., 47* (9): 844–847, 1967.

Becker twister
>A standard twister cable device made by the Becker Company.

Beeger bridge cast
>Plaster corset to immobilize the cervical spine. Schanz (17), p. 136.

Beely splint
>Pelvic band with single thigh uprights and cuffs to pull knees apart. Hohmann (10), p. 147.

Bell back brace
>Lumbosacral posture brace. Hines in Licht (13), p. 4.

Bell-Grice splint
>A bilateral shoe clamp spreader bar. Bell, J. F., and Grice, D. S. Treatment of congenital talipes equinovarus with modified Denis Browne splint. *J. Bone Joint Surg., 26:* 799–811, 1944.

Bender splint
>Fifth-finger adduction splint with spring wire. Bender, F. L. Prevention of deformities through orthotics. *J. A. M. A., 183:* 946, 1963. See Chapter 8 and Fig. 8.31.

Benesh shoe
>A shoe for the equinus foot made by the M. J. Markell Company.

Bennett, Robert L. Physiatrist, Warm Springs, Georgia, under whose direction various orthoses were developed which were most often labeled Warm Springs (*q.v.*); see also Chapter 8 of this book.

Bennett finger splints
>Simple orthoses for the digits of the hand to control instabilities and deformities commonly encountered in rheumatoid arthritis. These

are mostly metal devices to be slipped on a digit ("slip-on splints"), occasionally also with a strap of metal or textile material. Bennett, R. L. Orthetic devices to prevent deformities of the hand in rheumatoid arthritis. *Arthritis Rheum.*, *8:* 1006–1018, 1965.

Bennett reacher or feeder

A device to assist or provide functional motion of the shoulder joint. Bennett, R. L. Orthetic devices for weakness of the upper extremity. *South. Med. J.*, *50:* 791–795, 1957. Bennett, R. L., and Stephens, H. R. Assistive and adaptive apparatus for upper extremities: feeders. *Phys. Ther. Rev.*, *35:* 626–640, 1955.

Bennett spinal brace

A Knight brace modified by the addition of a horizontal band over the iliac crests to obtain a firm grip of the pelvis. Bennett, George E. (Baltimore orthopedic surgeon). The treatment of tuberculosis of the spine in children. *Surg. Clin. North Am.*, *16*(5): 1321–1335, 1936.

Biesalski-Eckhardt brace

Hip stabilization splint used in arthritis. Biesalski, K. Neue Modelle aus der orthopädischen Werkstatt. *Arch. Orthop. Unfallchir.*, *28:* 163, 1930. Hohmann (10), p. 131.

Bigg, Henry H. London surgeon, 1826–1881.

Bigg spinal braces

Some such braces were made of steel. Thomas in *Orthopaedic Appliances Atlas* (1), p. 183. Schanz (17), p. 185.

Bigg splint for Volkmann's contracture

Wrist-hand orthosis devised in 1869, illustrated in Boyes (6), p. 154.

Bisgrove hand or splint

Tenodesis wrist-hand orthosis. Doman, R. J., *et al. Nonsurgical central approach to the central problem. Part II. Reflex therapy.* Hemiplegia School Lecture Course. Rehabilitation Center of Philadelphia, Winter 1957, in Hoerner, E. F. Rehabilitation of the amputee, the hemiplegic and the quadriplegic. *Clin. Orthop.*, *12:* 96–123, esp. 117–118, 1958; see Chapter 8 of this book.

Blanchard hip splint

Orthosis reaching from the ankle to a chest band in order to immobilize a fractured femur. Used in conjunction with a patten under the other shoe to avoid weightbearing. Devised in the 1860s by Wallace Blanchard, Chicago surgeon. Alldredge and Snow in *Orthopaedic Appliances Atlas* (1), pp. 351, 354.

Blenke dropfoot brace

High shoe with calf band attached to it by posterior upright. Schanz (17) in *Orthopaedic Appliances Atlas* (1), p. 426.

Blucher (blucher) shoe

Front-laced shoe of the Oxford type (*q.v.*), in which the lace stays extend forward over the vamp; since they are not stitched to it, they remain loose and can be fully opened, leaving more room to the entering foot. Named after the Prussian field marshal Gebhard von Blücher (1742–1819), who in 1810 introduced a high boot of this pattern.

Bluhm clubfoot splint

A modification of footplates to provide a corrective force in adduction deformity of the forefoot. Bluhm, Michael. Modification of the Denis Browne splint. *J. Bone Joint Surg., 29:* 248–249, 1947.

Böhler, Lorenz. Vienna orthopedic surgeon, 1885–1973.

Böhler arm splint

A piece of wood, measuring 30 × 15 × 5 cm, rounded at the upper end to fit the axilla. *Dorland's Illustrated Medical Dictionary* (9).

Böhler finger splint

Wire incorporated in plaster for finger fixation. Boyes (6), p. 153.

Boldrey cervical immobilizer

A cervical orthosis; see Chapter 5 and Fig. 5.14.

Bonnet torticollis support

Cervical collar with large shoulder harness. Schanz (17), p. 160.

Borggreve brace

Hip-knee-ankle-foot orthosis, including pelvic girdle, for paraplegics. Hohmann (10), p. 169.

Boston arch support

Arch support constructed of light metal with metatarsal support and slightly cupped leather-covered heel. Jahss in *Atlas of Orthotics* (2), p. 277.

Boston brace or corset

A prefabricated molded plastic thoracolumbosacral orthosis for the treatment of scoliosis; see Chapter 7 and Fig. 7.14.

Bosworth hip abduction splint

Bosworth, D. M. A hip brace. *J. Bone Joint Surg., 18:* 238, 1936.

Bouvier brace

A torticollis brace with a pelvic belt. Schanz (17), p. 157.

Braaz corset

A corset made of felt dipped in water glass and covered with shellac. Schanz (17), p. 148.

Brackett brace

Thoracolumbosacral orthosis of the shorter type. Attached to the posterior uprights, which are longer than the lateral uprights, is a thoracic strap. Devised by Elliott G. Brackett, Boston orthopedic surgeon, 1860–1942. Thomas in *Orthopaedic Appliances Atlas* (1), p. 211–213; see Fig. 6.11 of this book.

Bradford-Graham spinal brace

A modification of the Hoadley anterior hyperextension brace. Bradford, Charles H., and Graham, Walter C. Hyperextension back brace for treatment of compression fractures of vertebrae. *Mil. Surg., 98:* 40–42, 1946.

Bradford-Lovett bowleg braces
> Bilateral lower-limb braces with single medial uprights which curve anteriorly and upward to join a pelvic band. Knee caps and leg straps provide corrective force. Braces attach to shoes and have free ankle joints and no knee joints. Bradford, Edward Hickling (Boston orthopedic surgeon, 1848–1926) and Lovett, Robert W. (Boston orthopedic surgeon, 1859–1924). *A Treatise on Orthopedic Surgery*, ed. 5, New York, 1915, in *Orthopaedic Appliances Atlas* (1), p. 419.

Breidbach bandage
> Leather bandage for dropfoot. Rabl (15), p. 291.

Brewster jacket
> A hinged plaster jacket with turnbuckle composed of two girdle-like sections. The hinge is on the side of the convexity and the turnbuckle on that of the concavity. Shands, A. R., and Raney, R. B. *Handbook of Orthopaedic Surgery*, ed. 5, p. 431. St. Louis, 1957.

Brian Thomas splint
> See Thomas, F. Brian.

Brodie scoliosis brace
> Thomas in *Orthopaedic Appliances Atlas* (1), p. 184.

Browne, Sir Denis John. London orthopedic surgeon, 1892–1967.
> Denis Browne boot, bootie, or shoe
>> Pre-walker clubfoot shoe used in conjunction with the Denis Browne splint. It laces to the toe, and there is no toe box.

> Denis Browne splint
>> A bilateral shoe clamp spreader bar: two steel plates securely attached to a child's shoes and connected by a crossbar to keep the lower limbs abducted and the feet in a position to correct talipes equinovarus. Browne, D. J. Talipes equino-varus. *Lancet, 2:* 969–974, 1934. Moore in *Orthopaedic Appliances Atlas* (1), p. 485. Staros and LeBlanc in *Atlas of Orthotics* (2), p. 205.

Bruns Collar
> Cervical brace with four upright posts, used in torticollis. Schanz (17), p. 156.

Bryant splint
> A splint to keep lower limbs parallel and to obviate necessity for perineal band in treatment of hip disease and hip injuries. Bryant, Thomas (London surgeon, 1828–1914). On the value of parallelism of the lower extremities. . . . *Lancet, 1:* 159–160. 31 Jan. 1880, in Kelly (12).

Buckminster-Brown brace
> A head support. Mentioned in Clark, M. Melvin. An adjustable torticollis brace for postoperative use. *J. Bone Joint Surg., 13:* 613–615, 1931.

Bunge splint or radial glove
> Laced forearm cuff for radial nerve palsy. Hohmann (10), p. 107.

Bunnell, Sterling. San Francisco hand surgeon, 1882–1957. Original author of a comprehensive textbook, later edited by Joseph H. Boyes: *Bunnell's Surgery of the Hand*, ed. 5. Philadelphia, 1970, in which a great number of orthoses are discussed and illustrated. See Boyes (6) and Bunnell in *Orthopaedic Appliances Atlas* (1), pp. 277–326; Splinting of the hand, in *Instructional Course Lectures, 9:* 233–243, 1952; see also Chapter 8 of this book.

Burman forearm brace
An orthosis to correct pronation contracture. Burman, Michael S. A brace for the correction of spastic pronation contracture of the forearm. *J. Bone Joint Surg., 19:* 838–839, 1937.

Burnham splints
Dynamic finger splints. Bloomberg (5), p. 117.

Burns cockup splint
A posterior forearm-hand splint with wrist hinge adjusted by a turnbuckle. Burns, R. E. A corrective cock-up splint. *J. Bone Joint Surg., 11:* 94, 1929.

Butte scoliosis jacket
Plaster wedging jacket for scoliosis. Butte, F. F. Scoliosis treated by wedging jacket. *J. Bone Joint Surg., 20:* 1, 1938.

Butterworth back brace
A Taylor type of brace with buckles in front and shoulder straps which attach at about the 12th thoracic vertebra. A pelvic band is sometimes added at level of greater trochanter. Butterworth, R[eynoldson] D[uke]. Modification of Taylor back brace. *Virg. Med. Monthly, 91:* 385, 1964.

C

Cabot splint
Posterior wire splint for lower limb. *Dorland's Illustrated Medical Dictionary* (9).

Cadenza girdle
A girdle for abdominal and low back support made by the Camp Company.

California brace
A back brace resembling the Taylor brace. Bloomberg (5), p. 155.

California crutch
Synonym of Canadian crutch. Suggested term: wooden triceps crutch.

Callahan back brace
Thoracolumbosacral brace which covers the inferior angles of the scapulae and includes shoulder straps. Hines in Licht (13), p. 5.

Calot jacket
A plaster jacket, formerly used for tuberculosis of the spine, with extension to chin and occiput; in fact, a Minerva jacket. Named after

Jean-François Calot, French surgeon, 1861–1944. Calot, F. *Traité Pratique de Technique Orthopédique.* Paris, 1906. See also Ritchie jacket.

Calot leg splint

Manufactured by the Orthopedic Equipment Company.

Campbell-Mitchner knee extension apparatus

Thigh and calf cuffs incorporated in a complex lever system. Campbell, W. C., and Mitchner, J. M. An apparatus for the correction of flexion contracture of the knee. *J. Bone Joint Surg., 8:* 416, 1926.

Camp-Varco pelvic traction belt

A device designed by Dr. S. Varco and made by the Camp Company.

Camp-Zieman arm sleeve

Laced sleeve for treatment of edema; made by the Camp Company.

Canadian crutch

Wooden crutch, resembling an axillary crutch, but slightly shorter and ending by a leather cuff at or slightly above mid-arm level, which prevents flexion (buckling) of the elbow. Hence, its indication for triceps weakness. Also called California crutch. Suggested term: wooden triceps crutch.

Canty long leg brace

Knee-ankle-foot orthosis with ischial seat and a knee joint with axis posterior to weightbearing line, used in flaccid paralysis and fractures of lower limb. Canty, Thomas J. Functional full length leg brace. *Am. J. Surg., 81:* 474–480, 1951.

Carr splint

A wooden hand splint used in Ireland.

CARS-UBC knee orthosis

Named after the Canadian Arthritis and Rheumatism Society-University of British Columbia, it consists of two plastic cuffs, one for the thigh, one for the leg, connected by a telescoping rod. It is designed to correct a valgus or varus deformity of the knee, providing freedom to the flexed knee and a force to straighten it upon extension, as in the stance phase of gait. Reed, B. An evaluation of the C.A.R.S.-U.B.C. knee orthosis. *Orthotics Prosthet., 33*(1): 25–38, 1979.

Chambers, E. Francis S. American orthopedic surgeon, 1885–1962.

Chambers knee cap

Orthotic kneecap attached in a way that avoids pressure on the knee during flexion. Chambers, F. S. New method of attaching knee cap to caliper type of brace with lock knee joint by means of swiveled levers. *J. Bone Joint Surg., 16:* 212–213, 1934.

Chambers scoliosis brace

Chambers, F. S. A corrective appliance for scoliosis. *J. Bone Joint Surg., 17:* 219–224, 1935.

Chandler felt collar

A felt collar, usually covered with stockinet, a machine-knitted, washable cloth. Illustrated in *Dorland's Illustrated Medical Dictionary* (9) under splints.

Charnley caliper

A short-term adjustable caliper to be used immediately after the removal of plaster applied for a fractured tibia. Nangle (14), p. 148.

Chatfield-Girdlestone splint

See under Girdlestone.

Chatterton clubfoot splint

A modified Denis Browne splint. It can be mounted on, and easily removed from, shoes which at other times are used for weight bearing. Chatterton, C. C., and Blaisdell, J. A modification of the Denis Browne splint. *J. Bone Joint Surg.*, 27: 518–519, 1945.

Clark torticollis brace

A head-supporting brace comprising a pelvic band, two anterior uprights extending over the shoulders, and an occipitomental support. Clark, M. Melwin. An adjustable torticollis brace for postoperative use. *J. Bone Joint Surg.*, 13: 613–615, 1931.

Cloran mouthstick

Motor-operated telescoping stick held in the mouth by means of a custom-fitted mouthpiece. Developed by Ohio dentist Arthur J. Cloran. Telescoping mouth instruments for severely handicapped patients. *J. Prosthet. Dent.*, 32(4): 435–438, 1974.

Cole knee hinge

Apparatus incorporated in plaster to mobilize knee flexion contracture. Cole, J. P. A new type of knee hinge and cast for the correction of knee flexion deformities. *J. Bone Joint Surg.*, 19: 196, 1937.

Collin collar

A four-post cervical brace. Schanz (17), p. 156.

Collins spring splint

A spring splint for paralysis of the long extensors of the fingers, leaving the finger pads and the palm of the hand free. Murdoch, G. (ed.) *Prosthetic and Orthotic Practice*, p. 480. London, 1970.

Colonel Humphrey splint

A finger splint distributed by the Devonian Orthopedic Association, 59 Wonford Road, Exeter, England.

Colorado College knee brace

A knee cage with a posterior bar added to the usual two side bars. Woodward, H. W. A new knee brace. *J. Bone Joint Surg.*, 15: 1024, 1933.

Comarr clamp

A carbon dioxide actuated clamp for bladder training. Comarr, A. Estin, and Snelson, R. Carbon dioxide actuated clamp for quadriplegic bladder training. *Arch. Phys. Med. Rehabil.*, 42: 614–615, 1961.

Compère hip abduction splint

Compere, Edward L. *Pictorial Handbook of Fracture Treatment.* Chicago, 1947.

Cook anterior heel

Metatarsal bar placed between the inner and outer soles. Shands, A. R., and Raney, R. B. *Handbook of Orthopaedic Surgery*, ed. 5, p. 538. St. Louis, 1957.

Cook shingle

Pressure pad used as an accessory to a flexible orthosis (corset). It is of rectangular shape, about 8 cm high and between 25 and 35 cm long, and is most often applied to the lumbosacral area.

Cook walking caliper

An ischial weight-bearing brace manufactured by the Zimmer Manufacturing Company.

Coonse hip splint

Coonse, G. Kenneth. A simple modification of Putti's splint for the early treatment of congenital dislocation of the hip. *J. Bone Joint Surg., 13:* 602–605, 1931.

Corret splint

Used for the treatment of Volkmann's contracture, it consists of palmar and dorsal valves, covering forearm and hand and laced to each other. Corret, P. Nouvel appareil redresseur pour rétraction de Volkmann. *Presse Méd. 46:* 748, 1938. *Orthopaedic Appliances Atlas* (1), p. 326.

Cotrel cast

Body cast made with slow-setting plaster during cephalopelvic traction while the patient is suspended by derotation slings applied to the outside of the cast. Developed for the treatment of scoliosis by Yves Cotrel *et al.* at Berck-Plage, France. It is also called EDF cast, for Elongation, Derotation and [lateral] Flexion. Cotrel, Y. La technique de l'E.D.F. dans le traitement de la scoliose. *Entretiens Bichat.* Expansion Scientifique Française. Paris, 1962. Keim, H. A. Scoliosis. *Ciba Clin. Symp., 24*(1): 21, 27, 1972.

Coughlin shoulder splint

A body harness with outrigger arranged so that patient receives assisted abduction by actively extending shoulder. Coughlin, Edward J., Jr. An abduction exercise splint for the shoulder. *J. Bone Joint Surg., 31A:* 438–439, 1949. An improved abduction exercise splint for the shoulder. *J. Bone Joint Surg., 33A:* 267, 1951.

Craig bar or (hip) splint

Spreader bar to which shoes are attached. Used in the treatment of Legg-Calvé-Perthes disease with permission of weight-bearing. Similar to Ilfeld abduction splint.

Craig-Scott orthosis
>See Scott-Craig orthosis.

Cramer wire splint
>A flexible splint, consisting of two stout wires, parallel, with fine cross wires, resembling a ladder. *Stedman's Medical Dictionary* (18). Illustrated in Noall (1), pp. 327, 328.

Cravener knee extension apparatus
>A leg-thigh double lever system controlled through a ratchet mechanism. Cravener, E. K. Device for overcoming non-bony flexion contractures of the knee. *J. Bone Joint Surg., 12:* 437, 1930.

Cuban heel
>A heel that is higher than the heel of an Oxford shoe (ca 3 to 5 centimeters) and less large. Usually only found in women's shoes, the heel is still large and low enough to admit a standard ankle-foot orthosis.

Cullen abduction splint
>An adjustable orthosis for shoulder abduction. Noall in *Orthopaedic Appliances Atlas* (1), p. 330.

Curry walking splint
>Duralumin splint to afford large weight-bearing surface in walking, made by the Zimmer Company.

Curtillet dropfoot brace
>Ankle-foot orthosis. A spring connects the upper part of the upright to a steel plate under the sole of the shoe at about the mid-part of the foot. Mouchet, A., and Anceau, G. *Revue d'Orthopédie 6:* 278, 1919, in Alldredge and Snow (1), p. 425.

D

Dabney splint
>Modification of an orthosis designed by Engen (Engen reciprocal finger prehension unit). Dabney, Ray, *et al.* A modified reciprocal wrist-extension, finger-flexion orthosis: the radial W.E.F.F. splint. *Arch. Phys. Med. Rehabil., 45:* 239, 1964.

Dane long leg brace
>Hip-knee-ankle-foot orthosis with pelvic band and hip joint allowing wide abduction of thigh. Dane, J. *Trans. Am. Orthop. Assoc., 10:* 233–235, 1897, in Alldredge and Snow (1), p. 355.

Davis splint
>A simple upright with straps, used in the treatment of coxalgia. Kolbe, D. W. & Son. *Apparatus for Deformities of the Lower Extremities.* ed. 6, 1879, in Alldredge and Snow (1), p. 348.

Deaver double-ring lock or two-position lock.
>A lock which allows to lock the hip or knee joint of an orthosis not only in extension (standing position) but also in flexion (sitting

position). Thus, the lower limb of an athetoid child is stabilized, and sliding forward in a chair is prevented. Devised by George G. Deaver, New York physiatrist, 1890–1973. Deaver in Licht (13), pp. 261–262.

Delbet walking cast

Walking cast applied during traction and made of a series of overlapping plaster splints molded for weight bearing on the tibial condyles. Used in fractures of the leg, according to Pierre Delbet, French surgeon, 1861–1925. Roux, G. *Petite Chirurgie et Technique Médicale Courante*, ed. 2, p. 217, 1941.

Delitala splint

Adjustable hip abduction splint. Hohmann (10), p. 144. See also Ref. 8.

DeLorme brace

Knee-ankle-foot orthosis with adjustable uprights and shoe clamp by which it is attached to the heel of the shoe. DeLorme, Thomas L., *et al.* An adjustable lower-extremity brace. *J. Bone Joint Surg.*, 43A: 205–210, 1961.

Denis Browne splint

See Browne, Sir Denis John.

Denver bar, Denver heel

A variant of the metatarsal bar, it is attached to the outsole of the shoe but is usually thinner and extends farther posteriorly, to about the level of the tarsometatarsal joints. Used to relieve pressure on the metatarsal heads. See Fig. 11.27. An internal Denver bar is inserted between outsole and insole. Jahss in *Atlas of Orthotics* (2), pp. 268, 276. Anderson (3), p. 23. The origin of its name is, according to Joseph E. Milgram and Malcolm A. Jacobson (Footgear: therapeutic modifications of sole and heel. *Orthop. Rev.*, 7 (11): 57–62, 1978), the following. H. Sonnenschein, a New York orthopedist, referred to it as the Denver bar, since he had seen it used, in the late 1930's, by Dr. Lyle Packard in Denver. The latter had seen it used by Dr. Arthur Steindler, who had brought it to Iowa City after having seen it first used by Sir Robert Jones in England.

De Puy splint

One of several orthoses, particularly for the wrist and hand. Example: resting cockup wrist-hand orthosis made of canvas reinforced with metal stays. It is meant to allow very slight motion in the wrist. Thus, the patient can use the wrist to a limited extent, as is often allowed in rheumatoid arthritis. De Puy Manufacturing Company. *Fracture Appliances and Methods of Use.* Warsaw, Indiana, 1928, in *Orthopaedic Appliances Atlas* (1), pp. 289, 293, 328, 330.

Derby (derby) shoe

Men's shoe with low heel, with the quarters overlapping the vamp, usually with buckle, for outdoor use. Named after Edward Stanley,

12th earl of Derby, England (1752–1834). Similar to the blucher shoe.

Digby splint

A traction orthosis for fractures of the femoral shaft. Digby, Kenelm H[enry]. A flexible-knee traction splint for the lower limb. *Surg. Gynecol. Obstet., 43:* 207–214, 1926.

Diveley, Rex L. Orthopedic surgeon, Kansas City, Missouri, 1892–

Diveley dropfoot brace

Ankle-foot orthosis with posterior upright attached to molded foot plate entering the shoe, preventing footdrop. Dickson, F. D., and Diveley, R. L. *Functional Disorders of the Foot.* Philadelphia 1939. *Orthopaedic Appliances Atlas* (1), p. 431. See also Diveley (1), pp. 439–478.

Diveley lumbosacral support

A rectangular lumbar steel frame enclosed in a lumbosacral corset with perineal straps. Diveley, R. A lumbosacral support. *J. Bone Joint Surg., 31A:* 441, 1949.

Dollfus elastic splint

Elastic cables and webstraps to provide hip and knee extension and foot dorsiflexion, also to be used in conjunction with metal orthoses, to replace weak muscles. Dollfus, P. H., Lund, T., and Lygind, F. Elastic splints for patients with paralysis of the lower extremities. *Arch. Phys. Med. Rehabil., 36:* 564–566, 1955.

Dollinger hip brace

Designed to eliminate motion at a hip joint, it consists of a corset, double-upright thigh and leg parts and a high shoe, all four parts laced. Dollinger, Julius (Budapest). *Z. Orthop. Chir. Heilgymnastik Massage, 7:* 20, 1900. Alldredge and Snow (1), p. 355.

Donaldson-Engh scoliosis jacket

Combined plaster jacket and corset distracted by double-threaded tubes fastened to metal bands. Donaldson, J., and Engh, O. A. Correction of scoliosis by a distractor apparatus. *J. Bone Joint Surg., 20:* 405, 1938.

Dorinson hand splint

Dorsal hand splint to extend wrist and counteract ulnar deviation, and with thumb cuff to keep thumb abducted. Used in cerebral palsy. Dorinson, S. Malvern, *et al.* A functional hand splint for the cerebral palsied child. *Arch. Phys. Med. Rehabil., 35:* 711–713, 1954.

Dowse splint

An extension splint with steel upright and knee joint posterior to the weight-bearing line. Used for hip disease, it was "devised by Taylor of New York and called by him Dowse splint." Brackett, E. G. The experimental value of the Dowse splint. *Boston Med. Surg. J., 117:* 321–325, 1887.

Doyle head support
   A head halter for torticollis. Schanz (17), p. 165.
Duchenne scoliosis brace
   A back brace with straps and levers attached to a midline posterior
   upright. Thomas in *Orthopaedic Appliances Atlas* (1), p. 184.
Ducroquet cervicodorsal corset
   In Delitala (8), p. 80.
Dumoulin hand splint
   Glove with distal straps which, when attached to a forearm cuff, pull
   the digits into flexion. Dumoulin and Roederer. *Rev. Orthop.*, *29*: 259,
   1922, in Bunnell (1), p. 314.
Dutchman
   A beveled piece of leather inserted between layers of heel or sole
   (Lewin, P. *The Foot and Ankle*, ed. 4, p. 54. Philadelphia, 1959).
   Usually, it is a lateral sole wedge under the fifth metatarsal bone.
   Anderson (3), p. 17.

E

Eckhardt ischial seat
   A seating support placed under the ischial tuberosity of the unin-
   volved side but attached to a thigh corset of the involved side, thus
   relieving some of its weight. Eckhardt, Hellmut. Die Anwendung des
   Gegentuberhaltes bei orthopädischen Erkrankungen. *Z. Orthop.
   Chir. Heilgymnastik Massage*, *47*: 139, 1925–1926. *Orthopaedic Appliances Atlas* (1), p. 400.
Ellis splint
   A digital support reaching from the palm to the fingertip and being
   attached by straps to hand and finger. After J. D. Ellis (1928), in
   Orthopaedic Appliances Atlas (1), p. 306.
Engen, Thorkild J. Prosthetist-orthotist at Texas Institute for Rehabilita-
   tion and Research, where he developed orthoses also labeled TIRR
   (*q.v.*). See especially Engen, T. J. Development of upper extremity
   orthotics. Part I. *Orthotics Prosthet.*, *24* (1): 12–29, March 1970. Part
   II. *Orthotics Prosthet.*, *24* (2): 1–31, June 1970. See also Chapter 8 of
   this book.
Engen extension orthosis
   Orthosis based on the three-point pressure principle to correct joint
   deformities such as knee-, elbow-, or wrist flexion contractures or
   genu valgum. Engen, T. J. Adjustable knee or elbow extension
   orthosis: a new orthotic development. *Orthop. Prosthet. Appl. J.*, *15*:
   45, 1961.
Engen reciprocal finger prehension unit
   A flexor tenodesis splint. Engen, T. J. A modification of a reciprocal

wrist extension, finger flexion orthosis. *Orthop. Prosthet. Appl. J.,* *14:* 39, 1960.

Engen wrist splint
A palmar wrist splint; see Chapter 8.

English cane
Forearm crutch: usually made of aluminum, it has a single upright, a hand piece, and a hinged open cuff at the upper end of the forearm extension.

Erlacher, Philipp J. Vienna orthopedic surgeon.

Erlacher hand splint
Glove-like covering anchored to wrist band, keeping fingers in flexion. Hohmann (10), p. 114.

Erlacher scoliosis brace
Back brace with incorporated weight-and-pulley system for the correction of spinal deformities. Developed in 1928. Blount in Licht (13), p. 308.

Ernst cervical support
In Ernst, F. G. *Orthopaedic Apparatus,* p. 26. London, 1921.

Eschbaum collar
A four-post cervical brace. Schanz (17), p. 155.

Eschbaum corset
An aluminum corset laced in front. Schanz (17), p. 196.

Esmond walking brace
An ambulation training device which connects the lateral borders of the shoes of a child with the medial borders of the shoes of an adult. The child walks between the legs of the adult. Esmond, William G. Assisted walking brace for a cerebral palsied child. *Arch. Phys. Med. Rehabil.,* *44:* 463–465, 1963.

Eulenburg brace
A torticollis brace with pelvic belt and mandibular supports. Schanz (17), p. 157.

Everett crutch
Synonym of Warm Springs crutch (*q.v.*). A metal triceps crutch, named after Charles E. Everett, a patient at Georgia Warm Springs Foundation, Warm Springs, Georgia, for whom the first crutch of this type was made. Personal communication, Robert L. Bennett, M.D., Warm Springs. See also Irwin, C. E. Apparatus for the upper extremity disabled by poliomyelitis. *Instructional Course Lectures,* *9:* 208–221, esp. p. 219, 1952.

Ewing long leg brace
Orthosis including a modification of the upper portion of the medial thigh upright, aimed at decreasing the bulkiness in the crotch, particularly in bilateral orthoses. The upright is bent posteriorly and slightly spiraled to conform to the contour of the thigh. Ewing, Marlin

B. Long leg brace modification. *Arch. Phys. Med. Rehabil., 44:* 656, 1963.

Exeter wrist splint

A spring splint for the wrist, which allows active wrist and finger movements. Nangle (14), p. 104. Muckart, R. D., in Murdoch, G. *Prosthetic and Orthotic Practice*, pp. 478–479. London, 1970.

F

Faber brace

A trunk brace for paralyzed trapezius muscles. Hohmann (10), p. 92.

Fabricius finger flexor

A complicated brace, reaching to the arm, designed to flex the fingers. The fingertips are covered by long thimbles which, by means of strings, are pulled toward the forearm. Devised by Hieronymus Fabricius ab Aquapendente, Italian anatomist and surgeon, 1537–1619. Fabricius. *Opera Chirurgica*, 1647, in *Orthopaedic Appliances Atlas* (1), p. 326.

Fillauer bar or splint

Abduction bar, made of steel, on which the shoes of a child are attached, his lower limbs in abduction, for the correction of internal or external tibial torsion. Similar to a Denis Browne bar, the Fillauer bar has clamps which allow easy attachment and removal of the shoes. Devised by Carlton Fillauer (Durr-Fillauer Orthopedic, Chattanooga, Tennessee). Turek (19), p. 270.

Fink corset

Celluloid corset including chin and occiput support. Schanz (17), p. 205.

Fisher spinal brace

A Knight type of brace with a double pelvic band, molded corset, two lateral uprights, axillary crutches, and posterior uprights. Nangle (14), p. 121.

Flagstad equinus mobilization apparatus

A wedged plaster of Paris boot with a turnbuckle in front which pulls the foot into dorsiflexion. Flagstad, A. E. Traction apparatus used in correcting equinus deformities. *J. Bone Joint Surg., 8:* 718, 1926.

Florida brace

Thoracolumbosacral orthosis which, applying the three-point principle, restricts in particular flexion of the vertebral column. Manufactured by the Florida Brace Corporation, Winter Park, Florida.

Florida collar

A two-poster cervical orthosis. See Fig. 5.12.

Foerster splint

Bilateral thigh braces supported by shoulder straps. Hohmann (10), p. 172.

Forrester collar

A collar consisting of four pieces, two for the front and two for the back, each pair being spread apart by a pair of turnbuckles, to distract the cervical vertebrae. Such a collar may be connected to a spinal brace which in turn may be stabilized by a pelvic band. Wegner, W., and Munro, D. Cervical-spine brace which reduces use of plaster casts. *N. Engl. J. Med., 223:* 458–460, 1940. *Orthopaedic Appliances Atlas* (1), pp. 224–226.

Frejka pillow

A down- or kapok-filled pillow between the thighs, held in place by shoulder straps. It maintains the lower limbs of an infant flexed and abducted while allowing them to move. Used in congenital dislocation of the hip. Developed by Bedrich Frejka, orthopedist of Brünn, Czechoslovakia. Hart, V. L. Congenital dysplasia of the hip joint. *J. Bone Joint Surg. 31A:* 357–372, 384, 1949. *Orthopaedic Appliances Atlas* (1), p. 436. Hensinger, R. N. Congenital dislocation of the hip. *Ciba Clin. Symp., 31* (1): 15–16, 1979.

French lock

Also called Swiss lock (*q.v.*) and bail lock. See Fig. 9.17.

Fulton splint

A splint used in the treatment of dislocation of the radius. *Blakiston's Gould Medical Dictionary*, ed. 3. New York, 1972.

Funsten forearm splint

Arm, forearm, and handcuffs held in position by a medial iron, designed to immobilize forearm. Funsten, Robert V. (American orthopedic surgeon, 1892–1949). Suggestions from the brace shop. *J. Orthop. Surg., 2:* 345, 1920.

G

Gaenslen splint

A device for the treatment of clubfoot.

Gaines scoliosis brace

Spinal orthosis with thigh corset and large shoulder strap on the side of the convexity in order to give better support to the transverse strap applied directly over the convex hemithorax. After Gaines, in *Orthopaedic Appliances Atlas* (1), p. 236.

Galeazzi jacket

A corrective plaster jacket, applied with the patient standing, the spine in flexion and its curves and torsion corrected by mechanical means. Galeazzi, Riccardo. The treatment of scoliosis. *J. Bone Joint Surg., 11:* 81–86, 1929.

Galland back brace

Frame-like thoracolumbosacral brace with sternal and suprapubic pressure pads and counterpressure by large lumbar pad connected to the frame by three horizontal straps. It restricts, in particular, flexion of the spine. Hines in Licht (13), p. 4.

Galland ischial seat brace

An improved ischial seat brace. Galland, W. J. The ischial seat brace: a substitute for the Thomas ring brace. *J. Bone Joint Surg.*, *18:* 790, 1936.

Gaugele splint

Used to stabilize hip with congenital dislocation. Hohmann (10), p. 118.

Gauvain mitre

Headband used for cervical traction. Wilkinson, H. *Orthopaedics for Nurses.* London, 1961.

Gaylord sling

Upper limb sling with straps over both shoulders, for the suspension of a flail upper limb and shoulder. Developed at Gaylord Hospital, Wallingford, Connecticut. See Fig. 1.8.

Gaynor knee brace

Uses continuous elastic tension as a corrective force against contracture. Gaynor, Sidney S. A simple method for the ambulatory correction of flexion contracture of the knee. *J. Bone Joint Surg.*, *18:* 766–768, 1936.

Gazeley shoulder abduction brace

Harness with shoulder straps and support for the upper limb connected by a universal joint in the axilla permitting shoulder motions in all directions. Elevation is assisted by an adjustable spring. Developed for the rehabilitation of weak shoulders, to replace the use of an overhead sling. Gazeley, William E., and Dunham, W. A. A new type of brace for the rehabilitation of the weakened shoulder. *J. Bone Joint Surg.*, *34A:* 228–229, 1952.

Georgia Warm Springs

See Warm Springs.

German crutch

Metal forearm crutch.

Giannestras elbow support

An elbow support attached to a shoulder saddle by adjustable straps held in place by a strap around the arm and another around the thorax. Giannestras, Nicholas J. (Greek-born Cincinnati orthopedic surgeon, 1909–1978). A method of immobilization of acute acromioclavicular separation. *J. Bone Joint Surg.*, *26:* 597, 1944.

Gibney splint

An ankle plaster for early ambulation after sprain. Gibney, Virgil P. Sprained ankle. *N. Y. Med. J.*, *61:* 193–197, 1895.

Gibson femoral torsion splint

A development of the mermaid splint for knock knees designed by Dr. D. A. Gibson of Toronto, Canada.

Gibson shoe
> Men's shoe with low heel, with the quarters overlapping the vamp. Similar to the derby or blucher shoe.

Gibson splint
> A form of Thomas splint. *Dorland's Illustrated Medical Dictionary* (9).

Gillette sitting support orthosis
> Custom-molded plastic shell conforming to the sitting body posteriorly and laterally from the knees to the upper thorax. It is mounted on a base to be put on a wheelchair or any other seat. Developed for nonambulatory children with severe cerebral palsy or muscular dystrophy at Gillette Children's Hospital, St. Paul, Minnesota. Carlson, J. M., and Winter, R. The "Gillette" sitting support orthosis. *Orthotics Prosthet.*, *32*(4): 35–45, 1978.

Girdlestone, Gathorne Robert. Oxford orthopedic surgeon, 1881–1950.

Girdlestone mermaid splint
> Consists of two metal gutter splints riveted back to back, used for the treatment of genua valga. The gutters reach from the perineum to the medial aspect of the heels and are used only during the night. Girdlestone, G. R. Night splint for knock-knees: The Mermaid. *Lancet*, *1*: 312, 1944. Powell, M. *Orthopaedic Nursing*, ed. 6, pp. 79–80, 309–310. Edinburgh, 1968.

Chatfield-Girdlestone splint
> An apparatus which allows a person with bilateral deltoid paralysis to use crutches. *Dorland's Illustrated Medical Dictionary* (9).

Glimcher orthosis
> Orthosis relieving weight bearing of a hip affected by Legg-Calvé-Perthes disease. Allowing walking, it consists of a steel bar for the lower limb, ending in a small stilt under the shoe. Its upper end is attached to an ischial ring which is held in place by a strap over the opposite shoulder. A shoe lift is used on the uninvolved side. Developed by Melvin J. Glimcher (Boston orthopedic surgeon), Radin, E. L., and Amrich, M. M. The design of a new style ischial weight-bearing brace for use in the treatment of Legg-Perthes disease. *Orthotics Prosthet.*, *24*(3): 11–20, 1970.

Glisson, Francis. Cambridge and London physician, 1597–1677.

Glisson sling
> Head halter, first made of leather, used for cervical traction. The same sling was also used to correct torticollis. Russe, O. *Atlas Orthopädischer Erkrankungen*, p. 156. Stuttgart, 1964.

Gocht splint for radial palsy
> Wrist-hand orthosis with springs bridging the metacarpophalangeal joints. Developed in 1917 by Hermann Gocht (German orthopedic surgeon, 1869–1938). Illustrated in Boyes (6), p. 154.

Goff, Charles Weer. Hartford, Connecticut, orthopedic surgeon, 1897–1975.

Goff plantar splint

A metal plantar splint for fractures of the phalanges of the foot. Goff, C. W. An improved plantar splint. *J. A. M. A.*, *90:* 1536, 1928.

Goff shoe lift

Goff, C. W. An improved shoe lift. *J. Bone Joint Surg.*, *16:* 209, 1934.

Goldenberg knee straps

Goldenberg, Raphael R. Elastic straps to prevent slipping of a knee cage. *J. Bone Joint Surg.*, *21:* 797–798, 1939.

Goldschmidt dropfoot brace

Ankle-foot orthosis including single upright with wire spring bringing the attached shoe into dorsiflexion. Schanz (17), p. 102. *Orthopaedic Appliances Atlas* (1), p. 426.

Goldthwait, Joel E. American orthopedic surgeon, 1866–1961.

Devised several orthoses, particularly for the trunk. See especially Goldthwait, J. E., *et al. Diseases of the Bones and Joints*, p. 543. Boston, 1909. *Body Mechanics in the Study and Treatment of Disease*, pp. 80, 168–171. Philadelphia, 1934.

Goldthwait back brace

Thoracolumbosacral orthosis of leather-covered flexible steel molded to give firm support on the pelvis and some pressure on the lower part of the sacrum; it reaches to just below the scapulae. Straps below the buttocks and over the shoulders help to keep the orthosis in place. It is used to correct excessive lumbar lordosis and to restrict trunk motions in back pain.

Goldthwait sacroiliac brace

Lumbosacroiliac orthosis with firm dorsal and abdominal shield-like pads connected by three pairs of lateral straps and kept low by a pair of perineal straps. Called also Osgood sacroiliac brace. See Fig. 6.15.

Gooch splint

A splint of long, thin strips of wood attached to canvas or leather. Devised by Benjamin Gooch, Norwich, England, surgeon, 1700–1776. Gooch, B. *Cases and Practical Remarks in Surgery.* [England] 1758 (12).

Goodyear welt shoe

A shoe in which insole, outsole, and upper are stitched together, including an 8-mm wide strip of leather called a welt, along the border, except for the heel. Manufacture used since the 18th century, and improved since the 1860's by the Goodyear welt machine, which was perfected in the 1870's by Charles Goodyear, Jr. This construction facilitates certain orthotic modifications, notably those between outsole and insole (*cf.* McKay-stitched shoe).

Gordon-Barach belt

Emphysema belt. Suprapubic pad on which are placed two elastic metal bands connected to a canvas belt, about 20 cm large. It compresses the abdomen and thus pushes the diaphragm slightly higher. Both abdomen and diaphragm assume positions closer to expiration, which is thus facilitated, notably in pulmonary emphysema. Devised by Burgess L. Gordon (The mechanism and use of abdominal supports and the treatment of pulmonary diseases. *Am. J. Med. Sci., 187:* 692, 1934.), and modified in 1950 by Alvan L. Barach. *A Treatment Manual for Patients with Pulmonary Emphysema,* pp. 24–25, 32. New York, 1969. Illustrated in Licht (13), pp. 23, 144.

Granger, Carl V. Jr. American physiatrist.

Granger feeder

A standard feeder attached to bed frame for use in supine position. Granger, C. V., and Day, D. J. Feeder apparatus for the supine quadriplegic. *Am. J. Phys. Med., 38:* 89–94, 1959.

Granger knee splint

An adjustable knee-ankle-foot orthosis with shoe attachment for temporary use in ambulation training of patients with paresis of muscles supporting the knee. Granger, C. V. The adjustable knee splint. *Phys. Ther. Rev., 41:* 516–519, 1961.

Gray knee splint

Gray, H. A. An improved knee splint. *Lancet, 1:* 902, 1922.

Greenville spinal orthosis

Vacuum-formed polypropylene body cast including neck and pelvis for immobilization after spinal fusion. Developed at the Shriners Hospital for Crippled Children and manufactured by Greenville Orthopaedic Appliance Company, both in Greenville, South Carolina. Friddle, W. D., and Brown, L. P. Greenville Spinal Orthosis—Polypropylene. *Inter-Clinic Information Bulletin 15*(9–10): 7–12, 1976.

Griswold back brace

An anterior hyperextension orthosis, modified Hoadley type. Devised by Rettig Arnold Griswold, Kentucky surgeon. Griswold, R. A. A three-point hyperextension back brace. *J. Bone Joint Surg., 18:* 784, 1936.

Gross extension apparatus

Hip-knee-ankle orthosis for the extension of the lower limb, devised by Samuel David Gross, Philadelphia surgeon, 1805–1884. Kolbe, D. W. & Son, 1879, in *Orthopaedic Appliances Atlas* (1), p. 349.

Guilford cervical orthosis

A two-poster cervical orthosis with one anterior and one posterior poster, shoulder straps, and axillary straps attached to a breast plate. Named after its designer, a Cleveland, Ohio, orthotist (G. A. Guilford & Sons). See Fig. 5.10 of this book. Hartman, J. T., *et al.* Cineradiography of the braced normal cervical spine. *Clin. Orthop., 109:* 97–102, 1975.

H

Hallam gag

Jaw-like device kept between the teeth in reduced range of the temporomandibular joints. A screw spreads the two parts of the device, thus opening the patient's mouth. Cyriax, J. H. *Text-Book of Orthopaedic Medicine*, vol. I: *Diagnosis of Soft Tissue Lesions*, p. 193. London, 1962.

Hammond cockup splint

A palmar splint for temporary use which requires little or no fitting. Held in place by adhesive straps or elastic bandage. Hammond, T. E. The non-operative treatment of nerve lesions involving the upper extremity. *J. Orthop. Surg.*, *1*: 320–335, 1919.

Harris back brace

A chairback type of lumbosacral brace used in Toronto, Canada, where it was devised by Dr. R. I. Harris of the Hospital for Sick Children.

Hart finger splint

Rigid aluminum finger traction device made by the Zimmer Company.

Hass abduction splint

Used in treatment of dislocated hips after reduction. Hass, Julius. *Congenital Dislocation of the Hip*. Springfield, Ill., 1951.

Hauser bar, Hauser comma bar

Comma-shaped forefoot support: a metatarsal bar applied to the outsole of a shoe, proximally to the metatarsal heads I–IV. Being higher laterally, the forefoot is put into slight pronation. Hauser, Emil D. *Diseases of the Foot*. Philadelphia, 1939, 1950. Jahss in *Atlas of Orthotics* (2), pp. 272, 276. Anderson (3), p. 27.

Heald ulnar deviation splint

A plastic ribbon wound around hand and forearm to counteract ulnar deviation of the fingers. Heald, C. B., *et al. Lancet*, *1*: 396, 1949, in *Orthopaedic Appliances Atlas* (1), p. 319.

Heidelberg corset

Used in the treatment of spondylitis. Hohmann (10), p. 55.

Heinecke back brace

Spinal support used in treatment of spondylitis. Schanz (17), p. 184.

Helfet heel cup or insole

Shoe insert to improve posture. Helfet, A. J. A new way of treating flat feet in children. *Lancet*, *1*: 262, 1956. Roaf and Hodkinson (16), p. 28.

Herrick splint

Herrick, F. C. A flexible metal splint adaptable to any angle of the knee or elbow. *Cleve. Med. J.*, *13*: 706, 1914.

Herzmark masseter helmet

> Plaster of Paris cup and jaw piece with elastic bands to assist the pull of weakened masseters. Herzmark, Maurice H. Masseter paralysis in anterior poliomyelitis treated by a specially constructed helmet. *J. Bone Joint Surg.*, *14:* 962–964, 1932.

Herzog finger extension splint

> Wrist-hand orthosis with straps for the extension of all digits. After M. B. Herzog, 1944. Illustrated in Boyes (6), p. 154.

Hess finger splint

> A finger traction splint for fractures, held in place by a padded collar around the hand. Hess, Henry L. Metacarpal and phalangeal traction splint. *J. Orthop. Surg.*, *1:* 302–303, 1919.

Hessing brace

> One of various braces with steel skeleton and molded leather encasing the neck, trunk, a limb, or any body segment. Designed by Friedrich von Hessing, Augsburg, Germany, orthopedic surgeon and outstanding brace maker, 1838–1918. His braces became models for many decades to come. Hessing, F., and Hasslauer, L. *Orthopädische Therapie*. Berlin, 1903.

Heusner external rotation serpent

> Foot night splint for children. Rabl (15), p. 252.

Heusner knee cap

> A spring to reinforce an elastic knee bandage used in severe instability. Heusner, L. Über die Dauerresultate der Sehnenüberpflanzung bei arthrogener Kniecontractur. *Arch. Klin. Chir.*, *67:* 6, 1902.

Hewitt knee brace

> Long elastic knee brace with front lacing. Designed in 1939 by E. R. Hewitt, engineer. Jordan (11), p. 136.

Highet splint

> One of several orthoses, such as finger splints and a shoulder abduction brace, with adjustable shoulder and elbow. Highet, W. Bremmer. Splintage of peripheral nerve injuries. *Lancet, 1:* 555–558, 1942.

Hittenberger shoulder splint

> A splint including thoracic bands and shoulder straps, which holds the arm in abduction, the forearm at a right angle, and the hand in the neutral position. Used in the treatment of Erb's palsy. Noall in *Orthopaedic Appliances Atlas* (1), p. 332.

Hoadley spinal brace

> The first anterior hyperextension brace. A steel rod frame which forms two lateral uprights; an anterior bar across the pelvis, and another across the upper anterior thorax, held in place by a dorsal apron which attaches to the lateral uprights and pulls the spine into hyperextension. Hoadley, A. E. Spine brace. *Trans. Am. Orthop. Assoc.*, *8:* 164, 1895.

Hobble splint

An abduction bar for talipes equinovarus. Nangle (14), p. 172.

Hodgen, John T. Kentucky-born surgeon in St. Louis, 1826-1882.

Hodgen splint or apparatus

Suspension splint consisting of two sturdy wires continuous at their lower ends and a padded ischial ring, similar to a Thomas splint, but with four loops, two at the proximal, two at the distal parts. Ropes leading from these loops to another rope and a pulley allow the limb (usually fractured at the lower or middle third of the femur) to be suspended, while the patient is supine. Traction can also be applied. A similar wire suspension splint was devised for fractures of the forearm. Hodgen, J. T. On the treatment of gunshot fractures of the femur and tibia. *Am. Med. Times*, 7: 169-170, 1863.

Hoefftcke splint

Splint for non-union of the femur. Hoefftcke, Carel A. *The Ambulatory Treatment of Fractures and Diseased Joints.* pp. 18-25. London, 1923 (12).

Hoffa, Albert. Berlin orthopedic surgeon (1859-1907) who devised several orthoses discussed in his *Lehrbuch der orthopädischen Chirurgie.* Stuttgart, 1898; ed. 6, 1924.

Hoffa brace

One of several braces molded on the body part according to the principles of Hessing (leather with steel reinforcement).

Hoffa knock-knee splint

A knee orthosis consisting of two long cuffs, one for the thigh, the other for the leg, articulated with each other and connected by a turnbuckle on the convex (medial) side. See also Alldredge and Snow in *Orthopaedic Appliances Atlas* (1), p. 422.

Hoffa wrist dorsiflexion splint

A wrist-hand orthosis in which a sling embracing metacarpals II-V pulls the hand toward a rigid bar attached to the dorsal aspect of a forearm cuff and extending distally. Bunnell in *Orthopaedic Appliances Atlas* (1), p. 326.

Hohmann, Georg. Munich orthopedic surgeon (1880-1970) who devised several orthoses, among which were the following.

Hohmann clubfoot splint

A night splint acting especially upon the forefoot in clubfoot deformities. Hohmann (10), p. 192.

Hohmann cockup splint

A wrist-hand cockup orthosis with extension to the proximal phalanx of the middle finger. Bunnel in *Orthopaedic Appliances Atlas* (1), p. 293.

Hohmann scoliosis brace

A spinal orthosis with pelvic support and adjustable lever arms attached posteriorly for corrective pressure through lateral pads. Hohmann (10), p. 101.

Hohmann shoulder control brace

Shoulder harness with pressure pads to hold head of humerus against glenoid fossa to prevent recurrent dislocation. Hohmann (10).

Hohmann spiral leg and foot brace

An ankle-foot orthosis with single spiral upright attached to an inlay with arch support. Hohmann (10), p. 163. Alldredge and Snow in *Orthopaedic Appliances Atlas* (1), p. 427.

Hoke corset

High-fitting thoracolumbosacral corset of cotton or similar material with multiple stays, front opening, and perineal straps. Introduced by Michael Hoke (1874–1944), chief surgeon at the Georgia Warm Springs Foundation, in about 1930. See Chapter 4.

Hook cervical brace

Cervical brace with chin-piece attached to a sternal plate and occipital piece attached to a dorsal plate. Developed by F. R. Hook, Jr., *et al.* Bloomberg (5), p. 186.

Hoover cane

Long light aluminum cane used by a blind person when walking and probing for his way. Developed during World War II by Richard E. Hoover (a medical student who later became an ophthalmologist) and his associates.

Horwitz, M. Thomas. American orthopedic surgeon, 1909–1977.

Horwitz knee extension apparatus

An apparatus to be incorporated in plaster for the correction of knee flexion contracture complicated by posterior tibial luxation. Horwitz, M. T. Conservative method of correcting flexion deformity of the knee complicated by posterior luxation of the tibia. *J. Bone Joint Surg.*, 19: 522–523, 1937.

Horwitz scoliosis brace

Horwitz, T. An active three-point-pressure scoliosis brace. *J. Bone Joint Surg.*, 22: 1085–1087, 1940.

Horwitz thumb opposition splint

Opponens thumb splint made from one continuous piece of clotheshanger wire and either held by a strap across dorsum of hand or incorporated in a cockup splint. Horwitz, T. Opponens thumb wire splint. *Am. J. Surg.*, 58: 460, 1942.

Horwitz-Tocantins scapular palsy brace

An elbow rest supported on the pelvis, designed to lift humeral head up and back to derotate scapula and hold it against chest wall. Horwitz, M. T., and Tocantins, Leandro M. Isolated paralysis of the serratus anterior muscle. *J. Bone Joint Surg.*, 20: 720–725, 1938.

Howard tibial torsion splint

    A simple snap joins the shoes together at the toes or heels. Howard, Rex J., and Kleuser, L. P. Simple night splint for correction of tibial torsion in children. *J. Bone Joint Surg., 42A:* 177–178, 1960.

Hunter Negator (or Neg'ator) spring assist

    Spring wire with finger loop which can be attached to any hand brace to abduct index finger when first dorsal interosseus is weak. Manufactured by Hunter Spring Company of Lansdale, Pennsylvania. Werssowetz, O. F. von, *et al.* Supportive appliances in rehabilitation of the paralytic hand. *Arch. Phys. Med. Rehabil., 36:* 559–563, 1955.

I

Ilfeld, Frederic W. California orthopedic surgeon, 1907–

  Ilfeld abduction splint

    Abduction splint consisting of an adjustable spreader bar and two thigh cuffs, used for infants with dislocation of the hips. It gives the child much freedom to move. Ilfeld, F. W. The management of congenital dislocation and dysplasia of the hip by means of a special splint. *J. Bone Joint Surg., 39A:* 99–109, 1957. Also in Hensinger, R. N. Congenital dislocation of the hip. *Ciba Clin. Symp., 31*(1): 15–16, 1979. Older children, *e.g.*, with adductor tightness from cerebral palsy, may use the Ilfeld splint (also called Craig splint) which allows them to crawl. Scaramuzza, V. Control of lower extremity movement in cerebral palsy. *Phys. Ther., 47*(9): 831–837, 1967.

  Ilfeld half-ring splint

    Thomas splint modified to give more room and comfort in the groin. Ilfeld, F. W. A modified half-ring splint and combined foot support and exerciser. *J. Bone Joint Surg., 43A:* 139, 1961.

IPMR, IRM

    Abbreviations for Institute of Physical Medicine and Rehabilitation (IPMR), now Institute of Rehabilitation Medicine (IRM), of New York University Medical Center, New York City. Several orthoses and orthotic parts were developed there. They may be labeled by one of these abbreviations or by the name of Lehneis (*q.v.*).

  IPMR eccentric cam lock

    An adjustable cam which can be set at any angle to avoid fatigue or to maintain a tighter grasp when applied to a flexor hinge tenodesis splint. Designed by Hans Lehneis, prosthetist-orthotist at IRM. Illustrated in Licht (13), p. 710.

J

Jergesen clubfoot splint

    Modification of Denis Browne splint used for correction of unilateral talipes equinovarus. Jergesen, Floyd H. The treatment of unilateral congenital talipes equinovarus with the Denis Browne splint. *J. Bone Joint Surg.*, *25:* 185–187, 1943.

Jewett brace

Frame-like thoracolumbosacral orthosis, based on the three-point pressure principle, built to maintain an erect posture by means of a large pressure pad in the thoracolumbar area and counterpressure by a sternal pad and a suprapubic pad, with somewhat less pressure on both sides. It restricts, in particular, flexion of the vertebral column. Jewett, Eugene L. A light hyperextension back brace. *J. Bone Joint Surg.*, *19:* 1128–1129, 1937. Berger and Lusskin, in *Atlas of Orthotics* (2), p. 357.

Jobst sleeve, stocking, leotard

Soft elastic supports used to apply pressure in order to counteract a tendency to orthostatic hypotension or, most frequently, to decrease edema in a limb. In addition to these elastic garments, which may be worn the whole day or day and night, there are also inflatable sleeves, boots, and stockings for the application of greater pressure, also intermittently, during shorter periods. Manufactured by the Jobst Institute, Inc., Toledo, Ohio. See Chapter 4 and Figs. 4.9, 4.10, and 5.2.

Johns Hopkins Hospital brace

An aluminum long leg brace. *Proceedings, First Annual Symposium on Orthopedic Appliances*, p. 47. Orthopedic and Artificial Limb Manufacturers Association. Washington, 1950.

Jones, Sir Robert. British orthopedic surgeon, 1858–1933.

Jones cockup splint

A metal splint used to hold the wrist in dorsiflexion.

Jones frame

A metal frame for the mobilization of the hip.

Jones metatarsal bar

A metatarsal bar applied to the outsole of a shoe. Jones, R. *Notes on Military Orthopaedics*. London, 1917.

Jones spinal support

A metal and leather spinal brace. *British Medical Dictionary* (7).

Jordan, Henry H. German-born New York orthopedic surgeon, 1897–1970. Developed several orthoses discussed in his book (11).

Jordan abduction splint

Abduction splint consisting of a waist belt joined with thigh cuffs, for congenital dislocation of the hip. Jordan (11), p. 122.

Jordan active supporting spinal brace

Molded pelvic corset with lateral pressure pad used in scoliosis. Jordan (11).

Jordan cervical support

Padded shoulder yoke with two posterior uprights which maintain the position of a metal hinged chin-occiput support. Jordan (11), p. 126.

Jordan cockup splint

A metal splint applied to the anterior surface of the forearm and palm. Nangle (14), p. 102.

Jordan ischial weight-bearing brace

An "unweighting" brace in which the ischium rests on a soft leather strap and is assisted in its support by a lateral hip pad. Jordan, H. H. New ischial seat brace for elimination of weight bearing. *J. Bone Joint Surg.*, *22:* 1097, 1940.

Jordan passive supporting spinal brace

Molded pelvic corset for dorsolumbar immobilization. Jordan (11).

Jordan shoulder abduction apparatus

Fixed abduction brace anchored at the opposite shoulder rather than the pelvis; emphasizes external rotation of the shoulder. Jordan, H. H. An improved abduction splint for the upper extremity. *J. Bone Joint Surg.*, *26:* 600, 1944.

Jörg head halter

A torticollis brace with circular headband. Schanz (17), p. 163.

Judet corset

Thoracolumbosacral rigid orthosis which leaves the anterior chest-wall free, except for an extension on each side to the subclavicular areas (cowhorns). MacLean and Kamenetz in Licht (13), p. 712.

Judson brace

One of several knee-ankle-foot orthoses used to stabilize the knee. *Trans. 9th Internat. Med. Congress*, p. 645, 1887, in (1), p. 353. Delitala (8), p. 221.

Jungmann girdle

Lumbosacral orthosis with sacral pad for low back strain. Hohmann (10), p. 31.

K

Kanavel cockup splint

Wrist-hand orthosis with palmar support to keep wrist in dorsiflexion. Illustrated in *Dorland's Illustrated Medical Dictionary* (9), under "Splint."

Karewsky corset

A water glass corset reinforced with wire mesh. Schanz (17), p. 141.

Kawamura-Yanagida leg brace

Kawamura, B., *et al.* On the Kawamura-Yanagida brace for the leg joints in poliomyelitis. *J. Jap. Orthop. Assoc.*, *38:* 635, 1964.

Keller splint

A hinged half-ring splint for the lower limb, a modification of the Thomas splint. *Splints and Appliances of the U. S. Army*, ed. 2. 1918, in (1), p. 399.

Keller-Blake splint
> Similar to the Keller splint. *Dorland's Illustrated Medical Dictionary* (9).

Kelly hip splint
> A steel band which passes from 5 cm above the patella along the middle of the anterior aspect of the thigh to the hip joint and then diagonally to the opposite nipple. It is held in place with straps and used in conjunction with non-weight-bearing in the treatment of unilateral arthritis of the hip. Kelly, Michael. Splint for arthritic hip joint. *Lancet, 1:* 150–151, 1964.

Kelton axillary crutch
> An axillary support similar to that of a crutch, kept in place by one pelvic and two chest straps, designed to elevate the scapula in acromioclavicular separation. Kelton, W. Treatment of fractures of the clavicle. *J. A. M. A., 68:* 1814–1815, 1917, in (1), p. 338.

Kendall hand splints
> Plaster of Paris orthoses for peripheral nerve lesions: opponens cuff, lumbricales cuff, opponens-lumbricales cuff, cockup splint. Kendall, Henry O. (1898–1979) and Kendall, Florence P. (Baltimore physical therapists). *Care during the Recovery Period in Paralytic Poliomyelitis.* Public Health Bulletin No. 242, revised. Washington, 1939.

Kenny crutch
> Double-upright wooden forearm crutch with leather cuff. Suggested for patients with poliomyelitis by Elizabeth Kenny, Australian nurse and physical therapist who later came to the U. S. (Sister Kenny, 1886–1952).

Keropian splint
> Universal hand splint made by Keropian of San Francisco.

Kerr-Lagen abdominal belt
> A wide partly elastic belt around the trunk from the pubis to above the umbilicus to control abdominal ptosis and to aid in case of respiratory insufficiency. Kerr, William J., and Lagen, John B. The postural syndrome related to obesity leading to postural emphysema and cardiorespiratory failure. *Ann. Intern. Med., 10:* 569–595, 1936.

King hip brace
> Pelvic band with two thigh cuffs to control hip rotation. Used in painful hip osteoarthritis. King, Don. A brace for arthritic hip joints. *J. Bone Joint Surg., 19:* 836–837, 1937.

Klein scoliosis brace
> Metal frame stabilized at pelvis, extending to axilla with lateral correction applied through canvas swathe. Klein, A. Treatment of structural scoliosis. *J. Bone Joint Surg., 6:* 858, 1924.

Kleinberg brace
> Modified Abbott brace for scoliosis. Kleinberg, Samuel. *Scoliosis . . .* , pp. 233–245. New York, 1926, in Kelly (12).

Kleinknecht back brace
Spinal support with pelvic band and laced chest belt. Schanz (17), p. 184.

Klenzak, J. Designer and machinist (died 1956) at Pope Brace Company, Kankakee, Illinois. Representing the team, his name was used to designate several orthotic spring-loaded joints such as mentioned below. See also Pope joint. *Orthopaedic Appliances Atlas* (1), pp. 391–392, 406–415, 429.

Klenzak ankle joint
Spring-loaded ankle dorsiflexion-assisting joint with spring adjustment and plantar flexion stop.

Klenzak brace
Without further designation, this is most commonly a double-upright ankle-foot orthosis with Klenzak ankle joint and double stirrup attachment to a steelplate between sole and heel of the shoe.

Knight, James C. Maryland physician, 1810–1887.
Devised in 1874 one of the most frequently used types of back braces, described below, still extensively used 100 years later. Knight, J. *Orthopaedia, or a Practical Treatise on the Aberrations of the Human Form* (see pp. 181, 184). New York, 1874, in Kelly (12).

Knight brace
Thoracolumbosacral brace (rather short, also called chairback brace), restricting flexion, extension, and lateral motions of the lumbar spine. It consists of a posterolateral metal frame and a full-front abdominal flexible support. The frame (now aluminum) is made of four uprights (two lateral and two lumbosacral posterior) and two bands (one pelvic, one thoracic), all connected with each other. Prototype of one of the most frequently used back orthoses. Berger and Lusskin in *Atlas of Orthotics* (2), p. 352. See Fig. 6.10 of this book.

Knight-Taylor brace
Thoracolumbosacral orthosis which combines features of the Knight brace and the Taylor brace (*q.v.*). Consisting of a metal frame (with paraspinal and lateral uprights, pelvic and thoracic bands), shoulder straps, and abdominal support, it restricts, in particular, flexion and extension in the thoracolumbar and upper lumbar joints. Berger and Lusskin in *Atlas of Orthotics* (2), p. 355.

Koch functional hand splints
A variety of aluminum and leather glove splints for hand injuries and deformities. Koch, Sumner L., and Mason, M. L. Purposeful splinting following injuries of the hand. *Surg. Gynecol. Obstet.*, 68: 1–16, 1939.

Kolbe, D. W. Designer of several orthoses for various parts of the body, described in his book, which saw several editions (later by Kolbe, D. W. & Son): *Orthopaedic Apparatus and Description of the Mechanical Appliances Employed in the Treatment of Deformities and*

Deficiencies of the Body. Philadelphia, 1868. See also *Orthopaedic Appliances Atlas* (1), *passim.*

Kolbe torticollis brace

A headpiece which applies corrective forces to the occipitotemporal region on the affected side and upon the mandible of the opposite side is attached to a trunk brace which is supported on the pelvis.

Kölliker corset

Thoracic corset made of soluble sodium and potassium silicate, also known as soluble glass or water glass. It was used for the treatment of pectus excavatum. Kölliker. Ein Wasserglasskorsett. *Zentralbl. Orthop. Chir. 3:* 1886. Schanz (17), Fig. 8. Bick (4), p. 465.

Kosair orthosis

A metal orthosis for scoliosis, developed at the Kosair Crippled Children's Hospital, Louisville, Kentucky. See Chapter 7.

Koven pelvic brace

Koven, B., and Koven, M. J. Spinal pelvic compression brace. *J. Bone Joint Surg., 17:* 800, 1935.

Kramer hip splint

Used extensively in Switzerland for congenital hip dislocation, but of German origin.

Kraus splint

A footdrop splint with shoe inlay. Rabl (15), p. 296.

Krida foot plate

A metal plate shaped to a molded plaster model of the foot used as a foot support in the treatment of osteoarthritis. Krida, A. Foot plate for treatment of osteoarthritis. *J. Bone Joint Surg., 7:* 730, 1925.

Krukenberg-Thomsen splint

Fingers are pulled into flexion by elastics anchored at elbow. Hohmann (10), p. 110.

Kyle metatarsal bar

A metatarsal bar on the shoe sole. Kyle, B. H. A simple method for elevating the depressed metatarsal arch. *J. Bone Joint Surg., 7:* 722, 1925.

L

Lackum jacket

A plaster jacket for the treatment of scoliosis, applied under cephalopelvic traction and over muslin surcingle straps correcting the deformities. Called also surcingle cast. Devised by William von Lackum, New York orthopedic surgeon. Lackum, W. H. von, and Miller, J. P. Critical observations of the results in the operative treatment of scoliosis. *J. Bone Joint Surg., 31A:* 102, 1949. Keim, H. A. Scoliosis. *Ciba Clin. Symp., 30*(1): 24–26, 1978.

Lambrinudi foot plate
    Shoe insert to be used after surgery for claw toes. Named after
    Constantine Lambrinudi, London surgeon, 1890–1943. Nangle (14).
    British Medical Dictionary (7).
Lange, Fritz. Munich orthopedic surgeon (1864–1952) who devised various
    orthoses.
    Lange arch support
        Arch support made of celluloid. Lange, F. Neue Plattfusseinlagen aus
        Celluloid-Stahldraht. *Münch. Med. Wochenschr.*, 7: 1903. Delitala
        (8), p. 253.
    Lange clubfoot brace
        A night brace. Jordan (11), p. 148.
    Lange scoliosis brace
        Metal and leather brace for scoliosis. Lange. F. *Lehrbuch der Ortho-
        pädie.* Jena, 1928. Blount in Licht (13), p. 308.
Langenbeck brace
    A scoliosis brace. Schanz (17), p. 161.
Larrey bandage
    A many-tailed bandage with the edges glued together. Named after
    Dominique Jean Baron de Larrey, French surgeon (1776–1842) and
    the greatest military surgeon of his time. *Dorland's Illustrated
    Medical Dictionary*, ed. 24, 1965.
Lasher elbow splint
    Arm and forearm cuffs connected by two steel bars with holes for
    easy adjustment of angulation of elbow. Lasher, Willis W. A reversible
    and adjustable elbow splint. *J. A. M. A.*, 72: 1282, 1919.
Lavoie splint
    Lavoie, Zenon Annable (New Hampshire surgeon, 1872–1950), and
    Foster, G. S. The Lavoie splint in fracture of the humerus. *Am. J.
    Surg.*, 17: 444–447, 1932, in Kelly (12).
Lehneis, Hans Richard. Prosthetist-orthotist at Institute of Rehabilitation
    Medicine, where he developed orthoses also labeled IPMR or IRM
    (*q.v.*).
    Lehneis spiral orthosis
        Plastic ankle-foot orthosis that slings around the leg in a spiral
        fashion and cradles the heel. The foot part is applied inside the shoe.
        It is used in footdrop and similar conditions. Sarno, J. E., and Lehneis,
        H. R. Prescription considerations for plastic below-knee orthoses.
        Arch. Phys. Med. Rehabil., 52: 503–510, 1971. Lehneis, H. R. New
        developments in lower-limb orthotics through bioengineering. *Arch
        Phys. Med. Rehabil.*, 53: 303–310 and 322, 1972. Lehneis, H. R., *et al.*
        Bioengineering design and development of lower-extremity orthotic
        devices. *Bull. Prosthet. Res.*, 10–20: 132–221, 1973. See Fig. 9.12 of
        this book.

Lenox Hill orthosis
> Double anterior-loop knee orthosis for the protection of relaxed medial and lateral ligaments of the knee while allowing full knee flexion. Used generally during sports activities. *The Lenox Hill Derotation Brace.* Lenox Hill Brace Shop, Inc., New York. Staros and LeBlanc in *Atlas of Orthotics* (2), p. 218.

Levis splint
> A splint of perforated metal which extends from below the elbow to the palm. *Dorland's Illustrated Medical Dictionary* (9).

Levy inlay or mold
> Mold made from sawdust and latex or similar material, used as a full-extension inlay in a shoe, destined to increase the weight-bearing area of the foot. It includes a longitudinal arch, a metatarsal support, and a toe crest. Developed by Benjamin Levy, Schenectady, New York, podiatrist. Levy, B. An appliance to induce toe flexion on weightbearing. *J. Natl. Assoc. Chirop., 40*(6): 24, 1950.

Lewin crescent
> A metatarsal bar that is slightly convex anteriorly, concave posteriorly. After Philip Lewin. *The Foot and Ankle*, ed. 4, p. 53. Philadelphia, 1959.

Lewin finger splint
> Extends the terminal phalanx of the fourth digit. Lewin, Philip. A simple splint for baseball finger. *J. A. M. A., 85:* 1059, 1925.

Lewin Stern thumb splint
> A splint, anchored to a wristband and holding the thumb hyperabducted. Owen, H. R. Fractures of the bones of the hand. *Surg. Gynecol. Obstet., 66:* 500–505, 1938.

Lionel hand
> Wrist-hand orthosis providing digital prehension in a completely paralyzed hand, the activating force being electric current through an electric motor and rheostat mechanism. Hoerner, E. F. Rehabilitation of the amputee, the hemiplegic and the quadriplegic. *Clin. Orthop., 12:* 96–123, esp. 118, 1958.

Lipscomb brace
> Lumbosacral orthosis in which the lateral uprights are connected to the pelvic band by movable joints. Four straps hold an apron in place. Called also Wilcox brace. Thomas in *Orthopaedic Appliances Atlas* (1), p. 213. See Fig. 6.14 of this book.

Liston, Robert. Scottish surgeon in London, 1794–1847.

Liston gum splint
> Splint made of two or three layers of lint soaked in a strong solution of gum acacia and laid on in strips. Liston, R. *Practical Surgery*, p. 144. London, 1837.

Liston splint or "long Liston"

A simple straight splint made of wood and padded with cotton, applied to the side of the body from the axilla to the foot; most often used for fractures of the femur. *Orthopaedic Appliances Atlas* (1), p. 345.

Littler thumb abduction splint

A forearm cuff with a wire extension to provide traction on the first metacarpal with counterpressure at the second metacarpal. Used for contracture of first webspace. Littler, J. W., and Tobin, W. J. Thumb abduction splint. *J. Bone Joint Surg., 30A:* 240, 1948.

Littler-Jones shoulder abduction splint

Light metal framework anchored to the pelvis by a webbing strap and extending halfway around the arm to support the humerus in abduction (16), p. 292. Murdoch, G. *Prosthetic and Orthotic Practice,* p. 475. London, 1970.

Ljubljana FEPB (functional electronic peroneal brace)

Knee-ankle-foot orthosis combined with a system of electric stimulation. The latter includes a stimulator, electrodes inside an elastic stocking, and a switch on the shoe heel, which initiates a modulated train of electric impulses. Developed at the Rehabilitation Institute Ljubljana, Yugoslavia, published in 1966. Gračanin, F. Electrical stimulation as orthotic aid: experiences and prospects, in Murdoch, G. *Prosthetic and Orthotic Practice,* pp. 503–511. London, 1970.

Lofstrand crutch

Metal forearm crutch designed and brought on the market *ca.* 1944 by Adolf Lofstrand (*ca.* 1894–*ca.* 1974) in collaboration with George C. S. Woodward. Also called in some areas English cane.

Long, Charles

See Chapter 8.

Lorenz torticollis bandage

Long elastic webbing which circles a thigh and opposite shoulder. Schanz (17), p. 164.

Lovett, Robert W. Boston orthopedic surgeon (1859–1924).

Lovett-Brewster jacket

A plaster jacket fitted with patient in hanging traction, split horizontally; turnbuckle correction. Lovett, R. W., and Brewster, A. H. The treatment of scoliosis by a different method from that usually employed. *J. Bone Joint Surg., 6:* 847, 1924.

Bradford-Lovett bowleg braces

See under Bradford.

Lowman rocker sole

A rocker bottom added to a shoe to smoothen the gait, notably in weakness of the triceps surae. Lowman, Charles LeRoy (Los Angeles orthopedic surgeon, 1879–1977). The rocker soled shoe. *Orthop. Prosthet. Appl. J., 15:* 178–180, 1961.

Lusskin varus brace

Foot orthosis made of leather and stainless steel, to be attached to the foot by means of two straps. Lusskin, Harold. Brace to correct varus of the fore part of the foot. *J. Bone Joint Surg., 33A:* 269, 1951.

Lyman-Smith dropfoot brace

Manufactured by the Zimmer Manufacturing Company.

Lyons corset

Corset with cervical extension, originally made of plastic and leather, for the treatment of scoliosis. It has mobile parts, anterior and posterior uprights and small transversal bars. Devised in the 1960's by Pierre Stagnara, physician, in Lyons, France.

M

MacAusland back brace

Thoracolumbosacral brace with clock-spring posterior uprights, a pelvic and a thoracic band, and an apron kept in place by three straps attached to the back frame. Used mostly as a postural orthosis, allowing lateral motions. Designed by W. Russell MacAusland, Boston orthopedic surgeon (1882–1965). See Fig. 6.13 of this book.

Magnuson brace

Trunk support with a large pelvic belt and a narrower thoracic band, the latter extending anteriorly and upward to end close to the manubrium sterni. The two transverse bands are connected by two pairs of rigid uprights, one in the back, one in front. Thomas in *Orthopaedic Appliances Atlas* (1), pp. 215, 218. See Fig. 6.17 of this book.

Marino-Zuco hip brace

An orthosis that permits ambulation while affording immobilization and traction of the hip joint. Named after Carlo Marino-Zuco, Italian orthopedic surgeon. Del Torto, U. Realizzazione di una trazione continua sull'arto inferiore. *Orizzonti Ortoped., 4:* 1, 1959.

Marquardt shoe insert

Used in Germany to improve foot stability. Lange, M. *Lehrbuch der Orthopädie*, p. 228. Stuttgart, 1960.

Martin ischial-bearing brace

Possibly the first example of ischial weight-bearing by an orthosis with crutch-like support: a hip-knee-ankle orthosis including a pelvic band. Devised in 1841 by M. Ferdinand Martin, from Bonnet, A. *Traité de Thérapeutique des Maladies Articulaires.* Paris 1853, in Alldredge and Snow (1), pp. 350, 352, 397.

Maseritz foot plate

Metal plate shoe insert to correct forefoot varus and heel pronation. Maseritz, J. H. A simple brace for the treatment of pigeon-toe in children. *J. Bone Joint Surg., 22:* 216, 1940.

Mathieu brace

A torticollis brace which includes a pelvic belt. Schanz (17), p. 159.

Mayo bar

Metatarsal bar, about 2.5 to 4 cm wide, with a convex anterior border. Named after the Mayo Clinic in Rochester, Minnesota, where it was first used. Brachman, P. R. *Shoe Therapy*, p. 72. Chicago, 1951.

Mayo sacroiliac belt

A sacroiliac support with front- and back reinforcement and perineal straps. *Orthopaedic Appliances Atlas* (1), p. 244.

McBride foot plate

A leather-covered metal foot plate insert used to correct pronated or everted foot. McBride, E. D. A brace for foot correction in children. *J. Bone Joint Surg.*, 12: 177, 1930.

McCurdy hip brace

Long traction hip splint with pelvic belt, perineal straps, and waistbelt for traction and immobilization of the hip joint. McCurdy, Steward Leroy. Combination traction and immobilization hip-joint brace. *Trans. Am. Orthop. Assoc.*, 8: 37, 1895. *Orthopaedic Appliances Atlas* (1), p. 354.

McIntyre splint

A metal orthosis in the form of two inclined planes, used to support the leg and thigh. Named after William McIntyre (7).

McKay-stitched shoe

A shoe whose sole is constructed in a relatively simple way. Developed around 1860 by Gordon McKay. This construction is less well suited for orthotic modifications between outsole and insole than the Goodyear welt construction (*q.v.*).

McKibben muscle

Also called pneumatic, or artificial, muscle, this is an inflatable rubber tube in a woven nylon cover, used to supply external power for an orthosis. Developed in 1957 for his disabled daughter by Los Alamos physicist Joseph L. McKibben, in conjunction with Vernon L. Nickel, orthopedic surgeon. See Chapter 8 of this book. Barber, L. M., and Nickel, V. L. Carbon dioxide-powered arm and hand devices. *Am. J. Occup. Ther.*, 23(3): 215–225, 1969. Murphy and Burstein in *Atlas of Orthotics* (2), p. 29.

Mermaid splint

See under Girdlestone.

Metcalfe back brace

Thoracolumbosacral brace with thoracic and pelvic bands, four anterior bands, and sternal pad, restricting in particular flexion of the spinal column. Hines in Licht (13), p. 5.

Meyer arch support

Arch support, particularly for the metatarsal arch. Named after Georg Hermann von Meyer, Zurich anatomist (1815–1892) and author of *Die richtige Gestalt der Schuhe.* Zurich, 1858. English translation, Edinburgh, 1864. In Kelly (12). von Meyer, G. H. *Ursache und Mechanismus der Entstehung des erworbenen Plattfusses.* Jena, 1883.

Meyerding-Krusen splint

1. Simple splint made of ordinary wooden tongue depressors applied to the dorsum of the digits II–V of the hand, also extending to the wrist and retained by circular bands of adhesive tape. Thus, it maintains the digits, hand, and forearm in the same plane. 2. A banjo-type splint to maintain extension of the wrist and all digits in the plane of the forearm with adhesive tape and rubber bands. Meyerding, Henry W., and Krusen, Frank H. The treatment of Volkmann's ischemic contracture. *Ann. Surg., 110:* 420–426, 1939.

Michigan feeder

Control mechanism of an elbow support. Smith, E. M., and Juvinall, R. C. (Ann Arbor, Michigan). Design refinement of the linkage feeder. *Arch. Phys. Med. Rehabil., 44:* 609, 1963.

Milgram bar

A long rocker bar under a shoe, starting its curve at the posterior margin of the heel block extending to behind the metatarsal heads. The bar may consist of two parts with an interruption under the shank. Designed by Joseph E. Milgram. Milgram, J. E., and Jacobson, M. A. Footgear: therapeutic modifications of sole and heel. *Orthop. Rev., 7*(11): 57–62, 1978.

Milici hand splint

Banjo splint for Volkmann's contracture. Milici, A. Treatment of Volkmann's ischemic paralysis by elastic traction. *J. Bone Joint Surg., 15:* 516, 1933.

Miller twister

A torsion cable which, when fixed to a belt at one end and to a shoe at the other, implies a rotation to the lower limb. Used alone or in combination with a hip-knee-ankle-foot orthosis for correction of internal or external rotation. See Fig. 10.1 of this book.

Milwaukee brace

Orthosis reaching from the occiput and chin to the pelvis, it is built to counteract the effect of gravity, to encourage certain motions of trunk muscles, and to improve spinal alignment in scoliosis, lordosis, and kyphosis. Developed by Walter P. Blount and coworkers in Milwaukee *ca.* 1945. Blount, W. P., Schmidt, A. C., *et al.* The Milwaukee brace in the operative treatment of scoliosis. *J. Bone Joint Surg., 40A:* 511–525, 1958. Blount, W. P., *et al.* Making the Milwaukee brace. *J. Bone Joint Surg., 40A:* 526–528, 624, 1958. Blount, W. P., and Moe, J. H. *The Milwaukee Brace.* Baltimore, 1973. See Chapter 7.

Minerva jacket

A jacket of plaster of Paris (or, today, of any other rigid material), enveloping the trunk, iliac crest, and chin; it may even extend to incorporate a helmet. Used for vertebral fractures. Named after the Roman goddess, often shown armor-clad.

Minerva type of (cervical) orthosis, Minerva extension

Any cervical orthosis or cervical part of a larger orthosis that extends superiorly to enclose the occiput; it may embrace a larger part of the skull or only include a band around the forehead.

Mitchner back support

Mitchner, J. M. A double-bar plaster back support. *J. Bone Joint Surg., 22:* 456, 1940.

Mixter collar

Mixter, W. J. Fractures and dislocations of the spine. In *Nelson's New Loose Leaf Surgery,* New York, 1930.

Moore ulnar splint

Splint of vulcanized wood fiber, secured to the palmar aspect of the fingers by adhesive tape. Moore, Stuart A. Myological principles: a new ulnar splint. *Br. Med. J., 1:* 41–42, 1919.

Morton, Dudley J. American orthopedist, 1884–1960.

Morton extension (pad), toe extension or shelf

Metatarsal support extending an arch support medially to the distal phalanx of the first toe and laterally to the fifth metatarsophalangeal joint. Thus its medial part prolongs, as it were, the short first metatarsal bone of a "Morton's toe." See Fig. 11.26 of this book.

Morton insert, insole or support

Arch support with extension pad (see preceding entry). Morton, D. J. Physiological consideration in the treatment of foot deformities. *J. Bone Joint Surg., 19A:* 1052, 1937. Jahss in *Atlas of Orthotics* (2), p. 275. Anderson (3), p. 147.

Muller arch support

Arch support made from nonmetallic material after casting during weight bearing, according to Robert Muller, M.D. Muller, R. The arthritic foot: A method of taking weight-bearing impressions for the making of supports. *Arch. Phys. Med. Rehabil., 36:* 244–248, 1955.

Murray shoe

The first type of so-called space shoes, it is molded directly over a cast of the individual foot. Used for various types of foot deformities. Developed *ca.* 1940 by Allan E. Murray, later manufactured by the Murray Space Shoe Company in Bridgeport, Connecticut.

N

Nachlas splint

Orthosis with rigid part to hold the wrist in dorsiflexion while elastic parts pull the metacarpophalangeal joints II–V into flexion. Nachlas,

I. W. A splint for the correction of extension contractures of the metacarpophalangeal joints. *J. Bone Joint Surg.*, *27:* 507, 1945. *Orthopaedic Appliances Atlas* (1), p. 310.

Napier hand splint

A strap pulling the thumb into opposition, combined with a sponge rubber wedge placed between thumb and index finger. Napier, J. Russel. A corrective splint for paralysis of the thenar muscles. *Br. Med. J., 1:* 15, 1946.

NCH

Abbreviation for Newington Children's Hospital. See under Newington.

Neapolitan tap

A lift under the sole of a shoe, almost, but not quite, as large as the regular sole; used for a small elevation. See Fig. 11.28*H* of this book.

Negator (or Neg'ator) spring assist

See Hunter Negator spring assist.

Neil clubfoot splint

The first clubfoot abduction splint, it was made of wood, to be attached to the heels of a child's shoes. Devised by Henry Neil of Philadelphia in 1825. Moore in *Orthopaedic Appliances Atlas* (1), p. 485.

Neill splint

A straight splint for the lower limb. Neill, John (American surgeon, 1819–1880) *New Means for Making Extension and Counter-Extension in Fracture of the Leg and Thigh.* Philadelphia, 1855, in Kelly (12).

Neviaser splint

Adjustable hand splint with double bars, locking wrist joint, palm support, and two outriggers for traction in separate planes (with adhesive strapping on fingers). Neviaser, Julius S. Splint for correction of claw-hand. *J. Bone Joint Surg., 12:* 440–443, 1930.

Newington Children's Hospital, formerly Newington Home and Hospital for Crippled Children, Newington, Connecticut.

Newington ambulation-abduction brace

Bilateral knee-ankle-foot orthosis similar to the Toronto Legg-Perthes brace, with spreader bar at the level of the feet and spreader device protecting the knees against valgus deformity. Curtis, B. H., *et al.* Treatment for Legg-Perthes disease with the Newington ambulation-abduction brace. *J. Bone Joint Surg., 56A:* 1135–1146, 1974. Staros and LeBlanc in *Atlas of Orthotics* (2), p. 229. See Fig. 10.3 of this book.

Newington brace for cerebral palsy

Orthosis reaching from lower trunk to both feet. It combines four separate sections: trunk, pelvis, lower limbs, and shoe assembly, allowing gradual withdrawal of the brace piece by piece as the child is trained in controlling the body segment. A single upright is used per limb. Fuldner, R. V., and Rosenberger, J. The Newington brace for cerebral palsy. *Clin. Orthop.*, *12:* 151–158, 1958.

Nickel splint

One of several splints such as a finger-driven flexor-hinge splint, a wrist-driven flexor-hinge splint, devised by Vernon L. Nickel, orthopedic surgeon at Rancho Los Amigos Hospital (*q.v.*). Nickel, V. L., Perry, J., and Garrett, A. Development of useful function in the severely paralyzed hand. *J. Bone Joint Surg.*, *45A:* 933–952, 1963.

Nigel splint

Posterior spinal support for scoliosis. Roaf and Hodkinson (16), p. 290.

Nitschke brace

Single-bar knee-ankle-foot orthosis with knee lock. Nitschke, Robert O. A single-bar above-knee orthosis. *Orthotics Prosthet.*, *25* (4): 20–25, 1971. *Atlas of Orthotics* (2), p. 224.

Noble Smith brace

Spinal support with pelvic belt and axillary straps. Schanz (17), p. 184.

Norton-Brown brace

Thoracolumbosacral brace restricting flexion, extension, and lateral motions. Norton, Paul L., and Brown, Thornton. The immobilizing efficiency of back braces: their effect on the posture and motion of the lumbosacral spine. *J. Bone Joint Surg.*, *39A:* 111–138, 1957. See also three articles in *Orthop. Prosthet. Appl. J.*, *20*(4): 299–312, 1966 (Norton, P. L., p. 299; Buschenfeldt, K. W., p. 305; and Brook, D. L., p. 310).

Nussbaum bracelet

Cuff-like self-help device for holding a pencil in cases of writer's cramp. Hohmann (10), p. 114.

Nutt wedge

Short wedge constructed of leather positioned posterior to the first metatarsal head. It prevents medial rotation of hallux and reduces medial plantar pressure associated with hallux valgus deformity. Nutt, J. J. An adduction shoe wedge. *J. Bone Joint Surg.*, *6:* 915, 1924. Jahss in *Atlas of Orthotics* (2), p. 276.

Nyquist hand splint

Forearm-hand splint with C-bar and opponens bar with an attachment device for adaptive equipment. Nyquist, Roy H. Special appliances for the disabled. *Arch. Phys. Med. Rehabil.*, *42:* 164–166, 1961.

Nyrop torticollis apparatus

Occipital support attached to a pelvic belt. Schanz (17), p. 160.

NYU

Abbreviation for New York University, New York City. Most orthoses developed at NYU are known under the name of IRM (*q.v.*).

NYU insert brace
> Molded plastic to be worn in the shoe, to support a dropfoot. Dolan, C. M. E., Mereday, C., and Hartmann, G. *Evaluation of NYU insert brace.* New York University Medical Center, New York, July 1969. Staros and LeBlanc (2), p. 208.

O

OCCC
> Abbreviation for Ontario Crippled Children's Centre Toronto, Ontario, Canada, where several orthoses were developed. See under Toronto orthoses.

Oppenheimer, Edgar D. New York orthopedic surgeon, 1883–1946. Devised several orthoses, among which were the following.

Oppenheimer finger splint
> A double springwire attached to the wrist extends over dorsum of hand and applies extension to fingertip. Oppenheimer, E. D. Splint for correction of finger contracture. *J. Bone Joint Surg., 19:* 247, 1937.

Oppenheimer radial palsy splint
> A torsion spring wrist cockup splint with outrigger for thumb extension. Oppenheimer, E. D. Splint for correction of finger contracture. *J. Bone Joint Surg., 19:* 247, 1937.

Ortolani pillow
> Abduction device for infant used in the treatment of congenital dislocation of the hips. Named after the Italian physician Marino Ortolani.

Osgood sacroiliac brace
> Same as Goldthwait sacroiliac brace. Named after Robert B. Osgood, Boston orthopedic surgeon, 1873–1956. Thomas in *Orthopaedic Appliances Atlas* (1), pp. 210–211. See Fig. 6.15 of this book.

Oxford (oxford) shoe
> Front-laced low shoe (for men and women) with firm only slightly flexible sole and low large heel. It may also have straps instead of laces. Named after the city in England where, in about the year 1715, scholars of the university changed from the high to a low shoe laced over the instep.

P

Pancoast extension apparatus
> A traction device for the hip joint by a waist belt, to which was attached a perineal strap to afford upward traction and a lateral upright attached to the shoe (combined with a medial upright from the thigh to the shoe) for countertraction. Devised by Professor J. Pancoast in 1879 (1), p. 349.

Paris, plaster of

White powder, consisting of calcinated gypsum. In the early period of its use, it was prepared from the gypsums of Montmartre, a suburb of Paris. It is never named thus in France. Baron Dominique de Larrey, French military surgeon (1766–1842), is reputed of having introduced it as a splinting material. Plaster of Paris bandages were introduced in 1851 by Antonius Mathijsen, Belgian military surgeon (1805–1878).

Patton hip orthosis

Bilateral hip-knee-ankle-foot orthosis with pelvic band and hip joints which permit only flexion and abduction from the neutral position. Patton, E. T. A pelvic band leg brace with two-way motion at the hip. *J. Bone Joint Surg.*, *18:* 794, 1936.

Pavlik harness or stirrup

A pair of straps attached to the legs like stirrups as far as the heels, suspended from a belt which in turn is attached to a pair of shoulder straps. The combination keeps the lower limbs of an infant flexed and abducted while allowing them to move. Developed in 1944 for the treatment of congenital dislocation of the hip by the Czechoslovakian orthopedic surgeon Arnold Pavlik, who died in 1961. Pavlik, A. Die funktionelle Behandlungsmethode mittels Riemenzügel als Prinzip der konservativen Therapie bei angeborenen Hüftgelenksverrenkungen der Säuglinge. *Z. Orthop.*, *89:* 341–352, 1957. Anderson (3), pp. 491–510. Hensinger, R. N. Congenital dislocation of the hip. *Ciba Clin. Symp.*, *31* (1): 16, 1979.

Pawl lock

A knee hinge lock similar to the Swiss lock. In Nangle (14), p. 145.

Peabody scoliosis brace

A trunk support including pelvic and thigh corsets. Peabody, C. W. A corrective support in scoliosis. *J. Bone Joint Surg.*, *13:* 177–180, 1931.

Peacock hand splint

One of different splints of plaster and wire for radial nerve palsy or index finger abduction. Peacock, Erle E., Jr. Dynamic splinting for the prevention and correction of hand deformities. *J. Bone Joint Surg.*, *34A:* 789–796, 1952.

Perlstein orthosis

Single-upright ankle-foot orthosis with a cam ankle joint for adjustment of the plantar flexion stop. Developed by Meyer Aaron Perlstein, Chicago pediatrician, 1902–1969. Anderson (3), pp. 284, 291.

Perthes sling

The eponym refers to Legg-Calvé-Perthes disease. The device consists of a pelvic belt, from the posterior part of which hangs a strap with a buckle, to which is attached an ankle cuff. In the latter is kept the ankle of the limb affected by the disease, thus preventing weight bearing on this side. Anderson (3), pp. 472–473.

Petrie casts
Bilateral lower limb casts with proximal and distal spreader bars for abduction and internal rotation of the lower limbs, used in the treatment of Legg-Calvé-Perthes disease with permission of weight bearing.

Phelps, Abel Mix. New York orthopedic surgeon (1851–1902) who devised several orthoses.

Phelps corset
The first all-aluminum jacket (in place of steel or plaster) for the treatment of vertebral tuberculosis. Phelps, A. M. The aluminium corset. *Trans. Am. Orthop. Assoc.*, 6: 236–237, 1894.

Phelps hip splint
Hip-knee-ankle-foot orthosis with pelvic band and single (medial or lateral) upright for immobilization of hip joint and non-weightbearing. *Trans. Am. Orthop. Assoc.*, 4: 84–87, 1891; *The Post Graduate*, 16: 89–91, 1901, in *Orthopaedic Appliances Atlas* (1), pp. 353–354.

Phelps splint
Metal splint used for talipes equinovarus. *British Medical Dictionary* (7).

Phelps, Winthrop Morgan. Baltimore orthopedic surgeon, 1894–1971. Developed several orthoses, especially for use in cerebral palsy. See also his chapter "Bracing in the Cerebral Palsies" (1), pp. 521–536.

Phelps orthosis
Single-upright round caliper adjustable ankle-foot orthosis with a stop behind the upright that can be more or less bent to adjust the degree of plantar flexion of the ankle. This and other orthoses designed by Phelps are illustrated in: Phelps, W. M. Braces—cerebral palsy, upper extremity. *Instructional Course Lectures*, 9: 244–246, 1952; Braces—lower extremity—cerebral palsy, 10: 303–306, 1953. Anderson (3), pp. 284–290.

Pipkin brace
Thoracolumbosacral orthosis which restricts, in particular, spinal flexion by application of the three-point pressure principle.

Pitzen abduction splint
Night splint for congenital dislocation of hip. Hohmann (10), p. 116.

Ponseti splint
Curved adjustable abduction bar attached to the soles of a child's shoes. Used in congenital dislocation of the hip. Ponseti, Ignacio. Causes and failure in the treatment of congenital dislocation of the hip. *J. Bone Joint Surg.*, 26: 775–792, 1944.

Pope joint
One of several orthotic joints for the ankle, knee, hip, or wrist with or without spring, stop, or lock, manufactured by the Pope Brace

Company, Kankakee, Illinois. Some of these may also be labeled Klenzak joints (*q.v.*). The term Pope brace commonly refers to an ankle-foot orthosis including a double adjustable ankle joint with two spring channels placed lateral to the uprights. See also Chaper 8 and Fig. 8.11 and 9.4 of this book.

Pruce splint

Wristband with strap holding the last two digits in flexion. Pruce, A. M. Splint to correct deformity resulting from injury to ulnar nerve. *J. Bone Joint Surg., 28:* 397, 1946.

Putti, Vittorio. Bologna orthopedic surgeon, 1880–1940.

Putti abduction splint

A triangular metal or wood splint with straps to fasten it to the abducted lower limbs of a child. Used in the treatment of congenital dislocation of the hip. Putti, V. Early treatment of congenital dislocation of the hip. *J. Bone Joint Surg., 11:* 798, 1929.

Putti-Forrester-Brown splint

A plaster splint to hold both hips in abduction. Roaf and Hodkinson (16), p. 308.

Q

Queen Anne collar

Cervical orthosis which is particularly high in its posterior part. It limits all motions of the cervical spine, most of all extension. See Fig. 5.4 of this book. Colachis, S. C., *et al.* Cervical spine motion in normal women. *Arch. Phys. Med. Rehabil., 54* (4): 162, 1973.

R

Rabl clubfoot splint

A duraluminum support for metatarsus varus. Devised by Carl Rudolf Hans Rabl, German orthopedic surgeon, 1894–   . Rabl (15), p. 252.

Radike splint for radial palsy

Gauntlet from mid-forearm to the proximal interphalangeal joints with reenforcements for extension. Developed by Radike *et al.* in 1919. Illustrated in Boyes (6), p. 154.

Raffler ulnar palsy splint

A band wrapped around the hand and over the dorsum of the proximal phalanges of the fourth and fifth fingers to hold them in mild flexion. Raffler, K. *Zentralbl. Chir., 70:* 764, 1943. *Orthopaedic Appliances Atlas* (1), p. 302.

Rainal back brace

Spinal support with oval uprights. Schanz (17), p. 184.

Rancho Los Amigos splint, system, etc.

The name refers to Rancho Los Amigos Hospital, Downey, California, where several orthoses and orthotic components were devised, including a system of upper limb orthotics. See Chapter 8 of this book. See also Nickel splint.

Rancho Golden Arm
　　Motor-driven elbow-wrist-hand orthosis for complete paralysis of upper limb. It can be operated by motions of the chin or shoulder.
Rancho tenodesis splint
　　Metal wrist-hand orthosis with single-axis hinges at the wrist and the metacarpophalangeal joints. Nickel, V. L., Perry, J., and Snelson, R. *Handbook of Hand Splints*. Rancho Los Amigos Hospital, Downey, California, 1960. See also Chapter 8 of this book.
R and C bar
　　A metatarsal bar whose anterior margin is wave-shaped, with a central convex and two lateral concave parts. Designed at and named after the old Hospital for the Ruptured and Crippled (now Hospital for Special Surgery), New York. Milgram, J. E., and Jacobson, M. A. Footgear: therapeutic modifications of sole and heel. *Orthop. Rev.*, 7 (11): 57–62, 1978.
Raney flexion jacket
　　Thoracolumbosacral orthosis applying flexion and abdominal compression; used in the treatment of low back pain. Developed by Dr. Frank L. Raney, manufactured by Camp International, Jackson, Michigan.
Rey finger extension brace
　　After J. Rey, 1927, in Boyes (6), p. 154.
Reynders brace
　　Composite brace for trunk and torticollis. Schanz (17), p. 159.
Rhinelander adjustable cast
　　Hinges for incorporation into plaster casts. Rhinelander, F. W., and Ropes, M. W. Adjustable casts in the treatment of joint deformities. *J. Bone Joint Surg.*, 27: 311, 1945.
RIC tenodesis splint
　　Functional wrist-hand orthosis providing a three-jaw-chuck type of grasp for a paralyzed hand with effective wrist extensors. Developed at the Rehabilitation Institute of Chicago (RIC). Sabine, Clark, *et al.* Report of development of the RIC plastic tenodesis splint. *Arch. Phys. Med. Rehabil.*, 40: 513–515, 1959. A plastic tenodesis splint. *J. Bone Joint Surg.*, 47A: 533–536, 1965.
Richard brace
　　A torticollis brace. Schanz (17), p. 159.
Richards frog splint
　　A splint for mallet finger. Made by the Richards Manufacturing Company.
Ridlon wedge
　　A medial wedge inserted between inner and outer sole of a shoe, under the heel and shank.

Risser jacket
> Body cast for scoliosis, applied during cephalopelvic traction. Also called localizer cast, because pressure pads are "localized" over the apices of the major curves for corrective lateral pressure. Risser, Joseph C. The application of body casts for the correction of scoliosis. *Instructional Course Lectures, 12:* 255, 1955. Keim, H. A. Scoliosis. *Ciba Clin. Symp., 24* (1): 21 and 27, 1972.

Ritchie jacket
> Ritchie, S. Modification of Calot plaster jacket for immobilization of the cervical spine. *J. Bone Joint Surg., 28:* 166, 1946.

Rizzoli splint
> Band of metal and leather which encircles leg at upper calf from which a rigid bar passes down back of leg in midline to insert in shoe. Named after the famous Italian surgeon Francesco Rizzoli (1809–1880). Roaf and Hodkinson (16), p. 312.

Roberts (foot) plate or arch support
> Metal arch support with a full heel and extending to just proximal to the metatarsal heads. Its medial flange is relatively high in its posterior portion and lower anteriorly. Primarily used for children, advocated by Percy Willard Roberts, New York orthopedic surgeon. Prevention and treatment of weakfoot in children. *J. A. M. A., 75* (4): 237–240, 1920.

Robin Aids hand splint
> One of several splints, notably flexor hinge splints, wrist, and finger extension splints, produced by Robin Aids (after George B. Robinson) Manufacturing Company, Vallejo, California. Anderson, M. H. *Functional Bracing of the Upper Extremities*, pp. 63–65. Springfield, Illinois, 1958.

Robin Aids hook
> Shoulder-elbow-hand orthosis that includes a prosthetic hook placed into the hand and operated by shoulder muscles pulling a cable by means of a shoulder loop.

Robinson torticollis support
> Three elastic bands attached to a curved rod supported in plaster. Schanz (17), p. 165.

Rodopri brace
> Leather sling attached to a wheelchair and passed around the chest of a patient so as to exert pressure against the convexity of a scoliosis. Dorando, C., and Newman, M. K. Bracing for severe scoliosis of muscular dystrophy patients. *Phys. Ther. Rev., 37:* 230–231, 1957.

Roger Anderson
> See Anderson, Roger.

Rosen splint
> Device made of one piece of flat metal in the form of the letter H, in which the three bars are bent and molded at their ends to be hooked from the back of an infant over his shoulders, around his thorax (the transverse bar extends beyond the longitudinal bars) and his flexed and abducted thighs. Used for children with congenital dislocation of the hip. Rosen, Sophus von (Malmö, Sweden). Diagnosis and treatment of congenital dislocation of the hip joint in the new-born. *J. Bone Joint Surg., 44B:* 284–291, 1962. Hensinger, R. N. Congenital dislocation of the hip. *Ciba Clin. Symp. 31* (1): 15–16, 1979.

Rosenauer elastic thumb assist
> A rubber-covered piano wire loop around the proximal phalanx of the thumb and attached by an elastic band to a wristlet. Werssowetz, O. F. von, *et al.* Supportive appliances in rehabilitation of the paralytic hand. *Arch. Phys. Med. Rehabil., 36:* 559–563, 1955.

S

Salter bow-leg splint
> Designed by Dr. R. B. Salter of Toronto, Canada.

Sam Browne belt
> Synonym of Perthes sling (*q.v.*). Anderson (3), p. 472.

Sayre, Lewis A. American surgeon, 1820–1900.

Sayre dropfoot bandage
> Sling under foot supported by rubber bands. Schanz (17), p. 105.

Sayre head sling
> A soft (usually textile) mandible-occiput support for distraction of the cervical vertebrae.

Sayre jacket
> A plaster of Paris jacket used to immobilize the vertebral column. It is applied with the help of a Sayre apparatus for the suspension of the patient by the head and the axillae. Sayre, L. A. *Spinal Disease and Spinal Curvature, their Treatment by Suspension and the Use of the Plaster of Paris Bandage.* Philadelphia, 1877.

Sayre knee bandage
> Miller, H. G. Surgical note on Sayre knee joint splint. *Edinb. Med. J., 21:* 816, 1875.

Sayre head halter
> A mandible-occiput ring support held in place by a posterior extension from a back brace. Sayre, Reginald H. Spondylitis of second cervical vertebra with report of cases and instrument for treatment. *Trans. Am. Orthop. Assoc., 5:* 250–257, 1892.

Scarpa shoe
> A right-angled metal splint that restricts flexion of the foot; used in equinus deformity of the foot. Developed in 1803 by Antonio Scarpa,

Italian surgeon and anatomist (1747–1832), it was modified many times. Moore in *Orthopaedic Appliances Atlas* (1), pp. 479–495.

Schanz, Alfred. Dresden, Germany, orthopedic surgeon, 1868–1931. Developed several orthoses discussed in his book (17).

Schanz artificial quadriceps

Rubber bands or elastic webbing connecting thigh and leg parts of brace, used in paralysis of quadriceps. Schanz (17), p. 105.

Schanz collar

A filled tube of soft material, usually narrow stockinet stuffed with cellulose, slung three times around the neck; used to reduce motions of cervical vertebrae. Schanz (17), p. 162. See also in Delitala (8), p. 89.

Schanz splint for Volkmann's contracture

See also Boyes (6), p. 154.

Schaubel finger splint

Schaubel, H. J. Splint for the treatment of mallet finger. *J. Bone Joint Surg.*, *28*: 394, 1946.

Schede, Franz. German orthopedic surgeon (1882–1976) who described several orthoses in his book *Orthopädische Konstruktionen.* Stuttgart, 1962.

Schede corset

A scoliosis corset. See also Hohmann (10), p. 47.

Schede hand splint

A splint keeping the metacarpophalangeal joints II–V in flexion. *Münch. Med. Wochenschr.*, *66*: 998, 1919, in *Orthopaedic Appliances Atlas* (1), p. 311.

Schildbach back brace

Elastic straps extending spine. Schanz (17), p. 187.

Schulze-Gosler bandage

Leather bandage for dropfoot. Rabl (15), p. 293.

Schwartz, R. Plato. Rochester, N. Y., orthopedic surgeon, 1892–1965.

Schwartz (heel) meniscus

Shoe insert, sickle-shaped and made of leather, to support the heel of the foot and correct pronation. Devised, but apparently not published, by R. P. Schwartz; discussed in Rose, G. K. Correction of the pronated foot. *J. Bone Joint Surg.*, *44B*: 642–647, 1962.

Schwartz hip splint

A plaster splint for maintaining reduction of congenital dislocation of the hip. *J. Bone Joint Surg.*, *27*: 166, 1945.

Scott brace

Knee-ankle-foot orthosis for traction of the hip joint, *e.g.*, in osteoarthritis. Suggested in 1962 by Bryan O. Scott, physiatrist, and Anne Neilson Hollins, physical therapist, at United Oxford Hospitals in Oxford, England. Hollins, A. N. *Physiotherapy, 48:* 65, 1962.

Scott-Craig orthosis

Hip-stabilizing knee-ankle-foot orthosis with offset knee lock. Originated by Bruce A. Scott, orthotist at Craig Rehabilitation Hospital, Englewood, Colorado. Scott, B. A. Engineering principles and fabrication techniques for the Scott-Craig long leg brace for paraplegics. *Orthotics Prosthet.*, *25*(4): 14–19, 1971. *Atlas of Orthotics* (2), p. 222. See Fig. 9.24 of this book.

Scultetus bandage or binder

Many-tailed bandage: five or six strips of bandage, laid parallel and slightly overlapping, are sewn together in their midportions. The loose ends (tails) are applied alternately from right and left (usually over the abdomen), each one being held in place by the following one. Named after Johann Schultes, latinized Scultetus, German surgeon, 1595–1645. Scultetus, J. *Armamentarium Chirurgicum.* Ulm, 1653.

Seaman cervical collar

Electric heating pad constructed in the shape of a soft cervical collar. Seaman, George J. Cervical collar for treatment and immobilization. *J. A. M. A.*, *173:* 661, 1960.

Seattle orthosis

One of several orthoses developed at the University of Washington, Seattle, Washington, Department of Rehabilitation Medicine. See also Chapter 9, especially Fig. 9.12 of this book.

Seiger genu valgum splint

Bilateral knee-ankle-foot orthosis with lateral uprights, thigh band, knee band, and ankle band fixed by metal linkage at the ankle. Seiger, H. W. A night splint for the correction of genu valgum. *J. Bone Joint Surg.*, *28:* 178, 1946.

Shaffer (foot) plate or arch support

Metal arch support with heel seat and a high medial flange. Originally made in two adjustable portions, it was later constructed in one piece, and the metal may also be replaced by another rigid material. Shaffer, Newton M. Flatfoot, its causes and treatment. *N. Y. Med. J.*, pp. 717–721, May 29, 1897. Jahss in *Atlas of Orthotics* (2), p. 277.

Shnayerson finger splint

Metal splint which has a corresponding joint for each joint in the finger. Shnayerson, Ned. A finger splint for extension or flexion. *J. A. M. A.*, *110:* 2070–2071, 1938.

Shrewsbury paraplegic walker

A swivel walker for a paraplegic child or adult, comparable to a standing brace or parapodium (see also Toronto standing brace). It extends from two separate shoe plates to a chest strap, allows sitting as well as a swiveling displacement by appropriate trunk motions. Developed at Robert Jones and Agnes Hunt Orthopaedic Hospital, Shrewsbury, England, in the early 1970's. Rose, G. K., and Henshaw,

J. T. Swivel walkers for paraplegics. *Bull. Prosthet. Res.*, *10–20:* 62–74, 1973.

Silesian bandage or belt

Belt, usually of webbing, attached to a lower limb orthosis or prosthesis as a means of suspension. Staros and LeBlanc in *Atlas of Orthotics* (2), p. 194.

Smith dropfoot brace

An ankle-foot orthosis with calf band, weighing only 150 g. Its double upright with coils is made of one piece of wire. Smith, Lyman. A simplified brace for drop-foot. *J. Bone Joint Surg.*, *30A:* 788–789, 1948.

Smith knee extension apparatus

Leverage system operated by elastic tubing for mobilization of flexion contractures of the knee applied with horizontal traction and overhead suspension. Used to counteract tendency to subluxation of tibia on femur from hamstring action. Smith, L. D. A knee straightening device. *J. Bone Joint Surg.*, *7:* 206, 1925.

Snow long leg brace

Temporary brace of tubular double uprights, half-ring ischial seat, posterior thigh and calf cuffs, kneecap, and a weight-bearing footplate. Snow, William Benham. Multipurpose brace: a useful adjunct in rehabilitation. *J. A. M. A.*, *150:* 687, 1952.

Snyder sling

Sling supported on the shoulder opposite the involved hip, attached to the involved limb just above the ankle, with the length adjusted to hold knee in flexion and prevent weight bearing during ambulation. Snyder, C. H. A sling for use in Legg-Perthes disease. *J. Bone Joint Surg.*, *29:* 524, 1947.

Sofield clubfoot apparatus

Wedging plaster cast including rubber bands for traction. Sofield, H. A. Elastic traction assisting correction of clubfeet. *J. Bone Joint Surg.*, *13:* 283–286, 1931.

Spiers back brace

Spiers, H. W. A new spring back brace for fractured clavicles. *J. Bone Joint Surg.*, *12:* 663, 1930.

Spitzy, Hans. Vienna orthopedic surgeon, 1872–1956.

Spitzy button or spike

Pointed button, the size of half a marble which, fixed at a strategic place on an orthosis, forces its wearer to make a muscular effort in order to avoid a painful contact. As examples, see the two following articles.

Spitzy scoliosis brace

Thoracolumbosacral orthosis with chin piece on which is placed a painful button; another button is placed under the occiput, both buttons reminding the child to elongate his spine.

Spitzy shoe inlay or arch support

Removable innersole of a shoe with Spitzy button at the place of the longitudinal arch to stimulate the wearer with flatfoot to supinate the foot and elevate the arch.

Spitzy splint

A wrist-hand orthosis for radial palsy. Hohmann (10), p. 106.

Steeper splint

One of several orthoses manufactured by Hugh Steeper, Ltd., of Roehampton, England. Example: the Five Finger (Spider) splint extends all five digits of the hand by wires positioned over the dorsum of the hand. Steeper hand splints. *Bull. Prosthet. Res.*, *10–12:* 347–348, 1969.

Steindler, Arthur. Iowa orthopedic surgeon, 1878–1959.

Steindler back brace

High and rigid trunk support comprising a double pelvic band, a high thoracic band which ends anteriorly in infraclavicular pressure pads, three pairs of uprights (posterior, lateral, and anterior), and shoulder straps. Used for strong reduction of trunk motions in all directions. Steindler, A. *Diseases and Deformities of the Spine and Thorax.* St. Louis, 1929. See Fig. 6.19 of this book.

Steindler hand splint

Cockup hand splint with springs, elastics, and other variations. Steindler, A. Arthritic deformities of the wrist and fingers. *J. Bone Joint Surg.*, *33A:* 849–862, 1951.

Steindler heel spur correction

Replacement of the middle third longitudinal section of the shoe heel by sponge rubber and other remodeling of the heel aimed at the protection of a calcaneal spur. Jahss in *Atlas of Orthotics* (2), p. 278.

Sterling long leg brace

Hip-knee-ankle-foot orthosis including nonlocking knee joint with constant spring extension assist. Sterling, Harold M., and Kottke, F. J. Constant tension springs on long leg braces to assist the quadriceps femoris. *J. A. M. A.*, *172:* 1268–1270, 1960.

Stewart opponens splint

Molded opponens splint using a plastic material. Stewart, J. E. A plastic opponens splint for the thumb. *J. Bone Joint Surg.*, *30A:* 783, 1948.

Stracathro splint

Abduction splint made of polythene for congenital dislocation of the hip in the infant. Developed in 1960 at Stracathro Hospital in Scotland. MacKenzie, I. G. Congenital dislocation of the hip. *J. Bone Joint Surg.*, *54B:* 18–39, 1972.

Stryker cervical immobilizer

See Chapter 5 and Fig. 5.15 of this book.

St. Vincent skeleton splint

This is essentially a leather-covered metal pad applied to press against a rib hump in a scoliosis. The pad is kept in place by a framework consisting of a front and back upright anchored to a pelvic band and an oblique band over one shoulder and under the opposite axilla. Powell, M. *Orthopaedic Nursing.*, ed. 6, pp. 74, 296. Edinburgh, 1968.

Swanson night splint

Pancake-shaped orthosis, to be worn at night, for the stretching of flexion contractures in spastic hands. Made of aluminum and covered with leather, it allows stretching of the contracted wrist and finger flexors. The orthosis can be bent at the wrist. After Dr. Alfred B. Swanson, in Turek (19), p. 531.

Swedish knee cage

Orthosis to control genu recurvatum, consisting of two aluminum uprights connected posteriorly by a semicircular transverse bar, two webbing straps, above and below the knee, and an adjustable fluid-filled pad in the popliteal space. Designed in Sweden in 1966, reported by Hans Richard Lehneis in *Artificial Limbs 12* (2): 54–57, 1968. *Atlas of Orthotics* (2), pp. 217, 244. Anderson (3), p. 441.

Swiss lock

This lock, also called French lock and bail lock, works on the mechanical principle of the cam. As used in orthotics, it is most often a double knee lock. A semicircular steel handle in the popliteal space disengages a bolt from a notch in each of the two joints, thus opening them and allowing knee flexion. See Fig. 9.17 of this book.

T

Tachdjian orthosis

So-called trilateral socket hip abduction orthosis for unilateral Legg-Calvé-Perthes disease. A jointed medial steel bar connects a thigh socket to a support which avoids contact of the shoe with the ground while keeping the limb in abduction and internal rotation, allowing ambulation. A lift is required under the opposite shoe. Tachdjian, Miran A., and Jouett, L. D. Trilateral socket hip abduction orthosis for the treatment of Legg-Perthes disease. *Orthotics Prosthet.*, 22 (2): 49–62, 1968. *J. Bone Joint Surg.*, 50A (6): 1272–1273, 1968. *Atlas of Orthotics* (2), p. 228.

Taylor, Charles Fayette. New York orthopedic surgeon, 1827–1899. Devised in 1863, the spinal brace that became one of the most widely used over the next 100 years.

Taylor brace, also called the "spinal assistant"

Thoracolumbar hyperextension orthosis with two paraspinal steel bars reaching to the scapular spines. Their upper ends are prolonged by shoulder straps whereas the lower ends are attached to a pelvic band. Attached to the metal frame is a corset or full-front abdominal support reaching to the inguinal area and covering the lower ribs. It may be with or without perineal straps. It restricts motions of the thoracolumbosacral joints, notably flexion and extension. Taylor, C. F. On the mechanical treatment of Pott's disease of the spine. *Trans. Med. Soc. State N. Y.*, 67–87, 1863. The spinal assistant. *Trans. Am. Orthop. Assoc.*, *12:* 15, 1899. See Fig. 6.16 of this book.

Knight-Taylor brace

See under Knight, James C.

Taylor brace

Designed by Henry Ling Taylor in 1887, this thoracolumbosacral orthosis reenforces the hyperextension effect of the classical Taylor spinal brace (see Taylor, Charles Fayette). Taylor, H. L. A case of Pott's disease with an unusual deformity—description of improved spinal apparatus. *Med. Record*, *32:* 647–649, 1887.

Taylor inflatable collar

Inflatable soft cervical orthosis, consisting of a front section and a back section. Devised by Arabion N. Taylor, Alabama orthopedic surgeon. Taylor, A. N. An inflatable neck support. *Clin. Orthop.*, *81:* 87, 1971. See Fig. 5.2*B* of this book.

Terhune knee apparatus

Terhune, S. R. Apparatus for correction of flexion deformity of the knee. *J. Bone Joint Surg.*, *30A:* 244, 1948.

Teufel orthosis

Plastic posterior leaf-spring ankle-foot orthosis, to be worn inside the shoe, used to support the ankle in footdrop and similar conditions. Developed by Wilhelm J. Teufel, Stuttgart, Germany. Rubin, G., and Dixon, M. The modern ankle-foot orthoses. *Bull. Prosthet. Res.*, *10–19:* 20–41, esp. p. 23, 1973. See Fig. 9.12 of this book.

Thilo corset

Plaster of Paris corset with wire reinforcement. Schanz (17), p. 132.

Thomas, F. Brian. British orthopedic surgeon.

Brian Thomas radial palsy splint

Wrist-hand cockup orthosis with dorsal spring wire suspension for the digits, for the treatment of radial paralysis. Thomas, F. B. A splint for radial (musculospiral) nerve palsy. *J. Bone Joint Surg.*, *26:* 602–605, 1944; An improved splint for radial (musculospiral) nerve paralysis. *J. Bone Joint Surg.*, *33B:* 272–273, 1951. See Fig. 8.26 of this book.

Thomas, Hugh Owen. Liverpool orthopedic surgeon, 1834–1891.

Thomas abduction arm splint

It consists of a felt-lined aluminum section which embraces one hemithorax (with straps for closure on the opposite side) and joined with a padded trough for the arm, which in turn is joined with another trough for the forearm. Used to keep the arm in abduction. Powell, M. *Orthopaedic Nursing*, ed. 6, p. 89. Edinburgh, 1968.

Thomas arm splint

Consists of two steel bars connected by a crossbar distal to the elbow and a padded ring encircling the root of the limb. Similar to the splint for the lower limb (see Thomas splint, knee splint, or caliper), but the ring is hinged at its junction with the bars in the arm splint.

Thomas bar

Metatarsal bar.

Thomas collar

Molded collar originally made of perforated leather, with strap and buckle at the back. See Fig. 5.3 of this book.

Thomas heel

Medially extended heel of a shoe: heel whose anterior border (heel breasting) is extended forward in its medial third or half by *ca.* 1 to 2 cm, in order to better support the navicular bone and sustentaculum tali. Also called orthopedic heel. Occasionally, it is understood that the heel is not only extended but also higher (see Thomas wedge). Thomas, H. O. *Contributions to Medicine and Surgery*. London, 1874 *et seq.*, in Bick (4), p. 454. Anderson (3), p. 28.

Thomas heel, reversed

Laterally extended heel, *i.e.*, a left Thomas heel applied on a right shoe or *vice versa*. Also called reversed orthopedic heel.

Thomas hip splint or posterior splint

Splint that consisted of a flat metal bar reaching from the scapula to the ankle, being carefully molded over the back, buttocks, thigh, and calf; it was held in place by shoulder straps and circular bands at the chest, waist, thigh, and leg. To prevent weight bearing, the other foot was raised by a patten. Used in the treatment of arthritis. Thomas, H. O. *Diseases of the Hip, Knee, and Ankle Joints with Their Deformities, Treated by a New and Efficient Method*. London, 1875. Bick (4), p. 462. *Orthopaedic Appliances Atlas* (1), p. 351.

Thomas splint, knee splint, or caliper

Knee-ankle-foot orthosis consisting of two straight steel bars connected distally by a crossbar beyond the foot and proximally by a padded ring fitting tightly to the perineum and ischium. For emergency splinting, transportation, and traction in fractures of the thigh or leg. Weight bearing is transferred from the knee and foot to the pelvis.

Thomas wedge, Thomas heel wedge

Heel that is medially extended forward (like a Thomas heel) and medially higher (by 2 to 10 mm). Also called orthopedic heel wedge.

Thomsen finger splint

A splint with an outrigger to extend one or more fingers. Hohmann (10), p. 112.

Thomson clubfoot splint

A modification of the Denis Browne splint giving the infant freedom to kick while his lower limbs are in the abducted and corrected position. Thomson, Stuart A. Treatment of congenital talipes equinovarus with a modification of the Denis Browne method and splint. *J. Bone Joint Surg., 24:* 291–298, 1942. *Orthopaedic Appliances Atlas* (1), pp. 487, 495.

Thorndike shoulder harness

Shoulder orthosis combining shoulder strap, chest strap, and arm cuff attached to the latter. Used to prevent recurrent dislocation of the shoulder joint. Thorndike, Augustus. *Athletic Injuries, Prevention, Diagnosis and Treatment.* Philadelphia, 1942. *Orthopaedic Appliances Atlas* (1), p. 335.

TIRR

Abbreviation for Texas Institute for Rehabilitation and Research, Houston, Texas, where several orthoses were developed. See also Engen.

TIRR dropfoot brace or posterior leaf orthosis

Molded plastic to be worn in the shoe to support a dropfoot. See Fig. 9.12 of this book.

Tobruk splint

A modification of the Thomas splint in which the limb is partially encased together with the splint by circumferential plaster bandages to prevent lateral displacement; named after the port of Tobruk in North Africa, during the siege of which, in 1942, it was used by the British Army to immobilize the limb for easy and safe transportation. Bristow, W. R. Some surgical lessons of the war. *J. Bone Joint Surg., 25:* 524, 1943. Bick (4), p. 288.

Toronto attachment or splint

Arm or leg splint made for attachment to a Bradford frame and used in poliomyelitis. *British Medical Dictionary* (7).

Toronto orthoses

The name refers to the Ontario Crippled Children's Centre, Toronto, Canada, where several orthoses were developed which may also be named by the abbreviation OCCC.

Toronto Legg-Perthes orthosis

Bilateral knee-ankle-foot orthosis holding the lower limbs of a child in abduction and slight internal rotation, while allowing sitting as well as ambulation with crutches. Used in the treatment of Legg-Calvé-Perthes disease. Bobechko, W. P., McLaurin, C. A., and Motloch, W. M. Toronto Orthosis for Legg-Perthes disease. *Artif. Limbs, 12* (2): 36–41, 1968. See Fig. 9.45 of this book.

Toronto orthopodium or parapodium

A standing device for children, similar to the standing orthosis (see below), but also allowing unlocking for sitting. Motloch, W. The parapodium: an orthotic device for neuromuscular disorders. *Artif. Limbs*, *15* (2): 36–47, 1971. See Fig. 10.2 of this book.

Toronto standing orthosis

A standing device for children, stabilizing all joints from the feet to the hips in neutral position, allowing pivoting gait and swing-through crutch gait. Hamilton, E., and Motloch, W. M. The Toronto standing brace. *Inter-Clinic Information Bull.*, *8* (7): 12–13, 1969; *9* (10): 10–13, 1970. Staros and LeBlanc in *Atlas of Orthotics* (2), p. 233.

Truslow scoliosis brace

Resembles a Knight spinal brace. Truslow, W. A. A self-correcting brace for lateral curvature of the spine. *J. Orthop. Surg.*, *1:* 547, 1919.

Tubby splint

A palmar orthosis with extension to one digit, developed by Alfred Herbert Tubby (London orthopedic surgeon, 1862–1930) in 1896 for the treatment of Dupuytren's contracture. Illustrated in Boyes (6), p. 155. Tubby, A. H. *Deformities Including Diseases of the Bones and Joints.* London, 1912.

Tuck dropfoot brace

Ankle-foot orthosis with spring totally concealed in the heel of the shoe. Tuck, W. H. Dropfoot appliance with rubber torsion socket. *J. Bone Joint Surg.*, *44B:* 896–898, 1962.

Turner corset

A corset made with impregnated stockinette. Schanz (17), p. 143.

U

UC, UCB, UCBL, UC-BL

Abbreviations for University of California, Berkeley, or University of California Biomechanics Laboratory, San Francisco and Berkeley, where various orthoses and orthotic components were developed.

UC brace

Knee-ankle orthosis with single (lateral) upright attached to the back of the heel. Gucker in Licht (13), p. 361.

UC-BL dual-axis ankle-control system. Inman, V. T., *et al.* UC-BL dual-axis ankle-control system and UC-BL shoe insert. *Bull. Prosthet. Res.*, *10–11:* 130–214, 1969. See Fig. 9.15 of this book.

UCB (or UC-BL) shoe insert

Plastic laminate shoe insert (arch support) for flatfoot. Henderson, W. H., and Campbell, J. W. UC-BL shoe insert. *Bull. Prosthet. Res.*, *10–11:* 215–235, 1969. See also preceding reference. Jahss in *Atlas of Orthotics* (2), p. 273.

UCLA

Abbreviation for University of California, Los Angeles

UCLA functional long leg brace

Knee-ankle-foot orthosis with plastic thigh and pretibial shells, double uprights, offset ball-bearing knee joints, and an ankle hydraulic cylinder control. Strohm, B. R., Bray, J., and Colachis, S. C. The UCLA functional long leg brace: biomechanics and fabrication. *J. Am. Phys. Ther. Assoc.*, *43* (10): 713–716, 1963. See Fig. 9.31 of this book.

Ulrich finger flexion splint

Arm and forearm plaster, cockup wire from palm; plaster and skin traction to pull fingers into flexion. Ulrich, F. F. A. A splint for treatment of stiff fingers. *J. Orthop. Surg.*, *2:* 32, 1920.

University of California brace

See UC, UCB.

USAMBRL or AMBRL

Abbreviation for United States Army Medical Bioengineering Research and Development Laboratory, where several orthoses and prostheses were developed.

V

VAPC

Abbreviation for Veterans Administration Prosthetics Center, New York, a Federal agency of the U. S. The abbreviation is attached to the names of various orthoses and orthotic components, as well as to other devices and control systems.

VAPC shoe clasp or posterior clasp

A clasp which is attached to a single posterior bar of an ankle-foot orthosis and held in place by being clipped to the upper border of a low shoe. It allows easy change of the orthosis from one shoe to another. See Fig. 9.13 of this book.

Varney harness

Varney, J. Howard, *et al.* Treatment of acromioclavicular dislocation by means of a harness. *J. Bone Joint Surg.*, *34A:* 232–233, 1952.

Velpeau bandage

Bandage immobilizing a forearm in front of and close to the chest, *e.g.*, in injuries of the shoulder or upper limb. Named after the Paris surgeon Alfred Velpeau, 1795–1867. Later, the eponym was at times used to designate any elastic textile bandage.

Verth dropfoot brace

Ankle-foot orthosis in which the stirrup has a short, forward-pointing lever, to which is attached a spring coming from the proximal end of the upright andlifting the forepart of the shoe. *Orthopaedic Appliances Atlas* (1), p. 427.

Victoria collar

A poster-type cervical orthosis. See Fig. 5.6 of this book.

Vincent apparatus

Brace for correction of pectus carinatum. Schanz (17), p. 167.

Volkmann splint

> Knee-ankle-foot orthosis in which a fractured lower limb rests like in a gutter with a footpiece, protected from sideward motions by a medial and a lateral support. Designed by Richard von Volkmann, Halle, Germany, surgeon, 1830–1889.

Vulpius corset

> Cellulose corset covered with textile. Schanz (17), p. 197.

W

Ward arm brace

> A complicated orthosis designed to improve upper limb function in a patient with a lesion of the fifth cervical nerve root or the upper brachial plexus. Ward, G. E. *et al.* A device in which springs replace the action of paralyzed muscles of the arm. *J. Bone Joint Surg., 30A:* 987, 1948.

Warm Springs

> The name refers to Georgia Warm Springs Foundation, Warm Springs, Georgia, where several orthoses and orthotic devices were developed, among which is a system of upper limb orthotics with a basic opponens orthosis. See also Bennett, R. L., and Hoke in this chapter and Chapter 8 of this book.

Warm Springs crutch

> Aluminum variety of Canadian crutch, in which the metal band, at or slightly above the midlevel of the arm, is open laterally, but whose posterior portion prevents flexion of the forearm. Developed for poliomyelitis patients with weakness of triceps brachii at Georgia Warm Springs Foundation, Warm Springs, Georgia. Also called Everett crutch. Suggested term: metal triceps crutch. See Fig. 12.3*B.*

Warm Springs forefoot splint

> An orthosis for correction of forefoot adduction and equinus. Herring, J. M. Correction of deformity with orthetic devices. *Arch. Phys. Med. Rehabil., 44:* 537–540, 1963.

Warm Springs (scoliosis) corset

> A high canvas corset with flexible stays. Described in the same article.

Wegner-Munro cervical brace

> Shoulder collar with uprights to mandible and occiput supports attached posteriorly to a back brace. Wegner, Walter, and Munro, Donald. A cervical-spine brace which reduces the use of plaster casts. *N. Engl. J. Med., 233:* 458–460, 1940.

Wellington boot

> A square-tipped boot. Originally the term (after Arthur Wellesley, 1st Duke of Wellington, 1769–1852) referred to a riding boot for men which reached above the knee and also to a similar shorter boot.

Werssowetz, Odon F. von. American physiatrist (1910–1971). (See also Rosenauer.)

Werssowetz antilordosis brace

Lumbosacral brace with paravertebral and lateral uprights built to reduce lordosis. Hines in Licht (13), p. 4.

Werssowetz hyperextension brace

Thoracolumbosacral brace with frontal extensions joined by a sternal pressure pad. It is built to restrict flexion of the vertebral column. Hines in Licht (13), p. 5.

Wheeler finger splints

Extension splints made of wire and elastoplast, an elastic bandage. Wheeler, W. I. de Courcy. Splints for fingers and thumb. *Lancet, 2:* 546–547, 1940.

White thumb extension apparatus

Wrist cuff with elastic band looped around thumb to hold it in extension. White, J. Warren, and Jensen, W. E. The infant's persistent thumb-clutched hand. *J. Bone Joint Surg., 34A:* 680–688, 1952.

Whitman, Royal. Boston and New York orthopedic surgeon (1857–1946) who devised several orthoses discussed in his *Treatise on Orthopaedic Surgery.* Philadelphia, 1919 (ed. 9, Philadelphia, 1930).

Whitman arch support, (foot) plate or splint

Metal arch support with medial flange under the longitudinal arch and lateral flange at the heel. It stops just behind the metatarsal heads. Whitman, R. Observations on forty-five cases of flat-foot with particular reference to etiology and treatment. *Boston Med. Surg. J., 118:* 598–601, 616–620, 1888. The importance of positive support in the curative treatment of weak feet and a comparison of the means employed to assure it. *Am. J. Orthop. Surg., 11:* 215–230, 1913. *Orthopaedic Appliances Atlas* (1), pp. 456–460. Jahss in *Atlas of Orthotics* (2), pp. 272, 277.

Combination Whitman

Metal shoe inlay similar to a regular Whitman arch support but extending forward to include support to the metatarsal area.

Whitman twister

A spiral band from the pelvic band to the outer border of the shoe used to correct rotation of the lower limb. See Fig. 10.1 of this book.

Whittemore tip

Metal-and-rubber crutch tip, consisting of a metal base into which is screwed a small rubber tip. Used for adaptation to various surfaces. See Fig. 12.2*C* of this book.

Wilbur Coon shoe

Shoe of extra depth so that it can accommodate an inlay and interior bracing. It is therefore of the blucher type and has a strong counter. Manufactured by Wilbur Coon in Rochester, N. Y., until the 1950s, later by P. W. Minor & Son, Inc., Batavia, N. Y.

Wilcox brace

Lumbosacral orthosis in which the lateral uprights are connected to the pelvic band by movable joints. Four straps hold an apron in place. Called also Lipscomb brace. Thomas in *Orthopaedic Appliances Atlas* (1), p. 213. See Fig. 6.14 of this book.

Williams lordosis brace

Thoracolumbosacral orthosis based on the three-point pressure principle, restricting in particular extension of the lumbar spine and to some extent lateral motions, while allowing flexion. Two posterior transverse bars, one at the lower thoracic level and another over the buttocks, exert forward pressure, while a corset-type front with low abdominal pad presses backward. The lateral uprights pivot in their attachment to the pelvic band. Devised by Paul C. Williams, Dallas, Texas, orthopedic surgeon (1900–1978). Williams, P. C. Conservative management of lesions of the lumbosacral spine. *Instructional Course Lectures, 10:* 90–121 (p. 112), 1953. See Fig. 6.12 of this book.

Willock jacket

A sort of jacket used to aid respiratory movements in pulmonary emphysema. *Dorland's Illustrated Medical Dictionary* (9).

Wilson collar

An orthosis for rigid immobilization of the entire cervical spine. See Chapter 5 and Fig. 5.7 of this book.

Wilson splint

An elastic splint cut from rubber gloves to prevent claw toes. Wilson, William J. A simple and effective splint for use in the treatment of clawing of the toes. *J. Bone Joint Surg., 31A:* 198–199, 1949. See also illustration in Boyes (6), p. 155.

Wingfield-Morris shoulder abduction splint

A modification of the Littler-Jones shoulder abduction splint. Nangle (14), p. 117. Murdoch, G. *Prosthetic and Orthotic Practice*, p. 475. London, 1970.

Wolf, Josef. Iowa orthopedic surgeon (1899–1970).

Wolf serratus palsy apparatus

Wolf, J. The conservative treatment of serratus palsy. *J. Bone Joint Surg. 23:* 959–961, 1941.

Wolf shoulder apparatus

Wolf, J. An appliance for the prevention of recurrent dislocation of the shoulder. *J. Bone Joint Surg., 21:* 472–474, 1939.

Y

Young ischial ring

Modification of original H. O. Thomas ischial ring. Young, Charles S. A study in fitting the ring of the Thomas splint. *J. A. M. A., 93:* 602–604, 1929.

Z

Zanoli corset

Corset with rigid posterior pelvic band, paraspinal uprights with lateral extensions to the subclavicular areas (cowhorns), and a single posterior extension to the level of the neck, ending in a narrow collar. It was popular in Italy during the first half of the 20th century. Illustrated in Licht (13), p. 727.

Zimmer braces, splints

Orthoses of various types made by the Zimmer Manufacturing Company.

REFERENCES

Books

1. AMERICAN ACADEMY OF ORTHOPAEDIC SURGEONS. *Orthopaedic Appliances Atlas.* Vol. I. *Braces, Splints, Shoe Alterations.* Ann Arbor, Michigan, J. W. Edwards, 1952.
2. AMERICAN ACADEMY OF ORTHOPAEDIC SURGEONS. *Atlas of Orthotics. Biomechanical Principles and Application.* St. Louis, C. V. Mosby Co., 1975.
3. ANDERSON, M. H. *A Manual of Lower Extremities Orthotics.* Springfield, Illinois, Charles C Thomas, 1972, 1977.
4. BICK, E. M. *Source Book of Orthopaedics,* ed. 2. Baltimore, Williams & Wilkins Co., 1948.
5. BLOOMBERG, M. H. *Orthopedic Braces.* Philadelphia, J. B. Lippincott Co., 1964.
6. BOYES, J. H. *Bunnell's Surgery of the Hand,* ed. 4. Philadelphia, J. B. Lippincott Co., 1964.
7. *British Medical Dictionary.* Philadelphia, J. B. Lippincott Co., 1963.
8. DELITALA, F. *Gli Apparecchi Ortopedici.* Bologna, L. Cappelli, 1921.
9. *Dorland's Illustrated Medical Dictionary,* ed. 25. Philadelphia, W. B. Saunders, 1974.
10. HOHMANN, G. *Orthopädische Technik,* ed. 3. Stuttgart, Ferdinand Enke, 1951.
11. JORDAN, H. H. *Orthopedic Appliances,* ed. 2. Springfield, Illinois, Charles C Thomas, 1963.
12. KELLY, E. C. *Encyclopedia of Medical Sources.* Baltimore, Williams & Wilkins Co., 1948.
13. LICHT, S. (Ed.) *Orthotics Etcetera.* New Haven, Connecticut, Elizabeth Licht, 1966.
14. NANGLE, E. J. *Instruments and Apparatus in Orthopaedic Surgery.* Oxford, Blackwell, 1951.
15. RABL, C. R. H. *Orthopädische Schuhe.* Stuttgart, Ferdinand Enke, 1963.
16. ROAF, R., AND HODKINSON, L. J. *Textbook for Orthopaedic Nurses.* Philadelphia, J. B. Lippincott Co., 1964.
17. SCHANZ, A. *Handbuch der Orthopädischen Technik,* ed. 2, Jena, Gustav Fischer, 1923.
18. *Stedman's Medical Dictionary,* ed. 23. Baltimore, Williams & Wilkins Co., 1976.
19. TUREK, S. L. *Orthopaedics: Principles and Their Application,* ed. 3. Philadelphia, J. B. Lippincott Co., 1977.

Serials

Archives of Physical Medicine and Rehabilitation
Bulletin of Prosthetics Research (U. S. Veterans Administration)
Clinical Orthopaedics and Related Research (The Association of Bone and Joint Surgeons)
Instructional Course Lectures (American Academy of Orthopaedic Surgeons)
Journal of Bone and Joint Surgery
Orthopedic and Prosthetic Appliance Journal (continued as *Orthotics and Prosthetics*)
Orthotics and Prosthetics: The Journal of The American Orthotic and Prosthetic Association

Acknowledgment

I wish to acknowledge Dr. Ian MacLean's contribution to the first edition of this chapter.

Index